Dr. T. W. Greenwood MA. MB. FRCP.
West Middlesex University Hospital
Twickenham Road
Isleworth
Middlesex TW7 6AF

PERSPECTIVES IN CARDIOLOGY 1988

Editors:

Burton E. Sobel
Professor of Medicine and Director, Cardiovascular Division,
Washington University School of Medicine, St Louis, MO, USA

Desmond G. Julian
Medical Director, British Heart Foundation, London, UK

Paul G. Hugenholtz
Professor of Cardiology, Thoraxcentrum, Erasmus University,
Rotterdam, Netherlands

Coordinating Editor:

S.R. Underwood
National Heart and Chest Hospitals, London, UK

Associate Editors:

R.H. Anderson
Cardiothoracic Institute, London, UK

N.H. Brooks
Wythenshawe Hospital, Manchester, UK

K.M. Fox
National Heart Hospital, London, UK

E. Rowland
Cardiothoracic Institute, London, UK

A.D. Struthers
Ninewells Hospital, Dundee, UK

R.K. Walesby
London Chest Hospital, London, UK

Published by Current Medical Literature Ltd.
40–42 Osnaburgh Street, London NW1 3ND, UK.

ISBN 1 85009 013 0

Printed by The Eastern Press, London and Reading.

Preface

Since the publication of *Perspectives in Cardiology 1984*, cardiovascular medicine has seen many important developments. New hypotheses have been evolved to expound the pathogenesis of cardiac disease; established diagnostic techniques have been refined and new ones introduced; drugs and surgical procedures are available in greater number than ever before; and the optimal forms of management and rehabilitation continue to be the subjects of controversy.

In order to examine the relevance of all this new information, we believe it is time once again to step back and take a broad view of the literature. Retaining the formula of its predecessor, *Perspectives in Cardiology 1988* presents a compendium of reviews and comment encompassing most of the current cardiovascular literature. It highlights influential articles and discusses the contribution they have made from a detached and expert point of view.

The content of the book is presented in two ways. First, the Editors have identified forty topics of current importance and commissioned review articles from leading authorities in each field. The reviewers were asked to provide an account of both the present status of the topic and the prospects for future development. Second, groups of selected references dealing with all remaining topics are accompanied by a specialist editor's commentary that compares and contrasts the findings of the different authors, and places them in perspective. A system of cross-referencing and a detailed index allows the reader to locate any required information with speed and precision.

Since any selection must be subjective, and given that the choice of articles is enormous, we hope that readers will bear with us in what they consider to be omissions and misjudgements. On the positive side, we hope that *Perspectives in Cardiology 1988* will, like its predecessor, become a valuable addition to the library of clinicians and researchers alike — not only as an authoritative source of reference but also as an enjoyable and stimulating account of the changing field of modern cardiology.

B.E.S.
D.G.J.
P.G.H.
London 1988

List of Contributors

Philip C. Adams BA(Oxon), MB BS, MRCP
British-American Research Fellow of the American Heart Asssociation and the British Heart Foundation
Department of Medicine
Mount Sinai Medical School of the City University of New York
New York, NY 10029
USA

Robert H. Anderson BSc, MD, MRCPath
Joseph Levy Foundation Professor in Paediatric Cardiac Morphology
Cardiothoracic Institute
University of London
London SW3 6HP
UK

Edward J. Baker MD, MRCP
Senior Lecturer in Paediatric Cardiology
Guy's Hospital
London SE1 9RT
UK

Stephen G. Ball MA, MB BChir, PhD, MRCP
Professor of Cardiovascular Studies
The University
Leeds LS2 9JT
UK

Lionel M. Bargeron Jr MD
Division of Pediatric Cardiology
School of Medicine and Medical Center
University of Alabama at Birmingham
Birmingham, AL 35294
USA

Eugene H. Blackstone MD
Division of Cardiothoracic Surgery
School of Medicine and Medical Center
University of Alabama at Birmingham
Birmingham, AL 35294
USA

Michael E. Cain MD
Assistant Professor of Medicine
Director, Clinical Electrophysiology Laboratory
Washington University School of Medicine
St Louis, MO 63110
USA

James H. Chesebro MD, FACC
Professor of Medicine
Division of Cardiology
Mayo Clinic and Medical School
Rochester, MN 55095
USA

S.M. Cobbe MD, FRCP
Walton Professor of Medical Cardiology
Royal Infirmary
Glasgow, G31 2ER
UK

C. Richard Conti MD
Professor of Medicine
Chief, Division of Cardiology
Department of Medicine
University of Florida
Gainesville, FL 32610
USA

James L. Cox MD
Professor of Surgery
Chief, Division of Cardiothoracic Surgery
Washington University School of Medicine
St Louis, MO 63110
USA

A. David Cunningham BSc
Principal Physicist
The National Heart Hospital
London W1M 8BA
UK

Henry J. Dargie MB ChB, FRCP
Consultant Cardiologist
Western Infirmary
Glasgow, G11 6NT
UK

Graham J. Davies MB ChB, MD, MRCP
Senior Lecturer in Cardiovascular
Medicine
Royal Postgraduate Medical School
Consultant Cardiologist
Hammersmith Hospital
London, W12 0HS
UK

Michael J. Davies MD, FRCPath
British Heart Foundation Professor
of Cardiovascular Pathology
St George's Hospital Medical School
University of London
London SW17 ORE
UK

John S. Douglas Jr MD
Associate Professor of Medicine
(Cardiology) and Radiology
Emory University School of Medicine
Atlanta, GA 30322
USA

Myrvin H. Ellestad MD, FACC
Chief, Division of Cardiology
Memorial Medical Center of Long Beach
Long Beach, CA 90801-1428, and
Clinical Professor of Medicine
University of California at Irvine
California College of Medicine
Irvine, CA 92664
USA

Valentin Fuster MD, FACC
Arthur M. and Hilda A. Master Professor
of Medicine
Chief of Cardiology
Department of Medicine
Mount Sinai Medical School of the City
University of New York
New York, NY 10029
USA

A.M. Heagerty MB BS, MRCP
Lecturer in Medicine
University of Leicester
Leicester LE2 7LX
UK

Paul G. Hugenholtz MD, FACC
Professor of Cardiology
President, European Society of
Cardiology
Thoraxcentrum
Department of Medicine
Erasmus University
3000 DR Rotterdam
Netherlands

Stuart W. Jamieson MB BS, FRCS,
FACS
Professor and Head
Cardiovascular and Thoracic Surgery
University of Minnesota
Director, Minnesota Heart & Lung
Institute
Minneapolis, MN 55455
USA

Spencer B. King III MD
Professor of Medicine (Cardiology) and
Radiology
Emory University School of Medicine
Coronary Angioplasty Division
Emory University Hospital
Atlanta, GA 30322
USA

John W. Kirklin MD
Professor and Surgeon
Division of Cardiothoracic Surgery
Department of Surgery
University of Alabama at Birmingham
Birmingham, AL 35294
USA

Francis J. Klocke MD
Albert and Elizabeth Rekate Professor of
Medicine
Chief, Division of Cardiology
State University of New York at Buffalo
Buffalo, NY 14215
USA

Daan Kromhout PhD, MPHEpidemiol
Professor in Human Nutrition and
Nutritional Epidemiology
Institute of Social Medicine
University of Leiden
2300 RC Leiden
Netherlands

Kennedy R. Lees BSc, MB ChB, MRCP
Lecturer in Materia Medica
University of Glasgow, and
Honorary Senior Registrar
Stobhill General Hospital
Glasgow G21 3UW
UK

Floyd D. Loop MD
Cleveland Clinic Foundation
Cleveland, OH 44106
USA

Philip A. Ludbrook MB BS, FRACP
Professor of Medicine and Radiology
Washington University School of
Medicine
Cardiovascular Division
St Louis, MO 63110
USA

Averil O. Mansfield ChM, FRCS
Consultant Vascular Surgeon
St Mary's Hospital Medical School,
Royal Postgraduate Medical School, and
Hammersmith Hospital
London
UK

Michael G. Marmot PhD, MB BS, MPH
Professor of Community Medicine
University College London and
Middlesex Hospital Medical School
London WC1E 6EA
UK

Christopher G.A. McGregor MB ChB,
FRCS
Consultant Cardiothoracic Surgeon
Freeman Hospital
Newcastle upon Tyne NE7 7DN
UK

John McMurray BSc, MRCP
Research Fellow
Department of Clinical Pharmacology
Ninewells Hospital & Medical School
Dundee DD1 9SY
UK

Anthony W. Nathan MD, MRCP, FACC
Department of Cardiology
St Bartholomew's Hospital
West Smithfield
London EC1A 7BE
UK

D. John Parker MB ChB, FRCS, FRCP
Consultant Cardiac Surgeon
St George's Hospital
London SW17 0QT
UK

John O. Parker MD, FRCP(C)
Professor and Chairman
Division of Cardiology
Queen's University
Kingston, Ont. K7L 3N6
Canada

E. John Perrins MD, BSc, MRCP, FACC
Consultant Cardiologist
General Infirmary
Leeds, LS1 3EX
UK

Arshed A. Quyyumi BSc, MB BS, MRCP
Associate in Cardiology
Department of Health & Human Services
National Institutes of Health
Bethesda, MD 20205
USA

A.P. Rae BSc, MB ChB, MRCP
Consultant Cardiologist
Royal Infirmary
Glasgow G31 2ER
UK

John L. Reid MA, DM, FRCP
Regius Professor of Materia Medica
University of Glasgow, and
Consultant Physician
Stobhill General Hospital
Glasgow G21 3UW
UK

Gary S. Roubin MB, PhD
Assistant Professor of Medicine
(Cardiology) and Radiology
Emory University School of Medicine
Atlanta, GA 30322
USA

Maarten A.D.H. Schalekamp MD
Erasmus University
3000 DR Rotterdam
Netherlands

A.G. Shaper MB ChB, FRCP, FRCPath,
FFCM
Professor of Clinical Epidemiology
Regional Heart Study
Royal Free Hospital School of Medicine
London NW3 2PF
UK

Pamela J. Shaw MB BS, MRCP
Registrar in Neurology
University of Newcastle upon Tyne and
Royal Victoria Infirmary
Newcastle upon Tyne NE1 4LP
UK

Michael B. Simson MD
Samuel Bellet Associate Professor of
Medicine
Director, Medical Intensive Care Unit
Cardiovascular Section
Hospital of the University of Pennsylvania
Philadelphia, PA 19104
USA

Peter Sleight MD, DM, FRCP, FACC
Field Marshall Alexander Professor
of Cardiovascular Medicine
University of Oxford
Cardiac Department
John Radcliffe Hospital
Oxford OX3 9DU
UK

Burton E. Sobel MD, FACC
Lewin Professor of Medicine
Director, Cardiovascular Division
Department of Internal Medicine
Washington University School of
Medicine
St Louis, MO 63110
USA

Allan D. Struthers MD, MRCP
Consultant Physician
Department of Clinical Pharmacology
Ninewells Hospital & Medical School
Dundee DD1 9SY
UK

J. D. Swales MA, MD, FRCP
Professor of Medicine
University of Leicester
Leicester LE2 7LX
UK

Michael Tynan MD, FRCP
Joseph Levy Professor of Paediatric
Cardiology
Guy's Hospital
London SE1 9RT
UK

S. Richard Underwood MA, BM BCh,
MRCP
Senior Lecturer
Magnetic Resonance Unit
National Heart and Chest Hospitals
London SW3 6NN
UK

Thomas von Arnim MD
Lecturer
Ludwig Maximilians University
8000 Munich 70
FR Germany

Neil Wilson MB BS, DCh, MRCP
Consultant Paediatric Cardiologist
Killingbeck Hospital
Leeds LS14 6UQ
UK

Contents

1. ISCHEMIC HEART DISEASE

EPIDEMIOLOGY   1

Understanding Trends in Coronary Heart Disease Mortality   1
    Review: Michael G Marmot

Risk Factors for Coronary Heart Disease   12
    Review: AG Shaper

Lipids and Fish Oils in Ischemic Heart Disease   25
    Review: Daan Kromhout

PATHOPHYSIOLOGY   31

The Development, Progression and Regression of Atherosclerosis   31

Evaluation of the Physiologic Significance of Coronary Artery Stenosis   35
    Review: Francis J Klocke

Hemodynamic Significance of Coronary Artery Stenosis   40

Coronary Artery Spasm   42
    Review: C Richard Conti

STABLE AND UNSTABLE ANGINA PECTORIS   55

Pathophysiology   55

Diagnosis and Assessment   57

    Chest Pain With Normal Coronary Arteries   57

    Left-ventricular Function in Angina   58

    Ambulatory ST-segment Monitoring   61

    Exercise Testing: Current Trends   62
        Review: Myrvin H Ellestad

    The Effect of Cigarettes and Coffee on Angina   67

CONTENTS

Silent Ischemia   68
    Review: Thomas von Arnim

Therapy   72

    Beta-blockers and Calcium Antagonists in Angina   72

    Nitrates and Nitrate Tolerance in Angina Pectoris   77
        Review: John O Parker

    The Treatment of Unstable Angina   83
        Review: Paul G Hugenholtz

New Agents in Angina   98

Percutaneous Transluminal Coronary Angioplasty   99
    Review: Spencer B King III, John S Douglas Jr & Gary S Roubin

Laser Angioplasty   106

Current Aspects of Coronary Artery Surgery   109
    Review: D John Parker

Syndrome X   113
    Review: Graham J Davies

MYOCARDIAL INFARCTION   118

The Pathology of Acute Myocardial Infarction and Sudden Ischemic Death   118
    Review: Michael J Davies

Techniques for Use in the Diagnosis of Myocardial Infarction   126

Reciprocal ST-Segment Depression During Myocardial Infarction   127
    Review: Arshed A Quyyumi

Non-Q Wave Myocardial Infarction   133

Recent Advances in Coronary Thrombolysis   134
    Review: Philip A Ludbrook & Burton E Sobel

PROGNOSIS OF ANGINA PECTORIS AND MYOCARDIAL INFARCTION   150

2. CONGENITAL HEART DISEASE

Simplifying the Description of the Morphology of Congenitally Malformed Hearts   159
    Review: Robert H Anderson

Catheter Treatment in Congenital Heart Disease   163
    Review: Michael Tynan & Edward J Baker

Transposition of the Great Arteries   170
    Review: John W Kirklin, Lionel M Bargeron Jr & Eugene H
        Blackstone

Complete Transposition   174

The Role of Doppler Echocardiography in Congenital Heart Disease   179
    Review: Neil Wilson

Cross-sectional Echocardiography and Doppler Techniques   184

The Arterial and Venous Ducts: Closure, Persistent Patency and Pharmacologic Manipulation   188

Defects of the Atrial, Atrioventricular or Ventricular Septal Structures   191

Tetralogy of Fallot   196

Common Arterial Trunk ('Truncus Arteriosus')   201

Pulmonary and Aortic Stenosis   203

Hearts with a Univentricular Atrioventricular Connection   204

Coarctation of the Aorta   213

Pulmonary Vascular Disease   218

Miscellaneous Conditions and Other Topics   219

3. VALVE DISEASE

Mitral Valve Prolapse   226

Aortic Valvuloplasty   227

Mitral Valvuloplasty   229

Nutritional Status   230

Mechanical Valves   230

Miscellaneous   232

4. ENDOCARDIAL, MYOCARDIAL AND PERICARDIAL DISEASE

HYPERTROPHIC CARDIOMYOPATHY   235

Pathophysiology   235

Arrhythmias   236

Drug Therapy   238

Inheritance   239

Hypertrophic Cardiomyopathy in Childhood   240

INFECTIVE ENDOCARDITIS   241

Incidence and Etiology   241

Antibiotic Prophylaxis   242

5. HEART FAILURE

Current Concepts in Cardiac Failure   244
Review: Henry J Dargie

The Neuroendocrine Axis in Heart Failure   253

ACE Inhibitors in Heart Failure   254

6. ELECTROPHYSIOLOGY, HEART RATE AND RHYTHM

Electrophysiologic Stimulation Protocols for the Evaluation and Management of Ventricular Arrhythmias   258
Review: Anthony W Nathan

Value of Electrophysiologic Testing   268

Electrophysiologic Studies in Patients After Myocardial Infarction   272
Review: AP Rae & SM Cobbe

Indications for the Treatment of Ventricular Arrhythmias   281
Review: Michael E Cain

The Surgical Approach to the Treatment of Arrhythmias   301
Review: James L Cox

Antiarrhythmic Drug Therapy   308

The Physical Aspects of Catheter Ablation   313
Review: A David Cunningham

Current Status of Late Potentials   323
Review: Michael B Simson

Physiologic Rate-responsive Pacing   331
Review: E John Perrins

Pacing   334

Atrial Fibrillation   338

Arrhythmogenic Right-ventricular Dysplasia   340

Arrhythmias in Congenital Heart Disease   341

7. EXAMINATION AND DIAGNOSTIC PROCEDURES

Magnetic Resonance Imaging of the Cardiovascular System   344
     Review: S Richard Underwood

Doppler Ultrasound   359

Positron Emission Tomography   361

8. SURGERY

HEMODYNAMICS   363

Pharmacologic Agents   363

Cardiac Physiology   364

TECHNIQUES OF PRESERVATION   365

Myocardial Preservation   365

    Clinical   365

    Experimental   367

Spinal Cord Preservation   370

CORONARY ARTERY BYPASS SURGERY   372

Coronary Artery Bypass Surgery in Mild Angina   372

Internal Thoracic (Mammary) Artery Grafts in Coronary Artery Surgery   372
     Review: Floyd D Loop

Aspirin and Vein Grafts 379
Review: Philip C Adams, James H Chesebro & Valentin Fuster

Atherosclerosis in Coronary Bypass Grafts 390

Coronary Surgery at Life's Extremes 392

Left Main Stem Lesions 393

Significance of New Q Waves After Bypass Surgery 394

VALVE SURGERY 395

Mitral Valve Repair 395

Risks of Mitral Valve Replacement 396

Anticoagulation and Mechanical Valves 397

PERICARDIECTOMY 399

COMPLICATIONS OF CARDIAC SURGERY 399

Cerebral Complications of Cardiac Surgery 399
Review: Pamela J Shaw

Bleeding After Cardiopulmonary Bypass 413

TRANSPLANTATION 414

Combined Heart and Lung Transplantation 414
Review: Stuart W Jamieson

Prospects for the Artificial Heart 420
Review: Christopher GA McGregor

CAROTID ENDARTERECTOMY 425

Carotid Endarterectomy With or Without Coronary Artery Bypass Grafting 425
Review: Averil O Mansfield

9. PHYSIOLOGY

Atrial Natriuretic Peptide: Pharmacology, Physiology and Clinical Significance in Man   432
  Review: John McMurray & Allan D Struthers

Dopamine in Cardiovascular Medicine   442
  Review: Stephen G Ball

Cardiovascular Peptides   451

Intracellular Calcium   452

Prostaglandins   453

Angiotensin II Responsiveness in Hypertension   454

10. HYPERTENSION

Ion Transport and Hypertension   455
  Review: JD Swales & AM Heagerty

The Sympathetic Nervous System and Essential Hypertension   464
  Review: John L Reid & Kennedy R Lees

The Treatment of Mild Hypertension   470
  Review: Peter Sleight

Angiotensin Converting Enzyme Inhibitors in Hypertension: Recent Developments   475
  Review: Maarten ADH Schalekamp

Treatment of Hypertension   480

   Dietary Manipulation   480

   Diuretics   481

   Alcohol Reduction   482

   Other Treatment Strategies   483

Hypertension in Pregnancy   484

Renovascular Hypertension   485

Pulmonary Hypertension   487

11. THROMBOSIS AND EMBOLISM

Atrial Fibrillation and Stroke   489

Anticoagulation for Embolic Stroke   490

Venous Thrombosis   491

Oral Contraceptives   492

INDEX   493

1. Ischemic Heart Disease

EPIDEMIOLOGY

UNDERSTANDING TRENDS IN CORONARY HEART DISEASE MORTALITY

Review: MICHAEL G. MARMOT

In 1980, discussing the American decline in coronary heart disease (CHD) mortality rates, *The Lancet* commented: "Sceptics say that when John Snow removed the handle from the Broad Street Pump the cholera epidemic which he was seeking to abort was already on the wane" [1]. There are any number of claimants for the removal of the CHD pump handle, all of whom are supposedly responsible for the wane of the epidemic in the USA and elsewhere – surgeons doing coronary artery bypass grafts, cardiologists with PTCA, lysis and coronary care units, as well as beta-blockers, or public health campaigners for a healthy lifestyle. Certainly, the epidemic is waning, to some extent, and the challenge is to determine which, if any, of these factors or agents has been responsible.

In interpreting mortality trends, one must remember that if two phenomena co-vary it does not necessarily imply a causal relationship. Other factors may be involved: for example, a change in dietary fat consumption with a concurrent change in heart disease mortality rates is not evidence *per se* that the diet change led to the disease change. Applying the same principle, anomalies in the data do not on their own refute a theory of causation. In other words, data on trends should not be used in isolation to test etiologic hypotheses.

International Trends in CHD Mortality

Figures 1 and 2 show trends in CHD mortality for selected countries [2]. The data for these figures come from successive World Health Statistics Annuals [3], and 1968 was chosen as a starting point because the 8th Revision of the International Classification of Diseases (ICD) was introduced in this year. Age adjustments were performed by the direct method, using the England and Wales population as standard.

The most dramatic decline in CHD mortality from 1968 to 1982 took place among men and women in the USA. Compared with results in England and Wales, for example, the CHD mortality rate of men in the USA in 1968 was more than one-third higher. By 1978, the US rate had actually dropped to below the England and Wales figure. Finland appears to have passed the dubious distinction for the highest male CHD rates on to Scotland and (not shown) Northern Ireland. But data from South Africa make it likely that Indians in that country have among the highest rates in the world, for reasons that are not readily apparent [4].

The downward trend in England and Wales and Scotland, which we have been watching cautiously since the peak in 1978, appears to have continued to 1982, but 1983 figures were marginally higher. The percentage change in CHD mortality for England

1

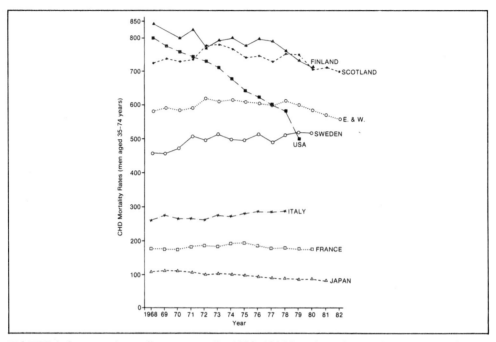

FIGURE 1: Coronary heart disease mortality 1968–1982 in selected countries: men aged 35–74 years. Age-adjusted rates/100 000 [2]. E. & W. = England and Wales.

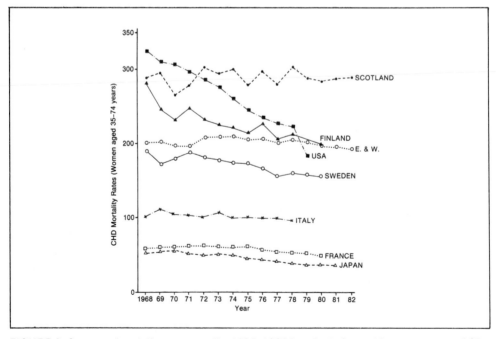

FIGURE 2: Coronary heart disease mortality 1968–1982 in selected countries: women aged 35–74 years. Age-adjusted rates/100 000 [2]. E. & W. = England and Wales.

and Wales is shown in Figures 3 and 4 separately by age, taking 1968–1970 as a baseline of 100 for each age. The decline is proportionately greater at younger than at older ages – a similar picture to that seen in Scotland.

The latest figures are possibly affected by the change to the 9th Revision of the ICD, which occurred in 1978 in Italy, and in 1979 in Scotland, England and Wales, the USA, France and Japan. The effect of the change is seen most dramatically in the USA: 1979 is sharply down compared with 1978. The same discontinuity between rates coded under the 8th and 9th Revisions is not seen in other countries. This is shown by the so-called 'comparability ratios'. In the USA [5] and England and Wales [6], samples of deaths are coded according to both the 8th and 9th ICD Revisions. For example, in the USA, the ratio for ischemic heart disease was 0.878, i.e. 12.2% fewer certificates were classified as ischemic heart disease under the 9th than under the 8th Revision. By contrast, in England and Wales, it was 0.956, i.e. only 4.4% fewer. In analyses of subsequent years, adjustments must be made to take account of these differences.

Similarly, to go further back before the 8th Revision (1968) poses problems, as the category 'heart disease' was treated differently in the 6th and 7th Revisions. In an earlier report, we went back to the 1950s by combining all non-rheumatic heart disease and hypertension [7]. The breadth of this category reduced the likelihood that international differences in CHD rates were due to diagnostic or coding differences, although it may have masked differing changes in subcategories. This is the approach taken by Thom *et al* [8]: age-adjusted mortality rates among men and women aged 45–64 years from non-rheumatic heart disease and hypertension (heart disease) were plotted for 26 countries (Fig. 5). There are several notable points:

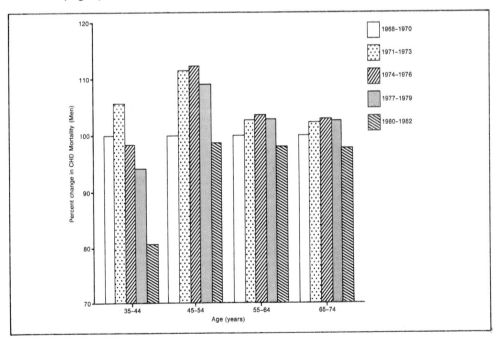

FIGURE 3: Percent change in CHD mortality in men in England and Wales, by age, taking 1968–1970 as 100.

3

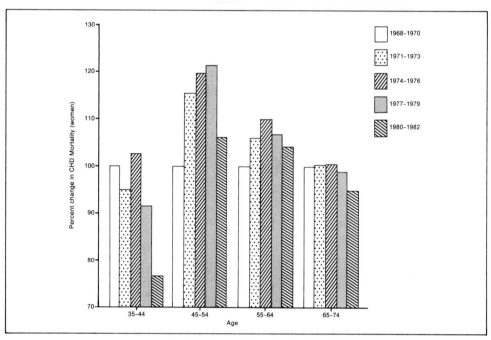

FIGURE 4: Percent change in CHD mortality in women in England and Wales, by age, taking 1968-1970 as 100.

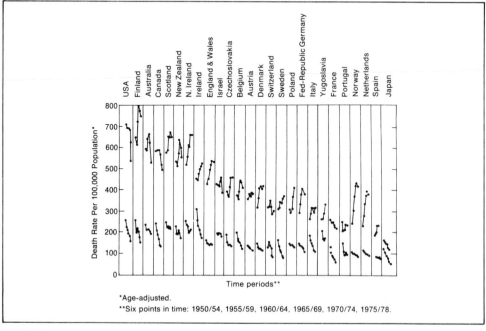

FIGURE 5: Death rates from non-rheumatic heart disease and hypertension in men and women aged 45-64 years in 26 countries, 1950-1978 [8].

(i) heart disease mortality declined earlier, and in more countries, in women than in men;

(ii) as a result, the M/F ratios of death rates for heart disease increased;

(iii) among men, there were sharp declines in heart disease mortality in some high-rate countries (the USA, Finland, Australia, Canada and New Zealand), in some 'intermediate'-rate countries (Israel, Belgium and Switzerland) and in some low-rate countries (France and Japan). Decline in mortality cannot therefore be attributed to some kind of regression to the mean;

(iv) several countries – Ireland, Sweden, Czechoslovakia, Poland and Yugoslavia – showed a continued upward trend; and

(v) perhaps the most notable was the persisting international differences in heart disease rates: although the dramatic decline in the USA brought it 'down' in the international rankings and the rise in Norway and the Netherlands brought them 'up', the differences between countries, in general, were more dramatic than the time trends within single countries. It should not be assumed that these persisting international differences are genetic, as migrants from one country to another experience changes in disease rates [9].

Trends within Great Britain and the USA

A disadvantage of international comparisons is that they mask a great deal of diversity within countries. In Great Britain, for example, between the 1950s and 1960s, heart disease changed from being more common in social classes I and II to being more common in classes IV and V [10]. This trend has become more exaggerated in the last decade (Fig. 6) [11]. CHD mortality declined by 15% in men in non-manual classes, but rose by 1% in manual classes; a similar divergence is seen in women. Table I shows that this difference by social class obtains in every region of the country, and that long-standing regional inequalities persist.

Similarly, in the USA, insurees with the Metropolitan Life Insurance Company had a steeper decline in heart disease mortality than the US average, as did Californian white male physicians – both groups presumably being more affluent than the average [12].

Decline in Incidence or Case-Fatality?

A decreased mortality rate could result from a decreased incidence and/or a decrease in case-fatality rates. The latter, in turn, could result from an improvement in treatment, or a change in the natural history, or from other less well-identified influences, or a combination of all these. It could also be artefactual: an apparent decline in the age-specific hospital case-fatality rate could result from increased admission of milder cases. It is not known how much each of these has played a role. However, figures from the WHO myocardial infarction registries show a high correlation between acute myocardial infarction attack rates and mortality from acute myocardial infarction (as gleaned from national vital statistics records). This suggests that differences between countries in CHD mortality rates are unlikely to be due to differences in case-fatality rates.

More direct evidence comes from the USA [13]. Among the 75 000–94 000 male employees of the Du Pont Corporation from 1957 to 1983, there was a 28% decline in

5

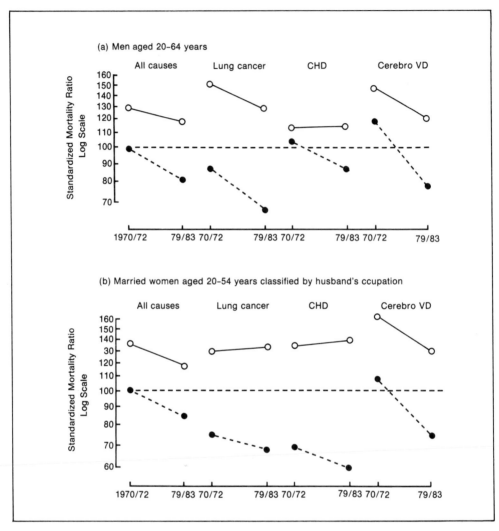

FIGURE 6: Standardized mortality ratios (SMR) for select causes of death in Great Britain 1970–1972 and 1979–1983 for manual (o---o) and non-manual (●---●) groups [11]. For each cause the SMR in 1979–1983 is 100 for each sex.

the incidence of CHD events, which was steeper among salaried (white-collar) employees than among production workers. There was also a small decline in case-fatality rates beginning in 1969, with a marked drop after 1975. Pell and Fayerweather conclude that improved medical care may have made some contribution to the decline in CHD mortality, but the decline in incidence, which had begun earlier, was more important [13].

Factors Responsible for Improvement
If decreased mortality from CHD in the USA, Finland, Australia and Canada is partly

Table I: Standardized mortality ratios* for coronary heart disease 1970–1972 and 1979/83 for manual and non-manual occupations by region in England and Wales and Scotland: men aged 20–64 years [11]

	Non-manual		Manual	
	1970–1972	**1979/83**	**1970–1972**	**1979/83**
North West	121	104	129	131
Wales	117	93	140	125
Yorkshire and Humberside	114	97	120	120
North	111	100	132	129
West Midlands	100	86	108	112
East Midlands	96	87	101	106
South West	93	79	103	100
South East	90	76	95	98
East Anglia	86	69	82	81
Central Clydeside Conurbation		110 ⎫		163 ⎫
Strathclyde (excluding Clydeside)	103	105 ⎬ 100	137	166 ⎬ 144
Rest of Scotland		94 ⎭		125 ⎭

*SMR for all men in Great Britain in 1979/83 = 100. The 1970–1972 figures are standardized using the 1979/83 rates. The two time periods are therefore directly comparable.

or mostly a reflection of decreased incidence, it is important to try to determine the factors responsible. The quality of the data available on trends in incidence and risk factors does not allow the testing of causal hypotheses.

Smoking

Smoking is strongly related to cardiovascular disease in high-risk countries. There are a number of reasons, however, why trends in smoking may not correlate strongly with trends in CHD mortality: international data on tobacco consumption may not be comparable; smoking is less strongly related to CHD in countries where the disease is less frequent; and factors other than smoking may account for the disease trends. Despite this, there is evidence that smoking influences CHD trends on an international scale. In the USA and Australia, tobacco sales have declined since 1960, which is consistent with the decline in CHD; but there has also been a drop in tobacco sales in the UK, which had no decrease in CHD until 1979, and in Sweden, which had an *increase*. In the USA and Finland, surveys have shown a decrease in the prevalence of smoking among men but not women, although both sexes had reduced coronary mortality.

Taking data from 21 countries, there was a small positive correlation between changes in consumption of cigarettes 1968–1977 and changes in heart disease mortality over the same period (Fig. 7) [14]. Building in a time-lag did not improve the correlation. To put the apparently low correlation of 0.17 in perspective, the highest correla-

7

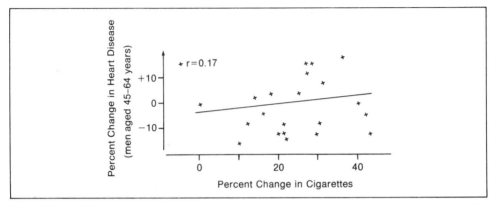

FIGURE 7: Correlation of percent changes in mortality from non-rheumatic heart disease, 1968–1977, with percent changes in cigarette consumption, 1968–1976 [14]. Data taken from 21 countries.

tion between smoking and lung cancer in these 21 countries was 0.32 (taking smoking and cancer in the same year); the correlation between changes in lung cancer and changes in cigarette consumption was even weaker than with heart disease. In the Soviet Union, where heart disease mortality has increased, smoking has been increasing and a causal connection is possible.

Diet
The contribution to dietary calories by fat in the USA increased from 32% in 1909–1913 to 41% in 1957–1959, and has stayed at this level ever since (in 1981, for example, reaching 42%). But the type of fat in the food supply has changed: although the *per capita* amount of saturated fat has changed little since 1935, the amount of linoleic acid has increased, particularly since the 1960s. Table II shows the ratio of linoleic acid to saturated fat in the US food supply [2]. Between 1925–1929 and 1957–1959, it moved

Table II: US food supply [2]: food energy as saturated fatty acids and linoleic acid*

Year	Food Energy (% of calories)		Linoleic Acid
	Saturated	**Linoleic**	**Saturated**
1909–1913	12.9	2.3	0.18
1925–1929	13.9	2.9	0.21
1935–1939	14.6	3.1	0.22
1947–1949	15.2	3.8	0.25
1957–1959	15.5	4.5	0.29
1967–1969	15.5	5.4	0.34
1975	14.1	6.2	0.43
1981	14.2	6.8	0.48

* Most of the remainder of the fat is made up by oleic acid.

only from 0.21 to 0.29, but by 1981 it had increased to 0.48. Dietary cholesterol decreased. These data pertain to food available for consumption but not necessarily eaten. In contrast, Table III, using data from food-consumption surveys, shows that there has been a reduction in the intake of milk, eggs, beef, pork and visible fats. Overall, this amounts to a decline of 17% in total fat consumed.

As they stand, the above data are more consistent with the idea of a protective effect of essential fatty acids (linoleic acid) or a high ratio of essential to saturated fatty acids than with a harmful effect of saturated fats. Evidence that increased linoleic acid consumption may have contributed to the favorable CHD trend in the USA compared with the UK comes from a survey of reported analyses of adipose tissue biopsies [15]. In the USA, since the mid-1960s there has been a progressive increase in the proportion linoleic acid makes up of total fatty acids in adipose tissue; in the UK, with no decline in CHD until 1979, the proportion of linoleic acid in the diet remained unchanged [15]. It is now known that there is an inverse relationship between adipose linoleic acid and CHD.

Interestingly, in the UK, the type of fat in food may at last be changing [16]. Between 1975 and 1980, the consumption of soft margarine more than doubled, and the consumption of vegetable and salad oils increased by 66%; saturated fat decreased by 7% (Table IV).

Data from several countries substantiate the importance of changes in dietary pattern. In Australia, the decline in CHD has occurred against the background of a 21% reduction in carcass meat, a 65% reduction in butter and an 11.2% reduction in milk consumption; margarine consumption increased by 450%. In Finland, dairy fat but not total animal fat had decreased by 1975. These data from the USA, Australia, Finland and the UK are broadly in line with the idea of a protective role for essential fatty acids and a harmful role for saturated fats – perhaps more the former than the latter.

Nevertheless, there are significant exceptions which do not easily fit the dietary hypothesis. Sweden reports similar dietary changes to the USA, but an increase in CHD mortality. Japan has had an increase in fat consumption and a decrease in mortality from CHD. Israel, too, appears to have decreased CHD mortality and increased

Table III: Intake of foods and nutrients (g/day) 1965 and 1977, and % change, men aged 35–50 years: US nationwide food-consumption surveys

Food or Nutrient	1965	1977	% Change*
Milk and milk drinks	236	203	−14
Cheese	13	18	+38.5
Eggs	51	41	−19.6
Beef	102	79	−22.5
Pork	82	52	−36.6
Fish	13	17	+30.8
Fats and oils	39	19	−51.3
Total fat	132.4	109.3	−17.4

* (1977–1965)/1965.

9

Table IV: Fatty acids (g/person/day) and ratio of polyunsaturated/saturated fatty acids (P/S ratio) in the average household diet (in 1974, changes in methods resulted in two estimates) [16]

Year	Saturated	Monounsaturated	Polyunsaturated	P/S ratio
1959	53.0	43.0	9.2	0.17
1969	56.7	46.5	11.0	0.19
1972	52.0	42.9	11.5	0.22
1973	51.5	41.9	11.5	0.22
1974	51.4	41.2	10.8	0.21
1974	50.7	39.8	10.6	0.20
1975	51.7	39.8	10.1	0.19
1976	50.1	39.7	10.5	0.20
1977	47.5	39.0	10.4	0.21
1978	47.2	39.3	10.6	0.22
1979	47.8	39.7	10.7	0.22
1980	46.8	39.6	11.3	0.24
1981	45.6	38.9	11.4	0.25
1982	44.4	38.7	12.1	0.27

saturated fat consumption. As is always the case with CHD, a one-factor explanation will simply not fit all the observed trends.

Blood Pressure
It is difficult to determine whether blood pressure levels have decreased over time because of the ever-present differences in the techniques and frequency of measurements. Mortality from cerebrovascular accident (stroke) has been declining in many Western countries, and this started long before the CHD decline. If, as has been suggested, a decrease in blood pressure were responsible for the decline in mortality from stroke, it follows that a decrease in blood pressure could not by itself account for the CHD decline – otherwise, CHD and stroke would have followed the same time curve.

The US decline in mortality from stroke began in the 1930s, well before there were effective drugs available and before they were used extensively in the population. Nevertheless, in both New Zealand and the USA there has been an accelerated decline in stroke mortality in the later 1960s and 1970s, suggesting that the treatment of blood pressure may have made some contribution. In Japan, where there has been active treatment of elevated blood pressure, stroke and CHD mortality have declined. Once again, Sweden provides the exception to the trend.

Physical Activity
Despite the American enthusiasm for jogging, it is difficult to obtain evidence on the magnitude of the US increase in physical activity, and hence whether it has contributed substantially – or even at all – to the decrease in CHD.

Stress is excluded from discussions of trends in mortality because of conceptual, definitional and measurement difficulties. It is mentioned here only as a reminder that, although trends over time cannot be charted, something important may have been missed.

An Overview?

The lack of data on trends in CHD incidence and coronary risk factors in most countries has prompted the World Health Organization to coordinate the MONICA studies (Monitoring Trends and Determinants in Cardiovascular Diseases). In the meantime, a series of reports from 11 countries were brought together in 1985 in one issue of *Cardiology*, and summarized by Pyörälä *et al* (Table V) [17]. Their impression is that primary prevention has contributed to a decline in CHD mortality, but they have difficulty in explaining the anomalies - the rise in CHD mortality in certain countries.

The Lancet concluded in 1980: "Despite the inconsistencies, it is tempting to believe that a combination of [...] changes – diet, smoking, physical activity, treatment of blood pressure – have contributed to the improved heart disease pattern" [1]. It is still tempting, although the whole story is not yet in.

Table V: CHD mortality trends in the 1970s – contributory influences [17]

Trends	USA	Australia	New Zealand	Finland	Norway	Belgium	Israel	Sweden	Poland	Italy	Spain
CHD mortality trends*	↓	↓	↓	↓	↓	↓	↓	↑	↑	↑	↑
National preventive efforts+	++	++	+	++	++	++	0	+	0	+	0
Trend toward better dietary habits+	++	++	+	+	+	++	0	0	0	0	0
Risk factors*											
Serum cholesterol	↓	?	(↓)	↓	↓	↓	ø	ø	(↑)	(↑)	(↑)
Blood pressure	↓	(↓)	↓	↓	↓	(↓)	↓	(↓)	(↓)	(↓)	(↓)
Smoking	↓	↓	↓	↓	↓	↓	ø	↓	?	(↑)	(↑)
Physical inactivity	↓	?	↓	↓	↓	?	?	↓	?	(↓)	?
Improvement in the treatment of CHD+	++	++	+	+	+	++	++	+	+	+	+

* ?=no data; ↓=decline; ø=no change; ↑=increase; ( )=possible change.
Scale of 0 to ++.

References

[1] Anonymous.
Why the American decline in coronary heart disease? [Editorial].
Lancet 1986; i: 183–6.

[2] Marmot MG.
Interpretation of trends in coronary heart disease mortality.
Acta Med Scand 1985; **701** (Suppl): 58–65.

[3] World Health Statistics Annuals, 1965–1983. Geneva: WHO.

[4] Wyndham CH.
Mortality from cardiovascular diseases in the various population groups in the Republic of South Africa.
S Afr Med J 1979; 56: 1023–30.

[5] National Center for Health Statistics. Monthly vital statistics report.
Estimates of selected comparability ratios based on dual coding of 1976 death certificates by the 8th and 9th Revisions of the International Classification of Diseases. US Department of Health, Education and Welfare, Vol. 28, no. 11, 1980.

[6] Office of Population Censuses and Surveys. Mortality statistics.
Comparison of 8th and 9th Revisions of the International Classification of Diseases. London: HMSO, series DH1 no. 10, 1983.

[7] Marmot MG, Booth M, Beral V.
Changes in heart disease mortality in England and Wales and other countries.
Health Trends 1981; 13: 33–8.

[8] Thom TJ, Epstein FH, Feldman JF, Leaverton RF.
Trends in total mortality and mortality from heart disease in 26 countries from 1950 to 1978.
Int J Epidemiol 1985; 14: 510–20.

[9] Marmot MG, Adelstein AM, Bulusu L.
Lessons from the study of immigrant mortality.
Lancet 1984; i: 1455–7.

[10] Marmot MG, Adelstein AM, Robinson N, Rose GA.
Changing social class distribution of heart disease.
Br Med J 1978; ii: 1109–12.

[11] Marmot MG, McDowall ME.
Mortality decline and widening social inequalities.
Lancet 1986; ii: 274–6.

[12] Stamler J.
The marked decline in coronary heart disease mortality rates in the United States, 1968–81: Summary of findings and possible explanations.
Cardiology 1985; 72: 11–22.

[13] Pell S, Fayerweather WE.
Trends in the incidence of myocardial infarction and in associated mortality and morbidity in a large employed population, 1957–1983.
N Engl J Med 1985; 312: 1005–11.

[14] Marmot MG.
Epidemiology of cardiovascular disease in different countries in relation to smoking. In: Schettler FG et al, eds. Atherosclerosis. Berlin: Springer Verlag, 1983; pp. 888–92.

[15] Katan MB, Beynen AC.
Linoleic acid consumption and coronary heart disease in USA and UK.
Lancet 1981; ii: 371.

[16] Committee on Medical Aspects of Food Policy - DHSS Diet and Cardiovascular Disease.
Report on Health Social Subjects. London: HMSO, no. 28, 1984.

[17] Pyörälä K, Epstein FH, Kornitzer M.
Changing trends in coronary heart disease mortality: Possible explanations.
Cardiology 1985; 72: 5–10.

RISK FACTORS FOR CORONARY HEART DISEASE

Review: A.G. SHAPER

Since the last review of the epidemiology of coronary heart disease (CHD) in this series of volumes [1], a number of important publications have emerged (see also review by M.G. Marmot, this volume), attempting to make comprehensible the decrease in CHD mortality in some countries (e.g. the USA [2], Finland and Australia) and the increase in CHD mortality in others (e.g. Sweden, Bulgaria and Romania).

Possible explanations for changing trends in CHD mortality were fully reviewed in 1985 in a special issue of *Cardiology*, with papers from 11 countries [3]: in seven of these (the USA, Australia, New Zealand, Finland, Norway, Belgium and Israel), the CHD mortality rate declined during the 1970s; in four countries (Sweden, Poland, Italy and

Spain), the prevailing trend in the 1970s was a rise in male mortality. In six of the seven countries showing decline, national efforts for CHD prevention proceeded throughout the 1970s, with a trend towards better dietary habits, more physical activity, less cigarette smoking and lower serum total cholesterol concentrations. In the four countries with rising CHD mortality rates, no definite change has occurred in dietary habits, and in three of these the serum total cholesterol levels appear to have been rising; in two of these four countries, the prevalence of cigarette smoking has increased.

Overall, there is a strong message that declining rates of CHD have run parallel to the improvements in CHD risk-factor status. While most countries with a declining CHD mortality rate attribute the decline to better medical and surgical care, Israel considers that improved treatment of hypertension and symptomatic CHD has made the greatest contribution, since no changes have occurred there in dietary or smoking habits. It is of interest that Sweden, a country with highly advanced medical and surgical treatment of symptomatic CHD, is amongst the group with increasing mortality rates for CHD. If changes in risk-factor levels can be firmly associated with changes in CHD mortality rates, this would strongly support both the hypothesis relating the major risk factor (serum total cholesterol) to CHD and the case for primary prevention. The WHO Monitoring the Trends and Determinants in Cardiovascular Diseases (MONICA) research project is attempting to measure, over a 10-year period, changes in CHD morbidity and mortality as well as changes in risk factors, lifestyle and medical care, in 30 participating countries using standardized methods [4].

A very useful, up-to-date comparison using WHO data of CHD mortality rates in 29 countries from 1968 to 1981 has been published by the Cardiovascular Research Unit in Dundee, Scotland [5].

Prevention Trials
The major trial of prevention to be reported in the last two years is that of the Lipid Research Clinics Program in the USA [6]. This trial has obtained considerable publicity, and its findings have been widely discussed in terms of appropriate strategies for the prevention of CHD. Essentially a 'high-risk' trial, the study screened 480 000 American men aged 35–39 years, yielding 18 000 with serum total cholesterol levels of at least 6.85 mmol/l. After excluding those men (80%) whose serum total cholesterol levels responded to dietary measures over four months, 3806 men (1% of the screened population) remained to take part in a trial designed to test whether reducing serum total cholesterol concentrations would lead to a decline in CHD events.

Subjects were randomized into two groups, one receiving six packets of cholestyramine a day, the other receiving a placebo. The procedure was double-blind, and both groups were also on a moderate cholesterol-lowering (increased polyunsaturated/saturated (P/S) fat ratio) diet. After a seven-year follow-up, in comparison to the placebo group, the drug-treated group showed the following: (i) 9% lower serum total cholesterol levels; (ii) a 19% lower incidence of fatal and non-fatal CHD events; (iii) 20% fewer cases of angina; and (iv) 21% fewer coronary bypass operations.

It must be noted, however, that over the follow-up period definite CHD developed in 9.8% of the placebo group and in 8.1% of the cholestyramine group. Although the difference between groups satisfies the minimum criterion for statistical significance ($P<0.05$), the magnitude of the difference is small in view of the large numbers of subjects involved. It is certainly not of an order to inspire confidence in the ability of this regimen to affect CHD on a community level.

The findings of this study have encouraged enthusiasm for the identification and drug treatment of those with considerably elevated levels – i.e. the 'high-risk' approach. The authors estimate that a 25% reduction in serum total cholesterol levels would lead to a 50% reduction in CHD incidence [6], but there has been considerable argument as to whether the findings in this rigorously selected 'high-risk' group can readily be extrapolated to men with lower serum total cholesterol levels.

National Institutes of Health Consensus Development Conference (USA) has recommended that "all physicians should be encouraged to include, whenever possible, a blood cholesterol measurement on every adult patient when that patient is first seen [7]." In the UK, it has been suggested that "we should aim at identifying those above the eightieth percentile of serum cholesterol concentration and blood pressure measurement [8]." Case finding by the widespread use of serum cholesterol measurement, and consequently the development of more lipid clinics, has been proposed as a complement to population measures [9,10]. These suggestions imply the need to measure serum total cholesterol in the whole adult population, albeit on an opportunistic basis.

It is clear that the Lipid Research Clinics trial has had a major impact on attitudes to risk for CHD, yet there is considerable evidence to suggest that this may not be a particularly cost-effective approach. In countries such as the USA and the UK, identification of the top 20% of the serum total cholesterol distribution in middle-aged men identifies a group in whom less than one-third of the cases of acute myocardial (fatal or non-fatal) and sudden cardiac death will occur over the ensuing five years of observation [11]. One could achieve a higher percentage of 'cases' occurring in this period of time by identifying the top 20% of the blood pressure distribution (either systolic or diastolic) or the top 20% of the distribution of number of cigarette-smoking years. Indeed, even the top 20% of the age distribution in these middle-aged men will give the same yield of 'cases'!

We have long known that the multifactorial approach is by far the strongest method of predicting risk for CHD. It is therefore interesting that only the MRFIT (Multiple Risk Factor Interventional Trial) has used this approach in selecting subjects for an intervention study [12]. In the MRFIT study, only those men in the upper range of a risk-score distribution (based on cigarette smoking, blood pressure and plasma cholesterol concentration) were entered. It should, however, be noted that none of the 12 866 men showed any evidence of CHD, either clinically or on ECG. This latter point is made because it is well established that evidence of pre-existing coronary heart disease is the strongest predictor of a major CHD event (acute myocardial infarction or sudden cardiac death). There is also good evidence that men with evidence of pre-existing CHD may show the greatest response to preventive measures. In the Belgian Heart Disease Prevention Project, multifactorial intervention (diet, cigarette smoking, obesity, exercise and blood pressure control) was strikingly more effective in men with an ischemic electrocardiogram at initial examination than in men with a normal ECG at baseline [13]. Indeed, 46% of the total benefit in reducing the incidence of CHD occurred in the 7% of men with an ischemic ECG at entry.

From these issues, it can be concluded that, if a 'high-risk' approach is to be adopted at a community (primary care) level, 'high risk' should be determined in *all men*, rather than only in those men free of all evidence of CHD. As it is estimated that perhaps one-quarter of middle-aged men in the UK have some evidence of CHD [14], it makes little sense to exclude them from any proposed strategy for prevention, and the results of the Belgian study strongly suggest that the benefits may be proportionately greater in this group [13].

A strategy for identifying men at high risk of heart attacks, suitable for the primary care setting but equally applicable to more specialized situations, has been proposed, based on the findings of the British Regional Heart Study [11]. A risk score is derived using cigarette smoking, blood pressure, recall of a doctor-diagnosis of CHD and/or diabetes mellitus, questionnaire evidence of current angina, and history of parental death from 'heart trouble'. The top 20% of the score distribution identified 53% of men who developed a major CHD event in the subsequent five years. The addition of serum total cholesterol and ECG evidence made only a modest improvement in prediction (to 59%), and measurement of these two factors would considerably increase the cost and effort of screening. The measurement of serum total cholesterol in this high-risk group, where facilities allow, would be of considerable additional help in *individual* management; likewise, in those in whom angina is revealed for the first time by questionnaire, an ECG would be useful.

New and Old Risk Factors

Lipids
It is now clear that risk for CHD is continuous over the whole range of cholesterol concentrations, the lowest mortality being among men with concentrations below the 20th percentile; the American MRFIT data [15,16] and the British Whitehall data [17] confirm this observation. It is also apparent that the average serum total cholesterol level in middle-aged British men carries a twofold risk of a major CHD event compared with men with lower levels [18]. Thus, at least 60% of middle-aged men in countries with total cholesterol distributions similar to Great Britain carry at least a two fold risk of CHD.

In disagreement with the above assumption is a study in 10 059 Israeli civil servants [19]. Coronary heart disease mortality did not increase at total cholesterol concentrations below 5.6 mmol/l, and an appreciable increase occurred only in the highest quintile of total cholesterol (>6.2 mmol/l). On the other hand, the inverse association between high-density lipoprotein (HDL) cholesterol and CHD was continuous. While these findings may seem to conflict with those of the British studies and the MRFIT, they may well be explained by the much lower levels of serum total cholesterol found in the Israeli men and the curvilinear relationship between total cholesterol and CHD risk.

One disturbing publication in the lipid field came from the British Regional Heart Study, concerning the role of HDL cholesterol in determining the risk of CHD [20]. While the mean HDL cholesterol concentration was lower in the 'cases' of CHD compared with other men, the differences became small and non-significant after adjustment for age, body mass index, blood pressure, cigarette smoking and non-HDL cholesterol concentration. Multivariate analysis showed that non-HDL cholesterol was a far more powerful predictor of risk for CHD than was the HDL/total cholesterol ratio. This finding has led to considerable discussion [21], and the matter has yet to be resolved. What is clear is that the widely accepted relationship between HDL cholesterol and CHD may well vary in different communities.

Hypertension
For a review of some important aspects of hypertension, also as a risk factor, see the article by P. Sleight in this volume.

Smoking
In a study of 119 British cigarette smokers who survived their first myocardial infarction for one month, subjects were followed for five years or until death [22]. Those who stopped smoking after their infarction had 55% of the age-sex corrected mortality of those who continued to smoke ($P<0.05$). This small study appears to confirm that it is important for a patient to stop smoking after a first myocardial infarction. Similar results come from a larger and more complex US study involving 1873 cases of first myocardial infarction in men aged 20–54 years, selected from 78 coronary care units [23]. A control group of 2775 men was drawn from those admitted to hospital for conditions unrelated to smoking. Current smokers in this case-control study had three times the risk for myocardial infarction of those who had never smoked. Men who had given up smoking 1–2 years previously had a relative risk of 2.0, while those who had given up more than two years previously had the same risk as non-smokers. While these results are of considerable comfort to ex-smokers, they are almost too good to be true.

There is growing evidence that the increased risk of CHD associated with cigarette smoking is not as rapidly or completely reversible as has been widely accepted [24].

Clotting
There has long been interest in the role of fibrinogen in coronary heart disease and stroke [25], but few major prospective studies have included measurement of fibrinogen or fibrinolysis. In a prospective study from Sweden, 792 randomly selected middle-aged men were followed for 13.5 years [26]. Univariate analysis revealed that serum cholesterol, blood pressure, smoking and plasma fibrinogen were associated with the subsequent occurrence of myocardial infarction. Fibrinogen and smoking were strongly interrelated. With multivariate analysis, the association between fibrinogen and myocardial infarction became much weaker and non-significant. Nevertheless, this remains an interesting area for future study.

One case-control study assessed fibrinolytic activity in 71 young (under 54 years of age) three-year survivors of myocardial infarction and compared it with that in 50 age-matched healthy subjects [27]. The patients had low tissue plasminogen activator (t-PA) activities after venous occlusion, associated with high circulating levels of a t-PA inhibitor and with reduced t-PA release from the vascular endothelium. These findings support the belief that reduced fibrinolytic activity might play a role in the development of myocardial infarction. However, studies of this kind require confirmation by more exactingly designed investigations.

A somewhat neglected area of coagulability is that of blood viscosity, and two recent studies draw attention to this mechanism. In one, plasma viscosity was measured in 108 patients with CHD [28]. The highest values were found in 'unstable angina'; lower values were found in patients with acute myocardial infarction and normal values in those with stable angina - suggesting that increased plasma viscosity may reduce myocardial blood flow and account for some manifestations of CHD. Once again, studies of this kind need to take careful account of possible confounding variables. A more experimental study in eight normal subjects showed that mild surface-cooling resulted in an increase in packed cell volume and whole blood viscosity, as well as in systolic and diastolic blood pressure and both high- and low-density lipoprotein cholesterol [29]. These changes could account in part for the increased mortality from CHD and stroke frequently observed in the winter months.

Sex Hormones
Despite the appearance of two somewhat contradictory sets of findings regarding the use of estrogen preparations to control postmenopausal symptoms, there is a consensus at present that hormone replacement therapy does not increase CHD risk and that it may even reduce risk. The Framingham Study, reporting on 1234 postmenopausal women over the age of 50 at their twelfth biennial examination, concluded that those using estrogen had a 50% higher incidence of cardiovascular morbidity and a twofold risk of stroke in the succeeding eight years compared with those who had not taken estrogen [30]. Increased rates for myocardial infarction were seen in estrogen users who smoked; amongst non-smokers estrogen use was associated only with increased evidence of stroke [30]. In a US postal questionnaire study among 32 317 postmenopausal women, the risk of CHD in estrogen users was half that of non-users, even when adjusted for other known risk factors [31]. It has been suggested that these discordant results may be a product of the different study designs and their very different methods of selecting subjects and acquiring information.

Consensus opinion at present considers that the combined (estrogen/progestogen) pill may cause an increase in arterial pressure even in the lower doses currently used; the progestogen-only pill does not appear to do so in normotensive women [32]. The progestogen-only pill also does not appear to predispose to venous or arterial thrombosis, and unlike the combined pill is not contraindicated in women with congenital or rheumatic heart disease.

Family History
Evidence continues to accumulate that a family history of heart disease is a risk factor for CHD independent of familial aggregations of cholesterol, blood pressure and cigarette smoking. A US study of 4014 men and women aged 40–79 years, followed for nine years, found that a positive family history of heart attack was independently predictive of death from cardiovascular and coronary heart disease in men, but not in women [33]. Significant differences were restricted to younger men (<60 years), in whom there was a fivefold *excess* risk of cardiovascular death in those with a positive family history. Interestingly enough, a family history of premature heart attack (<50 years of age) was not predictive of mortality in men or women. The degree of excess risk encountered here was far greater than that reported in most studies of family history.

Psychologic Factors

There is an increasing belief that personality, while not being a fundamental etiologic factor, is a factor likely to make CHD manifest in individuals with compromised coronary arteries. A Dutch study of 243 men followed for almost 10 years showed a significant association between the type A personality and fatal coronary events, but not all coronary events [34]. In a study as small as this, any association found is both remarkable and open to question. In an analysis of 2314 patients taking part in the Aspirin Myocardial Infarction Study, there was no correlation between type A score (using the Jenkins Activity Survey questionnaire) and recurrence of a CHD event [35]. In an Australian study of 92 patients admitted for coronary angiography, type A behavior as well as tension and anxiety indices were associated with severity of coronary artery disease, while depression and hostility were associated with severity and duration of angina [36]. It seems difficult in studies of this kind to separate cause from consequence, and there can be little doubt that the presence of CHD symptoms is likely to cause many of the above responses, and more so in individuals of a type A personality.

A study was carried out in the USA to determine whether type A behavior could be modified in survivors of a myocardial infarction and, if so, to see whether this would result in an improved prognosis [37]. Subjects (592 experimental, 270 control) without diabetes mellitus and who had not smoked for six months were involved. The experimental group, which received type A behavior counselling in addition to the general advice on diet, exercise and drugs given to both groups, showed a far greater reduction in type A behavior and a highly significant reduction in recurrence rate of CHD events (7.2% *vs* 13.2%), mainly due to a reduction in non-fatal reinfarction. There was no difference in mortality rates. These results seem to encourage type A behavior counselling for survivors of myocardial infarction. A similar study in 516 patients from the Multicenter Post-Infarction Research Group (USA), however, showed no relationship between type A score and survival over 1–3 years [38].

It would be of interest to examine risk-factor changes in the various groups studied before advocating counselling for type A behavior, although it seems perfectly reasonable to provide appropriate advice to postinfarction patients whose personality and behavior precipitate symptoms.

Many episodes of myocardial infarction are 'silent', and there is now good evidence that mental stress can precipitate silent myocardial ischemia. Regional myocardial perfusion and ischemia were assessed in 16 patients with stable angina and coronary artery disease using ^{82}Ru uptake after both mental arithmetic and physical exercise [39]. After mental arithmetic, 12 patients had abnormalities of regional perfusion, accompanied by ST-segment depression in 6, with angina in 4 of these 6. After exercise, all patients had abnormalities of regional perfusion in segments that were ischemic after mental arithmetic: 16 showed ST-segment depression, and 15 had angina. Painless episodes of ST-segment depression can thus be triggered by mental stress, and this ischemia may or may not be accompanied by angina.

Physical Exercise

It may never be possible to carry out a major trial of the hypothesis that exercise is protective against CHD, for ethical reasons as well as because of the effects of confounding variables. Nevertheless, Leon provides a valuable analysis of epidemiologic and supporting studies in this field [40], and the work of Paffenbarger *et al* on Harvard alumni strongly supports the protective hypothesis [41]. The 16 936 Harvard men were followed for 117 680 man-years, and it was clear that habitual exercise after leaving college predicted low risk of CHD, independently of smoking, obesity, weight gain, hypertension and adverse parental history of disease. An excellent review of the role of regular moderate exercise in the secondary prevention of CHD suggests an improved life-expectancy and reduced reinfarction rate [42], although differences of statistical significance have not consistently been demonstrated. Perhaps the fact that people feel better with regular moderate exercise is a sufficient justification for the effort: the quality, if not the length, of life is improved.

A Norwegian study of 122 cross-country skiers aged 26–64 years and 2014 apparently healthy men aged 40–59 years, the latter divided into four groups according to physical fitness, found a strong, graded association between physical fitness and lower prevalence of coronary risk factors, and an inverse relationship between high fitness and risk of CHD death [43]. The athletes and the top group of non-athletes had the same seven-year CHD mortality rate, suggesting that you do not have to ski to achieve protective levels of fitness.

Overweight and Obesity
Being overweight or obese in a Western society carries with it the likelihood of higher blood pressure, raised blood lipid concentrations and diabetes mellitus. Because of these associations, the relationship between obesity and CHD seen on univariate analysis loses statistical significance on multivariate analysis. Nevertheless, it is clear that overweight/obesity is an indicator of considerable importance in the natural history of CHD.

The Gothenburg Study (Sweden) has recently reported on risk factors for CHD in 792 men born in 1913 [44]. At 54 years of age (in 1967), they were examined and then followed up for 13 years in relation to stroke, CHD and death from all causes. A statistically significant association was found between the ratio of waist to hip circumference and stroke ($P<0.002$) and CHD ($P<0.04$). This association was *not* independent of smoking, systolic blood pressure and serum cholesterol.

A similar study from Gothenburg reported on a 12-year follow-up of 1462 women aged 38–60 years at initial examination [45]. Again, the ratio of waist to hip circumference showed a significant association with the incidence of myocardial infarction, angina, stroke and death. In multivariate analysis, only the relationship with myocardial infarction remained significant.

Dietary Factors
In a brief review of the dietary aspects of coronary heart disease, it is not possible for me to do more than refer to some of the more important issues that have been focused on in recent years, prefaced by one dogmatic statement: atherosclerosis and CHD are fundamentally nutritional/metabolic problems, and the necessary prerequisite for a high level of CHD in a population is a customary diet high in saturated fats and with a low P/S ratio. This *necessary* background may not be *sufficient* to produce clinical CHD, and cigarette smoking and raised blood pressure are critical factors in aggravating atherosclerosis and increasing the incidence of CHD. A large number of other aggravating or

'protective' factors play a role in increasing or decreasing the incidence of CHD in populations susceptible to the disease.

Linoleic Acid in Adipose Tissue
Population studies suggest that a low proportion of the essential fatty acid, linoleic acid (C18:2:n-6), in adipose tissue may be associated with an increased risk for CHD. The fatty acid composition of adipose tissue provides a stable indication of long-term dietary habits. This hypothesis has been studied in a cross-sectional survey of random population samples of apparently healthy men aged 40–49 years, taken from four European regions with differing mortality rates from CHD [46]. The proportion of linoleic acid in adipose tissue was lowest in men from North Karelia (Finland), where mortality from CHD is highest, and highest in men from Italy, where mortality is lowest. Men from Scotland and south-west Finland showed intermediate proportions and intermediate mortalities. The proportion of saturated fatty acid in adipose tissue was highest in Finland, intermediate in Scotland and lowest in Italy. The regional differences in adipose linoleic acid remained highly significant when observed differences in other known risk factors for CHD among the four areas were taken into account: serum cholesterol concentrations, obesity and blood pressure were *highest*, and HDL cholesterol was also *higher*, in Finland. This important study contains an informative table of correlations between the fatty acid composition of adipose tissue and classical risk factors for CHD in the four regions [46]. The most consistent and significant correlation is between the proportion of saturated fatty acids and body mass index, once again pointing up the importance of obesity despite its dismissal in multivariate analysis.

Fish and Fatty Acids
The low incidence of CHD in the Eskimo people has led to a considerable interest in their diet, and in particular to the marine polyunsaturated fats, with their long-chain n-3 polyunsaturated fatty acids (20:5-eicosapentaenoic; 22:6-docosahexaenoic). There has been a series of papers on the findings, and comment on their implications for research and clinical practice (*cf.* editorial review [47]).

In a small Dutch study of 852 middle-aged men followed up for 20 years, mortality from CHD was more than 50% lower among men who ate at least 30 g of fish/day than among those who did not eat fish [48]. The suggestion is made that eating fish once or twice a week may help to prevent CHD (see also review by D. Kromhout, this volume). A larger Swedish study classified fish consumption in 15 864 people in 1967/68 by self-administered questionnaire, and followed them for 14 years [49]. The results show a clear dose-response relationship, with the lowest risk for those who had a high fish consumption. The relative-risk patterns were similar for men and women. Adjustment for smoking, relative weight and social factors had little or no effect on the relative risks presented.

One cannot help reflecting that those who eat fish predominantly or regularly are very likely to eat fewer meat and dairy products, because of their environmental circumstances if for no other reason. So, while fatty acids from fish may be very beneficial in a multitude of ways, the key issue may still be the relatively low intake of saturated fatty acids and the consequent high P/S ratio. However, a recent study in a hyperlipidemic swine model challenges this interpretation of the findings [50]:

> Supplementation of an atherogenic diet with fish oil resulted in a marked reduction in the extent of coronary atherosclerosis in swine, despite the continued dietary intake of large amounts of saturated fats and the continued presence of severe hyperlipidemia.

These findings suggest a *direct* role for fish oils in the prevention of atherosclerosis and CHD, rather than the merely indirect effect of a fish diet leading to a low saturated fat intake.

Coffee and Cholesterol

The possible association between coffee drinking and CHD has been followed for over 15 years, and both the Framingham Study and the Boston Collaborative Drug Surveillance group have reported on the issue, with conflicting results. More recently, workers in Tromso (Norway) have reported that drinking six cups of coffee a day increased the serum total cholesterol concentration by 0.55 mmol/l in a small group of 17 volunteers [51]. From Jerusalem, a sample of 1007 men and 589 women aged 35–64 years showed an association between the intake of coffee (using dietary recall) and plasma cholesterol levels [52]. After controlling for a number of factors, it was found that men who drank five or more cups of coffee had plasma cholesterol concentrations about 0.5 mmol/l higher than those of non-coffee drinkers. The effect was less marked in women.

While there is still no clear evidence that coffee drinking is associated with an increased risk for CHD, it would be well for those doctors managing individuals with raised levels of serum total cholesterol to enquire about coffee intake and to assess the effects of curtailing it.

Alcohol

A recent Health Education Council survey in Great Britain revealed that half the population believed moderate drinking to be beneficial to the heart. Several reviews support this popular belief, and suggest that light or moderate drinking is 'protective' in relation to coronary heart disease [53,54]. These reviews are based on reports that non-drinkers – defined in a variety of ways – have a higher mortality overall and from CHD than those who drink lightly or moderately. In several studies, heavy drinkers have higher mortality rates than light or moderate drinkers, resulting in the 'U-shaped' curve of mortality first described by Pearl in 1904; however, others show the lowest rates of CHD mortality in heavy drinkers, so the findings are not consistent.

A recent prospective study of middle-aged British men showed no significant relationship between reported alcohol intake and the CHD event rate [55]. Light daily drinkers had the lowest CHD event rate, but they also had the lowest smoking rate, the lowest body mass index, the lowest blood pressures and the lowest proportion of manual workers. Unless one postulates that light daily drinking is responsible for all these findings, one must assume that the characteristics of men who drink regular but small amounts are more likely to account for a relatively low CHD rate than is the direct effect of alcohol. Another issue relates to the nature of 'non-drinkers', and the same study provides evidence that the majority of non-drinkers are ex-drinkers, and that they show considerable evidence of increased morbidity from cardiovascular disease and other causes, as well as increased rates of medication [55]. They should certainly not be used as a baseline from which to measure the effects of alcohol intake.

Prospects for the Future

Over the next few years there will be more data produced on the role of the apoproteins, on specific fatty acids in red cell membranes and plasma, and on the various fractions of HDL cholesterol. It is unlikely that this information will lead to improved prevention strategies, but it will probably improve the predictive power of our present screening methods, albeit at some cost. Considerable progress will be made in the field of thrombus formation and dissolution, stimulated by therapeutic endeavours in the thrombolysis field. It is to be hoped that there will be new studies using multifactorial methods of assessing and reducing risk, and focusing on subjects with and without existing evidence of CHD. Associated with these trials there should be detailed studies on the regression of atherosclerosis, using imaging to trace the changes in arterial lesions.

Mortality rates from CHD are likely to diminish in the Western world and to increase in many Eastern European countries. The arguments about risk factors will continue, in the vain belief that risk prediction should be perfect and pathogenesis completely explained before action can be justified.

References

[1] Marmot MG.
Epidemiology of coronary artery disease. In: Sobel BE, Julian DG, Hugenholtz PG, eds. *Perspectives in Cardiology 1984*. London: Current Medical Literature, 1984; pp. 1–10.

[2] Pell S, Fayerweather WE.
Trends in the incidence of myocardial infarction and in associated mortality in a large employed population, 1957–1983.
New Engl J Med 1955; **312**: 1005–11.

[3] Pyörälä K, Epstein FH, Kornitzer M, eds.
Changing trends in coronary heart disease mortality: Possible explanations.
Cardiology 1985; **72**: 5–104.

[4] World Health Organization.
Proposal for the multinational monitoring of trends and determinants in cardiovascular disease and provisional protocol *(WHO/MNC/ 821)*. Geneva: WHO, 1983.

[5] Tunstall-Pedoe H, Smith WCS, Crombie IK.
Levels and trends of coronary heart disease mortality in Scotland compared with other countries.
Health Bull 1986; **44**: 153–61.

[6] Lipid Research Clinics Program.
The Lipid Research Clinics coronary primary prevention trial results.
JAMA 1984; **251**: 351–64.

[7] National Institutes of Health Consensus Development Conference Statement.
Lowering blood cholesterol to prevent heart disease.
JAMA 1985; **253**: 2080–6.

[8] Oliver MF.
Strategies for preventing and screening for coronary heart disease.
Br Heart J 1985; **54**: 1–5.

[9] Lewis B, Mann JI, Mancini M.
Reducing the risks of coronary heart disease in individuals and in the population.
Lancet 1986; i: 956–9.

[10] Anggard EE, Land JM, Lenihan CJ et al.
Prevention of cardiovascular disease in general practice: A proposed model.
Br Med J 1986; **293**: 177–80.

[11] Shaper AG, Pocock SJ, Phillips AN, Walker M.
Identifying men at high risk of heart attacks: A strategy for use in general practice.
Br Med J 1986; **293**: 474–9.

[12] Multiple Risk Factor Intervention Trial Research Group.
Multiple Risk Factor Intervention Trial: Risk factor changes and mortality results.
JAMA 1982; **248**: 1465–77.

[13] Kornitzer M, De Backer G, Dramaix M et al. Belgian Heart Disease Prevention Project: Incidence and mortality results. Lancet 1983; i: 1066–70.

[14] Shaper AG, Cook DG, Walker M, Macfarlane PW. Prevalence of ischaemic heart disease in middle-aged British men. Br Heart J 1984; 51: 595–605.

[15] Neaton JD, Kuller LH, Wentworth D, Borhani NO. Total and cardiovascular mortality in relation to cigarette smoking, serum cholesterol concentration, and diastolic blood pressure among black and white males followed up for five years. Am Heart J 1984; 108: 759–70.

[16] Martin MJ, Hulley SB, Browner WS, Kuller LH, Wentworth D. Serum cholesterol, blood pressure and mortality: Implications from a cohort of 361,662 men. Lancet 1986; ii: 933–6.

[17] Rose G, Shipley M. Plasma cholesterol concentration and death from coronary heart disease: 10 year results of the Whitehall Study. Br Med J 1986; 293: 306–7.

[18] Shaper AG, Pocock SJ, Walker M, Phillips A, Whitehead TP, Macfarlane PW. Risk factors for ischaemic heart disease: The prospective phase of the British Regional Heart Study. J Epidemiol Community Health 1985; 39: 197–209.

[19] Goldbourt U, Holtzman E, Neufeld HN. Total and high density lipoprotein cholesterol in the serum and risk of mortality: Evidence of a threshold effect. Br Med J 1985; 290: 1239–43.

[20] Pocock SJ, Shaper AG, Phillips AN, Walker M, Whitehead TP. High density lipoprotein cholesterol is not a major risk factor for ischaemic heart disease in British men. Br Med J 1986; 292: 515–9.

[21] Anonymous. HDL and ischaemic heart disease in Britain [Editorial]. Lancet 1986; i: 481–2.

[22] Perkins J, Dick TBS. Smoking and myocardial infarction: Secondary prevention. Postgrad Med J 1985; 61: 295–300.

[23] Rosenberg L, Kaufman DW, Helmrich SP, Shapiro S. The risk of myocardial infarction after quitting smoking in men under 55 years of age. N Engl J Med 1985; 313: 1511–4.

[24] Cook DG, Shaper AG, Pocock SJ, Kussick SJ. Giving up smoking and the risk of heart attack: A report from the British Regional Heart Study. Lancet 1986; ii: 1376–80.

[25] Stone MC, Thorp JM. Plasma fibrinogen - a major coronary risk factor. J Roy Coll Gen Pract 1985; 35: 565–9.

[26] Wilhelmsen L, Svardsudd K, Korsan-Bengtsen K, Larsson B, Welin B, Tibblin G. Fibrinogen as a risk factor for stroke and myocardial infarction. N Engl J Med 1984; 311: 501–5.

[27] Hamsten A, Wiman B, de Faire U, Blomback M. Increased plasma levels of a rapid inhibitor of tissue plasminogen activator in young survivors of myocardial infarction. N Engl J Med 1985; 313: 1557–63.

[28] Fuchs J, Weinberger I, Rotenberg Z et al. Plasma viscosity in ischemic heart disease. Am Heart J 1984; 108: 435–9.

[29] Keatinge WL, Coleshaw SRK, Colter F, Matlock M, Murphy M, Chilliah R. Increases in platelet and red cell counts, blood viscosity and arterial pressure during mild surface cooling: Factors in mortality from coronary and cerebral thrombosis in winter. Br Med J 1984; 289: 1405–9.

[30] Wilson PWF, Garrison RJ, Castelli WP. Postmenopausal oestrogen use, cigarette smoking, and cardiovascular mortality in women over 50. The Framingham Study. N Engl J Med 1985; 313: 1038–43.

[31] Stampfer MJ, Willett WC, Colditz GA, Rosner B, Speizer FE, Hennekens CH. A prospective study of postmenopausal estrogen therapy and coronary heart disease. N Engl J Med 1985; 313: 1044–9.

[32] Wilson ESB, Cruikshank J, McMaster M, Weir RJ. A prospective controlled study of the effects on blood pressure of contraceptive preparations containing different types and dosages of progestogen. Br J Obstet Gynaecol 1984; 91: 1254–60.

[33] Barrett-Connor E, Khaw K. Family history of heart attack as an independent predictor of death due to cardiovascular disease. Circulation 1984; 69: 1065–9.

[34] Appels A, Mulder P.
Type A behaviour and myocardial infarction. A 9.5 year follow-up of a small cohort.
Int J Cardiol 1985; **8**: 465–70.

[35] Shekelle RB, Gale M, Norusis M.
Type A Score (Jenkins Activity Survey) and risk of recurrent coronary heart disease in the Aspirin Myocardial Infarction Study.
Am J Cardiol 1985; **56**: 221–5.

[36] Tennant CC, Langeluddecke PM.
Psychological correlates of coronary heart disease.
Psychol Med 1985; **18**: 581–8.

[37] Friedman M, Thorensen CE, Gill JJ *et al.*
Alteration of Type A behaviour and reduction in cardiac recurrences in postmyocardial infarction patients.
Am Heart J 1984; **108**: 237–48.

[38] Case RB, Heller SS, Case NB, Moss AL, Multicentre Post-Infarction Research Group.
Type A behaviour and survival after acute myocardial infarction.
N Engl J Med 1985; **312**: 737–41.

[39] Deanfield JE, Shea M, Kensett M *et al.*
Silent myocardial ischaemia due to mental stress.
Lancet 1984; ii: 1001–5.

[40] Leon S.
Physical activity levels and coronary heart disease. Analysis of epidemiologic and supporting studies. In: Goldberg L, Elliott DL, eds. *The Medical Clinics of North America*. Symposium on Medical Aspects of Exercise. Philadelphia: WB Saunders, 1985; pp. 3–20.

[41] Paffenbarger RS, Hyde RT, Wing AL, Steinmetz CH.
A national history of athleticism and cardiovascular health.
JAMA 1984; **252**: 491–5.

[42] Shephard RJ.
Exercise regimens after myocardial infarction: Rationale and results. In: Wenger NK, ed. *Exercise and the Heart*, 2nd edn. Philadelphia: Davis, 1985; pp. 145–57.

[43] Lie H, Mundal R, Erickssen J.
Coronary risk factors and incidence of coronary death in relation to physical fitness. Seven-year follow-up study of middle-aged and elderly men.
Eur Heart J 1985; **6**: 147–57.

[44] Larsson B, Svardsudd K, Welin L, Wilhelmsen L, Bjorntorp P, Tibblin G.
Abdominal adipose tissue distribution, obesity and risk of cardiovascular disease and death: 13 year follow-up of participants in the study of men born in 1913.
Br Med J 1984; **288**: 1401–4.

[45] Lapidus L, Bengtsson C, Larsson B, Pennert K, Rybo E, Sjostrom L.
Distribution of adipose tissue and risk of cardiovascular disease and death: A 12 year follow-up of participants in the population study of women in Gothenburg, Sweden.
Br Med J 1984; **289**: 1257–61.

[46] Riemarsma RA, Wood DA, Butler S *et al.*
Linoleic acid content in adipose tissue and coronary heart disease.
Br Med J 1986; **292**: 1423–7.

[47] Glomsett JA.
Fish, fatty acids and human health.
N Engl J Med 1985; **312**: 1253–4.

[48] Kromhout D, Bosschieter EB, de Lezenne Coulander C.
The inverse relation between fish consumption and 20-year mortality from coronary heart disease.
N Engl J Med 1985; **312**: 1205–9.

[49] Norell SE, Ahlbom A, Feychting M, Pedersen N.
Fish consumption and mortality from coronary heart disease.
Br Med J 1986; **293**: 426.

[50] Weiner BH, Ockene IS, Levine PH *et al.*
Inhibition of atherosclerosis by cod-liver oil in a hyperlipidemic swine model.
N Engl J Med 1986; **315**: 841–5.

[51] Arnesen E, Forde OH, Thelle DS.
Coffee and serum cholesterol.
Br Med J 1984; **288**: 1960.

[52] Kark JD, Friedlander Y, Kaufmann NA, Stein Y.
Coffee, tea and plasma cholesterol: The Jerusalem Lipid Research Clinic Prevalence Study.
Br Med J 1985; **291**: 699–704.

[53] Turner TB, Bennett VL, Hernandez H.
The beneficial side of moderate alcohol use.
Johns Hopkins Med J 1981; **148**: 53–63.

[54] Marmot MG.
Alcohol and coronary heart disease.
Int J Epidemiol 1984; 1?: 160–7.

[55] Shaper AG, Phillips A, Pocock AJ, Walker M.
Alcohol and ischaemic heart disease in middle-aged British men.
Br Med J 1987; **294**: 733–7.

LIPIDS AND FISH OILS IN ISCHEMIC HEART DISEASE

Review: DAAN KROMHOUT

It became clear in the early 1950s that specific fatty acids, not total fat intake, were the most important determinants of serum, or plasma, cholesterol [1]. Results in the 1960s showed that saturated fatty acids elevate and polyunsaturated fatty acids decrease plasma cholesterol [2,3]. Monounsaturated fatty acids did not influence plasma cholesterol, and dietary cholesterol had a small elevating effect. Comparative studies carried out among Eskimos and Danes in the early 1970s showed that the consumption of large amounts of marine products rich in *n*-3 polyunsaturated fatty acids reduced plasma total cholesterol and triglycerides and increased HDL cholesterol [4]. The renewal of interest in HDL as a protective moiety against coronary heart disease led to increasing evaluation of dietary determinants of HDL cholesterol concentrations in plasma [5,6].

Dietary Fatty Acids

Early in the study of diet and ischemic heart disease, a distinction was made between animal fat and plant fat. It was thought that animal fat contained mainly saturated fat and plant fat contained mainly unsaturated fat. This supposition was not sustained, however, because plant fats can contain large amounts of saturated fat (*viz.* coconut and palm oil). Fats were then classified based on the amounts of different fatty acids they contained.

The fatty acids can be divided into three main groups: saturated, monounsaturated and polyunsaturated. The most common saturated fatty acid in the diet is palmitic acid, the most common monounsaturated is oleic acid and the most common polyunsaturated is linoleic acid (Table Ia,b,c). Palmitic acid has 16 carbon atoms and no double bonds. Oleic and linoleic acid have 18 carbon atoms with one and two double bonds, respectively. The unsaturated fatty acids are classified by the number of carbon atoms, the number of double bonds and the location of the double bonds. Oleic acid is representative of the *n*-9 fatty acids, linoleic acid of the *n*-6 fatty acids, and eicosapentaenoic acid (Table Id) of the *n*-3 fatty acids. The different fatty acids have different effects on serum total and HDL cholesterol, and must therefore be discussed separately.

Table I: Structure of some common fatty acids

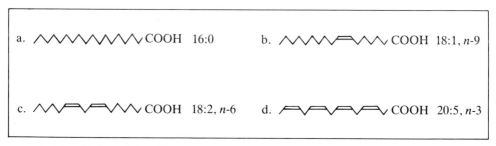

a = palmitic acid; b = oleic acid; c = linoleic acid; d = eicosapentaenoic acid.

25

Saturated Fatty Acids and Dietary Cholesterol
Results of metabolic studies in the 1950s and 1960s showed that saturated fatty acids elevate plasma cholesterol [2,3]. A change from the current Dutch diet containing 18% of energy from saturated fat to a Mediterranean-type diet with 10% of energy from saturated fat decreased cholesterol by about 0.6 mmol/l (22 mg/dl). The strong relationship between saturated fat and plasma cholesterol was supported by the results of the cross-cultural observational Seven Countries Study [7]. In the seven countries under study, saturated fat intake varied between 3% of total energy in Japan and 22% in eastern Finland. Average plasma cholesterol values in these populations amounted to 4.3 mmol/l (165 mg/dl) in Japan and to 7.0 mmol/l (270 mg/dl) in eastern Finland.

Results from studies of experimental animals beginning in 1910 have shown that it is virtually impossible to produce severe atherosclerosis in any species without increasing cholesterol in the diet [8]. Results from human subjects are less clear. Connor and co-workers have shown that the addition of 725 mg cholesterol a day to diets both high and low in saturated fat elevates plasma cholesterol by about 15%, compared with cholesterol-free diets [9]. Addition of cholesterol to the diet of more than 800 mg/day, however, does not lead to a further increase in plasma cholesterol levels [8]. Thus, dietary cholesterol influences plasma cholesterol when intakes between 0 and 800 mg/day are used. Generally, the plasma cholesterol-elevating effect of dietary cholesterol is less than that of saturated fat [2].

Information about the effect of dietary saturated fatty acids on HDL cholesterol is lacking. In most intervention studies, both saturated and polyunsaturated fat components are changed simultaneously, making it impossible to distinguish between the effects of the specific fatty acids on HDL cholesterol. In a cross-sectional study carried out in Caerphilly, Wales, an inverse association was found between saturated fat and HDL cholesterol [10]. Intervention studies with egg-yolk cholesterol showed a positive association between dietary cholesterol and HDL cholesterol [6]. Thus, dietary cholesterol increases plasma HDL cholesterol concentrations. However, the relationship between saturated fat and HDL cholesterol is not clear.

Monounsaturated Fatty Acids
Results of metabolic studies have shown that monounsaturated fats do not influence plasma cholesterol [2]. The role of monounsaturated fatty acids in relation to blood lipids and ischemic heart disease, however, remains controversial. Grundy and Mattson showed that diets with a high monounsaturated fat content do not lower HDL cholesterol, in contrast to diets with a high polyunsaturated fat or high carbohydrate content [11,12]. These results suggest that a diet with 35%–40% of total energy from fat and at least 50% of its fat content consisting of monounsaturated fatty acids may favorably influence blood lipids and lipoproteins. This diet would lower serum total cholesterol without lowering HDL cholesterol.

Polyunsaturated Fatty Acids
Polyunsaturated fatty acids lower plasma cholesterol. This effect is, however, more modest than the cholesterol-elevating effect of saturated fatty acids. It can be obtained both using vegetable oils rich in n-6 polyunsaturated fatty acids and using fish oils rich in n-3 polyunsaturated fatty acids in the diet [2,3,13,14].

Results of intervention studies with large amounts of dietary n-6 polyunsaturated fatty acids with P/S ratios of 4 or higher showed a significant reduction in plasma HDL cholesterol [11,15,16]. In short-term intervention studies (lasting about two weeks), a reduction in HDL cholesterol resulted from diets with 40% of energy from fat and P/S ratios of 1.0–2.0 [17–19]. No reduction in HDL cholesterol was seen with diets of the same total fat and fatty acid composition but consumed over 1–3 months [20–22]. In the Leiden Intervention Trial, a diet with a total fat content of 34% of total energy and a P/S ratio of 2 was used [23]. High-density lipoprotein cholesterol after two years of intervention was not significantly different from that at entry. Thus, diets with 40% of energy from fat and a P/S ratio of 4 or higher reduce HDL cholesterol; however, diets containing 35%–40% of energy from fat and with P/S ratios of 1.0–2.0 do not influence HDL cholesterol. Diets containing less than 30% of energy from fat decrease HDL cholesterol, probably because of their high carbohydrate content [6].

Eskimos have significantly higher plasma HDL cholesterol concentrations than Danes [4]. This may be because of the high content of n-3 polyunsaturated fatty acids in the Eskimo diet. Diets with 5–10 g n-3 polyunsaturated fatty acids elicited an increase of 11% in HDL cholesterol [24]. Elevations of this magnitude were not observed when smaller (2–4 g) or larger (13–29 g) amounts of these fatty acids were used. Regardless of the dietary content of n-3 polyunsaturated fatty acids, a significant reduction in plasma triglycerides occurred [14,24], in proportion to the amount of n-3 polyunsaturated fatty acids consumed.

Our group has recently completed a study of the effects of 26 years of habitual fish consumption on serum lipids and lipoproteins [24]. Two groups of 25 healthy men aged 67–82 years gave information on their fish consumption pattern over a 26-year period. During that period, the control group consumed an average of 3 g of fish/day, and the habitual fish consumers took an average of 33 g of fish/day. Total and intermediate-density lipoprotein (IDL) triglyceride levels were significantly lower and HDL_2 cholesterol levels were significantly higher among habitual fish consumers than among controls. Probably the most important HDL subfraction in relation to coronary sclerosis is HDL_2. The HDL_2 fraction is inversely related to coronary sclerosis, and the low-density lipoprotein (LDL) fraction is positively related to coronary sclerosis [25]. No difference in LDL cholesterol levels was observed between groups [24]. The LDL/HDL_2 cholesterol ratio was 17% lower among habitual fish consumers than among controls. These results suggest a strong inverse relationship of habitual fish consumption and n-3 polyunsaturated fatty acids with plasma triglycerides. High-density cholesterol can be increased by a habitual fish consumption of about 30 g/day or by 5–10 g n-3 polyunsaturated fatty acids, as has been seen in short-term intervention studies. Total plasma cholesterol can be decreased by the long-term consumption of at least 6 g n-3 polyunsaturated fatty acids/day.

Dietary Fatty Acids, Blood Lipids, Lipoproteins and Ischemic Heart Disease
Cross-cultural comparisons of the 15 cohorts in the Seven Countries Study have shown saturated fat intake to be strongly positively related to 15-year death from ischemic heart disease [26]. The 15-year mortality from ischemic heart disease was inversely related to the ratio of monounsaturated/saturated fat, suggesting that, apart from the positive association between saturated fat intake and ischemic heart disease, monoun-

saturated fat is inversely related to ischemic heart disease. Polyunsaturated fat intake was unrelated to ischemic heart disease mortality in the Seven Countries Study. Among Greenland Eskimos, the incidence of ischemic heart disease is very low (about 1/10) compared with that in Danes [27]. This may reflect the high intake among the Eskimos of n-3 polyunsaturated fatty acids. Mortality from ischemic heart disease is also very low in the Japanese [28], perhaps because of their low intake of saturated fat, their high consumption of fish and their accordingly high intake of n-3 polyunsaturated fatty acids.

Cross-cultural data strongly suggest that intake of the various fatty acids plays an important part in explaining the differences in ischemic heart disease mortality between countries. However, correlations observed in cross-cultural studies do not necessarily indicate that correlations are also present within populations. Positive associations have been found between saturated fat and/or dietary cholesterol and ischemic heart disease mortality in some prospective studies [29–31], but not in others [32–34]. Prospective studies on relationships between n-9, n-6 and n-3 polyunsaturated fatty acids and ischemic heart disease mortality have not been reported. In the Zutphen Study, we observed an independent inverse relationship between 20-year mortality from ischemic heart disease and consumption of fish [35]. Additional analysis showed that this relationship was attributable to the n-3 polyunsaturated fatty acid content of fish [36]. The inverse relationship between mortality and consumption of fish was confirmed in the prospective Western Electric Study carried out in Chicago but not confirmed in cohort studies carried out in Norway and Hawaii [37–39]. The inconsistency between results of prospective studies and those of cross-cultural studies appears to reflect difficulties in quantifying food intake, the narrow range in fatty acid intake in Western populations and the large intraindividual variation in fatty acid intake [40]. These factors impair accuracy of estimates of habitual fatty acid intake of individual subjects.

Controlled trials of the effects of different fatty acids on blood lipids, lipoproteins and ischemic heart disease are scarce. Among the best are the Los Angeles Trial and the Finnish Mental Hospitals Trial [41,42]. Both showed that changing from a high-saturated low-n-6 polyunsaturated fatty acid diet to a low-saturated high-n-6 polyunsaturated fatty acid diet led to a significant reduction in plasma total cholesterol of about 15%. In addition, a reduction was observed in mortality from ischemic heart disease but not in total mortality. These results suggest that a causal relationship exists between dietary fatty acids, blood lipids and mortality from ischemic heart disease.

In the early 1970s, it was thought impracticable to carry out large dietary intervention studies to estimate the effect of changes in fatty acid composition on mortality from ischemic heart disease. A large multi-center placebo-controlled intervention study was therefore carried out involving 3806 high-risk men aged 35–59 years [43,44]. All participants in the Lipid Research Clinics Primary Prevention Trial were advised to use a plasma cholesterol-lowering diet. The men in the experimental group were given an additional 24 g/day of the cholesterol-lowering drug, cholestyramine. Results of this trial showed that plasma total and LDL cholesterol lowering were followed by a significant reduction in the incidence and mortality attributable to ischemic heart disease [43,44]. An average reduction in plasma cholesterol of 1% was paralleled by a reduction of 2% in coronary heart disease incidence during the 7.4 years of follow-up. The lowering of plasma cholesterol did not appear to have any effect on total mortality.

An alternative strategy to evaluate the efficacy of lipid lowering is to use the rate of change in arterial lesions as an end-point. In seven of the nine small-scale studies using this type of approach, plasma cholesterol was related to changes in the arterial lesions [45]. Patients with a low plasma total/HDL cholesterol ratio (<6.9) before and during the Leiden Intervention Trial did not exhibit progression of coronary sclerosis during a follow-up period of two years [23]. A similar result was observed among the patients with high plasma total/HDL cholesterol ratios (>6.9) at entry and low ratios (<6.9) during the intervention period. The patients with high plasma total/HDL cholesterol ratio (>6.9) before and during the intervention period, however, showed significant progression. These results would seem to suggest that low plasma total/HDL cholesterol ratios may prevent progression of coronary sclerosis.

Overall, information available to date suggests that low plasma total/HDL cholesterol ratios are compatible with favorable cardiovascular effects. A low plasma total/HDL cholesterol ratio can be achieved with optimal dietary fatty acid composition – i.e. 30%–35% of energy from fat and not more than 10% of saturated fat. The 20%–25% of unsaturated fat should contain about 15% of monounsaturated fatty acids, leaving about 5%–10% for the n-6 and n-3 polyunsaturated fatty acids. It is not yet clear how much of the n-6 and n-3 polyunsaturated fatty acids an optimal diet should contain, although dietary intervention studies are planned to resolve the question.

References

[1] Groen J, Tjiong BK, Kamminga CE, Willebrands AF.
The influence of nutrition, individuality and some other factors, including various forms of stress, on the serum cholesterol: An experiment of nine months' duration in 60 normal volunteers.
Voeding 1952; 13: 556–87.

[2] Keys A, Anderson JT, Grande F.
Serum cholesterol response to changes in the diet. IV: Particular fatty acids in the diet.
Metabolism 1965; 14: 776–87.

[3] Hegsted DM, McGandy RB, Myers ML, Stare FJ.
Quantitative effects of dietary fat on serum cholesterol in man.
Am J Clin Nutr 1965; 17: 281–95.

[4] Bang HO, Dyerberg J, Brondum Nielsen A.
Plasma lipid and lipoprotein pattern in Greenlandic west-coast Eskimos.
Lancet 1971; i: 1143–6.

[5] Miller GJ, Miller NE.
Plasma-high-density-lipoprotein concentration and development of ischaemic heart disease.
Lancet 1975; i: 16–9.

[6] Katan MB.
Diet and HDL. In: Miller NE, Miller GJ, eds. Clinical and Metabolic Aspects of High-Density Lipoproteins. Amsterdam: Elsevier Science Publishers, 1984; pp. 103–31.

[7] Keys A.
Plasma-high-density-lipoprotein concentration and development of ischemic heart disease.
Coronary heart disease in seven countries.
Circulation 1970; 41 (Supp 1).

[8] Stamler J.
Diet. In: Tybjaerg Hansen A, Schnohr P, Rose G, eds. Ischemic Heart Disease. The Strategy of Postponement. Chicago: Yearbook Medical, 1977; pp. 132–62.

[9] Connor WE, Stone DB, Hodges RE.
The interrelated effects of dietary cholesterol and fat upon human serum lipid levels.
J Clin Invest 1964; 43: 1691–6.

[10] Fehily AM, Milbank JE, Yarnell JWG, Hayes TM, Kubiki AJ, Eastham RD.
Dietary determinants of lipoproteins, total cholesterol, viscosity, fibrinogen, and blood pressure.
Am J Clin Nutr 1982; 36: 890–6.

[11] Mattson FH, Grundy SM.
Comparison of effects of dietary saturated, monounsaturated, and polyunsaturated fatty acids on plasma lipids and lipoproteins in man.
J Lipid Res 1985; 26: 194–202.

[12] Grundy SM.
Comparison of monounsaturated fatty acids and carbohydrates for lowering plasma cholesterol.
N Engl J Med 1986; 314: 745–8.

[13] von Lossonczy TO, Ruiter A, Bronsgeest-Schoute HC, van Gent CM, Hermus RJJ.
The effect of a fish diet on serum lipids in healthy human subjects.
Am J Clin Nutr 1978; **31**: 1340–6.

[14] Herold PM, Kinsella JE.
Fish oil consumption and decreased risk of cardiovascular disease: A comparison of findings from animal and human feeding trials.
Am J Clin Nutr 1986; **43**: 566–98.

[15] Shepherd J, Packard CJ, Patsch JR, Gotto AM Jr, Taunton OD.
Effects of dietary polyunsaturated and saturated fat on the properties of high density lipoproteins and the metabolism of apoprotein A-I.
J Clin Invest 1978; **61**: 1582–92.

[16] Shepherd J, Packard CJ, Grundy SM, Yeshurun D, Gotto AM Jr, Taunton OD.
Effects of saturated and polyunsaturated fat diets on the chemical composition and metabolism of low density lipoproteins.
J Lipid Res 1980; **21**: 91–9.

[17] Ernst N, Fisher M, Bowen P, Schaefer EJ, Levy RI.
Changes in plasma lipids and lipoproteins after a modified fat diet.
Lancet 1980; **ii**: 111–3.

[18] Schaefer EJ, Levy RI, Ernst ND, Van Sant FD, Brewer HB Jr.
The effects of low cholesterol, high polyunsaturated fat, and low fat diets on plasma lipid and lipoprotein cholesterol levels in normal and hypercholesterolemic subjects.
Am J Clin Nutr 1981; **34**: 1758–63.

[19] Jackson RL, Kashyap RL, Barnhart RL, Allen C, Hogg E, Glueck CJ.
Influence of polyunsaturated and saturated fats on plasma lipids and lipoproteins in man.
Am J Clin Nutr 1984; **39**: 589–97.

[20] Thompson GR, Traynor I, Danford W, Mark F, Harrison R.
Plasma lipids and lipoproteins after modified fat diet [Letter].
Lancet 1980; **ii**: 421–2.

[21] Brussaard JH, Dallinga-Thie G, Groot PHE, Katan MB.
Effects of amount and type of dietary fat on serum lipids, lipoproteins and apoproteins in man.
Atherosclerosis 1980; **36**: 515–27.

[22] Schwandt P, Janetschek P, Weisweiler P.
High density lipoproteins unaffected by dietary fat modification.
Atherosclerosis 1982; **44**: 9–17.

[23] Arntzenius AC, Kromhout D, Barth JD, et al.
Diet, lipoproteins and the progression of coronary atherosclerosis: The Leiden Intervention Trial.
N Engl J Med 1985; **312**: 805–11.

[24] Kromhout D, Obermann-de Boer GL, Katan MB, et al.
The effects of 26 years' habitual fish consumption on serum lipids and lipoproteins.
Submitted for publication.

[25] Miller NE, Hammett F, Saltissi S, et al.
Relation of angiographically defined coronary artery disease to plasma lipoprotein subfractions and apoproteins.
Br Med J 1981; **282**: 1741–4.

[26] Keys A, Menotti A, Karvonen MJ, et al.
The diet and 15-year death rate in the Seven Countries Study.
Am J Epidemiol 1986; **124**: 903–15.

[27] Kromann N, Green A.
Epidemiological studies in the Upernavik district, Greenland.
Acta Med Scand 1980; **208**: 401–6.

[28] Keys A.
Seven Countries: A multivariate analysis of death and coronary heart disease.
Cambridge, MA: Harvard University Press, 1980.

[29] Shekelle RB, MacMillan Shryock A, Paul O, et al.
Diet, serum cholesterol and death from coronary heart disease: The Western Electric Study.
N Engl J Med 1981; **304**: 65–70.

[30] McGee DL, Reed DM, Yano K, Kagan A, Tillotson J.
Ten-year incidence of coronary heart disease in the Honolulu Heart Program.
Am J Epidemiol 1984; **119**: 667–76.

[31] Kushi LH, Lew RA, Stare FJ, et al.
Diet and 20-year mortality from coronary heart disease: The Ireland-Boston Diet-Heart Study.
N Engl J Med 1985; **312**: 811–8.

[32] Morris JN, Marr JW, Clayton DG.
Diet and heart: A postscript.
Br Med J 1977; **2**: 1307–14.

[33] Gordon T, Kagan A, Garcia-Palmieri M, et al.
Diet and its relation to coronary heart disease and death in three populations.
Circulation 1981; **63**: 500–15.

[34] Kromhout D, De Lezenne Coulander C.
Diet, prevalence and 10-year mortality from coronary heart disease in 871 middle-aged men: The Zutphen Study.
Am J Epidemiol 1984; **119**: 733–41.

[35] Kromhout D, Bosschieter EB, De Lezenne Coulander C.
Fish consumption and 20-year mortality from coronary heart disease.
N Engl J Med 1985; **312**: 1205–9.

[36] Kromhout D, Van 't Veer P, De Lezenne Coulander C, Bosschieter EB.
The intake of N-3 polyunsaturated fatty acids, selenium and 20-year mortality from coronary heart disease (The Zutphen Study).
Eur Heart J 1986; **7** (Suppl 1): 17.

[37] Shekelle RB, von Missell L, Paul O, MacMillan Shryock A, Stamler J.
Fish consumption and mortality from coronary heart disease [Letter].
N Engl J Med 1985; **313**: 820.

[38] Curb JD, Reed DM.
Fish consumption and mortality from coronary heart disease [Letter].
N Engl J Med 1985; **313**: 821.

[39] Vollset SE, Heuch I, Bjelke E.
Fish consumption and mortality from coronary heart disease [Letter].
N Engl J Med 1985; **313**: 820–1.

[40] Kromhout D.
Body weight, diet and serum cholesterol in 871 middle-aged men during 10 years of follow-up (The Zutphen Study).
Am J Clin Nutr 1983; **38**: 591–8.

[41] Dayton S, Pearce ML, Hashimoto S, Dixon WJ, Tomiyasu U.
A controlled clinical trial of a diet high in unsaturated fat in preventing complications of atherosclerosis.
Circulation 1969; **40** (Suppl II).

[42] Miettinen M, Turpeinen O, Karvonen MJ, Elosuo R, Paavilainen E.
Effect of cholesterol-lowering diet on mortality from coronary heart disease and other causes. A twelve-year clinical trial in men and women.
Lancet 1972; **ii**: 835–8.

[43] Lipid Research Clinics Program.
The Lipid Research Clinics Coronary Primary Prevention Trial Results I. Reduction in incidence of coronary heart disease.
J Am Med Ass 1984; **251**: 351–64.

[44] Lipid Research Clinics Program.
The Lipid Research Clinics Coronary Primary Prevention Trial Results II. The relationship of reduction in incidence of coronary heart disease to cholesterol lowering.
J Am Med Ass 1984; **251**: 365–74.

[45] Kromhout D, Arntzenius AC.
Use of diet to modify serum cholesterol, lipoproteins and progression of coronary atherosclerosis. In: Watson RR, ed. *Nutrition and Heart Disease*. CRC Press Inc, 1987.

PATHOPHYSIOLOGY

THE DEVELOPMENT, PROGRESSION AND REGRESSION OF ATHEROSCLEROSIS

[1] Increased prostacyclin biosynthesis in patients with severe atherosclerosis and platelet activation.
FitzGerald GA, Smith B, Pedersen AK, Brash AR, Vanderbilt Univ, Nashville, TN, USA.
N Engl J Med 1984; **310**: 1065–8.

[2] Fibrinopeptide A and sudden coronary death.
Meade TW, Howarth DJ, Stirling Y, Welch TP, Crompton MR, Northwick Park Hosp, Harrow, UK.
Lancet 1984; **ii**: 607–8.

[3] Relation of atherosclerosis to arterial wall shear in the left anterior descending coronary artery of man.
Sabbah HN, Khaja F, Hawkins ET *et al*, Henry Ford Hosp, Detroit, MI, USA.
Am Heart J 1986; **112**: 453–9.

[4] Localization of atherosclerotic lesions in the bifurcation of the main left coronary artery.
Grottum P, Svindland A, Walloe L, Oslo City Hosp, Norway.
Atherosclerosis 1983; **47**: 55–62.

[5] Protection against atherogenesis with the polymer drag-reducing agent Separan AP-30.
Faruqui FL, Otten MD, Polimeni PL, Univ Manitoba Fac Med, Winnipeg, Manitoba, Canada.
Circulation 1987; **75**: 627–35.

[6] Natural resistance to atherosclerosis exhibited by the first centimeter of left and right coronary arteries.
Velican C, Velican D, Colentina Hosp, Bucharest, Rumania.
Atherosclerosis 1984; **50**: 173–81.

[7] Collagen content of atherosclerotic arteries is higher in smokers than in non-smokers.
Ribeiro P, Jadhav AV, Walesby R *et al*, Royal Postgrad Med Sch, London, UK.
Lancet 1983; i: 1070–3.

[8] Cigarette smoke and carbon monoxide do not have equivalent effects upon development of arteriosclerotic lesions.
Penn A, Butler J, Snyder C, Albert RE, New York Univ Med Cent, New York, NY, USA.
Artery 1983; **2**: 117–31.

[9] Tobacco constituents are mitogenic for arterial smooth-muscle cells.
Becker CG, Hajjar DP, Hefton JM, Cornell Univ Med Coll, New York, NY, USA.
Am J Pathol 1985; **120**: 1–5.

[10] Effects of tobacco and non-tobacco cigarette smoking on endothelium and platelets.
Davis JW, Shelton L, Eigenberg DA, Hignite CE, Watanabe IS, VA Med Cent, Kansas City, MO, USA.
Clin Pharmacol Ther 1985; **37**: 529–33.

[11] Progression of coronary atherosclerosis. Clues to pathogenesis from serial coronary arteriography.
Singh RN, Montefiore Hosp, Pittsburgh, PA, USA.
Br Heart J 1984; **52**: 451–61.

[12] Clinical and angiographic factors associated with progression of coronary artery disease.
Moise A, Théroux P, Taeymans Y *et al*, Montreal Heart Inst, Montreal, Quebec, Canada.
J Am Coll Cardiol 1984; **3**: 659–67.

[13] Clinical and angiographic predictors of new total coronary occlusion in coronary artery disease: analysis of 313 nonoperated patients.
Moise A, Lespérance J, Théroux P, Taeymans Y, Goulet C, Bourassa MG, Montreal Heart Inst, Montreal, Quebec, Canada.
Am J Cardiol 1984; **54**: 1176–81.

[14] Factors associated with progression of coronary artery disease in patients with normal or minimally narrowed coronary arteries.
Moise A, Théroux P, Taeymans Y, Waters DD, Montreal Heart Inst, Montreal, Quebec, Canada.
Am J Cardiol 1985; **56**: 30–4.

[15] Accelerated progression of atherosclerosis in coronary vessels with minimal lesions that are bypassed.
Cashin WL, Sanmarco ME, Nessim SA, Blankenhorn DH, Univ Southern California Sch Med, Los Angeles, CA, USA.
N Engl J Med 1984; **311**: 824–8.

[16] Retarding effect of lowered heart rate on coronary atherosclerosis.
Beere PA, Glagov S, Zarins CK, Univ Chicago, Chicago, IL, USA.
Science 1984; **226**: 180–2.

[17] Mechanism of protection from atherosclerosis by verapamil in the cholesterol-fed rabbit.
Blumlein SL, Sievers R, Kidd P, Parmley WW, Univ California, San Francisco, CA, USA.
Am J Cardiol 1984; **54**: 884–9.

[18] Suppression of experimental atherosclerosis in rabbits by interferon-inducing agents.
Kuo PT, Wilson AC, Goldstein RC, Schaub RG, UMDNJ-Rutgers Med Sch, New Brunswick, NJ, USA.
J Am Coll Cardiol 1984; **3**: 129–34.

Comment. The endogenous production of prostacyclin under physiologic conditions is extremely low – far below the capacity of vascular tissue to generate this substance in response to stimulation *in vitro*. This may reflect a low frequency or intensity of stimulation of prostacyclin production. However, if prostacyclin does act as an endogenous inhibitor, it should be produced in large amounts in a clinical setting, where platelet-vascular interactions are likely to be increased. Fitzgerald *et al* examined prostacyclin biosynthesis in patients with severe atherosclerosis and evidence of platelet activation *in vivo* [1]. The authors concluded that prostacyclin production may be low in a healthy person because there is almost no stimulus for its production, but that it may be enhanced in patients with severe atherosclerosis as a result of platelet interactions with endothelium or other vascular insults. Their observations are clearly incompatible with a role for prostacyclin as a local regulator of platelet-vascular interactions.

The importance of thrombin production as a part of the sequence of events leading to sudden death in patients with ischemic heart disease was studied in 31 patients who had died suddenly of ischemic heart disease and eight patients who had died suddenly of other causes [2]. The authors found that fibrinopeptide A concentration was five times higher in those patients who had died suddenly of ischemic heart disease, suggesting that thrombin production causes or aggravates the sequence of events leading to sudden death, particularly in those who have a past history of the disease.

One of the factors put forward as leading to the development of atherosclerosis is that of mechanical force related to the dynamics of arterial blood flow. It has been suggested that vascular endothelial injury caused by high fluid shear stress is the focus for subsequent development of atheroma. In contrast, other workers have suggested that low fluid shear stress leads to the formation of atheroma because of an adverse effect on the mass transfer of lipids across the arterial wall. Sabbah *et al* have shown that atheroma occurs more frequently on the inner curve of the left anterior descending coronary artery where the fluid shear rate is lower [3]. Similar findings have been made in the left main coronary artery. Grottum *et al* made casts of the left main coronary bifurcation, and measured the curvature of the arteries and angles of the bifurcation [4]. Atherosclerotic lesions were found to have a distinct pattern, with a high frequency on the outer walls of the bifurcation and at the inner curvature downstream from the bifurcation. Agents that reduce turbulence and promote laminar flow reduce atherosclerosis [5].

In a combined gross and histologic study of 270 subjects, a natural resistance to intimal thickening and plaque development in the left main coronary artery and in the first centimeter of the right coronary artery was found [6]. The importance of this natural resistance in children, adolescents, young and mature adults (up to 55 years of age) was demonstrated by a comparative investigation, involving the degree of intimal thickness, the media to intima thickness ratio, and the percentage of subjects with atherosclerotic plaques. The first atherosclerotic lesions developed three decades later in the left main coronary artery than in the proximal segment of the anterior descending artery. In the 51- to 55-year age group, only 13.3% of subjects showed atherosclerotic plaques in the left main coronary artery, compared with 77.6% in the proximal segment of the anterior descending coronary artery; also, only 6.6% of subjects in this group showed atherosclerotic plaques at 5 mm distal to the aortic origin of the right coronary artery, compared with 55.5% at 30 mm.

An analysis of the content of atherosclerotic arteries showed that smokers have a higher collagen content in coronary endarterectomy specimens and a higher cholesterol content in the aorta than non-smokers [7]. Studies in cockerels showed that cigarette smoke accelerated the development of atherosclerotic lesions, but this effect could not be attributed entirely to the carbon monoxide in the smoke [8]. Tobacco smoke may be mitogenic for arterial smooth muscle cells [9], and the effects of tobacco smoke on vascular endothelium and platelet aggregation are greater than the effects of non-tobacco smoke [10].

Considerable work has been done recently on the progression of atherosclerosis. In a study of 52 patients with coronary artery disease who had repeat coronary arteriographies, it was concluded that atherosclerosis progresses episodically in the proximal segments of the coronary arteries, and in relation to the abrupt development of new symptoms or acute coronary events, such as unstable angina or myocardial infarction [11]. Evidence of progression was seen in one-third of pre-existing stenoses. New lesions frequently occurred in previously normal segments of the arteries, and rapid progression of mild and new lesions was seen to occur as smooth intimal protrusions into the arterial lumen. In another study, multivariate analysis identified four independent predictors associated with the progression of coronary artery disease: the interval between repeat angiographies; the development of unstable angina; the amount of disease, including minor narrowing, at initial investigation; and the presence of coronary artery disease at a young age [12]. In a further study from the same group [13], it was found that occlusion of the coronary artery was likely to occur if there was a long time between angiographic studies, particularly if a myocardial infarction had occurred. A new occlusion was also likely to develop in relation to a severe initial stenosis, in association with multiple arterial segments with significant narrowing, in smokers and in men in general. In patients with normal or minimally diseased arteries, progression is more likely to occur in the presence of the conventional risk factors: age, smoking and raised cholesterol [14].

The hazards of performing bypass grafting on arteries with minimal atherosclerotic lesions were highlighted in a study of 85 men undergoing coronary artery bypass graft surgery [15]. Cashin et al identified 37 arteries with minimal atherosclerosis in which grafts had been inserted. As a control in the same 85 patients, there were 93 coronary vessels with minimal atherosclerosis that had not been grafted. During a mean follow-up of 37 months, progression of atherosclerosis was found to be 10 times as frequent in the bypassed arteries with minimal atherosclerosis as in the comparable arteries that had not been bypassed.

Attempts to identify factors that will halt the development or even cause retardation of atherosclerosis have included studies of the effects of lowering the heart rate. In a study of 14 monkeys, 6 of whom had had ablation of the sinoatrial node, it was found that animals with a low postoperative heart rate had less atherosclerosis than either controls or animals with heart rates above the mean [16]. The monkeys did not differ in any other known risk factors, and it was suggested that heart rate may be of some significance in the development of atherosclerosis; this could be due to the effects of pulsatile flow on the development of atherosclerotic plaques. In a study of 72 cholesterol-fed rabbits, pharmacologic maneuvers, involving the use of no drug, sub-cutaneous verapamil, metoprolol, hydralazine, metoprolol plus hydralazine, or oral verapamil, showed that rabbits given verapamil had significantly less severe aortic atherosclerosis than the other groups [17]. The mechanism by which verapamil may protect against atherosclerosis in the cholesterol-fed rabbit is not known. In another study involving the cholesterol-fed rabbit, interferon-inducing agents significantly reduced the aortic intimal surface lesions, in spite of having no effect on the hyper-cholesterolemia induced by the diet [18]. Further studies are necessary to determine whether endogenous interferon provides protection against atherosclerosis, and whether verapamil may be used to prevent the development of atherosclerosis or to cause its retardation.

EVALUATION OF THE PHYSIOLOGIC SIGNIFICANCE OF CORONARY ARTERY STENOSES

Review: FRANCIS J. KLOCKE

Energy Losses across a Stenosis
Energy losses – and therefore drop in pressure – across a stenosis are influenced by viscous effects, flow separation and possibly turbulence [1,2]. Viscous losses are due to ordinary wall friction; in the stenotic area, viscous losses are accentuated because of increased blood velocity. Separation losses are due to the fact that flow downstream to the stenosis separates from the vessel wall, forming eddies which dissipate additional energy. Although the magnitudes of viscous and separation losses are both flow-dependent, separation losses are proportional to flow raised to the second power, and become increasingly prominent as coronary flow increases. For any given level of flow, the most important determinant of the severity of stenosis is the minimal cross-sectional area within the stenosis (which appears as a second-order term in the expression of both viscous and separation losses). Although cross-sectional area in the poststenotic region does influence separation losses, it is of relatively minor biological significance when stenosis exceeds 50% of luminal diameter. Thus, even though a variety of interventions can affect the diameter of a coronary artery just proximal or distal to a stenosis, to have any major effect, an intervention must have the capacity to alter dimensions within the stenotic segment. Also, since the effects of length of stenosis are manifest through viscous rather than separation losses, stenosis length probably plays a less crucial role clinically than does minimal cross-sectional area.

Two consequences of these relationships are of particular significance.
(i) Because the pressure drop across even an anatomically rigid stenosis increases non-linearly with flow, the effective resistance of the stenosis ($\Delta P/Q$) increases as coronary flow rises – i.e. the functional significance of the stenosis is augmented by interventions which increase myocardial oxygen demand. When an intervention which

increases flow is not accompanied by a corresponding increase in aortic pressure, poststenotic coronary pressure falls, and the fall in pressure can either produce or accentuate a supply-demand imbalance [3].

(ii) Because the relationship between the pressure gradient across a stenosis and the severity of stenosis is non-linear, small changes in the degree of stenosis can significantly alter the functional consequences at any given level of flow: for a concentric stenosis, it is not unreasonable to expect an aortic-coronary pressure gradient to *double* when the degree of diameter narrowing increases from 70% to 80%, or from 80% to 90% [2]. Such an increment might reflect progression of the underlying atherosclerosis, but could also reflect coronary spasm, platelet aggregation or hemorrhage in the vessel wall. Conversely, even small decreases in stenosis severity, whether static or dynamic, have a potentially important therapeutic effect. Because coronary stenoses are frequently eccentric, with vascular smooth muscle and a relatively normal wall thickness retained in portions of the stenotic segment, it seems probable that there exist either active or passive dynamic changes in minimal cross-sectional area.

The Interpretation of Coronary Arteriograms
Evaluating the clinical implications of coronary arteriograms requires consideration of the issues discussed above. Inter- and intraindividual variations in estimating degree of stenosis in routine clinical arteriograms continue to be widely acknowledged. Although there is less disagreement on nearly normal or almost completely occluded vessels, there are still serious doubts about assessing lesions estimated to narrow internal diameter in the range of 50%–90%. Few arteriographers would expect consistently to distinguish between diameter narrowings of 70% and 80%, or 80% and 90%. There also remains the question of whether the vessel diameter adjacent to the stenosis (used as a reference in the estimation of percentage narrowing) is itself normal. Finally, even if an exact definition of stenosis narrowing were possible, functional severity would vary with flow.

The general recognition of limitations of conventional methods for estimating the severity of an arteriographic lesion has stimulated new approaches. The 'quantitative coronary arteriography' pioneered by Brown [4] utilizes high-quality orthogonal views, and calculations of minimum cross-sectional area within a lesion based on an assumed elliptical (rather than concentric) geometry. This approach has demonstrated that clinically important lesions in proximal coronary arteries are usually associated with residual cross-sectional luminal areas of only a few tenths of a square millimeter. It has also documented important dynamic changes in minimal cross-sectional area in response to certain pharmacologic agents [5]. However, since the cross-sectional area of normal coronary arteries decreases progressively from the coronary ostia to the periphery, the interpretation of a specific value for a cross-sectional area must somehow take this variation into account. Even for a given vessel – e.g. the proximal anterior descending artery – normal cross-sectional area probably varies with the patient's gender and the mass of myocardium perfused. In addition, the cross-sectional area of a stenosis of markedly crescentic geometry can be underestimated by even the quantitative arteriographic approach [2].

An alternative approach currently under investigation in a few centers involves videodensitometric measurement of the amount of contrast agent within an area which includes the stenosed portion of the artery, and comparison with the amount within an adjacent non-stenosed region [6,7]. Although this method has the theoretical advantage of being independent of the assumed geometry of the stenosis, the technology is demanding. In addition, interpretation of the videodensitometric comparison depends upon the appropriateness of the reference area used for comparison.

Interactions between Coronary Stenoses and the Distal Coronary Bed: Measurements of 'Coronary Reserve'

Effects of coronary artery stenoses on coronary flow depend greatly on vasodilator reserve at the arteriolar level. The ability of the distal coronary bed to 'autoregulate' – i.e. to maintain flow unchanged in the face of a change in coronary arterial pressure – is well recognized, and has recently been reviewed [8,9]. Since the effects of epicardial stenoses are potentially counteracted by vasodilatation at the arteriolar level, cliaical manifestations are not expected during the initial phases of development of a stenosis. As the severity of a stenosis increases, autoregulatory vasodilatation fails to maintain flow at an appropriate level during stress - at first with marked exertion but subsequently with increasingly less severe provocation. This failure usually affects the subendocardium before the subepicardium [9]. A regional limitation of flow in viable myocardium has traditionally been taken to indicate maximal distal vasodilatation.

The advantages of defining functional severity of a coronary stenosis by measuring vasodilator 'coronary reserve' (the increment in coronary flow occurring during maximal distal vasodilatation) have long been recognized in clinical and experimental studies. Thallium myocardial perfusion scans can be helpful in defining regional variations in flow increment during stress, but have limited sensitivity and specificity [10]. In the early 1980s, Marcus and colleagues applied a Doppler flow velocity probe to a coronary artery at the time of open heart surgery to document that vasodilator reserve is normally of the same order of magnitude in humans as in experimental animals – i.e. approximately sixfold at normal aortic pressures [11]. Reports from these and other investigators confirm that vasodilator reserve can be significantly reduced when ventricular hypertrophy is marked or with severe coronary artery disease [12,13]. With the development of a catheter-tip flow velocity measurement capability, instantaneous measurements are now possible in closed-chest conscious humans as well as in patients undergoing open heart surgery [14]. Positron-tomographic and 'fast CT' techniques for flow measurements are particularly attractive: they are non-invasive and permit regional analysis [1,15]. However, they are expensive, complex, technically demanding and, as yet, incompletely validated.

Despite the conceptual attractiveness of measurements of flow reserve, a number of factors limit the interpretation of even methodologically adequate measurements [3,16]. Maximum vasodilatation is unlikely to be achieved in all layers of the myocardial wall with pacing or the administration of catecholamines or radiographic contrast agent. In a dosage sufficient to achieve maximum coronary vasodilatation, intravenous dipyridamole is likely to be accompanied by some reduction in systemic arterial pressure; peak coronary flow (and therefore measured reserve) varies considerably with the level of aortic pressure in this setting. Intracoronary papaverine may obviate these difficulties but requires catheterization [17]. Less generally appreciated but equally important in evaluating coronary reserve are the changes in minimum possible resistance of the distal coronary bed that accompany changes in heart rate, myocardial contractility, left-ventricular preload and viscosity [3,16]. In addition, total flow through a stenotic coronary artery can increase in the face of a reduction of subendocardial flow within the region supplied by the artery [3]. Effects of collateral flow and variations in the absolute prevasodilatation level of flow further complicate comparisons of flow at rest and during vasodilatation with at least some of the techniques mentioned above.

Thus, while the concept of progressive limitation of coronary reserve with a progressive increase in stenosis is established and useful for understanding pathophysiology, measurements in individual patients must be interpreted cautiously. A flow increment of greater than 3.5 times resting flow is probably uncommon in clinically important stenoses – unless spasm aggravates lesion severity intermittently [18]. The extent to which lesions with greater clinical impact can be subclassified on the basis of measurement of reserve remains to be seen.

Factors Modulating Autoregulatory Responses: Chronic vs Acute Adaptations to Regional Coronary Artery Pressure Reduction

As noted earlier, the traditional concept of coronary autoregulation has been that metabolic stimuli are the predominant factors underlying coronary flow regulation, and that a reduction in flow due to coronary artery constriction indicates that maximal vasodilatation of the distal vascular bed is present. However, four laboratories have recently reported that reductions in subendocardial flow occur regularly in anesthetized animals during spontaneous autoregulation at a time when vasodilator reserve can still be recruited pharmacologically [19–22]. In addition, Grover and Weiss have demonstrated that the level of subendocardial metabolism, which has been reduced in association with a stenosis producing a reduction in flow at rest, can increase in response to physiologic stress [23]. Intrinsic and/or extrinsic factors modulating coronary autoregulatory flow responses are therefore of considerable current interest. A number of studies over the past few years have demonstrated that adrenergic vasoconstrictor influences can limit flow during pharmacologic and other stresses in at least some experimental settings [8].

An additional consideration relates to the possibility that chronic adaptations are more complex than acute adjustments to reductions in regional coronary pressure and flow. Although the point is controversial, some results in humans have suggested that myocardial perfusion is reduced at rest under basal circumstances in viable myocardium supplied by a severely stenotic artery [2]. Possible metabolic adaptations to chronic pressure and flow reduction include a shift from utilization of free fatty acids to aerobic metabolism of glucose [24]. Improvements in wall motion have been reported following surgical revascularization of myocardial areas that were assessed prior to surgery by positron emission tomography as having reduced resting blood flow and increased glucose utilization [25]. Changes in local sympathetic responsiveness following acute myocardial ischemia [26] and experimental myocardial infarction [27] have been reported as well. Efforts to develop more appropriate animal models for the study of chronically reduced myocardial perfusion continue [28].

Comment

Although many advances have been made in recent years in our understanding of the physiologic behavior of coronary artery stenoses, the new insight has been less effective in solving individual patient problems. The limitations of even high-quality coronary arteriography and current techniques for evaluating coronary perfusion and coronary reserve emphasize the continuing importance of rigorous assessment of clinical status when classifying individual patients for therapy. It is not always true that a reduction in regional coronary flow implies exhaustion of vasodilator reserve and concomitant regional ischemia. Future research should address factors modulating autoregulation in coronary disease and chronic adaptations to coronary stenoses.

Acknowledgment
Supported by the National Heart, Lung and Blood Institute (2-PO1-HLB-15194).

References

[1] Gould KL.
Quantification of coronary artery stenosis in vivo.
Circ Res 1985; **57**: 341–53.

[2] Klocke FJ.
Measurements of coronary blood flow and degree of stenosis: Current clinical implications and continuing uncertainties.
J Am Coll Cardiol 1983; **1**: 31–41.

[3] Klocke FJ, Ellis AK, Canty JM Jr.
Interpretation of changes in coronary flow that accompany pharmacologic interventions.
Circulation 1987; **75** (Suppl V): 34–8.

[4] Brown BG, Bolson E, Frimer M, Dodge HT.
Quantitative coronary arteriography: Estimation of dimensions, hemodynamic resistance, and atheroma mass of coronary artery lesions using the arteriogram and digital computation.
Circulation 1977; **55**: 329–37.

[5] Brown BG, Bolson E, Petersen RB, Pierce CD, Dodge HT.
The mechanisms of nitroglycerin action: Stenosis vasodilatation as a major component of the drug response.
Circulation 1981; **64**: 1089–97.

[6] Nichols AB, Gabrieli CFO, Fenoglio JJ Jr, Esser PD.
Quantification of relative coronary arterial stenosis by cinevideodensitometric analysis of coronary arteriograms.
Circulation 1984; **69**: 512–22.

[7] Johnson MR, McPherson DD, Fleagle SR, *et al*.
Videodensitometric analysis of coronary stenoses: Validation using intraoperative high-frequency epicardial echocardiography [Abstract].
Circulation 1985; **72**: III–261.

[8] Feigl EO.
Coronary physiology.
Physiol Rev 1983; **63**: 1–205.

[9] Klocke FJ, Ellis AK.
Physiology of the coronary circulation. In: Parmley WW, Chatterjee K, eds. *Cardiology*. Philadelphia: JB Lippincott, 1986/7 (in press).

[10] Beller GA, Gibson RS, Watson DD.
Radionuclide methods of identifying patients who may require coronary artery bypass surgery.
Circulation 1985; **72**: V9–V22.

[11] Marcus M, Wright C, Doty D, *et al*.
Measurements of coronary velocity and reactive hyperemia in the coronary circulation of humans.
Circ Res 1981; **49**: 877–91.

[12] Kochsiek K, Cott L, Tauchert M, Neubaur J, Larbig D.
Measurement of coronary blood flow in various conditions using the argon technique. In: Kaltenbach M, Lichtlen P, eds. *Coronary Heart Disease*. Stuttgart: Georg Thieme Verlag, 1971; pp. 137–52.

[13] Marcus ML, Doty DB, Hiratzka LF, Wright CB, Eastham CL.
Decreased coronary reserve: A mechanism for angina pectoris in patients with aortic stenosis and normal coronary arteries.
N Engl J Med 1982; **307**: 1362–6.

[14] Wilson RF, Laughlin DE, Ackell PH, *et al*.
Transluminal, subselective measurement of coronary artery blood flow velocity and vasodilator reserve in man.
Circulation 1985; **72**: 82–92.

[15] Goldstein RA, Mullani NA, Fisher DJ, Marani SK, Gould KL, O'Brien HA.
Perfusion imaging with rubidium-82. II: Effects of pharmacologic interventions on flow and extraction.
J Nucl Med 1983; 24: 907–15.
[16] Hoffman JIE.
Maximal coronary flow and the concept of coronary vascular reserve.
Circulation 1984; 70: 153–9.
[17] Wilson RF, White CW.
Intracoronary papaverine: An ideal coronary vasodilator for studies of the coronary circulation in conscious humans.
Circulation 1986; 73: 444–51.
[18] Wilson RF, Marcus ML, Drews TA, White CW.
Relationship of coronary vasodilator reserve to quantitative lesion geometry in patients with single vessel coronary artery disease [Abstract].
Circulation 1985; 72: III–386.
[19] Canty JM Jr, Klocke FJ.
Reduced regional myocardial perfusion in the presence of pharmacologic vasodilator reserve.
Circulation 1985; 71: 370–7.
[20] Aversano T, Becker LC.
Persistence of coronary vasodilator reserve despite functionally significant flow reduction.
Am J Physiol 1985; 248: H403–11.
[21] Pantley GA, Bristow JD, Swenson LJ, Ladley HD, Johnson WB, Anselone CG.
Incomplete coronary vasodilation during myocardial ischemia in swine.
Am J Physiol 1985; 249: H638–47.
[22] Grattan MT, Hanley FL, Stevens MB, Hoffman JIE.
Transmural coronary flow reserve patterns in dogs.
Am J Physiol 1986; 250: H276–83.
[23] Grover GJ, Weiss HR.
Effect of pacing on oxygen supply-to-consumption ratio in ischemic myocardium.
Am J Cardiol 1985; 46: 67–72.
[24] Schwaiger M, Schelbert HR, Ellison D, et al.
Sustained regional abnormalities in cardiac metabolism after transient ischemia in the chronic dog model.
J Am Coll Cardiol 1985; 6: 336–47.
[25] Tillisch J, Brunken RB, Marshall R, et al.
Reversibility of cardiac wall-motion abnormalities predicted by positron tomography.
N Engl J Med 1986; 314: 884–8.
[26] Ciuffo AA, Ouyang P, Becker LW, Levin L, Weisfeldt ML.
Reduction of sympathetic inotropic response after ischemia in dogs: Contributor to stunned myocardium.
J Clin Invest 1985; 75: 1504–9.
[27] Barber MJ, Mueller TM, Davies BG, Gill RM, Zipes DP.
Interruption of sympathetic and vagal-mediated afferent responses by transmural myocardial infarction.
Circulation 1985; 72: 623–31.
[28] Canty JM Jr, Klocke FJ.
Reductions in regional myocardial function at rest in conscious dogs with chronically reduced regional coronary artery pressure.
Submitted for publication.

HEMODYNAMIC SIGNIFICANCE OF CORONARY ARTERY STENOSIS

[1] Quantitative evaluation of regional myocardial blood flow by videodensitometric analysis of digital subtraction coronary arteriography in humans.
Ikeda H, Koga Y, Utsu F, Toshima H, Kurume Univ Sch Med, Kurume, Japan.
J Am Coll Cardiol 1986; 8: 809–16.
[2] Comparative study of coronary flow reserve, coronary anatomy and results of radionuclide exercise tests in patients with coronary artery disease.
Legrand VL, Mancini GBJ, Bates ER, Hodgson JMcB, Gross MD, Vogel RA, VA Med Cent, Ann Arbor, MI, USA.
J Am Coll Cardiol 1986; 8: 1022–32.
[3] Coronary artery stenoses. Relationship between angiographic severity and impact on mean diastolic pressure gradient.
Bateman TM, Gray RJ, Raymond MJ et al, Cedars-Sinai Med Cent, Los Angeles, CA, USA.
J Thorac Cardiovasc Surg 1983; 85: 499–507.

[4] Variation in the size of jeopardized myocardium in patients with isolated left anterior descending coronary artery disease.
DePace NL, Iskandrian AS, Nadell R, Colby J, Hakki A-H, Hahnemann Univ, Philadelphia, PA, USA.
Circulation 1983; **67**: 988–94.

Comment. Evidence showing that the visual estimation of coronary arteriographic abnormalities is inaccurate and unreliable for determining the hemodynamic consequences of stenoses has been increasing. Methods of assessing the functional significance of coronary stenosis include exercise thallium scintigraphy, coronary flow reserve measured by digital angiography before and after vasodilatation, and the measurement of clearance half-times of contrast agent during coronary arteriography [1]. Legrand *et al* assessed regional coronary flow reserve, quantitative percentage diameter coronary stenosis and exercise-induced perfusion and wall motion abnormalities in 39 patients with coronary artery disease, 19 of whom did not have transmural infarction or collateral vessels and 20 of whom did have collateral vessels [2]. They drew the following conclusions: a general relation exists between quantitative percentage diameter stenosis and reactive hyperemia, but it is not sufficiently precise to enable an accurate prediction of coronary flow reserve in individual patients; a low coronary flow reserve is usually associated with abnormalities on exercise testing with thallium-201 scintigraphy – the relation between these two functional tests is stronger than that between exercise test results and quantitative percentage diameter stenosis; in patients with multivessel disease, the number of regions supplied by arteries with physiologically significant stenoses is underestimated using exercise scintigraphy; and finally, when collateral vessels are present, there are profound alterations in coronary flow dynamics that preclude the use of coronary flow reserve as a reliable indicator of the functional significance of stenoses except when flow reserve is severely impaired.

Bateman *et al* [3] investigated the relationship between angiographic severity of coronary stenoses and related this to the directly measured pressure gradient of the stenosis at coronary artery surgery. They found that lesions >90% had a wide range of gradients, whereas lesions <90% tended to have more predictable gradients. Major gradients in supply vessels had, not unnaturally, a high incidence of associated myocardial infarction. Surprisingly, the length of the stenosis was not an important influence on the gradient. In a complementary study by DePace *et al* [4] on the variation in the size of defects in 35 jeopardized patients with isolated left anterior descending coronary artery disease, exercise thallium scans were performed. Nine patients with a stenosis of <70% had smaller defects than 26 patients with a stenosis of >70%. In 12 of these 26 patients, the defect was >30% of the perimeter of the scan. Analysis of several variables showed that only age correlated with perfusion defect size, i.e. in patients aged 50 years or under the defects were larger than in those over 50. Significant stenosis of the left anterior descending artery (>70%) therefore can put at risk more than 30% of the heart muscle in a great number of patients. This appears to be more common in patients aged under 50.

CORONARY ARTERY SPASM

Review: C. RICHARD CONTI

The definition of large-vessel coronary artery spasm remains arbitrary. Coronary artery spasm (or, as some workers prefer, 'increased vasomotor tone') can be seen as a transient reduction in lumen diameter of an epicardial coronary artery, of sufficient degree to produce myocardial ischemia in the absence of any significant increase in heart rate or blood pressure. Using this definition, there are no limits set on the degree of lumen diameter reduction required for a diagnosis of coronary artery spasm, since the changes in vessel size must be accompanied by ischemia. Thus, patients with either normal or diseased coronary arteries may be said to experience spasm.

The perceived prevalence of coronary artery spasm depends on how one defines the condition. In my view, coronary angiography is essential in the confirmation of spasm in the individual patient. ST-Segment elevation does not prove that patients are undergoing coronary artery spasm – rather, it is suggestive that severe myocardial ischemia is present, and probably also a transient decrease in myocardial blood flow.

Physiologic Observations [1–14]
Physiologic changes are similar in patients with spontaneous or ergonovine-provoked coronary artery spasm [1]. Heart rate response is variable; inferior ischemia is often associated with a slight decrease in heart rate, whereas ischemia is associated with a slight increase.

Blood pressure may drop just before the onset of ST-segment elevation and rise later as pain develops, but this is not always the case: left-ventricular end-diastolic pressure rises uniformly during ischemia secondary to coronary artery spasm [2].

The earliest changes in ventricular function are prolonged diastolic relaxation followed by decreased regional wall motion. Coronary sinus blood flow declines by 10%–50% during coronary artery spasm [2].

Experimental modes of coronary artery spasm demonstrate that the vasoconstrictive responses of different arterial preparations to different agents are variable and complex [9].

It seems that the presence of atherosclerosis is an important precondition for the development of coronary artery spasm, and that serotonergic receptors are the primary mediators [10,14]. However, one must use caution when extrapolating data from animals or from isolated arteries to the intact human.

Pathology [15–19]
Although autopsy information on the status of major epicardial coronary arteries in patients with documented coronary artery spasm is limited, there have been cases reported in which there was autopsy evidence (postmortem angiography) of coronary artery spasm [15,16]. Most of the reported cases have been in association with coronary atherosclerosis, but El-Maraghi and Sealey failed to show atherosclerotic plaques or other fixed lesions in the epicardial coronary arteries [15]. The patient had 'contraction' rings in the right coronary artery when it was opened longitudinally at autopsy. This suggests that 'spasm' persisted after death in this patient, just as the contracted state of the ventricle persists after death [15].

Angiography [20–25]

Coronary artery spasm may be a focal or diffuse process involving the epicardial coronary arteries; it may also occur in multiple segments, in a migratory fashion.

Heupler has reported that spasm involves the right coronary artery more commonly than it does the anterior descending or circumflex arteries [23]. He notes that 60% of patients with ischemic spasm have fixed severe underlying coronary artery disease, whereas the others have normal or mildly abnormal arteriograms [23]. Several reports indicate that the coronary arteriograms are normal because they have no significant stenoses. In actual fact, many of these show atherosclerotic narrowings of 25%–30%. MacAlpin found that in 90% of cases the spasm causing ischemia was precisely superimposed on and limited to the site of a pre-existing organic lesion [20]. Most investigators believe that coronary artery spasm occurs only rarely in a completely normal artery. However, there seems to be a higher proportion of normal coronary angiograms in patients with coronary artery spasm reported from Japan [24].

Etiology [26–33]

No single cause for coronary artery spasm has been found, and basic as well as clinical investigations indicate that it is a heterogeneous entity. This may explain both the differences in therapeutic responses between patients with known coronary artery spasm and the difficulty in finding a perfect provocative agent. This disorder is possibly the result of multiple pathophysiologic mechanisms, which could include both passive and active influences on vessel caliber, acting singly or in concert at any given time in a given patient. Active influences may involve either endogenous vasoconstrictors or the loss, through a vascular injury, of endothelial-dependent vasodilator substances [28]. Spasm may involve both the large epicardial conduit vessels and the small resistance vessels, and may be associated with a fundamental change in the activational processes of vascular smooth muscle.

Provocative Testing

Ergonovine [34–37]

Most investigators report that ergonovine provocative testing is highly sensitive and specific in patients with the clinical syndrome of variant angina, especially if normal or near-normal coronary arteriograms are present. Bertrand reports a high degree of reproducibility of this test when the same patient is studied within a short period of time without any treatment [34]. Provocative testing is not without risks, but the risk is low [36]. The incidence of arrhythmias reported by Bertrand was 0.56%, and these arrhythmias were always observed in patients with coronary artery spasm [34]. The incidence of arrhythmias in patients with provoked spasm was 4.5%. Serious complications (myocardial infarction and death) have been described by Buxton, who observed three deaths from refractory spasm [35]. However, the spasm was treated only with sublingual nitroglycerin, not intracoronary nitroglycerin.

The most important clinical indication for ergonovine provocative testing is the presence of infrequent episodes of resting chest pain suggestive of angina but with no documentation of myocardial ischemia. Another indication would be to test the short- and long-term efficacy of spasmolytic drug therapy.

Although it is not a universal recommendation, many investigators suggest that this type of testing should be done in the catheterization laboratory: (i) to document the change in epicardial coronary artery calibre; and (ii) to allow the use of intracoronary nitroglycerin if necessary.

Cold Stimulation [38–41]

Cold stimulation has a moderate physiologic vasoconstrictor effect, which leads to enhanced norepinephrine and epinephrine release. It may provoke angiographic evidence of coronary artery vasoconstriction; however, only in a small proportion of patients with coronary artery spasm will cold exposure elicit substantial myocardial ischemia. While this limits its usefulness as a diagnostic tool, it does underscore the fact that the cause of coronary artery spasm must be multifactorial.

Exercise Testing [42–46]

Exercise testing in patients with variant angina results in ST-segment elevation in approximately 30% of patients, ST-segment depression in 30%, a mixed response in a few patients, and no ST-segment changes in about 40% of patients. In the individual patient, these changes appear to be of limited value for predicting the presence of fixed coronary artery stenoses, although ST-segment depression is more frequently associated with significant coronary artery stenoses. In patients with proven significant coronary artery disease, one-third will manifest ST-segment elevation during exercise, one-third ST-segment depression, and one-third no ST-segment changes. Of patients reported to have variant angina without significant coronary artery disease, 60% will have a normal exercise test, 30% will have ST-segment elevation, and 10%–20% ST-segment depression. The test's sensitivity for detecting coronary artery spasm is thus quite low. However, a finding of ST-segment elevation is specific when previous myocardial infarction has been ruled out. Théroux and Waters report that vasospastic angina is diagnosed in the exercise laboratory in about 10% of patients. The diagnosis is usually made by the recording of a 12-lead electrocardiogram during an episode of spontaneous angina.

Other Provocative Tests [47–51]

Other methods than ergonovine, exercise and cold may induce coronary artery spasm: these include hyperventilation, epinephrine, methacholine, histamine and alcohol. Hyperventilation is less sensitive in provoking coronary spasm but less risky than ergonovine, and may be used for provoking a mild degree of coronary spasm [47,48]. Epinephrine is less sensitive than ergonovine, hyperventilation and methacholine, and is not recommended as a routine test for coronary spasm. Methacholine is fairly sensitive, but the time interval between the injection of the drug and the appearance of the attack is usually 6–20 minutes, which makes this test less useful than ergonovine. Histamine may induce coronary spasm [50], but the use of this agent as a routine test for coronary spasm cannot be recommended until large groups of patients have been studied. Alcohol may also induce coronary spasm, but it cannot be recommended as a routine test for coronary spasm because the time interval between ingestion of the agent and appearance of the attack varies widely among patients, ranging from 1.5 to 12 hours [51].

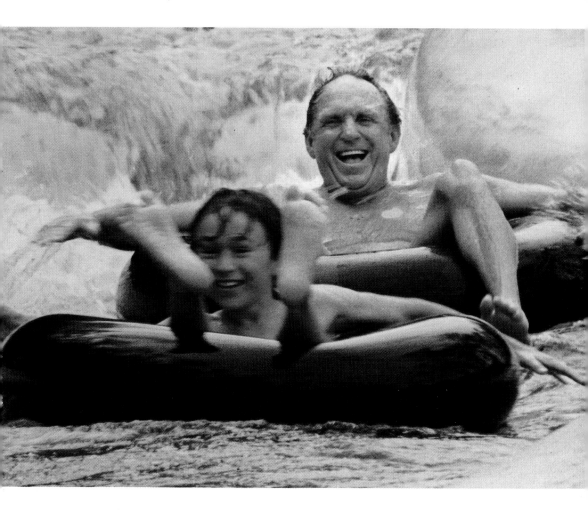

Transiderm®-Nitro

glyceryl trinitrate

Winning the hearts of patients everywhere

Presentation Transdermal therapeutic system containing glyceryl trinitrate, available in 2 strengths: Transiderm-Nitro 5 patches containing a drug reservoir of 25mg glyceryl trinitrate (average amount of glyceryl trinitrate absorbed per patch in 24 hours is 5mg). Transiderm-Nitro 10 patches containing 50mg glyceryl trinitrate (average of 10mg absorbed per patch in 24 hours).
Indications Prophylactic treatment of attacks of angina pectoris.
Dosage Individually variable: 1 Transiderm-Nitro 5 or 1 Transiderm-Nitro 10 daily. Tolerance: see full prescribing information.
Contra-indications Known hypersensitivity to nitrates, severe

hypotension, increased intracranial pressure, myocardial insufficiency due to obstruction.
Precautions Pregnancy and lactation. Recent myocardial infarction, arterial hypoxaemia due to severe anaemia, acute heart failure. Withdraw gradually when discontinuing treatment. Remove before cardioversion or DC defibrillation. Concomitant use of blood pressure lowering agents.
Side-effects Mostly mild and transient: e.g. headache, reflex-tachycardia. Occasionally skin reactions. Rarely after high doses: postural hypotension, dizziness, nausea and vomiting.

Packs and prices Boxes of 30 patches. Transiderm-Nitro 5 (PL0001/0094), basic NHS price 64.4p per day; Transiderm-Nitro 10 (PL0001/0095) 70.9p per day.
® denotes registered trademark. Full prescribing information is available on request from Ciba Laboratories, Horsham, West Sussex.

Ciba

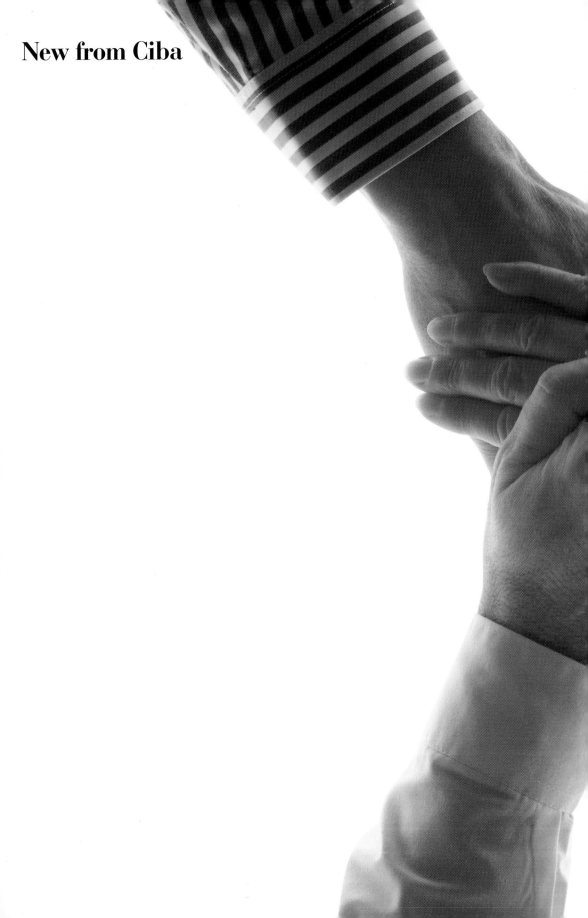

New from Ciba

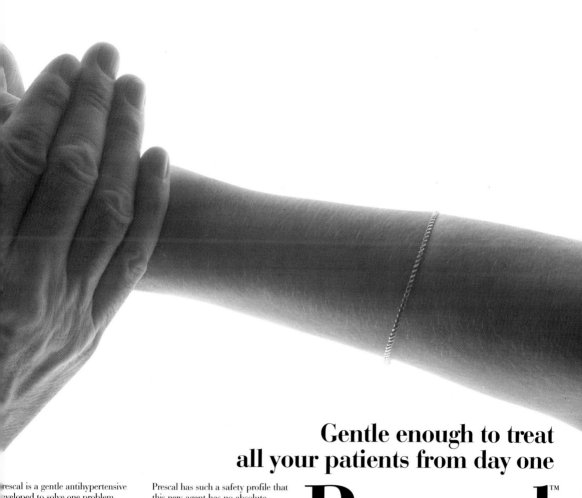

Gentle enough to treat all your patients from day one

Prescal™

isradipine calcium channel blocker

Prescal is a gentle antihypertensive developed to solve one problem without creating others.

It's "gentle" because it starts gradually, without a sudden first dose hypotension and because its effectiveness is not offset by a host of side-effects such as fatigue, breathlessness and cold hands and feet.[1] Side-effects are very mild with Prescal and their frequency is low – around the same as found with placebo.[2]

Prescal has such a safety profile that this new agent has no absolute contra-indications – not in asthma, not in diabetes, not in cardiac failure.[1]

Isn't it reassuring to know that you could prescribe Prescal for **anyone** with mild to moderate hypertension.

Because it is suitable for anyone and because it is so gentle, Prescal is one calcium channel blocker you could consider from the start for all your patients.

Prescribe Prescal for mild to moderate hypertension

Make infusion phlebitis a thing of the past

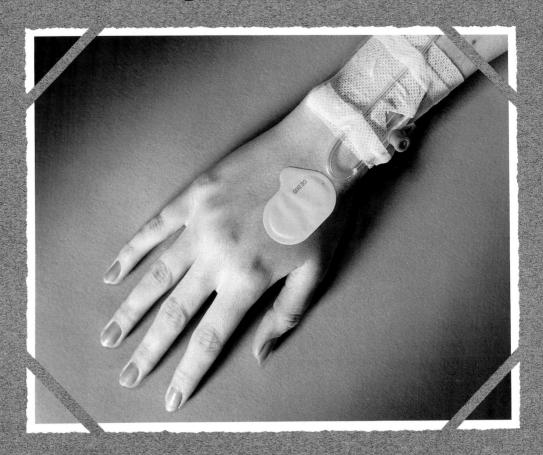

Transiderm®-Nitro

glyceryl trinitrate

Ciba

New effective prevention for infusion phlebitis and extravasation.[1,2]

Role of Spasm in Patients with Angina Pectoris [52,53]

The evidence for coronary artery spasm in patients with variant angina is strong. The ECG abnormality that is a hallmark of this syndrome, ST-segment elevation, resembles that seen when the coronary artery of an animal is ligated and, in many instances, when the human coronary artery is totally occluded by a balloon angioplasty catheter. In these patients, angina is not preceded by an increase in myocardial oxygen demand. Physiologic studies assessing continuous coronary sinus oxygen content have shown a decrease in coronary sinus oxygen preceding either ECG changes or chest pain, and regional blood flow changes have been reported in patients during chest pain.

The evidence supporting the presence of coronary artery spasm in patients with both angina at rest and effort angina is based on observations that indices of myocardial oxygen demand are often not increased prior to chest pain. The ECG shows ST-segment elevation in 25%–35% of patients during chest pain, coronary blood flow when measured has been shown to be decreased during chest pain, and provocative testing with ergometrine induces spasm in 15%–20% of patients tested.

There is a low prevalence of coronary artery spasm in patients with effort angina; however, spasm should be suspected in patients who have variable exercise tolerance, walk-through angina, ST-segment elevation associated with effort, and positive evidence of coronary artery spasm after provocative testing with ergonovine. In addition, at angiography some patients will develop spasm during spontaneous chest pain. There will be the occasional patient with an excellent response to calcium blockers and a poor response to beta-blockers.

Role of Spasm in Patients with Myocardial Infarction [54–57]

Everyone accepts that an occlusive thrombus is an integral part of the early phase of acute transmural myocardial infarction. However, there are no data to prove that thrombosis is the inciting event in acute infarction. There is some evidence to suggest that the clot may be secondary to coronary artery spasm [56]. Well-documented cases of myocardial infarction occurring with angiographically normal or near-normal coronary arteries imply the existence of a dynamic process that interrupts coronary blood flow long enough to cause ischemic necrosis without precipitating thrombosis. In a number of instances, occlusive coronary spasm has been visualized angiographically during the time-course of an evolving myocardial infarction. Careful studies of patients experiencing unstable angina which eventually culminates in myocardial infarction have led some investigators to incriminate vasospasm as a cause of infarction in all persons with high-grade fixed atherosclerotic coronary disease. However, most believe it is impossible to say whether vasospasm, when present in conjunction with advanced coronary lesions, is the cause or result of platelet aggregation. As aggregating platelets produce and release a variety of potent vasoactive agents, one can only infer that a dynamic interaction exists between vessel wall and platelets.

Role of Spasm in Precipitating Arrhythmias [58–60]

Reperfusion arrhythmias occur during the reflow following a temporary coronary artery occlusion. Interest in these arrhythmias grew with the recognition that coronary artery spasm could cause temporary total coronary occlusion, producing similar conditions to those under which reperfusion arrhythmias are experimentally produced. Although the occurrence of ventricular fibrillation during release of coronary spasm has not been documented except in animal data, it nevertheless has strong potential as a cause of death, as a significant proportion of sudden death victims have not suffered acute myocardial infarction. The data available at present indicate that reperfusion is attended by the highest risk of ventricular arrhythmias when a moderate to large ischemic region with incipient but incomplete necrosis is abruptly reperfused [60].

Small-Vessel Coronary Artery Spasm: Clinical Relevance [61–64]

Studies suggest that many patients with angina pain and normal epicardial coronary arteries may have chest pain precipitated by vasoconstriction or the inadequate vasodilatation, during stress, of coronary arteries too small to be visualized by coronary angiography [61]. The majority of these patients do have abnormal left-ventricular function during exercise, as assessed by radionuclide angiography; additionally, they benefit symptomatically from calcium antagonists – probably because of the coronary arterial or vasodilatory effects of these agents. The major remaining doubt pertains to the mechanism of small-vessel coronary artery spasm. Is this an abnormality of autoregulation, or is it spasm involving the smallest epicardial or intramyocardial arteries proximal to the usual sites for autoregulation? As to the prognosis of these patients, this is also uncertain; however, 17% of the patients studied by Cannon et al had regional wall motion abnormalities at rest, associated with reduced global ejection fraction – suggesting that myocardial necrosis can occur in these patients and, in some, result in a dilated cardiomyopathy [63]. Long-term follow-up studies are obviously required to define the natural history of this condition.

Prognosis [65–69]

Myocardial infarction probably occurs more frequently in patients with coronary spasm who also have severe organic coronary lesions [65]. In the study of Severi et al, patients with coronary stenoses greater than 50% in two or three vessels had a significantly higher incidence of infarction than the remainder of their patients [66]. In the series by Waters et al, the risk of infarction with survival for at least one month thereafter was 9.5% (6 out of 63) for patients with stenoses greater than 70%; 11.9% (7 out of 59) for patients with one-vessel disease; and 20% (8 out of 40) for those with multi-vessel disease [68].

The long-term prognosis of patients with coronary artery spasm who develop infarction, as with other patients with infarction, is determined primarily by the degree of left-ventricular dysfunction and the extent and severity of organic coronary disease. Patients with continuing evidence of coronary spasm after infarction probably have a very poor prognosis.

The syndrome of variant angina is frequently characterized by spontaneous exacerbations and remissions [69]. The cause of spontaneous coronary spasm and the reason why it often disappears are unknown. The clinical assessment of patients with variant angina is complicated by episodes of silent myocardial ischemia: these are quite common in patients with frequent symptomatic angina attacks, but can almost never be documented by ambulatory ECG monitoring in patients who have had no angina for many months. Thus, variant angina should be thought of as a temporary condition; the fact that many patients, particularly those with associated organic lesions, are asymptomatic without treatment for up to 1–5 years after diagnosis should be considered in the evaluation of the long-term results of treatment and when planning care for the individual patient [68].

Treatment

Nitrates [70–74]

Various nitrate preparations are available and, when used in adequate dosages, these have been shown to be effective therapy. Assessing the therapeutic effect of the different drugs on coronary artery spasm can be difficult, and therapy must be individualized – there is no one best way to monitor patient response. The treatment of acute attacks of coronary artery spasm is usually easy with either intravenous or sublingual nitroglycerin. Chronic therapy with various nitrate preparations, using a variety of methods, has also been shown to be effective. However, the effect of nitrates on long-term prognosis is unknown. Few studies reporting on patients with coronary artery spasm have used nitrate preparations alone as treatment, so the effect of these drugs alone on clinical outcome is difficult to ascertain.

The important aspects of initiating nitrate therapy include: (i) a program for acute attacks in all patients; (ii) use of a dosage high enough to have clinical efficacy and titration for the individual patient; and (iii) choice of a preparation that the patient can tolerate. The decision on how long to continue therapy should be based on a thorough knowledge of the individual patient, the duration and seriousness of symptoms, and the markers of disease activity. Coronary artery spasm is a potentially life-threatening disease, and the decision to withdraw therapy should not be taken lightly. Nitrates have been used for many years in the treatment of variant angina and coronary artery spasm; they have proven themselves useful and continue to be a mainstay of therapy. As for many other cardiac conditions, however, combination therapy – either with or without nitrates – will probably assume the major role in the prophylaxis and treatment of coronary artery spasm.

Calcium Antagonists [75]

The three calcium antagonists available in the USA, verapamil, nifedipine and diltiazem, either when used alone or in combination with long-acting nitrate preparations, are extremely effective in patients with variant angina pectoris. Many believe that, because of ease of administration and the relatively low reported incidence of adverse effects, these agents should be used as 'first-line' therapy in patients with coronary artery spasm. In many patients with variant angina who have remained pain-free on calcium antagonists for several months, these agents can be safely and successfully discontinued; this leaves the patient free of angina, without medical therapy.

Beta-Blockers [76]

Current data seem to contraindicate beta-blockade in patients with coronary artery spasm and mild underlying coronary atherosclerosis. Beta-blockade may be useful in patients with significant atherosclerotic narrowing, especially when spasm is exercise-induced. When there is a residual fixed stenosis producing exertional angina even when spasm is relieved, myocardial ischemia may be due primarily to decreased supply from the fixed obstruction, with vasomotor instability playing only a minor role. Beta-blockade, by reducing myocardial oxygen requirements, should theoretically be of benefit here. Patients with spasm who develop a marked sympathetic response, manifested by tachycardia and hypertension associated with ischemia or the onset of pain, may benefit from a combination of beta-blockade with nitrates or calcium antagonists. Another alternative, however, would be the sole use of calcium antagonists with negative chronotropic effects, which would have some ability to decrease myocardial oxygen consumption as well as providing epicardial coronary vasodilatation. Beta-blockade alone should be considered contraindicated in patients with coronary spasm who have mild fixed stenosis after spasm is relieved.

Alpha-Blocking Drugs [77]
Phentolamine cannot play a major role in the acute treatment of variant angina; its tendency to increase myocardial oxygen demand would therefore aggravate the condition of patients with advanced coronary artery disease.

Phenoxybenzamine may be used in patients with variant angina. However, because of its side-effects (such as nausea, weakness, palpitations and orthostatic hypotension) and because it is less effective than calcium antagonists, this drug will probably play no significant role in the treatment of variant angina.

Prazosin [78–80]
Winniford et al and Robertson et al found prazosin ineffective in patients with variant angina [78,79]. Tzivoni reports a favorable response, which may be explained by the difference in patient population (all of his patients had had acute transmural myocardial infarction), and may also be explained by the higher dose of prazosin used and the fact that all patients received nitrates and calcium antagonists in addition to the prazosin [80].

Anticholinergic Drugs [81]
Atropine, as reported by Yasue and co-workers, reversed coronary artery spasm in three patients with variant angina [81]; also, 1 mg atropine administered 20 minutes before the methacholine prevented coronary spasm in all three patients.

Labetalol [82]
An interesting drug, with both alpha- and beta-blockade properties, labetalol may prove to be effective mainly in patients with significant coronary artery disease, with its action of increasing coronary blood flow and simultaneously reducing myocardial oxygen demand [82]. To date, it has not been tested as a therapeutic agent in patients with proven coronary artery spasm.

Amiodarone [83]

Rutizky *et al* used large doses of amiodarone (800–1000 mg/day) to prevent variant angina attacks in three patients [83]. These investigators attribute the favorable response to the drug's non-competitive alpha-blockade causing coronary vasodilatation.

Drugs that Modify Platelet Function and Arachidonic Acid Metabolism [84–90]

The major drugs used to modify platelet function have been cyclo-oxygenase, thromboxane A_2, and serotonin inhibitors and prostacyclin. In two trials, aspirin was studied because of its platelet-inhibitory effects [84,85]; the dosage was kept small so as to inhibit thromboxane A_2 preferentially. Unfortunately, in spite of the inhibition of thromboxane A_2 formation, aspirin did not influence the frequency of transient ischemic episodes. In one of these studies, indomethacin was also used [84]. Again, there was no decrease in episodes of myocardial ischemia, although thromboxane A_2 synthesis was suppressed. In contrast to these studies, which showed no change in frequency of myocardial ischemia, Miwa *et al* found an increase in spontaneously occurring episodes of ST-segment elevation following administration of four grains of aspirin [86]. The worsening of ischemia in these patients could be explained at least in part by the diversion of arachidonic acid metabolism towards lipoxygenase products. The data from these trials lead one to conclude that cyclo-oxygenase inhibitors do not have salutary effects in patients with variant angina pectoris.

Studies with selective thromboxane A_2 synthetase inhibitors in patients with variant angina have also provided inconsistent data. Yui *et al* used O.K.Y.-046 in patients with vasospastic angina, and objectively evaluated ischemic episodes [87]: the number of these episodes was not significantly altered by therapy. Unpublished studies with other selective thromboxane A_2 inhibitors have also not shown significant benefit in patients with variant angina.

The concept of prostacyclin deficiency was examined by Chierchia *et al* in patients with variant angina [88]. They administered prostacyclin in the highest tolerated dosage to patients. This did not decrease the number, duration and severity of the episodes of ST-segment elevation. Moreover, prostacyclin did not prevent myocardial ischemia induced by ergonovine.

To examine whether coronary artery vasospasm was related at least in part to platelet serotonin release, a double-blind placebo-controlled study with ketanserin was conducted [89]. This study showed that ketanserin, in a dose sufficient to suppress serotonin-induced platelet aggregation, did not affect the number, severity and duration of episodes of variant angina [89]; moreover, in a dose sufficient to prevent the vasoconstrictor effects of serotonin, it did not abolish or decrease the threshold for myocardial ischemia induced by the administration of ergonovine [90].

Surgery for Patients with Coronary Artery Spasm [91–97]

Patients with proven coronary artery spasm and normal or near-normal coronary arteries are currently not candidates for routine coronary artery surgery. If fixed coronary obstruction involving proximal major coronary arteries is present, drug therapy is still the treatment of choice. If pain persists despite drug therapy, coronary artery surgery may then be considered. However, for this condition, the current results of surgery may not be as good as for patients with angina and no evidence of coronary artery spasm. This difference in operative results may be due in part to spasm occurring along the entire length of the coronary artery, proximal and distal to a fixed obstruction. If surgery is performed, coronary vasodilator therapy should be continued postoperatively.

Future Research into the Causes of Coronary Artery Spasm

There must be human and animal studies designed to evaluate the numerous conditions that might trigger coronary artery spasm in a normal or hypersensitive vessel. There is a possibility that inflammation, or immunologic processes involving the blood vessels, are in part responsible for abnormal vasoconstriction. It is also important to continue investigation of the role of the calcium ion at the cellular and subcellular level of normal or abnormally contracting vascular smooth muscles.

The study of the endothelium-dependent relaxant factor, the biologically active vasodilatory substance elaborated by endothelium in response to numerous stimuli, may prove fruitful. This substance could be the link between atherosclerosis and spasm, since atherosclerotic plaques disrupt endothelium and decrease endothelium-dependent relaxant factor.

More information must be gained about factors that determine prognosis in patients with proven coronary artery spasm; the systematic study of (i) clinical presentation, (ii) presence or absence of a previous myocardial infarction, (iii) state of the left ventricle, (iv) region of myocardial ischemia, and (v) relationship to the extent and location of coronary artery disease should provide important clinical information. Perhaps one or more of the clinical descriptors can shed light on why some patients with proven coronary artery spasm proceed to acute myocardial infarction or death, while others have long periods of remission or have their symptoms easily controlled by nitrates or calcium antagonists.

References

[1] Curry RC Jr, Pepine CJ, Sabom MB, Conti CR. Similarities of ergonovine-induced and spontaneous attacks of variant angina. *Circulation* 1979; **59**: 307–11.

[2] Feldman RL, Pepine CJ, Whittle JL, Curry RC, Conti CR. Coronary hemodynamic findings during spontaneous angina in patients with variant angina. *Circulation* 1981; **64**: 76–83.

[3] Feldman RL, Hill JA, Whittle JL, Conti CR, Pepine CJ. Electrocardiographic changes with coronary artery spasm. *Am Heart J* 1983; **106**: 1288–96.

[4] Curry RC, Pepine CJ, Sabom MB, Feldman RL, Christie LG, Conti CR. Effects of ergonovine in patients with and without coronary artery disease. *Circulation* 1977; **56**: 803–9.

[5] Feldman RL, Curry RC Jr, Pepine CJ, Mehta J, Conti CR. Regional coronary hemodynamic effects of ergonovine in patients with and without variant angina. *Circulation* 1980; **62**: 149–59.

[6] Curry RC Jr, Pepine CJ, Sabom MB et al. Hemodynamic and myocardial metabolic effects of ergonovine in patients with chest pain. *Circulation* 1978; **58**: 648–54.

[7] Goldberg S, Lam W, Mudge G et al. Coronary hemodynamic and myocardial metabolic alterations accompanying coronary spasm. *Am J Cardiol* 1979; **43**: 481–7.

[8] Orlick AE, Ricci DR, Cipriano PR, Guthaner DF, Harrison DC. Coronary hemodynamic effects of ergonovine maleate in human subjects. *Am J Cardiol* 1980; **45**: 48–52.

[9] Segal A, Pearle DL, Gillis RA.
Coronary spasm produced by picrotoxin in
cats.
Eur J Pharmacol 1981; **76**: 447–51.

[10] Brazenor RM, Angus JA.
Ergometrine contracts isolated canine coronary arteries by a serotonergic mechanism: No
role for alpha adrenoceptors.
J Pharmacol Exp Ther 1981; **218**: 530–6.

[11] Shimokawa H, Tomoike H, Nabeyama S *et al.*
Coronary artery spasm induced in atherosc-
lerotic miniature swine.
Science 1983; **221**: 560–2.

[12] Perez JW, Saffitz JE, Gutierrez FA, Henry PD.
Coronary artery spasm in intact dogs induced
by potassium and serotonin.
Circ Res 1983; **52**: 423–31.

[13] Henry PD, Yokoyama M.
Supersensitivity of atherosclerotic rabbit aorta
to ergonovine: Mediation by a serotonergic
mechanism.
J Clin Invest 1980; **66**: 306–13.

[14] Kawachi Y, Tomoike H, Maruoka Y *et al.*
Selective hypercontraction caused by ergonovine in the canine coronary artery under conditions of induced atherosclerosis.
Circulation 1984; **69**: 441–50.

[15] El-Maraghi NRH, Sealey BJ.
Recurrent myocardial infarction in a young man
due to coronary arterial spasm demonstrated
at autopsy.
Circulation 1980; **61**: 199–207.

[16] Maron BJ, Henry WL, Roberts WC, Epstein SE.
Comparison of echocardiographic and necropsy measurements of ventricular wall thickness in patients with and without disproportionate septal thickening.
Circulation 1977; **55**: 341–6.

[17] Conti CR, Pepine CJ, Curry BC Jr.
Coronary artery spasm: An important mechanism in the pathophysiology of ischemic heart
disease.
Curr Prob Cardiol 1979; **4**: 1–70.

[18] Conti CR, Curry RC Jr.
Coronary artery spasm and myocardial ische-
mia.
Mod Concepts Cardiovasc Dis 1980; **49**: 1–6.

[19] Conti CR, ed.
*Coronary Artery Spasm: Pathophysiology, Di-
agnosis and Treatment.* New York: Marcel Dekker, 1986.

[20] MacAlpin RN.
Relation of coronary arterial spasm to sites of
organic stenosis.
Am J Cardiol 1980; **46**: 143–53.

[21] MacAlpin RN.
Correlation of the location of coronary arterial
spasm with the lead distribution of ST segment
elevation during variant angina.
Am Heart J 1980; **99**: 555–64.

[22] Bertrand MD, LaBlanche J, Tilmant PY *et al.*
Frequency of provoked coronary arterial
spasm in 1089 consecutive patients undergoing coronary arteriography.
Circulation 1982; **65**: 1299–306.

[23] Heupler FA Jr.
Syndrome of symptomatic coronary arterial
spasm with nearly normal coronary arteriograms.
Am J Cardiol 1980; **45**: 863–80.

[24] Endo M, Kanda I, Hosoda S, Hayashi H, Hirosa-
wa K, Konno S.
Prinzmetal's variant form of angina pectoris:
Re-evaluation of mechanisms.
Circulation 1975; **52**: 33–7.

[25] Dhurandhar RW, Watt DL, Silver MD, Trimble
AS, Adelman AG.
Prinzmetal's variant form of angina with arter-
iographic evidence of coronary arterial spasm.
Am J Cardiol 1972; **30**: 902–5.

[26] Ezra D, Boyd LM, Feuerstein G, Goldstein RE.
Coronary constriction by Leukotrien C_4, D_4,
and E_4 in the intact pig heart.
Am J Cardiol 1983; **51**: 1451–4.

[27] Folts JD, Gallagher K, Rower GG.
Blood flow reductions in stenosed canine
coronary arteries: Vasospasm or platelet
aggregation?
Circulation 1982; **65**: 248–55.

[28] Furchgott RF.
Role of endothelium in responses of vascular
smooth muscle.
Circ Res 1983; **53**: 557–73.

[29] Ginsburg R, Bristow MR, Davis K, Diabase A,
Billingham ME.
Quantitative pharmacologic responses of nor-
mal and atherosclerotic isolated human epicar-
dial coronary arteries.
Circulation 1984; **69**: 430–40.

[30] Joris I, Majno G.
Endothelial changes induced by arterial
spasm.
Am J Pathol 1981; **102**: 346–58.

[31] Kawachi Y, Tomoike H, Maruoka Y *et al.*
Selective hypercontraction caused by ergonovine in the canine coronary artery under conditions of induced atherosclerosis.
Circulation 1984; **69**: 441–50.

[32] Logan SE.
On the fluid mechanics of human coronary
artery stenosis.
IEEE Trans Biomed Eng 1975; **22**: 327–34.

[33] Mehta JL.
Prostaglandin's regulatory role in cardiovascular system and implications in human ischemic
heart disease.
Int J Cardiol 1983; **4**: 249–59.

[34] Bertrand ME, LaBlanche JM, Tilmant PY *et al.*
Frequency of provoked coronary arterial
spasm in 1089 patients undergoing coronary
arteriography.
Circulation 1982; **65**: 1299–306.

[35] Buxton A, Goldberg S, Hishfeld J *et al.*
Refractory induced coronary spasm: Import-
ance of intracoronary nitroglycerin.
Am J Cardiol 1980; **46**: 329–34.

[36] Heupler FA.
Provocative testing for coronary arterial spasm.
Risk, method and rationale.
Am J Cardiol 1980; **46**: 335–7.

[37] Whittle JL, Feldman RL, Pepine CJ, Curry C,
Conti CR.
Variability of electrocardiographic response to
repeated ergonovine provocation in variant
angina patients with coronary artery spasm.
Am Heart J 1982; **103**: 161–7.

[38] Mudge GH Jr, Grossman W, Mills RM Jr, Lesch
M, Braunwald E.
Reflex increase in coronary vascular resist-
ance in patients with ischemic heart disease.
N Engl J Med 1976; **295**: 1333–7.

[39] Mudge GH, Mirsky I.
The clinical utility of cold pressor tests in assessing left ventricular dysfunction in patients with
coronary artery disease [Editorial].
Int J Cardiol 1983; **3**: 307–9.

[40] Mudge GH Jr, Grossman W, Mills RM Jr, Lesch
M, Braunwald E.
Evidence for reflex coronary artery spasm in
patients with ischemic heart disease.
Trans Assoc Am Physicians 1976; **89**: 225–36.

[41] Feldman RL, Whittle JL, Pepine CL, Conti CR.
Regional coronary angiographic observations
during cold stimulation in patients with exertional chest pain: Comparison of diameter
responses in normal and fixed stenotic vessels.
Am Heart J 1981; **102**: 822–30.

[42] Chaitman BR, Waters DD, Theroux P, Hanson
JS.
ST segment elevation and coronary spasm in
response to exercise.
Am J Cardiol 1981; **47**: 1350–7.

[43] DeFeyter PJ, Majio PA, Van Eenige MJ, Wardeh
R, Wempe FN, Roos JP.
Clinical significance of exercise-induced ST
segment elevation. Correlative angiographic
study in patients with ischaemic heart disease.
Br Heart J 1981; **46**: 84–92.

[44] Waters DD, Chaitman BR, Dupras G, Theroux
P, Mizgala HF.
Coronary artery spasm during exercise in pa-
tients with variant angina.
Circulation 1979; **59**: 580–5.

[45] Waters DD, Szlachcic J, Bourassa MG, Scholl
JM, Theroux P.
Exercise testing in patients with variant angina:
Results, correlation with clinical and angiog-
raphic features and prognostic significance.
Circulation 1982; **65**: 265–74.

[46] Waters DD, Szlachcic J, Bonan R, Miller DD,
Dauwe F, Theroux P.
Comparative sensitivity of exercise, cold
pressor and ergonovine testing in provoking
attacks of variant in patients with active disease.
Circulation 1983; **67**: 310–5.

[47] Girotti LA, Crosatto JR, Messuti H *et al.*
The hyperventilation test as a method for developing successful therapy in Prinzmetal's
angina.
Am J Cardiol 1982; **49**: 834–41.

[48] Yasue H, Nagao M, Omote S, Takizawa A,
Miwa K, Tanaka S.
Coronary arterial spasm and Prinzmetal's
variant form of angina induced by hyperventila-
tion and Tris-buffer infusion.
Circulation 1978; **58**: 56–62.

[49] Yasue H, Omote S, Takizawa A, Nagao M,
Nosaka K, Nakajima H.
Alkalosis-induced coronary vasoconstriction:
Effects of calcium ions, diltiazem, nitroglycerin
and propranolol.
Am Heart J 1981; **102**: 206–10.

[50] Ginsburg R, Bristow MR, Kantrowitz N, Baim
DA, Harrison DC.
Histamine provocation of clinical coronary
artery spasm: Implications concerning
pathogenesis of variant angina pectoris.
Am Heart J 1981; **102**: 819–22.

[51] Takizawa A, Yasue H, Omote S *et al.*
Variant angina induced by alcohol ingestion.
Am Heart J 1984; **107**: 25–7.

[52] Chierchia S, Brinelli C, Simonetti I, Lazari M,
Maseri A.
Sequence of events in angina at rest: Primary
reduction in coronary flow.
Circulation 1980; **61**: 759–68.

[53] Conti CR, Pepine CJ, Curry RC.
Coronary artery spasm: An important mechanism in the pathophysiology of ischemic heart disease. In: Harvey WP, ed. *Current Problems in Cardiology, Vol. 4.* Chicago: Year Book Medical Publishers, 1979.

[54] Oliva PB.
Pathophysiology of acute myocardial infarction, 1981.
Ann Intern Med 1981; **94**: 236.

[55] El-Maraghi NR, Sealy BJ.
Recurrent myocardial infarction in a young man due to coronary arterial spasm demonstrated at autopsy.
Circulation 1980; **61**: 199.

[56] Vincent GM, Anderson JL, Marshall HW.
Coronary spasm producing coronary thrombosis and myocardial infarction.
N Engl J Med 1983; **309**: 220.

[57] Maseri A, L'Abbate A, Baroldi G et al.
Coronary vasospasm as a possible cause of myocardial infarction. A conclusion derived from the study of "preinfarction" angina.
N Engl J Med 1978; **299**: 1271.

[58] Sheehan FH, Epstein SE.
Determinants of arrhythmic death due to coronary spasm: Effect of preexisting coronary artery stenosis on the incidence of reperfusion arrhythmia.
Circulation 1982; **65**: 259–64.

[59] Sheehan FH, Epstein SE.
The effect of calcium channel blocking agents on reperfusion arrhythmias.
Am Heart J 1982; **103**: 973–7.

[60] Sheehan FH, Epstein SE.
Determinants of arrhythmic death during coronary artery reperfusion: Effect of perfusion bed size.
Am Heart J 1983; **105**: 911–4.

[61] Cannon RO, Watson RM, Rosing DR, Epstein SE.
Angina caused by reduced vasodilator reserve of the small coronary arteries.
J Am Coll Cardiol 1983; **1**: 1359.

[62] Cannon RO, Rosing DR, Leon MB, Watson RM, Epstein SE.
Influence of vasodilator reserve and left ventricular filling pressure on coronary blood flow in hypertrophic cardiomyopathy.
Circulation 1985; **71**: 234.

[63] Cannon RO, Bonow RO, Bacharach SL, Green MV, Rosing DR, Epstein SE.
Left ventricular dysfunction in patients with angina pectoris, normal epicardial coronary arteries, and abnormal arteriolar vasodilator reserve [Abstract].
Circulation 1983; **68**: III–164.

[64] Cannon RO, Watson RM, Rosing DR, Epstein SE.
Efficacy of calcium antagonists therapy in patients with angina pectoris, normal epicardial coronary arteries, and abnormal vasodilator reserve.
Am J Cardiol 1985; **56**: 242.

[65] Bott-Silverman C, Heupler FA Jr.
Natural history of pure coronary artery spasm in patients treated medically.
J Am Coll Cardiol 1983; **2**: 200–5.

[66] Severi S, Davies G, Maseri A, Marzullo P, L'Abbate A.
Long-term prognosis of "variant" angina with medical treatment.
Am J Cardiol 1980; **46**: 226–32.

[67] Waters DD, Szlachcic J, Miller D, Theroux P.
Clinical characteristics of patients with variant angina complicated by myocardial infarction or death within 1 month.
Am J Cardiol 1982; **49**: 658–64.

[68] Waters DD, Miller DD, Szlachcic J et al.
Factors influencing the long-term prognosis of treated patients with variant angina.
Circulation 1983; **68**: 258–65.

[69] Waters DD, Bouchard A, Theroux P.
Spontaneous remission is a frequent outcome of variant angina.
J Am Coll Cardiol 1983; **2**: 195–9.

[70] Conti CR, Feldman RL.
The use of nitrates in the treatment of ischemic heart disease. In: Willis Hurst J, ed. *Clinical Essays of the Heart, Vol. 2.* New York: McGraw-Hill, 1984; pp. 3–24.

[71] Pepine CJ, Feldman RL, Conti CR.
Action of intracoronary nitroglycerin in refractory coronary artery spasm.
Circulation 1982; **65**: 411–4.

[72] Distante A, Maseri A, Severi S, Biagini A, Chierchia S.
Management of vasospastic angina at rest with continuous infusion of isosorbide dinitrate.
Am J Cardiol 1979; **44**: 533–9.

[73] Hill JA, Feldman RL, Pepine CJ, Conti CR.
Randomized double-blind comparison of nifedipine and isosorbide dinitrate in patients with coronary arterial spasm.
Am J Cardiol 1982; **49**: 431–8.

[74] Ginsburg R, Lamb IH, Schroeder JS, Hu M, Harrison DC.
Randomized double-blind comparison of nifedipine and isosorbide dinitrate therapy in variant angina pectoris due to coronary artery spasm.
Am Heart J 1982; **103**: 44–8.

[75] Winniford MD, Johnson SM, Mauritson DR *et al.*
Verapamil therapy for Prinzmetal's variant angina: Comparison with placebo and nifedipine.
Am J Cardiol 1982; **50**: 913–8.

[76] Robertson RM, Wood AJJ, Vaughn WK, Robertson D.
Exacerbation of vasotonic angina pectoris by propranolol.
Circulation 1982; **65**: 281–5.

[77] Chierchia S, Crea F, Davies G, Berkenboom G, Crean P, Maseri A.
Coronary spasm: Any role for alpha receptor? [Abstract].
Circulation 1982; **66** (Suppl 2): II–247.

[78] Robertson RM, Bernard Y, Carr RK, Robertson D.
Alpha adrenergic blockade in vasotonic angina: Lack of efficacy of specific alpha 1 receptor blockade with prazosin.
J Am Coll Cardiol 1983; **2**: 1146.

[79] Winniford MD, Filipchuck N, Hillis LD.
Adrenergic blockade for variant angina: A long-term, double blind, randomized trial.
Circulation 1983; **67**: 1185.

[80] Tzivoni D, Keren A, Benhorin J, Gottlieb S, Atlas D, Stern S.
Prazosin therapy for refractory variant angina.
Am Heart J 1983; **105**: 262.

[81] Yasue H, Touyana M, Shimanoto M, Kato H, Tanaka S, Akiyama F.
Role of autonomic nervous system in the pathogenesis of Prinzmetal's variant form of angina.
Circulation 1974; **50**: 534.

[82] Frishman W, Strom J, Kirschner M *et al.*
Labetalol therapy in patients with systemic hypertension and angina pectoris: Effects of combined alpha and beta adrenoceptor blockade.
Am J Cardiol 1981; **48**: 917.

[83] Rutizky B, Girotti A, Rosenbaum MB.
Efficacy of chronic amiodarone therapy in patients with variant angina pectoris and inhibition of ergonovine coronary constriction.
Am Heart J 1982; **103**: 38.

[84] Robertson RM, Robertson D, Robertson LJ *et al.*
Thromboxane A_2 in vasotonic angina pectoris. Evidence from direct measurements and inhibitor trials.
N Engl J Med 1981; **304**: _98–1003.

[85] Chierchia S, DeCaterina R, Crea F, Patrono C, Maseri A.
Failure of thromboxane A_2 blockade to prevent attacks of vasospastic angina.
Circulation 1982; **66**: 702–5.

[86] Miwa K, Kambara H, Kawai C.
Effect of aspirin in large doses on attacks of variant angina.
Am Heart J 1983; **105**: 351–5.

[87] Yui Y, Hattori R, Takatsu Y *et al.*
Is increased coronary sinus thromboxane A_2 production a cause or a result of vasospastic angina? [Abstract].
Circulation 1983; **68**: III–397.

[88] Chierchia S, Patrono C, Crea F *et al.*
Effects of intravenous prostacyclin in variant angina.
Circulation 1982; **65**: 470–7.

[89] DeCaterina R, Carpeggiani C, L'Abbate A.
A double-blind, placebo-controlled study of ketanserin in patients with Prinzmetal's angina.
Circulation 1984; **69**: 889–94.

[90] Freedman B, Chierchia S, Rodriguez-Plaza A, Bugiardini R, Maseri A.
Ergonovine-induced myocardial ischemia: No role for serotonergic (S-HT) receptors [Abstract].
Circulation 1983; **68**: III–257.

[91] Bertrand ME, LaBlanche JN, Rousseau MF, Waremberg HH, Stankautak C, Scots G.
Surgical treatment of variant angina: Use of plexectomy with aortocoronary bypass.
Circulation 1980; **61**: 877.

[92] Grondin C, Limet R.
Sympathetic denervation in association with coronary artery grafting in patients with Prinzmetal's angina.
J Thorac Cardiovasc Surg 1977; **23**: 111.

[93] Clark D, Quint R, Mitchell R, Dugell WW.
Coronary artery spasm: Medical management, surgical denervation and autotransplantation.
J Thorac Cardiovasc Surg 1977; **73**: 332.

[94] Pasternak RC, Hutter AM, DeSanctis RW, Jaro MF, Buckley M.
Variant angina.
J Thorac Cardiovasc Surg 1979; **78**: 614.

[95] Shick EL, David Z, Lavery RM *et al.*
Surgical therapy for Prinzmetal's variant angina.
Ann Thorac Surg 1982; **33**: 359.

[96] Bertrand ME, LaBlanche JN, Tilmant PY et al.
Complete denervation of the heart (autotransplantation) for treatment of severe, refractory
coronary spasm.
Am J Cardiol 1981; 47: 1375–8.

[97] Buxton AE, Goldberg S, Harken A et al.
Coronary artery spasm immediately after
myocardial revascularization.
N Engl J Med 1981; 304: 1249–53.

STABLE AND UNSTABLE ANGINA PECTORIS

PATHOPHYSIOLOGY

[1] Mechanisms of nocturnal angina pectoris: importance of increased myocardial oxygen demand in patients with severe coronary artery disease.
Quyyumi AA, Wright CA, Mockus LJ, Fox KM, Nat Heart Hosp, London, UK.
Lancet 1984; i: 1207–9.

[2] Role of heart rate in pathophysiology of chronic stable angina.
Chierchia S, Gallino A, Smith G et al, Royal Postgrad Med Sch, London, UK.
Lancet 1984; i: 1353–6.

[3] Nocturnal angina: precipitating factors in patients with coronary artery disease and those with variant angina.
Quyyumi AA, Efthimiou J, Quyyumi A, Mockus LJ, Spiro SG, Fox KM, Nat Heart Hosp, London, UK.
Br Heart J 1986; 56: 346–52.

[4] Angina pectoris-like pain provoked by intravenous adenosine in healthy volunteers.
Sylven C, Beermann B, Jonzon B, Brandt R, Danderyd Hosp, Danderyd, Sweden.
Br Med J 1986; 293: 227–31.

[5] Coronary angioscopy in patients with unstable angina pectoris.
Sherman CT, Litvack F, Grundfest W et al, Cedars-Sinai Med Cent, Los Angeles, CA, USA.
N Engl J Med 1986; 315: 913–9.

Comment. There is evidence in many patients with nocturnal angina that myocardial ischemia is caused by an increase in coronary vasomotor tone with a resultant decrease in coronary blood flow, and not by an increase in myocardial oxygen demand, as in the usual form of effort angina. The hallmark of this primary reduction in blood flow is that signs of ischemia, such as electrocardiographic ST-segment depression, appear before any increase in heart rate. In a study of 11 patients, careful analysis of the ambulatory electrocardiogram showed 16 of 17 episodes of nocturnal ischemia and all episodes of daytime ischemia to be preceded by an increase in heart rate [1]. In contrast, Chierchia et al, also studying 11 patients with severe coronary disease, found that an increase in heart rate of greater than 10 beats/min preceded the ST-segment changes in only a minority of subjects [2]. In a subsequent study by Quyyumi et al [3], the electrocardio-gram, electroencephalogram, electromyogram, chest wall movements, nasal airflow and oxygen saturation were monitored continuously during sleep. All episodes of myocardial ischemia (reflected by ST-segment depression on the ECG) in the patients with coronary disease were preceded by an increase in heart rate which resulted from arousal, body movements, rapid eye movement sleep, or in one case sleep apnea, whereas in the patients with variant angina episodes of ST-segment elevation or depression occurred without any such precedents in all but three of the 26 episodes that were recorded.

Although at first sight the findings of these groups would appear to be diametrically opposed, both groups acknowledge that changes in oxygen supply and demand are important, and these workers differ only in their perception of a dominant mechanism.

During ischemia, adenosine is formed from adenosine triphosphate and monophosphate within the ischemic cell; it is cleared by vascular elements and has a half-life of 10 seconds. It has been reported that increased concentrations of adenosine are present in the blood from the coronary sinus during ischemia. Adenosine has several cardioprotective effects during ischemia which are mediated by cell surface receptors. In a study by Sylven et al, the hypothesis that adenosine causes angina pectoris and thus further protects the myocardium against ischemia is examined [4]. They administered a bolus of adenosine into the peripheral vein of six healthy subjects aged 30–44 years. On the first day of the study, the maximum tolerable dose of adenosine for each subject was determined. On the second day, one-third, two-thirds and the full maximum tolerable dose of adenosine and three doses of saline were administered in a single-blind randomized order. Thereafter, aminophylline (5 mg/kg) was administered, and the procedure was repeated but in a different randomized order. On the third day, between two-thirds and the maximum tolerable dose was given, followed by intravenous dipyridamole (10 mg) and a second injection of the same dose of adenosine. Chest pain was scored one minute after each dose of adenosine. All of the subjects had central chest pain which radiated to the shoulders, the ulnar aspect of the arm, the epigastric area, the back and into the throat, and which also provoked anxiety. Pain began approximately 20 seconds after the administration of adenosine and lasted for 10–15 seconds. An increase in the dose of adenosine was found to increase the intensity of pain. The administration of aminophylline resulted in a significant reduction of the pain. This result suggests that adenosine released from the ischemic myocardium induces angina pectoris by stimulating theophylline-sensitive receptors.

The following have all been implicated as causes of unstable angina: coronary spasm, increasingly severe coronary stenosis and coronary thrombosis. The results of systematic angiographic studies have demonstrated coronary thrombosis in 1.3% to 52% of patients with unstable angina. In a recent study, 95% of patients who died within six hours of an ischemic event had coronary thrombus or ulcerated plaque at autopsy [5]. This suggests that the prevalence of acute intimal pathological processes is much higher in patients with unstable angina than is detected using coronary angiography. Sherman et al used the newly developed high-resolution flexible fiberoptic angioscope to visualize the intracoronary lesions of 10 patients with unstable angina and 10 patients with stable coronary disease who were undergoing coronary artery bypass grafting. Of 32 vessels, it demonstrated only one of the four complex plaques and only one of seven thrombi. Using angioscopy, it was shown that none of the 17 vessels in the patients with stable coronary disease had either a complex plaque or thrombus, and in those patients with unstable angina all three who had accelerated angina were shown to have complex plaques and in all seven with angina at rest thrombi were demonstrated. From these results it can be seen that angioscopy can demonstrate coronary lesions not detected on coronary angiography. They also indicate that angina refractory to medical treatment can be the result of unstable pathological processes in the intima: plaque ulceration may increase the frequency and severity of angina on effort; the subsequent development of partially occlusive thrombi may cause unstable angina at rest.

DIAGNOSIS AND ASSESSMENT

CHEST PAIN WITH NORMAL CORONARY ARTERIES

[1]   Atypical chest pain: coronary or esophageal disease?
      Conte MR, Orzan F, Magnacca M *et al*, Univ di Torino, Torino, Italy.
      Int J Cardiol 1986; **13**: 135–42.
[2]   The oesophagus as a cause of recurrent chest pain: which patients should be investigated and which tests should be used?
      de Caestecker JS, Blackwell JN, Brown J, Heading RC, Royal Infirm, Edinburgh, UK.
      Lancet 1985; ii: 1143–6.
[3]   Chest pain - esophageal, cardiac, or both?
      Lee MG, Sullivan SN, Watson WC, Melendez LJ, Victoria Hosp, London, Ontario, Canada.
      Am J Gastroenterol 1985; **80**: 320–4.
[4]   Does it help to undiagnose angina?
      Dart AM, Davies HA, Griffith T, Henderson AH, Welsh Nat Sch Med, Cardiff, UK.
      Eur Heart J 1983; **4**: 461–2.
[5]   False suspicion of coronary heart disease: a 7 year follow-up study of 36 apparently healthy middle-aged men.
      Erikssen J, Dale J, Rootwelt K, Myhre E, Rikshospitalet, Oslo, Norway.
      Circulation 1983; **68**: 490–7.
[6]   Seven year survival of patients with normal or near normal coronary arteriograms: a CASS registry study.
      Kemp HG, Kronmal RA, Vliestra RE, Frye RL, and participants in the Coronary Artery Surgery Study, CASS Coordinating Cent, Univ Washington, Seattle, WA, USA.
      J Am Coll Cardiol 1986; **7**: 479–83.
[7]   Prognostic implications of angiographically normal and insignificantly narrowed coronary arteries.
      Papanicolaou MN, Califf RM, Hlatky MA *et al*, Duke Univ Med Cent, Durham, NC, USA.
      Am J Cardiol 1986; **58**: 1181–7.

Comment.   It is widely known that esophageal disease can cause retrosternal chest pain similar to that of cardiac origin. Conte *et al* present the results of cardiac and esophageal investigations in 55 patients with atypical chest pain [1]. Forty-five per cent of patients were found to have isolated esophageal disease, 14.5% had significant coronary artery disease, 10.9% had both and 29% were found to have neither. Although esophageal disease was found to be very frequent in patients with atypical chest pain, it did not always account for the symptoms completely. de Caestecker *et al* undertook investigations of the esophagus in 50 consecutive patients with recurrent chest pain thought to be non-cardiac in origin following cardiologic investigation [2]. Sixty per cent of these patients were found to have an esophageal disorder: gastroesophageal reflux and diffuse esophageal spasm were the most common. On routine contrast radiology and upper gastrointestinal endoscopy, only a minority of these patients had abnormalities. Nonetheless, esophageal disorders are common and, unless an esophageal abnormality can be demonstrated during chest pain, it is difficult to be certain that the pain and abnormality are related.

In some patients, the esophageal origin of chest pain can be determined only by pharmacologic provocation during manometry. Lee *et al* reported on nine patients with chest pain that could be explained by disorders of the esophagus [3]. Methacholine was found to provoke the pain and manometric abnormalities in five patients who had normal baseline tracings; however, on provocation with methacholine, seven patients developed ST-segment changes on the ECG, one of whom had changes typical of Prinzmetal's angina. All abnormalities were reversed by intravenous atropine.

The importance of making a firm clinical diagnosis is emphasized in a study by Dart *et al* [4]. They demonstrate that, once a clinical diagnosis of angina has been made, it is hard to reassure the patient even when a non-cardiac cause of chest pain is identified.

The outcome of patients with chest pain and normal coronary arteries is unclear, and the study of Erikssen *et al* is therefore particularly interesting [5]. Latent coronary disease was suspected in 115 of 2014 apparently healthy middle-aged men after a positive stress test. Of the 115 men, 105 underwent coronary angiography, and 36 were found to have normal coronary arteries. A seven-year follow-up of these 36 patients revealed that three had died of sudden cardiac death, four had received a later diagnosis of cardiomyopathy, and one had developed aortic regurgitation. They had all experienced a significantly more rapid decline in physical performance and maximum heart rate than randomly selected controls. Technetium ventriculography revealed a subnormal increase in ejection fraction during exercise in 14 of 27 patients studied, but in only 4 of 26 controls. These results suggest that incipient heart disease may be present in subjects who complain of chest pain, even when coronary angiography is normal.

Even if this is the case, however, the medium term prognosis is good. Data from the CASS registry were analysed to examine the effect of a normal or near normal coronary arteriogram on seven-year survival [6]. Of 21 487 consecutive coronary arteriograms, 4051 were found to be normal or near normal and the patients had normal left ventricular function (no history of congestive heart failure, no reported segmental wall-motion abnormality, and an ejection fraction of at least 50%); 3136 arteriograms were normal and 915 showed mild disease with <50% stenosis in one or more segments. For those patients with normal arteriograms, the seven-year survival rate was found to be 96%, and for those with mild disease it was 92% ($P<0.001$). In another study, 1977 consecutive patients with normal coronary arteries or 'insignificant' disease (i.e. no major epicardial artery with 75% or greater luminal diameter narrowing) were followed up [7]. Overall cardiac survival was 99% at 5 years and 98% at 10 years. However, patients with normal coronary arteries had a myocardial infarction-free survival rate of 99% at 5 years and 98% at 10 years, compared with 97% and 90% respectively, in patients with insignificant disease. Despite this favorable outcome with regard to prognosis, patients in both groups continued to have cardiac symptoms that resulted in frequent hospitalization, medication and difficulty with work.

LEFT-VENTRICULAR FUNCTION IN ANGINA

[1] Asynchronous left ventricular wall motion early after coronary thrombosis.
Gibson D, Mehmet H, Schwarz F, Li K, Kubler W, Brompton Hosp, London, UK.
Br Heart J 1986; **55**: 4–13.

[2] Left ventricular mechanical efficiency in coronary artery disease.
Nichols AB, Pearson MH, Sciacca RR, Columbia Univ, New York, NY, USA.
J Am Coll Cardiol 1986; **7**: 270–9.

[3] Cardiac efficiency and coronary heart disease (Editorial).
Ross J, Univ California San Diego Sch Med, La Jolla, CA, USA.
J Am Coll Cardiol 1986; **7**: 280–1.

[4] Left ventricular mechanical efficiency in coronary artery disease (Editorial).
Karliner JS, VA Med Cent, San Fancisco, CA, USA.
J Am Coll Cardiol 1986; **7**: 282–3.

[5] Changes in diastolic properties of the regional myocardium during pacing-induced ischemia in human subjects.
Sasayama S, Nonogi IH, Miyazaki S *et al*, Kyoto Univ Hosp, Sakyo-ku, Kyoto, Japan.
J Am Coll Cardiol 1985; **5**: 599–606.

[6] Effect of postextrasystolic potentiation on amplitude and timing of regional left ventricular wall motion in ischaemic heart disease.
Gibson DG, Fleck E, Rudolph W, Brompton Hosp, London, UK.
Br Heart J 1983; **49**: 466–76.

[7] Atrial transport function in coronary artery disease: relation to left ventricular function.
Hamby RI, Noble WJ, Murphy DH, Hoffman I, St Francis Hosp, Roslyn, NY, USA.
J Am Coll Cardiol 1983; **1**: 1011–7.

Comment.   Conventional assessments of left ventricular function derived from single end-diastolic and end-systolic ciné-angiographic frames neglect the vast amount of information available from the intermediate frames; they also discount the timing of regional wall motion and, therefore, are liable to estimate wrongly the total amplitude of regional wall motion. The limitations of conventional assessments are demonstrated beautifully in the study by Gibson *et al* [1] of left ventriculograms carried out during evolving myocardial infarction and before attempted thrombolysis, 3.5 ±1.2 hours after the onset of chest pain in 24 patients. The analysis is derived from plots of left ventricular wall motion, digitized frame by frame for the entire cardiac cycle, for 40 points around the circumference of the right anterior oblique ventriculogram. The results are displayed as contour plots or, more graphically, as three-dimensional diagrams of motion against time for each point on the left ventricular free wall. In this group of patients, the mean values of end-diastolic volume, ejection fraction, peak ejection and filling rates, and changes in cavity shape were within two standard deviations of normal, although mean end-systolic volume was increased. The total amplitude of motion of the ischaemic region was within normal limits in all but seven patients, and the most common abnormality was of delayed inward movement during isovolumic relaxation accompanied by hypokinesia during the ejection phase, and outward motion during isovolumic contraction. As most of the inward motion occurred after closure of the aortic valve, a simple comparison of end-systolic and end-diastolic frames would have been interpreted as indicative of akinesia or hypokinesia. These findings call into question our concepts of the immediate mechanical consequences of myocardial ischemia, which must now undergo reappraisal. The results also point to a means for determining whether or not a region of myocardium is viable after a coronary arterial occlusion.

There have been few clinical studies of left ventricular pump performance as measured by mechanical efficiency because efficiency of a pumping chamber has to be measured by determining both the external work performed by the chamber and its energy expenditure. Angiographic and hemodynamic measurements will provide the necessary information of left ventricular work, and energy expenditure can be assessed by measuring myocardial oxygen consumption. These complicated measurements were undertaken by Nichols *et al* [2] on 36 patients undergoing coronary arteriography, eight of whom had normal coronary arteries and left ventricular function (two of this group had left bundle branch block and left ventricular hypertrophy), 15 of whom had coronary artery disease and exertional angina and 13 of whom had coronary heart disease with a previous myocardial infarction (>6 months) that was associated with segmental wall-motion abnormalities. They found that the patients with coronary artery disease who had *not* suffered a myocardial infarction showed normal left ventricular myocardial oxygen consumption and normal mechanical efficiency at rest. However, the patients who had had a previous myocardial infarction showed a significantly reduced efficiency because left ventricular work is diminished during normal myocardial oxygen consumption. The reduced efficiency after a myocardial infarction was found to correlate with reduced ejection phase indices of left ventricular performance. Myocardial blood flow was reduced at rest in the patients with coronary artery disease, but total left ventricular flow was not reduced because of the augmentation of left ventricular mass, which did result in there being a significant difference in myocardial oxygen consumption among the three study groups. Ross [3] and Karliner [4] discuss these results. Ross addresses the clinical significance of reduced efficiency of the left ventricular pump, and Karliner considers the implications of the findings for future work.

In a study using contrast ventriculography with simultaneous micromanometer recordings of the left ventricle in pacing-induced angina, it was found that pacing induced the expected rise in left-ventricular end-diastolic pressure, accompanied by a fall in left-ventricular ejection fraction averaging 11% [5]. In normal myocardial segments, end-diastolic length and stroke excursion were increased and the diastolic pressure moved higher up its normal curve; in an ischemic segment, the diastolic length was unchanged and stroke shortening was reduced. Postextrasystolic potentiation caused significant increases in end-diastolic volume, ejection fraction and peak ejection and filling rates in 30 patients with coronary artery disease [6]. The amplitude of normally moving segments increased, regardless of the initial amplitude. Hypokinetic segments moved normally if the initial amplitude was greater than 5 mm, and there was reduced or absent response if it was 4 mm or less. These results suggest that the response of local wall movement to postextrasystolic potentiation depends only on basal amplitude and the increased volume change in postextrasystolic beats.

In a further study, the atrial contribution to ventricular stroke volume was evaluated in normals and in 50 patients with diseased myocardium [7]. In normal subjects and in patients with coronary artery disease, the atrial contribution to stroke volume was 20 ±7% and 33 ±11%, respectively. The combination of congestive heart failure and cardiomegaly was the only clinical aspect associated with a significantly higher atrial contribution to stroke volume. No patient with an ejection fraction greater than 50% had an atrial contribution greater than 40% of the stroke volume, indicating that atrial contribution to stroke volume is inversely related to left-ventricular function. This study is clearly of particular importance to cardiac surgery, where the necessity of maintaining sinus rhythm in the postoperative phase in those with poor left-ventricular function has probably been underestimated.

AMBULATORY ST-SEGMENT MONITORING

[1]   Ambulatory electrocardiographic ST segment changes in healthy volunteers.
Quyyumi AA, Wright C, Fox K, Nat Heart Hosp, London, UK.
Br Heart J 1983; **50**: 460–4.

[2]   The role of ambulatory ST-segment monitoring in the diagnosis of coronary artery disease: comparison with exercise testing and thallium scintigraphy.
Quyyumi A, Crake T, Wright C, Mockus L, Fox K, Nat Heart Hosp, London, UK.
Eur Heart J 1987; **8**: 124–9.

[3]   Morphology of ambulatory ST segment changes in patients with varying severity of coronary artery disease. Investigations of the frequency of nocturnal ischaemia and coronary spasm.
Quyyumi AA, Mockus L, Wright C, Fox KM, Nat Heart Hosp, London, UK.
Br Heart J 1985; **53**: 186–93.

[4]   Simultaneous recording of continuous arterial pressure, heart rate, and ST segment in ambulant patients with stable angina pectoris.
Davies AB, Subramanian VB, Cashman PMM, Raftery EB, Northwick Park Hosp, Harrow, Middx, UK.
Br Heart J 1983; **50**: 85–91.

[5]   Alterations in myocardial perfusion during painless ST-segment depression in patients with angina pectoris.
Ando J, Yasuda H, Koya T *et al*, Hokkaido Univ Sch Med, Sapporo, Japan.
Jpn Heart J 1985; **26**: 179–90.

Comment.   Ambulatory ST-segment monitoring is now frequently used in patients with angina pectoris to detect the presence and significance of silent myocardial ischemia. In a study performed on 120 healthy volunteers, 28 subjects (mostly men) had episodes of ST-segment elevation, usually related to a slow nocturnal heart rate [1]. ST-segment depression was seen in 10 subjects, usually associated with a tachycardia, and was reproducible on exercise on a bicycle ergometer. Thus, an 'ischemic' ST-segment shift does occur in healthy volunteers, and this finding may be important when interpreting ST-segment changes in patients with coronary artery disease. The same group have subsequently compared sensitivity of ambulatory monitoring for the detection of coronary artery disease in 100 patients [2]. Ambulatory ST-segment depression was at least as sensitive and specific as conventional exercise testing. The technique was more likely to detect ischemia in patients with three-vessel coronary disease than in those with single-vessel disease. Thallium scintigraphy proved to be slightly more sensitive in this study, disclosing uptake defects in nine patients who did not have ambulatory ST-segment changes; most of the defects were small and localized to the inferior or posterior segments of the left ventricular wall. These findings indicate that ambulatory ST-segment analysis is as valuable as stress testing in the detection of coronary disease. The technique could be particularly useful in patients who, for one reason or another, are unable to carry out a stress test satisfactorily.

In a study of 100 consecutive patients with chest pain who had been referred for coronary arteriography, ST-segment depression was recorded in 51 of 74 patients with significant coronary artery disease [3]. ST-Segment changes were more frequent and of the greatest duration and magnitude amongst patients with more extensive coronary disease: 80% of patients with triple-vessel disease and all of those with left main stem stenoses had ST-segment changes during the monitoring period. Evidence of nocturnal ischemia occurred almost exclusively in patients with multiple-vessel disease. The ST-segment changes occurred most often in periods of maximal basal heart rate [3]. In another study, simultaneous recordings of blood pressure and heart rate with ST-segment changes invariably showed angina and ST-segment depression to be accompanied by an increase in heart rate, despite a considerable variation in blood pressure [4]. The authors concluded that heart rate changes were more important than blood pressure in determining ischemic episodes.

Using thallium-201 scintigraphy, regional myocardial perfusion was evaluated in 21 patients with angina pectoris who showed painless ST-segment depression during a treadmill exercise test [5]. Myocardial images obtained during painless ST-segment depression revealed perfusion defects in 15 patients (71%). Five patients who showed ST-segment depression with chest pain underwent the examination a second time. Perfusion defects were observed in all five patients during ST-segment depression with chest pain (three of whom showed no perfusion defects during painless ST-segment depression); moreover, ST-segment depression associated with chest pain was found to be significantly greater than that without chest pain. From these results, it would appear that the majority of episodes of painless ST-segment depression occurring during exercise are accompanied by abnormalities in regional myocardial perfusion, and that transient ST-segment depression in patients with angina pectoris might indicate less severe myocardial ischemia.

EXERCISE TESTING: CURRENT TRENDS

Review: MYRVIN H. ELLESTAD

As more and more large multicenter studies apply exercise testing to different cohorts of patients, the clinical usefulness and limitations of the procedure become more apparent. It should be emphasized that, when patients referred for coronary angiography (as in CASS [1]) are analyzed, the result will be very different (due to patient selection) from that provided by an epidemiologic approach (such as that in the Seattle Heart Watch). The goal of testing varies according to the interest of the investigators, study design, and criteria for abnormal findings. An example is exclusion of upsloping ST-segment depression as a criterion of abnormal response, despite its prognostic value to many [2]. Exclusion arbitrarily lowers sensitivity and increases specificity of ST-segment analysis. Other types of bias depend on selection of unusual cohorts of patients.

Computer Classification of ST-Segment Changes
The prognostic value of exercise testing in high-risk men has recently been reported from a cohort randomized in the Multiple Risk Factor Intervention Trial (MRFIT) [3]: the low prevalence of ST-segment depression in the immediate post-exercise period (less than 1%) appeared to preclude use of this finding for screening for any type of intervention. A recent analysis reports a computer-derived ST integral of greater than 16 V/s as abnormal. This was based on results in 734 men (12% of 5149) randomized to usual care who were able to reach the target heart rate of 85% of predicted maximum: there was an almost fourfold increase in seven-year coronary mortality in this group,

with a risk ratio of 3.8. Multivariate analysis indicated this finding to be a strong independent predictor for future death, which was in agreement with results of the Lipid Research Clinics study of 3800 asymptomatic men [4].

The use of the integral has special importance in the horizontal-versus-upsloping ST segment controversy. The original MRFIT required at least 1 mm of horizontal or downsloping ST-segment depression on visual analysis to be categorized as abnormal [5]. The vast majority of patients in the recently reported study had an upsloping ST segment, tending to confirm the findings in our 1976 study [2], in which patients with an upsloping pattern had a prevalence of coronary events similar to that among patients with a horizontal ST-segment depression.

The analysis supports the concept that exercise testing in asymptomatic men with multiple risk factors is clinically useful – as was suggested by Bruce in his study of asymptomatic subjects in the Seattle Heart Watch [6] – and indicates that computerized on-line electrocardiographic analysis during exercise testing is a useful procedure.

Exercise Scores

Routine use of computer analysis for exercise testing has led to the construction of various scores based on manipulation of multiple variables [7–9]. Recently, Hollenberg [10] has revised a scoring system (first proposed in 1980 [11]) that allows for a number of variables known to influence the reliability of ST-segment depression, including: the sum of the integrals in two leads; the duration of exercise workload; and the R-wave amplitude. He reports only one false-positive among 377 young asymptomatic men on active duty in the Armed Forces [10]. These remarkable results are of special interest to us all. Hollenberg also reports an 87% sensitivity and 92% specificity in symptomatic patients [11]. Although subsequent results might be less spectacular than these, analysis based on multiple variables seems to be useful, compared with the time-honoured 'eye-ball analysis' of the ST segment.

Stress Testing with Dipyridamole

Although stress testing with dipyridamole has been used in thallium studies for several years, especially in patients who for some reason were unable to undergo exercise, its use in combination with exercise has been reported only recently. Walker *et al* from Bristol recently reported results with 300 mg oral dipyridamole one hour prior to exercise testing in 87 patients [12]. The study excluded those with previous myocardial infarction and those with ST-segment depression or angina during the first six minutes of the Bruce Protocol. Thus, patients with only mild disease were included preferential-ly, and decreased sensitivity would be expected. However, pharmacologic coronary vasodilatation increased the sensitivity of ST-segment depression and thallium scin-tigraphy. With exercise alone, the sensitivity was 76%. After dipyridamole it was increased to 84%. When thallium scintigraphy and electrocardiographic changes were combined as end-points, sensitivity increased from 95% to 100%. In 23 normal sub-jects, the specificity was 92% and the predictive accuracy of a negative result 76%. Walker *et al* found that the best time to capitalize on the high blood level of dipyrida-mole after oral dosing was from 60 to 120 minutes after ingestion. As with those given intravenous dipyridamole, aminophylline was needed occasionally to terminate angina. Three of the 29 patients with irreversible thallium defects had angiographically normal coronary arteries. None of those selected for the study had clinical evidence of myocardial infarction. 'Irreversible' scintigraphic defects were interpreted as being indicative of slow washout associated with very severe ischemia.

Others have used oral dipyridamole (in 200-mg and 400-mg doses) prior to thallium scintigraphy [13]. Sensitivity based on scintigraphic end-points was 65% with 200-mg and 84% with 400-mg doses; specificity was 100% with both.

It appears that the use of dipyridamole in combination with exercise may increase sensitivity without reducing specificity. If this is upheld by other studies it may provide us with a significant adjunct for certain situations. False-negative exercise tests may be minimized with the use of this approach.

Time-Course Patterns in ST-Segment Analysis

The times of onset and disappearance of ST-segment depression during progressive exercise testing have been used for many years as criteria for the severity of coronary disease [14,15], as re-emphasized by Barlow of Johannesburg [16], whose diagrams of ST-segment changes according to workload warrant validation. His proposal, that ST-segment depression developing early and normalizing with increasing workload and depression occurring at near-maximal exercise and normalizing very quickly after exercise are not usually associated with significant myocardial ischemia, conforms with my personal experience. A few striking exceptions could be cited, but the need to characterize the time-course deserves emphasis. Sensitivity and specificity of specific temporal patterns in specific populations require vigorous analysis.

Exercise Echocardiography

Exercise elicits transient regional wall-motion abnormalities in zones of ischemia [17,18]. Since 1979, echocardiography has been used to identify such changes to detect coronary disease [19,20]. The technique has been plagued, however, by methodologic limitations. Wann, working in Feigenbaum's laboratory in 1979, reported an almost 30% failure to obtain satisfactory echoes [19]. Continued work and improved equipment in this laboratory and other centers [21], however, has increased enthusiasm for the approach.

Limacher et al compared the method of Wann et al with treadmill exercise and two-dimensional echo recorded in the left lateral decubitus before and immediately after exercise with nuclear gated blood pool imaging [21]. Exercise echocardiograms yielded a sensitivity of 91% (regional wall-motion abnormalities or abnormal ejection fraction in patients with coronary disease) and 95% (two- and three-vessel disease). This compares with the 71% and 80% sensitivity for equivalent arteriographic findings using radionuclide ventriculography. The sensitivity of ST-segment depression was 71% and 78% for the same lesions. Limacher et al were able to image all patients in at least the two views needed for satisfactory analysis.

In 1983 Robertson, also working in Feigenbaum's laboratory, reported 92% satisfactory echoes and detection of the involved coronary artery in most cases – as well as akinesis indicative of previous infarctions [22].

Echocardiographic images permit not only the study of regional wall motion and ejection fraction, but also measurement of the magnitude of wall thickening with systole – a parameter not measurable with other non-invasive procedures. As experience is accumulated and equipment improves, echocardiography may supplant radionuclide ventriculograms in many cases.

Heart-Rate Corrected ST-Segment Depression

'Normalization' of ST-segment depression for heart rate is well founded. Blomqvist's work in normal subjects clearly shows that some increase in ST-segment depression accompanies accelerated heart rate [23]. Simoons *et al* noted the same over 10 years ago [24]. Linden and Elamin from Leeds claimed that their variation of this approach provided 100% reliability in identifying coronary heart disease [25], and 100% reliability in differentiating patients with one-, two- and three-vessel disease. Their report was greeted with scepticism [26], but it refocused attention on the need for correcting the magnitude of ST-segment depression for heart rate.

At this point, no one has been able to reproduce fully the results from Leeds, but Kligfield *et al* from Cornell have reported that the specificity of ST-segment analysis can be improved by this approach [27]. They emphasize, as does Linden, that a more gradual increase in workload improves the utility of the measurements [27]. They were able to improve specificity over that with the standard approach of ST-segment analysis in patients with three-vessel disease and stable angina from 56% to 97%. This was achieved without reducing sensitivity.

Kligfield *et al*, like the group at Leeds, use an ST/HR slope criterion, and believe that a slope greater than 6 μV/beat/min identifies three-vessel disease. It appears from their work that the greater the ST/HR slope, the more extensive the ischemia.

Results to date in patients with stable angina must be recognized as incomplete. Kligfield and colleagues recognized many false-positives in subjects with aortic insufficiency and many false-negatives in those with myocardial infarction [28]. Results in asymptomatic subjects and in those with atypical symptoms may differ.

References

[1] Weiner DA, McCabe CH, Ryan TJ *et al*.
Assessment of the negative exercise test in 4373 patients from the coronary artery surgery study (CASS).
J Cardiac Rehab 1982; 2: 562–8.

[2] Stuart RJ, Ellestad MH.
Upsloping ST segments in exercise testing: Six year follow-up of 438 patients and correlation with 249 angiograms.
Am J Cardiol 1976; 37: 19–22.

[3] Rautaharju PM, Prineas RJ, Eifler WJ *et al*.
Prognostic value of exercise electrocardiogram in men at high risk of future coronary heart disease: Multiple Risk Factor Intervention Trial experience.
J Am Coll Cardiol 1986; 8: 1–10.

[4] Ekelund LG, Karon JM, Gordon DJ, Probstfield JL, Rubenstein C, Sheffield LT.
Prognostic value of the exercise tolerance test (ETT) for coronary heart disease (CHD) mortality in men: The Lipid Research Clinics (LRC) follow-up study. In: Abstracts of Proceedings, 24th conference on Cardiovascular Disease Epidemiology, Tampa, Florida, March 8–9, 1984. *CVD Epidemiology Newsletter* 1984; pp. 35–63.

[5] The Multiple Risk Factor Intervention Trial Group.
Exercise electrocardiogram and coronary heart disease mortality in the Multiple Risk Factor Intervention Trial.
Am J Cardiol 1985; 55: 16–23.

[6] Bruce RA, Hossack KF, DeRouen TA, Hofer V.
Enhanced risk assessment for primary coronary heart disease events by maximal exercise testing: 10 years' experience in the Seattle Heart Watch Study.
J Am Coll Cardiol 1983; **2**: 565–73.

[7] Simoons ML.
Optimal measurements for detection of coronary artery disease by exercise electrocardiography.
Comput Biomed Res 1977; **10**: 483–99.

[8] Ascoop CA, Distelbrink CA, DeLand PA.
Clinical value of quantitative analysis of ST slope during exercise.
Br Heart J 1977; **39**: 212.

[9] Kansal S, Roitman D, Bradley EL Jr, Sheffield LT.
Enhanced evaluation of treadmill tests by means of scoring based on multivariate analysis and its clinical application: A study of 608 patients.
Am J Cardiol 1983; **52**: 1155–60.

[10] Hollenberg M, Mateo GO Jr, Massie BM, Wisneski JA, Gertz EW.
Influence of R wave amplitude on exercise induced ST depression: Need for a 'gain factor' correction when interpreting stress electrocardiograms.
Am J Cardiol 1985; **56**: 13–7.

[11] Hollenberg M, Budge WR, Wisneski JA, Gertz EW.
Treadmill score quantifies electrocardiographic response to exercise and improves test accuracy and reproducibility.
Circulation 1980; **61**: 276–85.

[12] Walker PR, James MA, Wilde RPH, Wood CH, Rees JR.
Dipyridamole combined with exercise for thallium-201 myocardial imaging.
Br Heart J 1986; **55**: 321–9.

[13] Taillefer R, Lette J, Phaneuf DC, Leveille J, Lemire F, Essiambre R.
Thallium-201 myocardial imaging during pharmacologic coronary vasodilation: Comparison of oral and intravenous administration of dipyridamole.
J Am Coll Cardiol 1986; **8**: 76–83.

[14] Weiner DA, Ryan TJ, McCabe CH *et al*.
Prognostic importance of a clinical profile and exercise test in medically treated patients with coronary artery disease.
J Am Coll Cardiol 1984; **3**: 772–9.

[15] Goldschlager H, Selzer Z, Cohn K.
Treadmill stress tests as indicators of presence and severity of coronary artery disease.
Ann Intern Med 1976; **85**: 277.

[16] Barlow JB.
The 'false positive' exercise electrocardiogram: Value of time course patterns in assessment of depressed ST segments and inverted T waves.
Am Heart J 1985; **110**: 1328–36.

[17] Sharma B, Taylor SH.
Localization of left ventricular ischaemia in angina pectoris by cineangiography during exercise.
Br Heart J 1975; **37**: 963.

[18] Borer JS, Bacharach SL, Green MV, Kent KM, Epstein SE, Johnston GS.
Real-time radionuclide cineangiography in the non-invasive evaluation of global and regional left ventricular function at rest and during exercise in patients with coronary artery disease.
N Engl J Med 1977; **296**: 839.

[19] Wann LS, Faris JV, Childress RH, Dillon JC, Weyman AE, Feigenbaum H.
Exercise cross-sectional echocardiography in ischemic heart disease.
Circulation 1979; **60**: 1300–8.

[20] Mason SJ, Weiss JL, Weisfeldt ML, Garrison JB, Fortuin NJ.
Exercise echocardiography: Detection of wall motion abnormalities during ischemia.
Circulation 1979; **59**: 50–9.

[21] Limacher MC, Quinones MA, Poliner LR, Nelson JG, Winters WL Jr, Waggoner AD.
Detection of coronary artery disease with exercise two-dimensional echocardiography.
Circulation 1983; **67**: 1211–8.

[22] Robertson WS, Feigenbaum H, Armstrong WF, Dillon JC, O'Donnell J, McHenry PW.
Exercise echocardiography: A clinically practical addition in the evaluation of coronary heart disease.
J Am Coll Cardiol 1983; **2**: 1085–91.

[23] Blomqvist CG.
Heart disease and dynamic exercise testing.
In: Willerson JT, Sanders CA, eds. *Clinical Cardiology*. New York: Grune & Stratton, 1977; pp. 213–7.

[24] Simoons ML, Boom HBK, Swallenberg E.
Online processing of orthogonal exercise ECGs.
Comput Biomed Res 1975; **8**: 105.

[25] Elamin MS, Boyle R, Kardash MM *et al*.
Accurate detection of coronary heart disease by new exercise test.
Br Heart J 1982; **48**: 311–20.

[26] Fox KM.
Exercise heart rate/ST segment relation. Perfect predictor of coronary disease?
Br Heart J 1982; **48**: 309–10.

[27] Kligfield P, Okin PM, Ameisen O, Wallis J, Borer JS.
Correlation of the exercise ST/HR slope with anatomic and radionuclide cineangiographic findings in stable angina pectoris.
Am J Cardiol 1985; **56**: 418–21.

[28] Ameisen O, Okin PM, Devereux RB *et al*.
Predictive value and limitations of the ST/HR slope.
Br Heart J 1985; **53**: 547–51.

THE EFFECT OF CIGARETTES AND COFFEE ON ANGINA

[1] Acute coronary hemodynamic response to cigarette smoking in patients with coronary artery disease.
Klein LW, Ambrose J, Pichard A, Holt J, Gorlin R, Teichholz LE, Mount Sinai Med Cent, New York, NY, USA.
J Am Coll Cardiol 1984; **3**: 879–86.

[2] Cigarette smoking and the treatment of angina with propranolol, atenolol, and nifedipine.
Deanfield J, Wright C, Krikler S, Ribeiro P, Fox K, Nat Heart Hosp, London, UK.
N Engl J Med 1984; **310**: 951–4.

[3] Effect of coffee on exercise-induced angina pectoris due to coronary artery disease in habitual coffee drinkers.
Piters KM, Colombo A, Olson HG, Butman SM, Long Beach VA Med Cent, Long Beach, CA, USA.
Am J Cardiol 1985; **55**: 277–80.

Comment. Any workers who remain doubtful of the harm done by smoking to the coronary circulation or hopeful that drugs may prevent the ill-effects should be disabused by the following two studies. Klein *et al* studied the marked increase in coronary sinus blood flow and decrease in coronary resistance which occurred in response to smoking in six patients without angiographically detectable coronary artery disease, and contrasted it with the effects of cigarette smoking in two groups of patients with significant coronary artery disease [1]. Although there was an overall increase in coronary sinus blood flow in the coronary artery disease group, it fell during cigarette smoking, suggesting that smoking has adverse effects by increasing coronary artery tone at the site of stenosis and limiting coronary blood flow in proportion to the size of the affected vascular bed. The study of Deanfield *et al* provides a clinical corollary to the work of Klein *et al*. Deanfield *et al* examined the efficacy of anginal drugs (nifedipine, atenolol and propranolol) in patients before and after they stopped smoking [2]. All treatments were more effective when the patients stopped smoking, the change being most pronounced with nifedipine.

In a study of 17 men with coronary artery disease, it was found that the acute ingestion of one to two cups of caffeinated coffee did not have any effect on exercise-induced angina pectoris [3].

SILENT ISCHEMIA

Review: THOMAS VON ARNIM

Introduction

Silent myocardial ischemia, i.e. the demonstration of objective signs of ischemia that are not accompanied by anginal pain, is currently a topic of great interest although it is by no means a recently detected phenomenon. In the early 1970s, Lichtlen was able to demonstrate the occurrence of electrocardiographic and dynamic changes during exercise well before the occurrence of angina [1]; Guazzi and co-workers and Maseri and his colleagues in their studies of patients with variant angina revealed the occurrence of episodes of transient ischemia that were completely silent [2–4]. A high incidence of coronary artery lesions was found at autopsy in soldiers killed in the Korean War [6] and in several studies significant coronary artery lesions have been found in 2.5–9% of asymptomatic middle-aged men who have undergone angiography and exercise testing [7–10]. Erickssen performed careful follow-up examinations on these asymptomatic subjects who had demonstrable disease and found that manifestations of coronary heart disease first occurred 3–4 years after the initial study. For some of the subjects in Erikssen's study, death or myocardial infarction were the first manifestations of coronary heart disease that were recognised [7]. These observations are in accordance with the figure of 20% for the prevalence of unrecognised myocardial infarction as determined in the Framingham Study [11] and with the autopsy findings of 25–50% previously unrecognised coronary artery disease in victims of sudden death [12]. Thus, coronary artery disease can begin early in life and be silent; it may remain silent until irreversible manifestations, such as death or myocardial infarction, occur.

Pathophysiology

Specific cardiac noci-ceptors do not exist, and as yet the link between transient myocardial ischemia and pain remains elusive [13]. Some patients with silent myocardial ischemia seem to have increased thresholds for pain perception [14,15]; in some patients, the occurrence of angina is connected with special psychological traits [12,14]. Opioid peptides may be involved in the genesis of anginal pain [16]; peptidergic nerves are abundant in the heart [17]. Conflicting results have been obtained with respect to the influence of descending pain inhibition, for instance by beta-endorphins, some authors [18,20] were able to unmask angina with naloxone [14], whereas others could not [21]. A recent paper by Sylven draws attention to adenosine as a possible mediator of anginal pain [22]; angina pectoris-like pain was consistently provoked by the intravenous injection of adenosine in volunteers. This mechanism of action in patients with silent myocardial ischemia is plausible because adenosine is released in increased amounts during ischemia.

Detection of silent myocardial ischaemia

All of the methods used to demonstrate objective signs of ischemia can be used to demonstrate silent myocardial ischemia. Electrocardiographic exercise testing is the most widely used and most standardized method for the detection of ischemia. Patients with silent ischemia tend to have greater ST-segment depression [14], because they are not prevented from continuing exercise by the occurrence of pain.

Recently, the concept of silent ischemia has focussed attention on the use of ambulatory electrocardiography with ST-segment analysis [23] to monitor patients' normal daily activities; it has been found that ischemic episodes can occur quite freqently, they are similar irrespective of whether they are accompanied by pain, and sometimes they may be accompanied by arrhythmias [24]. Radionuclide studies, using rubidium-82, and emission computer tomography have been used to validate the results obtained by the electrocardiographic monitoring of ischemic episodes [23]. However, thallium exercise scintigraphy is frequently used as another method of verifying the presence of ischemia in asymptomatic patients before invasive diagnostic procedures are used [25,26]. Silent ischemia can be demonstrated frequently in patients undergoing PTCA, especially when extended electrocardiographic monitoring is used [27]. Modern software and solid state memories may extend the possibilities of electrocardiographic monitoring considerably [28].

When investigating the occurrence of ischemia in either symptomatic or asymptomatic subjects, the first line of approach remains the exercise test. When testing for silent ischemia, two groups of patients must be identified: those who are totally asymptomatic and those in whom coronary artery disease is symptomatic, i.e. those who are suffering from or who have suffered from angina or myocardial infarction. The low prevalence of coronary artery disease in totally asymptomatic subjects in conjunction with the low sensitivity and specificity of the exercise test give a high number of false-positive results. Consequently, exercise testing is not cost-effective in this group of patients. In order to avoid prohibitive costs, only subjects with a high number of known coronary risk factors should be tested, and also serial testing with an independent method like thallium scintigraphy should be performed [29]. In this group of subjects, ambulatory electrocardiographic monitoring is not useful for determining the presence of coronary heart disease [30], but it is useful in determining the activity of the disease, i.e. the occurrence of ischemia over 24 hours.

Prognosis

A disease process that does not cause pain is of importance only if it has implications for the patient's prognosis. The MRFIT and Lipid Research Clinics Study have shown that a positive exercise test result in an asymptomatic subject is predictive of the occurrence of future coronary events, especially cardiac death [31,32]: in both trials, a positive exercise test on entry was by far the strongest age-independent predictor of future cardiovascular death. In studies involving much smaller numbers of patients with unstable angina pectoris undergoing Holter monitoring, it has been shown that transient episodes of silent ischemia do influence the patients' prognoses [33,34]. However, studies of the prognostic implications of episodes of silent ischaemia involving larger numbers of patients with stable angina pectoris have yet to be performed, as are randomized trials of the treatment of such episodes.

Management

As stated above, there are as yet no data available from randomised trials of the treatment of patients with silent ischemia. However, as most patients have both silent and symptomatic episodes of ischemia, these episodes are usually treated together. All the evidence suggests that symptomatic and silent episodes of ischemia respond to treatment in a similar way. The results of several studies have shown that episodes of silent ischemia that occur throughout the day tend to occur at lower heart rates than exercise-induced ischemia does [35,36]. These results could be taken to suggest that a reduced coronary blood supply is the prevailing mechanism in the pathogenesis of silent ischemia which might be the result of inappropriate vasoconstriction. If this hypothesis is correct, then treatment with calcium antagonists should be the most effective, but beta-blockers and nitrates have also been shown to be effective in reducing the number of ischemic episodes that can be detected on Holter monitoring [37]. Drug trials in which the aim is to reduce the number of ischemic episodes as detected by Holter monitoring are subject to considerable difficulties because of the wide spontaneous variability of such episodes not only throughout the day, but also from day to day and over weeks and months. Careful measures have to be taken in the design of such studies and in the statistical evaluation of the results in order to separate the effects of treatment from spontaneous variability [38].

Conclusions

In view of the large number of patients for whom acute myocardial infarction and sudden death may be the first manifestation of coronary heart disease, it is important to extend our view of ischemic heart disease to all those manifestations that can be detected by any practicable means. However, it must be borne in mind that because of the low prevalence of active disease searching for silent ischemia is appropriate only in totally asymptomatic subjects who are at increased risk. As yet, there are no controlled randomized trials of the prophylactic treatment of such patients.

References

[1] Lichtlen P.
The hemodynamics of clinical ischemic heart disease.
Ann Clin Res 1971; 3: 333–43.

[2] Guazzi M, Fiorenti C, Polese A, Magrini F.
Continuous electrocardiographic recordings in Prinzmetal's variant angina pectoris. A report of four cases.
Br Heart J 1970, 32: 611–6.

[3] Guazzi M, Polese A, Fiorentini C.
Left ventricular performance and related haemodynamic changes in Prinzmetal's variant angina pectoris.
Br Heart J 1971; 33: 84–94.

[4] Maseri A, Mimmo R, Chierchia S, Marchesi C, Pesola A, L'Abbate A.
Coronary artery spasm as a cause of acute myocardial ischaemia in man.
Chest 1975; 5: 625–33.

[5] Maseri A.
Role of coronary artery spasm in symptomatic and silent myocardial ischemia.
J Am Coll Cardiol 1987; 2: 249–62.

[6] Enos WF, Holmes RH, Beyer J.
Coronary disease among United States soldiers killed in action in Korea. Preliminary report.
JAMA 1986; 256: 2859–62.

[7] Erikssen J, Thaulow E.
Follow-up of patients with asymptomatic myocardial ischemia. In: Rutishauser W, Roskamm H (eds). Silent Myocardial Ischemia. Berlin, Heidelberg, New York, Tokyo: Springer Verlag, 1984, pp 195–257.

[8] Froelicher VF, Thompson AJ, Longo MR, Triebwasser JH, Lancaster MC.
Value of exercise testing for screening asymptomatic men for latent coronary artery disease.
Prog Cardiovasc Dis 1976; 16: 265.

[9] Langou RA, Huang EK, Kelley MJ, Cohen LS.
Predictive accuracy of coronary artery calcification and abnormal exercise test for coronary artery disease in asymptomatic men.
Circulation 1980; 62: 1196–203.

[10] Erickssen J, Cohn PF, Thaulow E, Mowinckel P.
Silent myocardial ischemia in middle aged men: Long term clinical course. In: von Arnim Th, Maseri A (eds) *Silent Ischemia, Current Concepts and Management*. Darmstadt: Steinkopff Verlag; New York: Springer Verlag, 1987, pp 45–51.

[11] Kannel WB, Abbott RD.
Incidence and prognosis of unrecognized myocardial infarction: An update on the Framingham Study.
N Engl J Med 1984; **311**: 1144–7.

[12] Kuller LH.
Sudden death – definition and epidemiologic considerations.
Prog Cardiovasc Dis 1980; **23**: 1.

[13] Malliani A.
Pathophysiology of ischemic cardiac pain. In: von Arnim Th, Maseri A (eds) *Silent Ischemia, Current Concepts and Management*. Darmstadt: Steinkopff Verlag; New York: Springer Verlag, 1987, pp 19–24.

[14] Droste C, Roskamm H.
Experimental approach to painful and painless ischemia. In: von Arnim Th, Maseri A (eds) *Silent ischemia, Current concepts and management*. Darmstadt: Steinkopff Verlag; New York: Springer Verlag, 1987, pp 31–42.

[15] Glazier JJ, Chierchia S, Brown MJ, Maseri A.
Importance of generalized defective perception of painful stimuli as a cause of silent myocardial ischemia in chronic stable angina pectoris.
Am J Cardiol 1986; **58**: 667–72.

[16] Millan MJ.
Central mechanisms of pain control: a survey. In: von Arnim Th, Maseri A (eds) *Silent Ischemia, Current Concepts and Management*. Darmstadt: Steinkopff Verlag; New York: Springer Verlag, 1987, pp 1–6.

[17] Weihe E.
Peripheral innervation of the heart. In: von Arnim Th, Maseri A (eds) *Silent Ischemia, Current Concepts and Management*. Darmstadt: Steinkopff Verlag; New York: Springer Verlag, 1987, pp 7–18.

[18] Sheps DS, Adams KF, Hinderliter A, Price C, Bissette J, Orlando G, Margolis B, Koch G.
Endorphins are related to pain perception in coronary artery disease.
Am J Cardiol 1987; **59**: 523–7.

[19] Weidinger F, Hammerle A, Sochor H, Smetana R, Frass M, Glogar D.
Role of beta-endorphins in silent myocardial ischemia.
Am J Cardiol 1987; **58**: 428–30.

[20] Heller GV, Garber CE, Conolly MJ, Allen-Rowlands CF, Siconolfi SF, Gann DS, Carleton RA.
Plasma beta-endorphin levels in silent myocardial ischemia induced by exercise.
Am J Cardiol 1987; **59**: 735–9.

[21] Ellestad MH, Kuan P.
Naloxone and asymptomatic ischemia: Failure to induce angina during exercise testing.
Am J Cardiol 1984; **54**: 982–4.

[22] Sylven C, Beermann B, Jonzon B, Brandt R.
Angina pectoris-like pain provoked by intravenous adenosine in healthy volunteers.
Br Med J 1986; **293**: 227–93.

[23] Deanfield JF, Maseri A, Selwyn P, Ribeiro P, Chierchia S, Krikler S, Morgan M.
Myocardial ischemia during daily life in patients with stable angina: its relation to symptoms and heart rate changes.
Lancet 1983; **ii**: 753–8.

[24] von Arnim Th, Gerbig HW, Erath A.
Arrhythmien im Zusammenhang mit transienten St-Hebungungen bei Prinzmetal-Angina: Auslosung durch Okklusion und reperfusion.
Z Kardiol 1985; **74**: 585–9.

[25] Berman DS, Rozanski A, Knoebel SB.
The detection of silent ischemia: cautions and precautions.
Circulation 1987; **75**: 101–5.

[26] Rozanski A, Berman D.
The frequency, pathophysiology and prognosis in exercise-induced silent ischemia. In: von Arnim Th, Maseri A (eds) *Silent Ischemia, Current Concepts and Management*. Darmstadt: Steinkopff Verlag; Springer Verlag, New York: 1987, pp 96–106.

[27] von Arnim Th, Stäblein A, Höfling B.
Detection of ischemia during PTCA with extended electrocardiographic monitoring. In: Hofling B (ed) *Current Problems in PTCA*. Darmstadt: Steinkopff Verlag; New York: Spinger Verlag, 1985, pp 27–34.

[28] Krucoff MW, Pope JE, Bottner RK, Adams IM, Wagner GS, Kent KM.
Decidated ST-segment monitoring in the CCU after successful coronary angioplasty: incidence and prognosis of silent and symptomatic ischemia. In: von Arnim Th, Maseri A (eds) *Silent Ischemia, Current Concepts and Management*. Darmstadt: Steinkopff Verlag; New York: Springer Verlag, 1987, pp 140–6.

[29] Berman DS, Rozanski A, Knoebel SB.
The detection of silent ischemia: cautions and precautions.
Circulation 1987; **75**: 101–5.

[30] Crea F, Kaski JC, Fragasso G, Hackett D, Stanbridge R, Taylor KM, Maseri A.
Usefulness of Holter monitoring to improve the sensitivity of exercise testing in determining the degree of myocardial revascularization after coronary artery bypass grafting for stable angina pectoris.
Am J Cardiol 1987; **60**: 40–3.

[31] Multiple Risk Factor Intervention Trial Research Group.
Exercise electrocardiogram and coronary heart disease mortality in the Multiple Risk Factor Intervention Trial.
Am J Cardiol 1985; **55**: 16–24.

[32] Gordon DJ, Ekelund LG, Karon JM, Probstfield JL, Rubenstein C, Sheffield LT, Weissfeldt L.
Predictive value of the exercise tolerance test for mortality in North American men: the Lipid Research Clinics Mortality Follow-up Study.
Circulation 1986; **2**: 252–61.

[33] Gottlieb SO, Weissfeldt ML, Ouyang P, Melliths ED, Gerstenblith G.
Silent ischemia as a marker for early unfavorable outcomes in patients with unstable angina.
N Engl J Med 1986; **314**: 1214–9.

[34] von Arnim Th, Gerbig HW, Krawietz W, Höfling B.
Prognostic implications of transient spontaneous – predominantly silent – ischemia in patients with stable and unstable angina.
Circulation 1986; **74**(Suppl II): 359.

[35] Carboni GP, Lahiri A, Cashman PM, Raftery EB.
Ambulatory heart rate and ST-segment depression during painful and silent myocardial ischemia in chronic stable angina pectoris.
Am J Cardiol 1987; **59**: 1029–34.

[36] Campbell S, Barra J, Rocco MB, Nabel EG, Mead-Walters K, Rebecca GS, Selwyn AP.
Features of the exercise test that reflect the activity of ischemic heart disease out of hospital.
Circulation 1980; **74**: 72–80.

[37] Tzivoni D, Keren A, Gavish A, Benhorn J, Stern S.
Guiding anti-ischemic therapy by Holter monitoring. In: von Arnim Th, Maseri A (eds) *Silent Ischemia, Current Concepts and Management*. Darmstadt: Steinkopff Verlag; New York: Springer Verlag 1987, pp 177–83.

[38] Deanfield JE, Spiegelhalter D.
Variability of myocardial ischemia in chronic stable angina. In: von Arnim Th, Maseri A (eds) *Silent Ischemia, Current Concepts and Management*. Darmstadt: Steinkopff Verlag; New York: Springer Verlag, 1987, pp 203–7.

THERAPY

BETA-BLOCKERS AND CALCIUM ANTAGONISTS IN ANGINA

[1] A double blind placebo controlled comparison of verapamil, atenolol, and their combination in patients with chronic stable angina pectoris.
Findlay IN, MacLeod K, Gillen G, Elliott AT, Aitchison T, Dargie HJ, Western Infirm, Glasgow, UK.
Br Heart J 1987; **57**: 336–43.

[2] Comparison of verapamil and propranolol therapy for angina pectoris at rest: a randomized, multiple-crossover, controlled trial in the coronary care unit.
Parodi O, Simonetti I, Michelassi C *et al*, Univ Pisa, Pisa, Italy.
Am J Cardiol 1986; **57**: 899–906.

[3] Effect of the addition of propranolol to therapy with nifedipine for unstable angina pectoris: a randomized, double-blind, placebo-controlled trial.
Gottlieb SO, Weisfeldt ML, Ouyang P *et al*, Johns Hopkins Med Insts, Baltimore, MD, USA.
Circulation 1986; **73**: 331–7.

[4] Effects of combined alpha and beta adrenoceptor blockade in patients with angina pectoris. A double blind study comparing labetalol with placebo.
Quyyumi AA, Wright C, Mockus L, Shackell M, Sutton GC, Fox KM, Nat Heart Hosp, London, UK.
Br Heart J 1985; **53**: 47–52.

[5] Oral labetalol in the management of stable angina pectoris in normotensive patients.
Upward JW, Akhras F, Jackson G, King's Coll Hosp, London, UK.
Br Heart J 1985; **53**: 53–7.

[6] Improvement in angina pectoris with alpha adrenoceptor blockade.
Collins P, Sheridan D, Welsh Nat Sch Med, Cardiff, UK.
Br Heart J 1985; **53**: 488–92.

[7] Relation of antianginal efficacy of nifedipine to degree of coronary arterial narrowing and to presence of coronary collateral vessels.
Schulz W, Jost S, Kober G, Kaltenbach M, Univ Frankfurt/Main, Frankfurt/Main, GFR.
Am J Cardiol 1985; **55**: 26–32.

[8] The acute effects of nifedipine on red cell deformability in angina pectoris.
Waller DG, Nicholson HP, Roath S, Southampton Gen Hosp, Southampton, UK.
Br J Clin Pharmacol 1984; **17**: 133–8.

[9] Salutary effect of nifedipine in pacing-induced angina: relation to afterload reduction.
Tiefenbrunn AJ, Sobel BE, Ludbrook PA, Washington Univ Sch Med, St Louis, MO, USA.
Cathet Cardiovasc Diagn 1983; **9**: 583–9.

[10] Acute nifedipine withdrawal: consequences of preoperative and late cessation of therapy in patients with prior unstable angina.
Gottlieb SO, Ouyang P, Achuff SC *et al*, Johns Hopkins Hosp, Baltimore, MD, USA.
J Am Coll Cardiol 1984; **4**: 382–8.

[11] Evaluation of efficacy of a new calcium-antagonist drug, diltiazem, in patients with effort angina. Therapeutical comparison with nifedipine (In Italian).
Di Pasquale G, Lusa AM, Manini GL, Dominici P, Pinelli G, Ospedale Bellaria, Bologna, Italy.
G Ital Cardiol 1983; **14**: 32–9.

[12] Beneficial effects of diltiazem in coronary artery disease.
Kenny J, Daly K, Bergman G, Kerkez S, Jewitt DE, King's Coll Hosp, London, UK.
Br Heart J 1984; **52**: 53–6.

[13] Comparative effects of diltiazem, propranolol, and placebo on exercise performance using radionuclide ventriculography in patients with symptomatic coronary artery disease: results of a double-blind, randomized, crossover study.
Anderson JL, Wagner JM, Datz FL, Christian PE, Bray BE, Taylor AT, Univ Utah Coll Med, Salt Lake City, UT, USA.
Am Heart J 1984; **107**: 698–706.

[14] Pharmacodynamic aspects of intravenous diltiazem administration.
Joyal M, Pieper J, Cremer K, Feldman RL, Pepine CJ, Univ Florida, Gainesville, FL, USA.
Am Heart J 1986; **111**: 54–61.

[15] Hemodynamic effects of intravenous diltiazem in patients treated chronically with propranolol.
Rocha P, Baron B, Delestrain A, Pathe M, Cazor J-L, Kahn J-C, Cent Hosp Intercommunal, Poissy, France.
Am Heart J 1986; **111**: 62–8.

[16] Efficacy and safety of nicardipine for chronic, stable angina pectoris: a multicenter randomized trial.

Scheidt S, LeWinter MM, Hermanovich J, Venkataraman K, Freedman D, New York Hosp-
Cornell Med Cent, New York, NY, USA.

Am J Cardiol 1986; **58**: 715–21.

Comment.   Although beta-blockers are acknowledged as the mainstay of pharmacological treatment for patients with effort-induced angina pectoris, they can cause side-
effects, and in some patients they are only partially effective and may be contraindicated. Calcium antagonists have recently been shown to be of benefit in the treatment
of effort-induced angina, and although the combination of a beta-blocker and a calcium
antagonist may be complementary it may produce detrimental drug interactions. The
combination of nifedipine and a beta-blocker is considered safe in patients with normal
left ventricular function, but verapamil in combination with a beta-blocker should be
administered with caution because of possible mutual potentiation of effects on cardiac
conduction and contractility. In a placebo-controlled study, Findlay *et al* investigated
the effect and efficacy of three weeks' treatment with verapamil (120 mg three times a
day) and atenolol (100 mg once daily) singly and in combination on the cardiac function
of 15 patients with angina pectoris [1]. Four patients withdrew from the study while
receiving combination therapy. Only combination therapy was found to reduce significantly the episodes of angina and the consumption of glyceryl trinitrate. Evidence of
ischemia during exercise was seen in 7 of the patients on verapamil, in 10 on atenolol but
in only 4 on the combination therapy. ST-Segment depression at peak exercise was
reduced by all of the treatments, but the reduction was greatest with combination
therapy. Mean left ventricular ejection fraction was significantly reduced to 53% on
combination therapy; it remained unchanged when either agent was used alone. The
authors conclude that verapamil is an effective alternative to atenolol; the combination
of these two agents, however, was found to be the most effective treatment regimen,
although patients did experience considerable morbidity whilst taking it.

The theoretical increase in coronary tone produced by beta-blockers makes their
use in unstable angina controversial. In a study of ten patients admitted to the coronary
care unit because of frequent attacks of angina at rest, the effects of oral verapamil (400
mg/day), oral propranolol (300 mg/day) and placebo were compared in a randomized,
double-blind, multiple crossover manner [2]. There were eight consecutive treatment
periods of 48 hours; ECG monitoring and tape recording were performed throughout
the 16 days of the trial. When compared with the placebo period, it was found that the
average number of diagnostic ST-segment shifts per 24 hours was significantly reduced
during verapamil treatment but not with propranolol ($P<0.01$). Similar statistically
significant reductions in the numbers of angina attacks and nitroglycerin tablets consumed were also observed. Moreover, verapamil was found to reduce ischemic episodes in both active phases in all of the patients; propranolol was not found to be
effective in three patients who had severe limitation of exercise tolerance, but it did not
consistently increase the number or duration of episodes in three of the patients who
had variant angina.

The opposite conclusion was reached by Gottlieb et al in a double-blind randomized placebo-controlled trial of propranolol in patients with unstable angina [3].
Thirty-nine patients were assigned to placebo and 42 to propranolol (at least 160 mg

daily). All patients were also treated with nifedipine (80 mg daily) and long-acting nitrates. There was found to be no difference in the incidence of cardiac death, myocardial infarction and need for coronary artery bypass grafting or angioplasty between the two groups. However, the propranolol-treated group did have a lower cumulative probability of experiencing recurrent angina at rest than the placebo group. Moreover, during the first four days of the trial, the mean number of clinical episodes of angina, the duration of angina and the number of nitroglycerin tablets required were fewer in the propranolol-treated group. Continuous ECG monitoring for ischemic ST-segment changes revealed there to be fewer daily ischemic episodes and a shorter duration of ischemia in the propranolol-treated patients. Thus, in this study the administration of propranolol to patients with unstable angina, in the presence of nitrates and nifedipine, was not detrimental, and it reduced the frequency and duration of symptomatic and silent episodes of ischemia.

It is logical to anticipate that labetalol, which combines alpha- and beta-adrenergic properties, would be effective in the medical treatment of angina. However, in early studies, effort-induced hypotension limited its use. Quyyumi et al investigated the effects of labetalol in 10 patients with chronic stable angina, and identified a dose-related benefit [4]. Upward et al, in a single-blind dose-ranging study, also found a dose-related benefit with active treatment [5]. Indoramin, a selective alpha$_1$ antagonist, was found to prolong exercise duration and to increase oxygen consumption during exercise in patients with angina pectoris who were receiving beta-blockers and nitrates [6]. The increased exercise capacity was associated with a reduction in ST-segment depression during exercise. These studies seem to suggest that alpha$_1$ blockade does confer additional benefit.

Calcium antagonists have now become routine therapy in patients with stable angina pectoris. Doubt still exists as to the major site of action of the drugs. In a study of 36 patients with chronic stable angina, classified according to their coronary arteriographic findings, nifedipine failed to relieve myocardial ischemia when occluded but collateralized coronary arteries were present; a significant benefit in contrast was seen where stenosed coronary arteries were present [7]. These findings suggest that the antianginal effects of nifedipine may be influenced by the underlying pathomorphologic characteristics. In a double-blind study of eight patients, a single sublingual dose of nifedipine increased red-cell deformity when compared with placebo [8]. The authors suggest the possibility that nifedipine's effect on red-cell deformity contributes to the drug's beneficial effect in myocardial ischemia. Finally, in a study of pacing-induced angina, the mean paced heart rate at onset of angina was increased after nifedipine, and there was a decrease in systolic blood pressure [9]. Consequently, the double product, heart rate × systolic blood pressure, did not change significantly at onset of chest pain. Thus, nifedipine was considered to decrease myocardial oxygen demand at a given heart rate by reducing left-ventricular afterload, but not to increase the rate/pressure product for the development of ischemic pain.

There is convincing evidence that patients experience 'rebound' phenomena after the sudden withdrawal of a drug, such as seen in patients with angina being treated with beta-blockers. However, there is little evidence whether or not such an effect occurs following the withdrawal of a calcium antagonist. As part of a randomized controlled trial of calcium antagonist treatment of rest angina, 81 patients were withdrawn suddenly from treatment [10]. No evidence of an early adverse effect of acute nifedipine withdrawal was found, although there was a worsening of symptoms in four patients who continued to experience rest angina. This study shows that, in patients who have had rest angina and whose symptoms have been controlled by the addition of nifedipine to conventional therapy, it is safe to withdraw the calcium antagonist.

Newer calcium antagonists are now available in addition to nifedipine and verapamil; the most recent that has become available for clinical use is diltiazem. In a study of 12 patients with stable effort angina, it was found that nifedipine and diltiazem had similar therapeutic efficacy, although side-effects (headaches, rashes and peripheral edema) were more common with nifedipine [11]. A further study in 11 patients with stable angina studied at rest and during rapid atrial pacing showed improved pacing time to angina and significant improvement of myocardial lactate extraction during pacing after the use of intravenous diltiazem [12]. This study confirms the antianginal effects of diltiazem, but suggests that it may exert its beneficial effect not only by reducing afterload, but also by a direct metabolic effect on the myocardium. When diltiazem, propranolol and placebo were compared using a double-blind randomized cross-over protocol with radionuclide ventriculography [13], diltiazem tended to increase ejection fraction at both submaximal and maximal exercise, also in those patients with decreased ventricular function. Propranolol had no effect on exercise ejection fraction at any stage, even when patients with an ejection fraction of less than 50% were excluded. Indeed, diltiazem was found to increase exercise performance to a greater extent than either placebo or propranolol, and this effect was most marked in patients with decreased left-ventricular function.

Joyal et al [14] investigated the serum concentration, the magnitude and time-course of systemic and coronary hemodynamic changes and ECG responses to intravenous diltiazem (250 µg/kg iv bolus and 1.4 µg/kg/minute infusion) in 14 patients with chronic stable angina pectoris. The minimum effective serum concentration of diltiazem was found to be 96 ng/ml. The drug was found to reduce blood pressure, systemic resistance and coronary resistance promptly, with only a small and transient increase in heart rate at three minutes (which was found to have resolved by eight minutes). The drug was also well tolerated by the patients. Rocha et al [15] investigated the hemodynamic effects of intravenous diltiazem (0.25 mg/kg) in 16 patients with chronic coronary heart disease but no clinical signs of heart failure. Eight of these patients were receiving long-term oral propranolol (120–240 mg daily). A decrease in systemic vascular resistance and an increase in cardiac index were found to occur at five minutes in the patients *not* receiving propranolol. However, in the propranolol-treated group, despite a slight decrease in peak positive first derivative of left ventricular pressure, an increase in cardiac index and systolic index and a decrease in systemic vascular resistance and mean blood pressure occurred at five minutes; at 15 minutes, systemic vascular resistance remained decreased and cardiac index and systolic index remained increased. The results of this study confirm that the administration of intravenous diltiazem does not have deleterious effects in patients with chronic coronary heart disease receiving beta-blockers. Moreover, in this group of patients, diltiazem appeared to offset the deleterious effects of beta-blockers by increasing peripheral vascular resistance and decreasing cardiac output.

Nicardipine, another new calcium antagonist, is one of the dihydropyridine derivatives. In a randomized, double-blind, placebo-controlled trial conducted at four different centres, nicardipine (30 or 40 mg three times daily) was administered to 63 patients with chronic stable angina pectoris [16]. It was found to increase resting heart rate slightly. During treadmill exercise testing, nicardipine increased exercise time by 9%, time to 1 mm of ST-segment depression by 16% and oxygen consumption at peak exercise by 13% over values obtained with placebo. Mean anginal frequency and weekly sublingual nitroglycerin consumption declined, although these differences were not significant. Nicardipine caused more cardiovascular side-effects than placebo: three patients experienced more angina, which was thought to be related to the drug. Side-effects resulting from vasodilatation were also more frequent with the administration of nicardipine, although only one patient withdrew from treatment because of them. These results show nicardipine to be effective in patients with chronic stable angina pectoris, and in general the drug was well tolerated.

NITRATES AND NITRATE TOLERANCE IN ANGINA PECTORIS

Review: JOHN O. PARKER

The organic nitrates comprise the agents most commonly used in the management of patients with angina pectoris secondary to coronary artery disease. The first report of nitroglycerin being employed in angina pectoris was by William Murrell in 1879 [1]. While nitrates are acknowledged to be extremely effective in the treatment of episodes of angina pectoris, there has been concern regarding their efficacy in the prophylaxis of angina pectoris. Originally, this concern arose from the demonstration of extensive first-pass hepatic metabolism [2]: it was felt that after oral ingestion systemic availability was so low that no significant antianginal effects would be present. Subsequent studies following oral dosing with isosorbide dinitrate, however, have documented that despite extensive first-pass metabolism approximately 20% enters the systemic circulation which, with the oral doses employed, produces significant hemodynamic and antianginal effects [3,4].

The next issue encountered with the use of nitrates in angina pectoris was the potential development of nitrate tolerance. It was known from studies in animals that the hemodynamic effect of the nitrates was rapidly attenuated during sustained therapy [5–7]. Even the marked hypotensive effect of intravenous nitroglycerin could be rapidly attenuated: within very short periods of time it was possible to give progressively larger doses of intravenous nitroglycerin without further effects on systemic blood pressure. Regarding humans, it was recognized that the side-effects of nitrate exposure on workers in the munitions industry were transient [8]. On initial exposure in the work environment, it was common for workers to develop severe headaches secondary to the vasodilatory effects of the nitrates. The headaches cleared within a few days of continued exposure - a demonstration of tolerance. It was also discovered that tolerance to the headaches was rapidly lost out of the work environment: after a weekend, workers commonly developed intense headache on return to the work environment. This 'Monday headache' was clearly a manifestation of loss of nitrate tolerance during the short period of removal from exposure.

The development of tolerance was not considered to be a clinically relevant problem, however, until recent studies assessing the efficacy of various nitrate preparations used objective measurements of hemodynamic alterations and exercise performance! [3,4]. A study employing multiple single doses of isosorbide dinitrate (from 15 mg to 120 mg) demonstrated a dose-related decrease in resting systolic blood pressure and an increase in heart rate – changes that persisted throughout an eight-hour observation period [3]. Treadmill testing showed that with each dose of isosorbide dinitrate there was a significant increase in time to the end-point of angina, and that this improvement persisted throughout the eight-hour observation period [3]. In the sustained phase of this investigation, patients received each of the doses four times daily for one week, and underwent treadmill exercise before and after the last oral dose of each medication [4]; during this sustained phase, the hypotensive response to isosorbide dinitrate was diminished. Rather than lowering systemic blood pressure and raising heart rate for a period of eight hours, the effects during sustained therapy were less marked, and persisted for only four hours. Of greater importance, however, was the fact that walking time was increased at one and two hours after the morning dose but that no improvement was apparent subsequently. Not only was the improvement in walking time diminished in duration, but the magnitude of improvement in treadmill walking time at one and two hours was significantly less than that seen during the acute phase of this investigation. These alterations in the hemodynamic and antianginal effects of oral isosorbide dinitrate during the short period of sustained four-times-daily therapy were not related to altered bioavailability or metabolism of isosorbide dinitrate, because the plasma concentrations of isosorbide dinitrate and its metabolites were substantially higher during sustained four-times-daily therapy than following the initial oral dose.

These observations denoting the importance of tolerance during oral isosorbide dinitrate therapy were contrary to earlier studies demonstrating that, despite attenuated hemodynamic effects, antianginal effects were not altered after several months of four-times-daily therapy with this agent [9]. In a study by Lee and co-workers, patients received isosorbide dinitrate every six hours for one month and no attenuation of the antianginal effect was reported [10]. Our group, however, have shown in subsequent studies that, during sustained four-times-daily therapy with isosorbide dinitrate, no antianginal effect can be demonstrated beyond one or two hours after a given dose [11,12]. It is of interest that, despite tolerance to oral isosorbide dinitrate, following sublingual administration of 5 mg isosorbide dinitrate or 0.6 mg nitroglycerin there is a normal increase in treadmill walking time. The mechanism for the continued effect of sublingual medication is not clear, but may depend on rapidly rising nitrate levels. Plasma nitrate levels are substantially elevated for a short period of time after sublingual administration. The subsequent nadir may be such that the mechanisms responsible for nitrate tolerance do not come into play.

The transdermal nitrates are now being utilized with increasing frequency for the treatment of both angina and heart failure. Nitroglycerin ointment and patches are used commonly on a continuous basis to provide 24-hour protection, but with our current knowledge regarding nitrate tolerance this may not be the most effective therapeutic approach. Nitroglycerin ointment has been available for many years. An early report by Reichek *et al* employed a relatively small dose of nitroglycerin ointment – a dose selected on the basis of its hemodynamic effects (i.e. a decline in systolic blood pressure of 10 mmHg or increase in heart rate of 10 beats/min) [13]. This dose prolonged exercise time three hours after application, but no effects were apparent after five hours. Subsequent acute studies employing larger doses have shown improvement for as long as seven hours after application of nitroglycerin ointment [14,15].

In view of the problem of nitrate tolerance, there is a surprising lack of studies on the effects of sustained therapy with nitroglycerin ointment. Reichek *et al* gave the same dose of ointment three times daily for one month to six of their patients and found that the effects on exercise tolerance persisted [13]. More information is required regarding the sustained effect of nitroglycerin ointment when applied three or four times daily. It seems likely that such regimens will be asssociated with a development of tolerance to anti-anginal effects.

This concern would certainly by supported by results of studies employing isosor-bide dinitrate ointment [16]. We had the opportunity of assessing the effect of a transdermal isosorbide dinitrate ointment that was designed to provide therapeutic plasma levels throughout a 24-hour period after application. In acute studies, 100 mg isosorbide dinitrate ointment was applied over a 200-cm^2 area of the chest wall. Treadmill testing documented an improvement in walking time to the onset of angina and to the development of moderate angina at 2, 4 and 8 hours after application, but at 24 hours the effect was similar to placebo. This absence of effect at 24 hours occurred despite maintenance of plasma isosorbide dinitrate levels throughout the 24-hour period. In a sustained phase of this study, the ointment was applied once daily for 7–10 days, and compared with placebo ointment in a double-blind fashion. Treadmill exercise testing carried out over a 24-hour period before and after the morning dose showed no difference between active and placebo medication. This complete tolerance to transdermal isosorbide dinitrate was present despite substantially higher plasma concentrations of isosorbide dinitrate and its two metabolites, isosorbide-2-mononitrate and isosorbide-5-mononitrate, during the sustained phase of investigation.

Transdermal nitroglycerin patches are now widely accepted as a method of nitrate administration. The patch designs have become quite elegant and are clearly more acceptable to patients than nitroglycerin ointment. Pharmacokinetic studies have shown that absorption of nitroglycerin from these patches leads to sustained plasma nitroglycerin levels over the 24-hour period of patch application. Clinical studies using exercise testing have been carried out to assess the efficacy of these devices. Thompson reported that treadmill exercise time was increased for 26 hours after application during sustained therapy [17]. This was a remarkable observation, considering that only 5 mg of nitroglycerin were released over the 24-hour period, and studies have shown that with this dose plasma nitroglycerin levels are in the range of 0.1–0.2 ng/ml. Further acute studies with larger single doses have shown that exercise time was prolonged for 2–8 hours after patch application; however, no effects were apparent after 24 hours [18,19]. There are very few data relating to sustained once-daily therapy with nitroglycerin patches. In one study, where patches designed to deliver 15 mg for 24 hours were administered daily for 7–10 days, treadmill walking times at 2, 4 and 24 hours after application showed patches to be identical in effect to placebo [19]. The documentation that acute dosing produced effects at 2 and 4 hours but with sustained once-daily therapy the effects were completely gone indicates the development of tolerance. The extent of improvement during the acute phase at 2 and 4 hours was also clearly less than that seen after sublingual nitroglycerin administration.

It has become increasingly evident that dosing regimens designed to produce a nitrate effect throughout a 24-hour period are associated with the rapid development of tolerance. Thus, during acute studies with transdermal nitroglycerin and isosorbide dinitrate there are increases in exercise performance for several hours, but not after 24 hours. This deterioration can be demonstrated despite the maintenance of plasma nitrate levels throughout the 24-hour period. The attenuated effect is probably a manifestation of early tolerance. Of more importance is the documentation that sustained therapy with these agents is associated with the development of complete tolerance. A very important study employing intravenous nitroglycerin was recently reported by Zimrin et al [20]. These investigators determined an infusion rate of nitroglycerin that was sufficient to lower systolic blood pressure to 90 mmHg. In a subsequent placebo-controlled 24-hour infusion period, exercise testing was carried out. Exercise time was increased at 1, 4 and 8 hours by the nitroglycerin infusion, although the effect progressively diminished. Despite the continued infusion, there was no effect on exercise tolerance at 24 hours. This diminishing effect occurred despite constant plasma nitroglycerin concentrations throughout the 24-hour period. This acute study clearly charts the rapid onset of tolerance, which was complete after 24 hours of infusion.

Other clinical studies have documented the early onset of hemodynamic tolerance to oral isosorbide dinitrate [21]. We performed a study employing 5 mg isosorbide dinitrate sublingually as an indicator of nitrate responsiveness. The initial blood-pressure response was assessed and patients were then placed on oral isosorbide dinitrate, 15 mg every 6 hours. On the morning of day 2, before the scheduled oral dose of isosorbide dinitrate and after only three isosorbide dinitrate tablets had been administered, the hypotensive response to sublingual isosorbide dinitrate was reduced by 50%. Oral isosorbide dinitrate was then continued, and on day 3 the sublingual challenge produced identical effects. This demonstrated that hemodynamic tolerance had developed within 20 hours of the first dosing of isosorbide dinitrate. Patients were then given placebo tablets every six hours and the sublingual isosorbide dinitrate challenge was repeated on days 4 and 5. On the morning of day 4, 21 hours after the last dose of isosorbide dinitrate, the hypotensive response to sublingual isosorbide dinitrate was identical to that seen initially. This study showed that hemodynamic tolerance develops rapidly to oral nitrates and is reversed promptly by withdrawal.

Mechanism of Action of the Nitrates and Basis of Nitrate Tolerance
The mechanism of nitrate action is not completely understood. A specific nitrate receptor has been postulated, but no binding studies have been reported. The hypothesis currently favored suggests that the nitrates stimulate the production of cyclic guanosine monophosphate (cGMP) in vascular smooth muscle of arteries and veins. It is thought that the organic nitrates are converted to nitric acid, which reacts with sulfhydryl-containing compounds in vascular smooth muscle and thus produces nitrosothiols [22]. The nitrosothiols subsequently stimulate guanylate cyclase, leading to the production of cGMP. Because of the important role of calcium in vasodilatation, it is thought that cGMP leads either to decreased calcium entry into the cell or to increased uptake by sarcoplasmic reticulum. A previous hypothesis for nitrate action involved the

prostaglandin system [23]: it was suggested that the cyclo-oxygenase pathways were influenced by increased prostacyclin production and decreased thromboxane A_2 release. The evidence to date would support the suggestion that cGMP is the major factor involved in nitrate vasodilatation.

The mechanism of nitrate tolerance is even less well understood. It is suggested that nitrate exposure leads to diminished levels of reduced sulfhydryl groups [24] and subsequently to a deficiency of nitrosothiol production [22]. The administration of *N*-acetylcysteine, a sulfhydryl group donor, has been shown to increase vascular responsiveness to the nitrates [25–28]. Other possible explanations for nitrate tolerance include expanded plasma volumes during nitrate therapy, augmented catecholamine release, or activation of the renin-angiotensin system.

Therapeutic Strategies to Diminish Nitrate Tolerance

It has been postulated that the administration of nitrates should be intermittent, thus allowing periods with relatively low nitrate levels in the circulation. Studies where isosorbide dinitrate was administered once or twice daily have documented persisting improvement during prolonged therapy [29,30]. We have recently completed an investigation comparing the oral administration of 30 mg isosorbide dinitrate twice, three times and four times daily, allowing periods of 20, 14 and 8 hours between last dosing and morning medication [31]. In this placebo-controlled trial, patients maintained the schedules for one week and were tested before and after the morning medication. On the twice- or three-times-daily therapeutic program, exercise time was increased over the morning baseline for the five-hour testing period, although the effects at three and five hours were substantially diminished compared with those apparent at one hour. During the four-times-daily treatment program, exercise time was prolonged at one hour, but this was substantially diminished in magnitude when compared with the other dosing regimens and there was no improvement apparent at three and five hours.

The use of intermittent transdermal therapy with nitroglycerin has not been studied, although it would appear rational to leave the patches or ointment in place for periods of only 12–14 hours and thus provide a nitrate-free period. In a report by Reiniger *et al* with transdermal nitroglycerin patches, exercise testing was carried out during initial patch application and after the application of a second patch on the following day [32]. Although improvement was documented following the initial patch application, testing carried out 2½ hours after patch application on day 2 showed no effect. In a continuation of this study, after the patch had been left in place for 14 hours it was removed, and the effects of patch application on day 3 were assessed. When exercise testing was carried out 2½ hours after the third patch there was no improvement in performance, suggesting that a 10-hour nitrate-free period was inadequate to restore nitrate responsiveness. More investigations will have to be carried out with intermittent patch therapy to give a more complete assessment.

Summary

Although it has been clearly shown that the nitrates are effective in angina, there is increasing documentation of tolerance, which is particularly likely to occur in programs designed to provide nitrates at a therapeutic level throughout a 24-hour period. Although nitrate tolerance develops rapidly it can be reversed promptly, and intermittent therapy providing a nitrate-free period appears to be desirable in the management of angina. In cases where intermittent therapy does not give adequate protection, patients should probably be on additional antianginal medication.

References

[1] Murrell W.
Nitro-glycerine as a remedy for angina pectoris.
Lancet 1879; i: 80.

[2] Needleman P, Lang S, Johnson EM Jr.
Organic nitrates: Relationship between biotransformation and rational angina pectoris therapy.
J Pharmacol Exp Ther 1972; **181**: 489–97.

[3] Thadani U, Fung H-L, Darke A, Parker JO.
Oral isosorbide dinitrate in the treatment of angina pectoris. Dose-response relationship and duration of action during acute therapy.
Circulation 1980; **62**: 491–502.

[4] Thedani U, Fung H-L, Darke AG, Parker JO.
Oral isosorbide dinitrate in angina pectoris: Comparison of duration of action and dose-response relation during acute and sustained therapy.
Am J Cardiol 1982; **49**: 411–9.

[5] Bogaert MG, Deschaepdryer AF.
Tolerance towards glyceryl trinitrate (Trinitrin) in dogs.
Arch Int Pharmacodyn Ther 1968; **171**: 221.

[6] Bogaert MG.
Tolerance to glyceryl trinitrate (Trinitrin) in rabbits.
Arch Int Pharmacodyn Ther 1968; **172**: 228.

[7] Needleman P.
Tolerance to the vascular effects of glyceryl trinitrate.
J Pharmacol Exp Ther 1970; **171**: 98.

[8] Swartz AM.
The cause, relief and prevention of headache arising from contact with dynamite.
N Engl J Med 1946; **235**: 98–102.

[9] Danahy DT, Aronow WS.
Hemodynamics and antianginal effects of high dose oral isosorbide after chronic use.
Circulation 1977; **56**: 205–12.

[10] Lee G, Mason DT, DeMaria AN.
Effects of long-term oral administration of isosorbide dinitrate on the antianginal response to nitroglycerin.
Am J Cardiol 1978; **41**: 82–7.

[11] Dalal JJ, Yao L, Parker JO.
Nitrate tolerance: Influence of isosorbide dinitrate on the hemodynamic and antianginal effects of nitroglycerin.
J Am Coll Cardiol 1983; **2**: 115–20.

[12] Dalal JJ, Parker JO.
Nitrate cross-tolerance: Effect of sublingual isosorbide dinitrate and nitroglycerin during sustained nitrate therapy.
Am J Cardiol 1984; **54**: 286–8.

[13] Reichek N, Goldstein RE, Redwood DR, Epstein SE.
Sustained effects of nitroglycerin ointment in patients with angina pectoris.
Circulation 1974; **50**: 348–52.

[14] Karsh DL, Umback RE, Cohen LS, Langou RA.
Prolonged benefit of nitroglycerin ointment on exercise tolerance in patients with angina pectoris.
Am Heart J 1978; **96**: 587–94.

[15] Nyberg G, Panfilov V.
Effect of nitroglycerin ointment (Nitrong) on exercise tolerance and several circulatory parameters in patients with angina pectoris.
Eur J Clin Pharmacol 1983; **24**: 733–9.

[16] Parker JO, VanKoughnett KA, Fung H-L.
Transdermal isosorbide dinitrate in angina pectoris. Effect of acute and sustained therapy.
Am J Cardiol 1984; **54**: 8–13.

[17] Thompson RH.
The clinical use of transdermal delivery devices with nitroglycerin.
Angiology 1983; **34**: 23–31.

[18] Reichek N, Priest C, Zimrin D, Chandler T, St.John Sutton M.
Antianginal effects of nitroglycerin patches.
Am J Cardiol 1984; **54**: 1–7.

[19] Parker JO, Fung H-L.
Transdermal nitroglycerin in angina pectoris.
Am J Cardiol 1984; **54**: 471–6.

[20] Zimrin D, Reichek N, Bogin K, Cameron S, Douglas P, Fung H-L.
Antianginal effects of i.v. nitroglycerin [Abstract].
Circulation 1985; **72** (Suppl 3): III–460.

[21] Parker JO, Fung H-L, Ruggirello D, Stone JA.
Tolerance to isosorbide dinitrate: Rate of development and reversal.
Circulation 1983; 68: 1074–80.

[22] Ignarro LJ, Lippton H, Edwards JC *et al*.
Mechanism of vascular smooth muscle relaxation by organic nitrates, nitrites, nitroprusside and nitric oxide. Evidence for the involvement of S-nitrosothiols as active intermediates.
J Pharmacol Exp Ther 1981; 218: 739–49.

[23] Trimarco B, Cuoclo A, Van Dorne D *et al*.
Late phase of nitroglycerin-induced coronary vasodilatation blunted by inhibition of prostaglandin systems.
Circulation 1985; 71: 840–8.

[24] Needleman P, Jakschik B, Johnson EM Jr.
Sulfhydryl requirement for relaxation of vascular smooth muscles.
J Pharmacol Exp Ther 1973; 187: 324.

[25] Horowitz JD, Antman EM, Lorell BH, Barry WH, Smith TW.
Potentiation of the cardiovascular effects of nitroglycerin by N-acetylcysteine.
Circulation 1983; 68: 1247–53.

[26] Torresi J, Horowitz JD, Dusting GJ.
Prevention and reversal of tolerance to nitroglycerine with N-acetylcysteine.
J Cardiovasc Pharmacol 1985; 7: 777–83

[27] Winniford MD, Kennedy PL, Wells PJ, Hillis LD.
Potentiation of nitroglycerin-induced coronary dilatation by N-acetylcysteine.
Circulation 1986; 73: 138–42.

[28] Packer M, Lee WH, Kessler P, Medina N, Yushak M.
Induction of nitrate tolerance in human heart failure by continuous intravenous infusion of nitroglycerin and reversal of tolerance by N-acetylcysteine, a sulfhydryl donor [Abstract].
J Am Coll Cardiol 1986; 7: 27A.

[29] Blasini R, Reiniger G, Brugmann U.
Tolerance to the anti-ischemic effect of isosorbide dinitrate during continuous but not during intermittent oral therapy. In: Cohn JN, Rittenhausen R, eds. *Mononitrates*. Berlin: Springer-Verlag, 1985; pp. 124–9.

[30] Rudolph W.
Tolerance development during isosorbide dinitrate treatment. Can it be circumvented?
Kardiol 1983; 72: 203–10.

[31] Parker JO, Lahey KA, Farrell B, Moe G.
Tolerance to the organic nitrates. Importance of dosing intervals.
Submitted for publication.

[32] Reiniger G, Blasini R, Brugmann U, Rudolph W.
Nitroglycerin patches in coronary artery disease: Can tolerance development be avoided through an interval therapy? [Abstract].
Circulation 1985; 72: III–431.

THE TREATMENT OF UNSTABLE ANGINA

Review: PAUL G. HUGENHOLTZ

Any physician intimately involved in the care of patients with coronary artery disease knows from experience that the toughest cases – those who require the most careful decisions in terms of management and therapy – are those individuals who are temporarily on the watershed between angina pectoris and myocardial infarction: at the boundary between a manageable loss of tissue (by the patient) during angina and the unmanageable loss of tissue (by the doctor) that ensues once myocardial infarction has taken place.

While it is true that not every case of unstable angina will lead to myocardial infarction or prolonged ischemia, or even sudden death, it is also unclear in what number of people symptoms or signs of these unstable syndromes have actually preceded sudden death or acute myocardial infarction. In fact, we remain woefully short of a real understanding of the natural history of unstable angina in any given patient within or outside the hospital. It is this uncertainty of outcome which obliges us, urges us, and indeed forces us to provide maximal therapy for all.

No matter which approach one chooses – conservative [1], intensive pharmacologic [2] or invasive [3] – such therapy should result in prompt (that is, within 24 hours) relief of symptoms with a near-absence of such sequelae as myocardial infarction or death over a one-year period.

Pathophysiology

It is clear that, in contrast to those with stable angina, patients with unstable angina form a widely heterogeneous group in terms of the prevailing but often changing pathogenic mechanisms, the underlying state of the coronary arteriosclerosis, and the degree of associated impairment of left-ventricular function. As Maseri and Foale put it [4]:

> At one end of the spectrum are patients with extremely severe reduction of coronary flow reserve in whom even a modest increase in myocardial oxygen demand is sufficient to precipitate ischaemia. At the other end are patients in whom coronary flow reserve is only marginally impaired, or even completely normal, and in whom ischaemia is caused by a transient interruption of coronary blood flow. The fixed reduction of coronary flow reserve may result from old atherosclerotic plaques, with or without an additional component (such as rupture) [5,6], or recent thrombosis [7]. Transient impairment of flow may also result from spasm, from intravascular plugging at the site of a stenosis, from constriction of resistance vessels, or from a combination of the above factors [7].
>
> The majority of patients with unstable angina appear to be between these extremes: they have a variable degree of fixed reduction of their coronary flow reserve and a variable extent of transient impairment of coronary flow, which is responsible for the spontaneous, usually unpredictable onset of anginal episodes. This proposition is supported by the angiographic observation that the severity of coronary artery stenosis in general is not dissimilar from that commonly found in patients with stable angina, and by pacing studies indicating that unstable patients usually have a high threshold for tachycardia induced ischaemia. Therefore it may be reasonable to assume that most often angina becomes unstable because of the occurrence of dynamic stenosis superimposed on an old or fresh (caused by a recent thrombus) fixed stenosis of variable severity. This hypothesis seems to be gaining acceptance.

The significant aspect, dominant in all forms suspected of reflecting 'high-risk' unstable angina, is that the pain is continual or even progressive in severity and intensity, despite bedrest. We are not talking here about patients who have had an attack of pain which subsided spontaneously, but about those who are still considered unstable: i.e., patients whose pain is persistent (>48 hours) or recurrent, and in whom Gazes *et al* found a 20% one-month mortality and 43% one-year mortality [8]. Julian, averaging all series since 1970 with >100 cases each with severe pain and ECG changes, finds a one-month mortality of 4%, a one-year mortality of 12%, and an early myocardial infarction rate of 8% [9]. In such patients, it is more the timing, the progressiveness and persistence than the character or location of the pain which denotes the instability of the angina. As Balakumaran *et al* put it [10]:

> Unstable angina is doubly distressing. On the one hand the patient is confronted with the disturbing new symptomatology, namely unfamiliarised pain (crescendo angina), unprovoked pain (angina at rest) or pain returning on the heels of the major blow of myocardial infarction (early post-infarct angina), on the other hand the physician knows that something potentially dangerous is afoot.

Maseri feels it is important to establish first whether the ischemic episodes which characterize the instability of the syndrome are caused: (i) by an excessive increase in myocardial demand in the presence of fixed limitation of coronary blood supply, or (ii) via sudden and often transient impairment of coronary blood supply [4] – in other words, to distinguish whether the ischemic episodes represent primary or secondary angina. As a second step, it is necessary to assess the severity of the reduction of coronary flow reserve and the tendency to develop persistent episodes of impairment of coronary flow. Table Ia recognizes three groups which reflect the classification as a first step. Table Ib provides a guideline with which to classify the patient according to the assumed reduction of coronary flow reserve.

Table Ia: Guideline to the classification of patients with unstable angina according to extent of reduction of coronary flow reserve (see also Table 1b)

Group 1: Normal or only slightly reduced coronary flow reserve
Clinical correlates: No history of reduced effort tolerance.
Angiographic correlates: Absence of critical lesions or good collaterals.
Objective evidence: Negative maximal exercise stress test.*

Group 2: Moderately reduced coronary flow reserve
Clinical correlates: History of exertional angina, but moderate efforts usually well tolerated.
Angiographic correlates: Presence of one or more severe coronary obstructions.
Objective evidence: Exercise stress test* produces signs or symptoms of ischemia only above 5 METS.[†]

Group 3: Severely reduced coronary flow reserve
Clinical correlates: Severe exertional angina, even moderate efforts never tolerated.
Angiographic correlates: One or more severe coronary obstructions.
Objective evidence: Exercise stress test* produces signs or symptoms of ischemia even below 5 METS.[†]

---

* After acute administration of nitrates or calcium antagonists.
[†] METS = metabolic equivalents.

Table Ib: Subdivision of above groups according to persistence of ischemia

---

According to the tendency to develop persistent episodes of ischemia, each group should be subdivided into:

A: Moderate tendency to develop persistent ischemic episodes
– spontaneous ischemic episodes lasting less than 5 minutes or promptly relieved by sublingual nitrates.

B: Severe tendency to develop persistent ischemic episodes
–recurring ischemic episodes lasting more than 5 minutes and responding poorly to sublingual nitrates.

Accordingly, a patient who reported an attack of spontaneous chest pain and who was thought to be in Group 1A would be subjected to a maximal exercise test which would usually be negative, and that would be the end of the investigation; this corresponds to the type seen by Mulcahy [1] and recently described in the randomized metoprolol-nifedipine trial [11]. However, in the long term, these milder cases may still have increased mortality and late myocardial infarction: in Mulcahy's cases, this amounted to 7% and 15%, respectively. Conversely, a patient in Group 3B may have such persistent symptomatology that provocative testing with bicycle ergometry or ergonovine is contraindicated; this is the type described by de Feyter *et al*, refractory to triple pharmacologic therapy and still suffering from angina and ischemia [3]. It becomes evident that when patients demonstrate anginal pain lasting longer than 15 minutes, associated with ST- and T-wave changes, a much more aggressive approach is warranted than in those patients classified in Groups 1 or 2.

When Maseri's classification is combined with the scheme proposed by Goldman *et al* [12], the manner in which the patient responds to therapy is recognized as a major classification principle. As shown in Figure 1a, three kinds of response, from complete to inadequate, are distinguished. In the inadequate category, two subsets exist (Fig. 1b): patients with brief versus patients with prolonged pain at rest. It is in this latter group that the most aggressive therapy should be pursued. Thus, on the basis of an initial 'guesstimate' of the pathogenesis in a given case, combined with the evaluation of the early (i.e. within hours) response after administration of a vasodilatory, beta-blocking or cardioprotective agent, the proper course of action can be judged (Fig. 2). As pointed out by Conti, the impact of coronary obstruction on nutritive perfusion is not definable simply in terms of cross-sectional area reduction within a lumen [13]. The impact reflects also the length and distribution of lesions within a vessel, potential additive effects attributable to lesions in series, and the nature of lesions that may appear to be similar angiographically while differing morphologically with varying contributions of thrombosis, atherosclerotic obstruction, fissuring and hemorrhage in the plaque, and calcification. Superimposition of coronary vasospasm, both proximal and distal, may exacerbate the functional significance of lesions at different times within the same patient and may account for differing functional implications of similar lesions among different patients [13].

The scheme depicted in Figure 3 indicates quite clearly to what degree the pre-existing condition of the coronary artery tree can suddenly be aggravated by six major factors. These conditions include: (i) extracardiac aggravating factors; (ii) rapid progression of coronary atherosclerosis; (iii) rapid decrease in coronary lumen size secondary to hemorrhage into an atherosclerotic plaque; (iv) transient platelet aggregation in diseased vessels with intermittent distal embolization; (v) transient coronary artery thrombosis; and (vi) abnormal coronary artery vasoconstriction (spasm) in normal or diseased vessels.

It may not be possible to identify the appropriate mechanism responsible for unstable angina in every case, but the clinician must attempt to do so, since the correct selection of therapy depends on recognition of the pathophysiology responsible for the symptoms in that individual at that time.

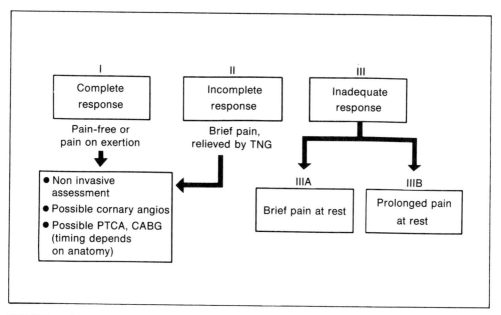

FIGURE 1a: Classification of patients with unstable angiography. Goldman *et al* [12] distinguish three types of patient response to therapy instituted on the basis of the scheme depicted in Table I. CABG, coronary artery bypass grafting.

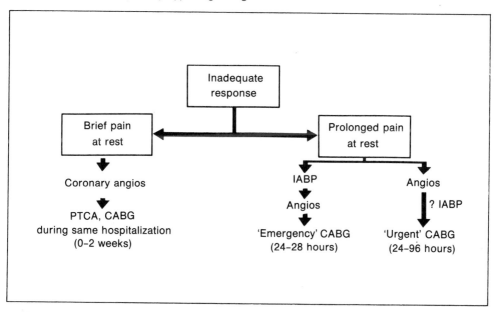

FIGURE 1b: If the response is inadequate (Figure 1a, III) and pain is prolonged at bedrest (IIIB), early angiography, with or without balloon pump support, would lead to emergency coronary artery bypass grafting (CABG) or PTCA. Thus, a combination of the scheme advocated by Maseri [4] with the therapeutic responsiveness of the patient as classified by Goldman [12] would allow for proper classification in most patients.

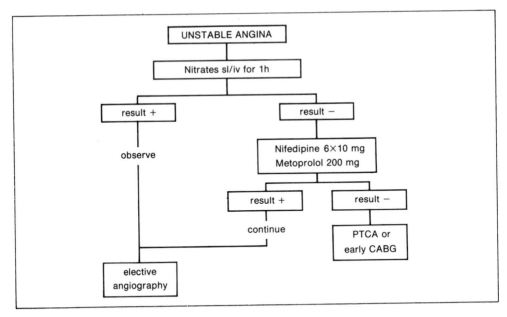

FIGURE 2: Schematic flow-chart showing the ideal management of a patient with acute unstable angina. Time intervals are obviously tentative, and depend on the responsiveness of the patient. CABG, coronary artery bypass grafting.

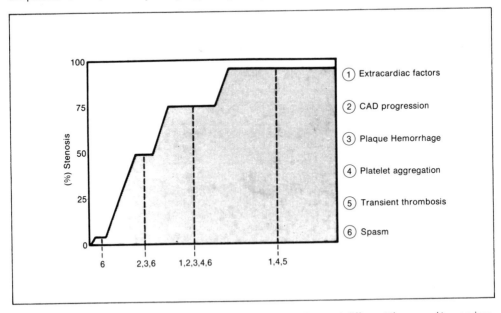

FIGURE 3: Unstable angina pathophysiology. Factors 1 to 6 can at different times and to varying extent be superimposed on the existing atherosclerotic fixed stenosis (vertical axis). For example, with only minimal coronary artery atherosclerosis, spasm may be a major cause of obstruction. Conversely, only minor platelet aggregation (factor 4), when fixed atherosclerosis has progressed to 95% stenosis, can cause occlusion. (After Conti [13].)

Thrombolytic Therapy, Anticoagulation

No well-designed studies are available to support the use of anticoagulants (such as warfarin-derived agents) in stable or unstable angina. On the other hand, heparin appears to be well accepted in the hospital environment, while aspirin has been advocated for the longer term. Since vasoactive substances, which may induce vasospasm, are released during platelet aggregation, platelet aggregation inhibitors could perhaps play a major role, although at present the usefulness of these drugs in unstable angina has not been established. In fact, no author has been able to show any clinical effect of prostaglandin derivatives and their blockers. As a consequence, short-term heparin (30 000 U/24 hours) is now advocated only in patients with prolonged bedrest or in those monitored with intravascular catheters to avoid deep-vein and pulmonary artery thrombosis.

Recently, intracoronary streptokinase has been advocated for patients with 'impending infarction', a clinical situation which may follow unstable angina pectoris. Fresh data from our institute and from the Netherlands Interuniversity Cardiology Institute have shown that, in 533 patients randomized either to standard therapy or to reperfusion by streptokinase (with PTCA and coronary artery bypass grafting in some), early reperfusion halves the death rate on an intention-to-treat principle (16.7% in controls *vs* 5.9% in lysed patients) [14,15]. Since 86 patients were included who progressed in hospital from unstable angina to acute infarction, and since the results in this subset were the best, a strong argument in favour of thrombolytic therapy can be made – when the suspected mechanism is indeed proven to be thrombotic obstruction. Earlier, Cowley *et al* had shown 40 out of 69 patients with unstable angina to have intraluminal filling defects or thrombolytic occlusion [16]. Similar findings have been described by Bresnahan *et al* [17], whose data have led some authors to infuse streptokinase, with success [18].

Nitrates

Nitroglycerin tablets, taken sublingually or in an intravenous solution, relieve most anginal attacks in two-thirds of cases. This agent's direct vasodilatory effect on the venous system lowers preload and, hence, wall stress and oxygen consumption of the left ventricle. An additional dilatory effect on the larger arteries may decrease afterload, and there may be a direct effect on coronary flow [19]. The latter has been repeatedly observed in Prinzmetal's angina where nitroglycerin, given directly into the coronary artery, was shown to relieve the obstruction caused by spasm. Recently, it has been indicated that nitrate may have an antiaggregatory action, affecting blood platelets and thus augmenting its efficacy. However, unwanted side-effects frequently occur and not all patients respond [20]. While hypotension and bradyarrhythmias can be managed by raising the legs to improve venous return and, if this is not sufficient, atropine (0.25–1 mg i.v.) is usually effective, sometimes plasma infusion has to be employed. While sublingual nitroglycerin acts within minutes, its duration of action is equally short. Nitroglycerin ointment for topical application has a prolonged effect, as has isosorbide dinitrate. These compounds are especially effective in preventing angina attacks at night. The 5-mg tablets of isosorbide dinitrate for sublingual use begin to act within minutes, and their action extends from one to three hours; the 20-mg tablets for oral administration provide an even longer-lasting effect. Even so, these drugs are not always effective, as their blood levels and metabolism vary widely from one individual to another. Molsidomin, a completely different compound in chemical terms, has a long half-life (>6 hours) and leads to a strong reduction in preload. It is completely absorbed, is at least as effective as the nitrates, and deserves further clinical evaluation in the context of unstable angina pectoris.

Beta-Blocking Agents

There is a vast literature on this subject and the reader is probably already partisan to one or more of these drugs. Beta-blocking agents reduce the action of catecholamines and therefore contractility and heart rate. However, when the heart is already enlarged, they may increase wall tension and hence oxygen consumption. The net effect upon the heart not in failure is usually a significant reduction in oxygen consumption, mainly via the induced bradycardia.

Beta-blockade has also been reported to redirect the limited blood supply from normal or overperfused areas to ischemic areas [21]; on the other hand, it may, by unbalancing the innervation of the coronary artery system, lead to increased receptor tone and hence reduced coronary blood flow. It is therefore quite understandable that this drug should not be given when true spasm, such as that seen in Prinzmetal's syndrome, is suspected [22]. When spasm is not suspected and one elects to use a beta-blocker, for the two reasons given above, the heart rate must be considerably slowed down for the drug to be effective. In acute ischemic conditions, propranolol (1–10 mg i.v., at 1 mg/min) will be most effective until a heart rate of 60 beats/min has been reached. Oral dosage in a range of 240–800 mg propranolol per 24 hours is then instituted. Although much higher dosages than 800 mg propranolol per 24 hours can be tolerated, we prefer to replace propranolol with acebutolol, metoprolol or atenolol when it is not effective as a first drug, although no convincing proof of the efficacy of the latter agents (except for that of metoprolol [11]) is available in randomized trials.

Recently, a large-scale trial (5778 patients) in acute myocardial infarction allocated 2877 patients to metoprolol and 2901 to placebo [21]. A small, statistically non-significant difference (4.3% vs 4.9%) was found in terms of reduction in 15-day mortality, although there was quicker pain relief and less arrhythmia in the treated group. This series included some patients with unstable angina, which suggests that no major impact on death rate or infarction rate can be expected from this beta-blocker. Data from Kudoch et al in a coronary-embolized dog model also failed to indicate a protective effect in terms of infarct size limitation [22]. Chamberlain, in a recent overview of all data available on beta-blockade in acute myocardial infarction, states [23]:

> The influence of beta-blockers on acute mortality is perhaps the area of greatest controversy. Some trials have shown decreased survival, while others have shown improvement. Many of these differences may be due to variations in protocol, but as yet no firm evidence of a therapeutic effect can be claimed.

Even so, most clinicians, when confronted with a patient with unstable angina obviously in sympathetic overdrive, will choose – next to the nitrate – a beta-blocker to reduce excessive oxygen consumption by the heart, and should persist with this therapy until heart rate has slowed down considerably.

Calcium Antagonists

Since their introduction in the early 1970s in Japan and Europe, calcium antagonists have enjoyed much attention from the cardiology community. This is undoubtedly due to the fact that one is dealing with a large group of compounds with a novel therapeutic principle. Experience has shown that they have great clinical efficacy for hitherto difficult-to-treat cases of angina [24]. The inhibition of smooth muscle excitation-contraction coupling in the coronary artery wall achieved by verapamil, nifedipine and diltiazem decreases contractile tone, resulting in vasodilatation and hence increased coronary blood flow. In the cardiac muscle cell itself, the inhibition of intracellular calcium activity reduces the contractile and mechanical function, and this diminishes myocardial oxygen demand. Calcium antagonists also appear to have an action on ischemic cells in protecting mitochondrial activity. These are highly desirable interventions when the myocardium is threatened by ischemia. On the other hand, inhibition of the cell membrane is also important in terms of treating cardiac arrhythmias. Here major differences exist between verapamil and nifedipine in antiarrhythmic properties. It may be that surface-binding properties and the specific availability of receptor sites determine the extent to which a specific calcium 'antagonist' antagonizes slow-channel Ca^{2+} transport.

In the clinical situation, the net hemodynamic and electrophysiologic effect of a given calcium antagonist remains the result of the complex interaction between its varying peripheral and central effects [24]. The degree of baroreceptor stimulation and reflex-mediated beta-adrenergic activity – which counteract and influence the intrinsic negative dromotropic, chronotropic and inotropic effects of the calcium antagonists – are related to the degree of peripheral dilatation, and the search for the ideal calcium antagonist, which would mainly affect the coronary arteries, continues. Nisoldipine may turn out to be this agent [25]. Currently, we share the view of Stone et al [26], that nifedipine is the most potent arterial vasodilator and is consequently associated with the most intense reflex adrenergic activity. The net effect of nifedipine is that of relatively pure vasodilatation, with little electrophysiologic or negative inotropic effect when given orally or intravenously. On the other hand, doses of verapamil and diltiazem which produce the same degree of vasodilatation as nifedipine have negative dromotropic effects, and the reflex-induced beta-adrenergic activity may not completely offset the direct electrophysiologic effects.

All three calcium antagonists discussed are effective in treating patients with coronary spasm or unstable angina, as well as in treating stable angina when increased vasomotor activity is the dominant underlying disorder. In patients with classic Prinzmetal's angina, an additional benefit might be expected (and has been demonstrated) from combined therapy of nifedipine with verapamil and diltiazem. In this laboratory, nifedipine has become a most useful adjuvant where beta-blockers and nitrates alone have not proved effective [27]. It has, in fact, changed our therapeutic approach in unstable angina, while in cases with proven spasm not responding to intracoronary nitroglycerin it has always relieved the spasm when given into the coronary artery. For Prinzmetal's angina, we begin short- and long-term therapy with nifedipine, and all patients with unstable angina receive nifedipine with a beta-blocker when a short-term trial (1–2 h) with nitrates proves unsatisfactory [27].

In some cases of unstable angina pectoris, the exact mechanisms of action will remain unclear because of uncertainty surrounding the cause(s) of the unstable angina. Thus, particularly when eccentric lesions are present which leave part of the circumference of the vascular wall intact, vasoconstrictive stimuli may cause marked change in the tone of the vessel wall and therefore in coronary blood flow. It can readily be understood why the combination of an eccentric, fixed endothelial lesion and a (hyper)sensitive, but otherwise healthy, vascular wall opposite will frequently lead to intermittent ischemic episodes. The fact that 42 of the 52 patients placed on nifedipine while maintaining beta-blocker therapy experienced early and complete relief of angina, which persisted for the entire period of observation, is indeed a strong argument in favour of the overriding vasodilatory effect of nifedipine even in beta-blocked coronary arteries [27]. Gerstenblith *et al* were able to duplicate our clinical observations in similar patients in a prospective randomized trial [28]: in 168 patients, nifedipine, when added to conventional therapy comprising beta-blockers and nitrates, was more effective than placebo in reducing the need for urgent surgery, and also demonstrated a reduction in subsequent myocardial infarction and the death rate. This was later substantiated by the data from the HINT study, involving over 500 patients [11]. So consistent was this subsequent response to nifedipine (and just as effective as had been pain relief by IABP in our previous experience in the same type of patient), and so comparable with that described by Parodi *et al* [29], that there can be little doubt that calcium antagonists in unstable angina with excess vasomotion are *the* agents which provide the extra factor. This is further confirmed by the nifedipine withdrawal study by Gottlieb [30]: of 81 patients whose pain was controlled by nifedipine, only four showed worsening after two years of therapy, or upon withdrawal prior to surgery. Braunwald reviewed these arguments, and stated that there might now very well be a preference for the primary use of calcium antagonists in patients suspected of having abnormally increased coronary vasomotor tone [31].

These expèriences have led to the designing of a prospective randomized trial in a category of patients with moderate unstable angina, in whom an attack of 15 minutes or more had taken place within six hours of admission, or who were observed after admission to have a pain episode with ECG changes [11]. Those in whom the severity was greater (persistent pain after nitrates or with enzyme elevation) or less (no recurrence of attacks) were excluded. A group of 338 patients not treated prior to admission with a beta-blocker were studied for their reaction to nifedipine, metoprolol, or a combination of the two, and all were compared to placebo. In 177 patients admitted while already on a beta-blocker, nifedipine was added in a random fashion. Three observations relevant for the clinician follow from this study [11]: (i) All non-responders to nitrates (p.o. and i.v.), most of whom were treated by PTCA or surgery, were excluded, thus, this study does not reflect on therapy in severe unstable angina; (ii) when nifedipine was added to the regimen of those patients experiencing unstable angina while on beta-blockade, the same effect was noted as in the earlier studies by Hugenholtz *et al* [27], Gerstenblith *et al* [28] and Moses [32] – the event rate ratio (where 1 = no effect) became 0.68 with confidence limits (0.47–0.97); and (iii) in the group not on prior beta-blockade, no great differences were seen between those primarily placed on nifedipine, metoprolol, a combination of the two or placebo, although a slightly favorable effect in terms of an event rate ratio of 0.76 (confidence limits 0.49–1.16) was seen when metoprolol was given first. This confirms the clinician's tendency to insist on slowing heart rate. The increased incidence of myocardial infarction in the nifedipine group of the trial [11] may be explained by the chance inclusion of more high-risk cases in this category, although the authors state that the exact onset of infarction could not be established in the study. Given the small sample and the logical inefficacy of nifedipine after infarction has occurred [33], it must follow that nifedipine alone, or for that matter any calcium antagonist, as a first-line therapy has little to offer this subset of patients.

Therapy by Mechanical Intervention
It is now clear that, while beta-blockers will reduce oxygen consumption, and vasodilators – in particular the nitrates and the calcium antagonists, nifedipine and diltiazem – have a major effect on symptoms as well as an impact on ischemia within the first few hours of administration, therapy-resistant cases will be identified after 8–12 hours. In these 'refractory' instances, the decision to proceed with further diagnostic investigations must be made early (Fig. 2). Usually, significant atherosclerotic narrowing is found with or without spasm and with or without intravascular thrombus. The latter can, according to the timing of the arteriography, be seen in up to 50% of cases.

Since this form of obstruction is most probably the major explanation for the persistence of the unstable state, mechanical recanalization must be undertaken either by means of percutaneous transluminal coronary angioplasty (PTCA) in the catheterization laboratory or by coronary artery bypass grafting in the operating room. One can argue, as de Feyter *et al* have done recently [3], that PTCA always has a place when optimal pharmacologic intervention has failed. A period of 24 hours would seem, in the view of Maseri [4] and Goldman [12] and their co-workers, to be almost too long to wait for any therapy to exert its optimal effect in the face of an ongoing loss of myocardial function and cell death: PTCA should not, as was coronary artery bypass grafting in the past, be seen as an emergency, 'last-ditch' treatment – rather as a semi-urgent elective procedure to be initiated early in the 'hot' stage of the disease, when the patient proves unresponsive to a triple pharmacologic therapy approach. This seems an essential and important step in the modern concept of the management of unstable angina pectoris.

Then, a combination of aspirin, calcium antagonists and perhaps heparin now seems most advisable for the period following such mechanical dilatation of the coronary artery. Many authors have argued that residual or returning spasm can occur during the healing phase of the distended atheromatous lesion, while it is also likely that recurrent thrombosis may take place on the denuded endothelium induced by the distending balloon; here, calcium antagonists would be indicated, given their potential healing effects [34]. The data of Cairns [35,36] and Lewis *et al* [37] suggest that aspirin plays a major role in preventing the acute recurrence of thrombocyte aggregation on top of the fissures and cracks which have been caused in the plaque. This is also in keeping with the findings of Born [7] and Becker [38].

The experience in Rotterdam with 139 patients with this type of unstable angina pectoris serves as a good example of the efficacy of PTCA [3]. Other data have recently been published by Meyer *et al*, in a series of 108 unstable angina pectoris patients treated with PTCA in two separate hospitals [39]. Both experiences indicate that with modern equipment (such as steerable catheters) the complication rate is around 5%, while the mortality rate ranges between 1% and 2%. Yet the majority of these vessels remained patent one year after the original procedure. Our group reports an initial success rate of 84% (89% with the new steerable systems) in 117 out of 139 patients [3]. In the 22 patients in whom the procedure was unsuccessful, coronary bypass grafting was carried out (as an emergency in 19). In the entire series, there was not a single death related to PTCA or coronary artery bypass grafting, although at one-year follow-up the cumulative mortality and myocardial infarction rate was 11.5% (the mortality component being one sudden cerebral death at eight months).

Thus, when unstable angina is refractory to triple therapy (nitrates, calcium antagonists and beta-blockers), major centers in Western Europe now resort early to mechanical dilatation which, if it proves unsuccessful, can be followed by coronary artery bypass grafting. The importance of the data reported thus far is that, while they do not form part of a randomized study design, they show a remarkably low complication rate and a virtual absence of mortality. Such findings are at striking variance with the early 1970s results of Gazes *et al* [8], or with those of conservative management [1]. Indeed, it can now be said that, when patients with unstable angina are properly managed, the mortality rate should be zero. Not only should unnecessary death be a thing of the past, but, from the data of de Feyter and Meyer *et al* [3,15,39], it appears likely that the infarction rate in the subsequent year should not exceed 10%. Goldman *et al*, in their carefully documented series of unstable angina pectoris, came to similar conclusions on properly timed coronary artery bypass grafting in patients unresponsive to pharmacologic therapy [12]. Using a univariate risk factor analysis in 299 patients with unstable angina coming to urgent surgery after failed pharmacologic therapy, the only difference from a similar analysis in 1003 patients with stable angina pectoris was in the functional class III and IV of the New York Heart Association and the higher prevalence of left main coronary artery stenosis. It seems therefore that, in these categories, CABG should be preferred over PTCA. Again, early recognition by coronary angiography would appear to provide for a good outcome, with an operative mortality of 5% and an incidence of perioperative myocardial infarction of 14%. Goldman also points to the significance of blood cardioplegia in patients with unstable angina pectoris [12], and current research at various clinics suggests a similar supportive role for cardioplegia with either nifedipine or diltiazem added as a cardioprotective agent during cardiopulmonary bypass.

For the period 1981–1983, Cohn *et al* report an operative mortality of 3% in 222 patients considered resistant to pharmacologic therapy, with a perioperative myocardial infarction rate of less than 1% [40]. Yet, over that period, there was a stronger trend towards complete revascularization, with multiple grafts being placed, a lower incidence of one- and two-vessel coronary disease requiring operation (undoubtedly reflecting the fact that PTCA was more often carried out in this subset of patients), and increased overall patient age – leading one to expect an increasing rather than decreasing mortality trend. The improved results also apply to patients with postinfarction unstable angina. Cohn further stresses the need for temporary intra-aortic balloon-pump support in patients who appear to be at excessive risk because of either main stem disease or severe ventricular dysfunction [40] – a point argued earlier from our laboratory [41]. The overall outcome of early bypass surgery after failure of PTCA has been outlined by Haalebos *et al* [41]: they indicate that in 53 patients who required coronary artery bypass grafting within 24 hours of a failed PTCA (out of 500 cases in which PTCA was attempted) there were signs of myocardial damage in roughly half, while an actual myocardial infarction could be demonstrated in a quarter of the cases. Apparently, very early reperfusion after a first failed PTCA cannot prevent loss of cardiac tissue, but early complete reperfusion by coronary artery bypass grafting does prevent death.

Aspirin

Ever since the VA studies reported by Lewis *et al* [37], aspirin has been featured as *the* new therapy for unstable angina. Despite additional evidence from Cairns [35] (ably condensed in a *Comment* in 1986 [36]), I must stress that aspirin as a general cyclo-oxygenase blocker (undoubtedly to be followed by more specific blockers for the synthesis of thromboxane A_2 or by stimulators of prostacyclin [42]) has as yet failed to be of help in acute cases.

In the study by Lewis *et al* on 1338 men, treatment did not begin until 51 hours after hospitalization [37], while Cairns *et al* entered 555 patients who began therapy within eight days of hospitalization [38]. Of the striking reductions of 41% at three months and 30% at 18 months, respectively, for cardiac death or non-fatal acute myocardial infarction (and even higher figures for three-month mortality: 51% and 56%, respectively), none apply to the acute situation. In contrast, they provide the best data to recommend aspirin as a secondary prevention after recovery from the leading attack of unstable angina. Thus, Cairns stated [36]:

> The present management of unstable angina includes bed rest and sedation, preferably in a coronary care unit, vigorous employment of nitrates, beta-blockers and calcium antagonists. Urgent cardiac catheterisation should be performed only in those patients who fail to respond to medical management. It is clear from two recent studies that aspirin should be added to the conventional therapy for unstable angina, with the anticipation of sharp reductions in cardiac death and non-fatal acute myocardial infarction. An initial dose of 1300 mg appears a reasonable choice for most patients, and for women it is the only dose of proven efficacy. In an attempt to minimise gastro-intestinal side-effects and enhance patient compliance, the administration of 650 mg of the enteric coated form twice daily is sound practice. The occurrence of side-effects or poor compliance should prompt dose reductions – in men 325 mg of aspirin daily may be equally efficacious. Therapy should be continued for at least two years, and it should be maintained in patients undergoing aorto-coronary bypass surgery.

Although it is clear that aspirin has no proven influence in the initial course of action and is truly a secondary prevention agent, the halving of the one-year late mortality with aspirin and the low initial death rate with triple pharmacotherapy and/or early PTCA indicate that unstable angina is now under control (Fig. 2).

Summary

Unstable angina presents itself to us as a continuous spectrum of ischemic syndromes. The disease is multifactorial, and within the same patient different pathophysiologic mechanisms may operate at different times and in succession. Consequently, there will never be *one* therapy for *every* case of unstable angina – nor will there ever be a best therapy for all. Rather, a stepped approach appears the most likely to succeed, beginning with bedrest, vasodilator therapy with nitrates and/or calcium antagonists *and* beta-blockade. If the triple therapy does not 'cool' the symptoms within 6–12 hours, semi-urgent arteriography is indicated. Depending on the pathophysiology, thrombolytic therapy, PTCA or coronary artery bypass grafting must be carried out early. Heparin in the short term and aspirin in the long term protect best against late complications. The moment is near when unstable angina resulting in infarction or death will be a rare occurrence.

References

[1] Mulcahy R, Al Awadhi AH, de Buitleon M. Natural history and prognosis of unstable angina. *Am Heart J* 1985; **109**: 753–8.

[2] Hugenholtz PG, Goldman BS, eds. *Unstable angina, current concepts and management*. Stuttgart: Schattauer Verlag, 1985; pp. 1–10.

[3] de Feyter PJ, Serruys PW, van den Brand M et al. Emergency coronary angioplasty in refractory unstable angina. *N Engl J Med* 1985; **313**: 342–6.

[4] Maseri A, Foale R. A pathophysiological classification of unstable angina. In: Hugenholtz PG, Goldman BS, eds. *Unstable angina, current concepts and management*. Stuttgart: Schattauer Verlag, 1985; pp. 71–8.

[5] Davies MJ, Thomas A. Thrombosis and acute coronary artery lesions in sudden cardiac ischemic death. *N Engl J Med* 1984; **310**: 1137–40.

[6] Falk E. Unstable angina with fatal outcome: dynamic coronary thrombosis leading to infarction and/or sudden death. *Circulation* 1985; **71**: 699–708.

[7] Born GVR. Pathogenetic possibilities. In: Hugenholtz PG, Goldman BS, eds. *Unstable angina, current concepts and management*. Stuttgart: Schattauer Verlag, 1985; pp. 13–8.

[8] Gazes PC, Mobley EM, Farris HM et al. Preinfarction (unstable) angina - a prospective study - ten year follow-up. *Circulation* 1973; **48**: 331–7.

[9] Julian DG. The natural history of unstable angina. In: Hugenholtz PG, Goldman BS, eds. *Unstable angina, current concepts and management*. Stuttgart: Schattauer Verlag, 1985; pp. 65–70.

[10] Balakumaran K, Fioretti P, Brower RW et al. Unstable angina and myocardial revascularisation. In: Hugenholtz PG, Goldman BS, eds. *Unstable angina, current concepts and management*. Stuttgart: Schattauer Verlag, 1985; pp. 309–7.

[11] Lubsen J, Tijssen JGP, Kerkkamp HJJ et al. Report of the Holland Interuniversity Nifedipine-metoprolol Trial (HINT) Research Group. Early treatment of unstable angina at the coronary care unit: A randomised, double blind, placebo controlled comparison of recurrent ischaemia in patients with nifedipine or metoprolol or both. *Br Heart J* 1986 **56**: 400–13.

[12] Goldman BS, Weisel RD, Christakis G et al. Predictors of outcome after coronary artery bypass graft surgery for stable and unstable angina pectoris. In: Hugenholtz PG, Goldman BS, eds. *Unstable angina, current concepts and management*. Stuttgart: Schattauer Verlag, 1985; pp. 319–30.

[13] Conti CR. Unstable angina: Thoughts on pathogenesis. In: Hugenholtz PG, Goldman BS, eds. *Unstable angina, current concepts and management*. Stuttgart: Schattauer Verlag, 1985; pp. 55–64.

[14] Simoons ML, Serruys PW, van den Brand M et al. Improved survival after early thrombolysis in acute myocardial infarction. A randomized trial conducted by the Interuniversity Cardiology Institute in the Netherlands. *Lancet* 1985; ii: 578–82.

[15] Serruys PW, Simoons ML, Suryapranata H et al. Preservation of global and regional left ventricular function after early thrombolysis in acute myocardial infarction. *J Am Coll Cardiol* 1986; **7**: 729–42.

[16] Cowley MJ, Disciascio G, Vetrovec GW.
Coronary thrombus in unstable angina: Angiographic observation and clinical relevance. In: Hugenholtz PG, Goldman BS, eds. *Unstable angina, current concepts and management*. Stuttgart: Schattauer Verlag, 1985; pp. 95–102.

[17] Bresnahan DR, Davis JL, Holmes DR Jr *et al*.
Angiographic occurrence and clinical correlates of intraluminal coronary artery thrombus: Role of unstable angina.
J Am Coll Cardiol 1985; **6**: 285–9.

[18] Zack PM, Ischinger T, Aker UT *et al*.
The occurrence of angiographically detected intracoronary thrombus in patients with unstable angina pectoris.
Am Heart J 1984; **108**: 1408–11.

[19] Parratt JR.
Coronary vascular endothelium, spasm and reperfusion arrhythmias; experimental approaches. In: Hugenholtz PG, Goldman BS, eds. *Unstable angina, current concepts and management*. Stuttgart: Schattauer Verlag, 1985; pp. 19–28.

[20] Furchgott RF.
Role of endothelium in responses of vascular smooth muscle.
Circ Res 1983; **53**: 557–3.

[21] The MIAMI Trial Research Group.
Metoprolol in acute myocardial infarction (MIAMI).
Eur Heart J 1985; **6**: 199–226.

[22] Kudoch Y, Maxwell MP, Hearse DJ *et al*.
Inability of metoprolol to achieve a sustained limitation of infarct size in 24 hours after coronary artery embolization in the closed chest dog.
J Cardiovasc Pharmacol 1984; **6**: 1201–9.

[23] Chamberlain DA.
In: Proceedings of the MIAMI Trial, section 1. *The Current Status of Beta Blockers in Acute Myocardial Infarction*. Auckland: Adis Press, 1985; pp. 4–14.

[24] Hugenholtz PG.
The calcium antagonists. In: *Handbook of Experimental Pharmacology, Vol. 76*. Berlin: Springer Verlag, 1985; pp. 459–538.

[25] Duncker DJ, Hartog JM, Hugenholtz PG *et al*.
The effects of nisoldipine (Bay K 5522) on cardiovascular performance and regional blood flow in pentobarbital-anaesthetized pigs with or without beta-adrenoceptor blockade.
Br J Pharmacol 1986; **88**: 9–18.

[26] Stone PH, Antman EM.
Use of the calcium channel blocking agents in unstable angina pectoris and acute myocardial infarction. In: Stone PH, Antman EM, eds. *Calcium Blocking Agents in the Treatment of Cardiovascular Disorders*. Mount Kisco, NY: Futura Publishing Company, 1983; pp. 321–46.

[27] Hugenholtz PG, Michels HR, Serruys PW *et al*.
Nifedipine in the treatment of unstable angina, coronary spasm and myocardial ischemia.
Am J Cardiol 1979; **47**: 163–75.

[28] Gerstenblith G, Ouyang P, Aschuff SC *et al*.
Nifedipine in unstable angina: A double blind randomized trial.
N Engl J Med 1982; **306**: 885–94.

[29] Parodi O, Maseri A, Simonetti D.
Management of unstable angina by verapamil.
Br Heart J 1979; **41**: 167–73.

[30] Gottlieb SO, Ouyang P, Achuff SC *et al*.
Acute nifedipine withdrawal: Consequences of preoperative and late cessation of therapy in patients with prior unstable angina.
J Am Coll Cardiol 1984; **4**: 382–8.

[31] Braunwald E.
Introduction: Calcium channel blockers.
Am J Cardiol 1980; **46**: 1045.

[32] Moses JW, Wertheimer JH, Bodenheimer MM *et al*.
Efficacy of nifedipine in rest angina, refractory to propranolol and nitrates in patients with obstructive coronary artery disease.
Ann Intern Med 1981; **94**: 425–32.

[33] Hugenholtz PG, Serruys PW, Fleckenstein A *et al*.
Why Ca^{2+} antagonists will be most useful before or during early myocardial ischemia and not after infarction has been established.
Eur Heart J 1986; **7**: 270–8.

[34] Hugenholtz PG, Lichtlen P, van der Giessen W *et al*.
On a possible role of calcium antagonists in atherosclerosis. A personal view.
Eur Heart J 1986; **7**: 546–60.

[35] Cairns JA, Gent M, Singer J *et al*.
Aspirin, sulfinpyrazone, or both in unstable angina. Results of a Canadian multicenter trial.
N Engl J Med 1985; **313**: 1369–75.

[36] Cairns JA.
Aspirin in unstable angina [Comment].
Cardiovascular Medicine 1986; **5**: 1–4.

[37] Lewis HD, Davis JW, Archibald DG et al.
Protective effects of aspirin against acute myocardial infarction and death in men with unstable angina: Results of a Veterans' Administration Cooperative Study.
N Engl J Med 1983; 309: 396–403.

[38] Becker AE.
Unstable angina revisited, the pathologist's view. In: Hugenholtz PG, Goldman BS, eds. Unstable angina, current concepts and management. Stuttgart: Schattauer Verlag, 1985; pp. 29–37.

[39] Meyer J, Erbel E, Schmitz HJ et al.
PTCA as emergency treatment in unstable angina. In: Hugenholtz PG, Goldman BS, eds. Unstable angina, current concepts and management. Stuttgart: Schattauer Verlag, 1985; pp. 239–52.

[40] Cohn LH, O'Neill A, Collins JJ Jr.
Surgical treatment of unstable angina up to 1984. In: Hugenholtz PG, Goldman BS, eds. Unstable angina, current concepts and management. Stuttgart: Schattauer Verlag, 1985; pp. 279–86.

[41] Haalebos M, Serruys PW, Luyten V et al.
Early coronary bypass surgery following unsuccessful percutaneous transluminal coronary angioplasty. In: Hugenholtz PG, Goldman BS, eds. Unstable angina, current concepts and management. Stuttgart: Schattauer Verlag, 1985; pp. 253–64.

[42] Ganz P, Alexander RW.
New insights into the cellular mechanisms of vasospasm.
Am J Cardiol 1985; 56: 11E–15E.

NEW AGENTS IN ANGINA

[1] Effects of L-carnitine on exercise tolerance in chronic stable angina: a multicenter, double-blind, randomized, placebo controlled crossover study.
Cherchi A, Lai C, Angelino F et al, Univ Cagliari, Cagliari, Italy.
Int J Clin Pharmacol Ther Toxicol 1985; 23: 569–72.

[2] Effects of coenzyme Q_{10} on exercise tolerance in chronic stable angina pectoris.
Kamikawa T, Kobayashi A, Yamashita T, Hayashi H, Yamazaki N, Hamamatsu Univ Sch Med, Hamamatsu, Japan.
Am J Cardiol 1985; 56: 247–51.

Comment. The rate of oxidation of fatty acids is decreased during hypoxia, and there is a consequent increase in long chain fatty acyl levels which induces an impairment of adenine nucleotide translocase activity responsible for the transfer of adenine nucleotide into and out of the mitochondria. l-Carnitine is the physiological carrier of acyl groups across the mitochondrial membrane; administration of this substance can reduce the concentration of acyl CoA by producing acyl carnitine which reduces the inhibition of adenine translocase. Moreover, the reduction of tissue carnitine levels observed during myocardial ischemia could cause an increase in ischemic damage by accelerating the accumulation of fatty acyl CoA esters. In a study of 44 men with chronic stable angina, l-carnitine (1 g twice daily) was administered in a double-blind, randomized, placebo-controlled crossover manner [1]. Each treatment period was for four weeks; an exercise test was performed at the end of a 10-day wash-out period with placebo and at the end of each treatment period. The mean exercise work load and the number of Watts to the onset of angina was found to increase after l-carnitine when compared with placebo. ST-segment depression was reduced after l-carnitine when compared with placebo at both maximum work load and maximum work load common to l-carnitine and placebo. Freedom from angina occurred in 22.7% of patients treated with l-carnitine compared with only 9.1% of those on placebo. Resting and exercise blood pressure, heart rate and the double product were not found to have been affected by the administration of *l*-carnitine. The results of this study demonstrate that treatment with *l*-carnitine can increase exercise tolerance and decrease the ECG indices of myocardial ischemia in patients with effort-induced stable angina pectoris.

Co-enzyme Q_{10} (CoQ_{10}), a lipid-soluble benzoquinone, is an essential component of the mitochondrial membrane. It is an intermediate between NADH or succinate dehydrogenase and cytochrome b in the human mitochondrial respiratory chain. There is evidence to suggest that CoQ_{10} may play an important part in the maintenance of normal heart function by regulating the energy metabolism of the myocardium. There have been other reports of the exogenous application of CoQ_{10} which suggest that it may be efficacious in the treatment of patients with coronary artery disease and exertional angina pectoris. Twelve patients with stable angina pectoris entered a randomized double-blind placebo-controlled crossover trial to examine the effects of CoQ_{10} (150 mg/day in three doses) on exercise performance [2]. Treatment was for four weeks. Although during treatment with CoQ_{10} the number of anginal attacks decreased, as did the quantity of nitroglycerin tablets consumed, these differences were not found to be significant. However, both exercise time and time to ST-segment depression (1 mm) were significantly increased during CoQ_{10} therapy ($P<0.05$ and $P<0.01$, respectively). It is clear that further investigations into the pathophysiological role of CoQ_{10} in angina, and the possible therapeutic implications this may have, are required.

PERCUTANEOUS TRANSLUMINAL CORONARY ANGIOPLASTY

Review: SPENCER B. KING III, JOHN S. DOUGLAS JR, GARY S. ROUBIN

The progress that has been made in percutaneous transluminal coronary angioplasty (PTCA) over the past few years has come as a result of increased operator experience, improvements in methods and equipment for performing the procedure, clinical research into the methodology of PTCA and prospective trials addressing the problems of restenosis. Following Gruentzig's development of PTCA in 1977 [1], experience in the procedure was so limited that almost all progress was able to be communicated at the semi-annual demonstration courses in Zurich in the early 1980s. At present, there are nearly 1000 operators in the USA alone, who performed an estimated 100 000 PTCA procedures in 1985 – half the number of coronary bypass operations performed in the same year. It is estimated that by 1990 PTCA and coronary bypass surgery will be performed in equal numbers.

The important questions now to be addressed are: (i) which patients should receive PTCA; (ii) who should be performing the procedure; (iii) what the correct roles are of PTCA and coronary bypass surgery; (iv) whether, on the basis of recent improvements in equipment and experience, the indications for the procedure can safely be broadened; and (v) what the long-term outlook is for patients selected for PTCA.

Selection
Selection for PTCA should be based on the demonstration of myocardial ischemia, the

presence of a lesion (or lesions) which can successfully be dilated, the expectation of an acceptable complication risk and a reasonable chance of continued success. Whereas most patients undergoing PTCA are symptomatic and would otherwise be candidates for coronary artery bypass graft surgery, other patients, i.e. those with silent ischemia documented by exercise stress-testing, may also be eligible. The potential benefit from the procedure must be weighed against the associated risk.

There is general agreement that patients with single-vessel disease who undergo revascularization should first be considered for PTCA. The controversy is over which patients with multi-vessel disease should also have PTCA. Acute complications are more common in multi-vessel disease, and long-term success is not equal to that found in single-vessel disease. There are, however, many patients with multi-vessel disease who can be treated successfully with PTCA with sustained improvement.

In over 6000 PTCA procedures performed at Emory University Hospital, mortality in 4500 cases of single-vessel disease was less than 0.1%, while in 1500 multi-vessel cases it was 0.5%. Restenosis rates in multi-vessel disease have been encouraging, since the per-lesion restenosis has been somewhat less than for single-vessel disease and the per-patient restenosis has not been significantly higher for those multi-vessel disease patients who have been selected. In the past, PTCA for multi-vessel disease was limited primarily to those patients who had discrete lesions of two or more arteries which had a reasonably high chance of PTCA success, and which did not pose a major threat to global left-ventricular function if acute closure occurred. PTCA was selected over coronary bypass surgery if a similar revascularization was possible with PTCA, leaving most patients with chronic total occlusion and diffuse disease, as well as all patients with left main stem disease, to be referred for bypass surgery. Gradually, there has been a shift towards PTCA for other multi-vessel disease patients, where the 'culprit' lesion or lesions (those believed to be responsible for the angina) have been dilated, leaving the less severe lesions and collateralized total occlusions undilated.

It remains unclear whether such cases of multi-vessel disease are best treated by PTCA or coronary bypass surgery. A prospective randomized trial has been funded by the National Institutes of Health, to be conducted at Emory, comparing PTCA and coronary bypass surgery in multi-vessel disease [2]. Another multicenter trial will follow [3]. Until the results of these trials have been evaluated, PTCA for multi-vessel disease should be limited to those low-risk patients who have a good chance of primary success without major complications.

PTCA Training and Performance
Although most physicians performing angioplasty have come from the ranks of trained angiographers without formal PTCA training, programs have now been established in the USA for formal training in PTCA after completion of the cardiology fellowship and angiography training. Demonstration courses are of significant value as an introduction to PTCA and even more useful as a continuing education device for experienced operators, but should not be construed as a substitute for 'hands-on' formal training. In our center, we consider one year's training in PTCA following a three-year cardiology fellowship to be adequate for the independent performance of the procedure. Only through performance of a large number of cases and through constant exposure to patients treated by medical therapy and coronary artery bypass surgery can one achieve

expertise in the selection for and performance of PTCA. There is no place for PTCA outside a surgical center.

Complications

Acute closure of the dilated artery is the principal complication of PTCA. Acute closure is defined as that resulting in cardiac ischemia, requiring either emergency catheterization to document and reverse closure or emergency coronary bypass surgery. If uncorrected, it leads to acute myocardial infarction or death. The NHLBI Registry initially reported a major complication rate of 9.1% [4,5]. As experience has increased, the rate has decreased to 5.8% in the 1985/86 cohort [6]. Complications in our first 3500 patients were reviewed by Bredlau *et al* in 1984 [7]. Only 19% of these patients had multi-vessel disease; prior myocardial infarction was present in 28% and unstable angina in 50%. Major complications occurred in 4.9%. With the shift towards treating more complex multi-vessel disease patients, the complication rate in 1985/86 increased to 5.7%. Mortality increased from 0.1% in the 1980–1984 series to 0.4% in the 1985/86 series.

The factors that predict the likelihood of acute closure have now been identified. With the more primitive equipment available in the early days of angioplasty, acute closure was found to be related to: female gender; unstable angina; right coronary artery dilatation; severe, eccentric and long stenoses; multi-vessel disease; calcification; and thrombus [5,7,8]. Many of these complications were related to the equipment used and, as techniques have changed [9], so have the predictors of acute closure. Ellis *et al* have reviewed the experience with acute closure at our hospital and found the independent preprocedural risk factors (ranked in order of importance) to be: length of lesion; female gender; a bend in the artery at the area of the stenosis; branch point location of stenosis; thrombus at the site of dilatation; and other stenoses in the same vessel [10]. Other factors found to be related to acute reclosure were: multi-vessel disease; hypertension; percentage of stenosis prior to PTCA; pre-PTCA gradient; and eccentricity of the lesion.

Powerful predictors of acute reclosure after PTCA have emerged, the most important being the presence of high translesional gradients and intimal tear or dissection. Oversizing of the balloon catheter can lead to increased incidence of dissection and acute closure rates. This was once felt to be the reason for the higher numbers of complications in women, although a recent analysis of complications indicates that women do have a higher acute reclosure rate, even when treated with balloons that have been properly sized.

The outcome of acute closure depends on the amount of myocardium served by the artery, the presence or absence of collaterals to that artery and the status of the remaining arteries and left-ventricular function. In a review of our experience with 215 acute reclosures, one-half of the acute closure cases occurred in the laboratory and one-half after patients had returned to their hospital rooms [11]. Among the latter, 42% were returned to the catheterization laboratory for attempted repeat dilatation; however, 69% of repeat closures required emergency bypass surgery. Factors associated with acute infarction or death after repeat closure were ST-segment elevation, a need for intra-aortic balloon counterpulsation and multi-vessel disease.

The risk of death following acute closure was also reviewed for the combined series of almost 9000 procedures from Emory University Hospital and the San Francisco

Heart Institute [11]. The most important predictors of death were: female gender; hypertension; left-ventricular hypertrophy; a large area of jeopardized myocardium; hypotension following closure; and prior myocardial infarction.

Long-Term Results

Restenosis following successful PTCA remains the major limiting factor for sustained success. Although reporting methods differ, it appears that the average restenosis rate for native coronary artery angioplasty remains approximately 25% [12–17]. Restenosis has been shown to result from a fibrocellular neointimal proliferation which partially fills the arterial lumen [18]. This process tends to reach a point of significant obstruction at between two and four months following the procedure. Angiographically, the recurrent stenosis is in the same location, with the same degree of obstruction as the original lesion [13]. If no significant restenosis has occurred at six months, the risk of restenosis is markedly reduced. A recent review of the patients treated by Gruentzig in Zurich, however, showed that a restenosis rate of between 7% and 15% occurs late (2–7 years after PTCA) [19].

A number of factors influence the likelihood of restenosis: patients with unstable angina, a short history of angina and total occlusion have a high restenosis rate [17]. Also, patients with total occlusion who have evidence of thrombus have a higher restenosis rate that those who do not [17,20]. These differences seem to point towards more aggressive restenosis in early and active atherosclerotic lesions than in old chronic stable lesions.

The location of the lesions significantly influences the chance of recurrence: restenosis of the left anterior descending artery is more common than of the right coronary artery, which is in turn more common than restenosis of the circumflex artery. The proximal left anterior descending artery shows a great propensity for restenosis at its origin from the left main stem [21]. Ostial lesions are structured differently from lesions in the shaft of an artery, and the right coronary artery ostium has a restenosis rate approaching 50% [22]. Vein grafts pose another problem: the distal vein graft anastomosis to the coronary artery has been found to restenose rarely, while the mid-portion of the graft or proximal anastomosis has a high rate of restenosis [23].

The initial effects of the procedure also influence restenosis. For example, a low final transluminal gradient and a low final diameter stenosis both diminish the chance of restenosis. The presence of an intimal tear, as indicated earlier, is a potent predictor of acute closure syndrome, but is actually associated with a *lower* restenosis rate if no in-hospital complication occurs. This apparent paradox – of more intimal disruption resulting in less restenosis – remains unresolved.

Modification of Restenosis

Many approaches to modifying the rate of restenosis have been tried, unfortunately with limited success. Coumadin (sodium warfarin) anticoagulation was used in the initial Zurich cohort [1]; the restenosis rate at six months was 30%. Later, Coumadin anticoagulation was compared with aspirin antiplatelet therapy, and no advantage for anticoagulation was found [24]. Antiplatelet agents comprising aspirin with or without dipyridamole are now used routinely, and prospective trials of various antiplatelet programs are underway. However, since most of these dose schedules have been used by one center or another without any dramatic effect on restenosis, more potent antiplatelet agents may be required for this approach to have a favorable impact on restenosis.

Other pharmacologic approaches to restenosis have been tried. Dextran was originally used, but has been abandoned by most. One study of dextran showed no effect on acute closure, and the restenosis data are only now being accumulated [25]. Heparin is used by some groups for 24 hours after PTCA, and a prospective trial of heparin therapy in the same early post-PTCA period is underway. The non-anticoagulant subfragments of heparin have an antimitogenic activity which may influence restenosis. Calcium antagonists are generally used for prevention of spasm and for a protective effect from ischemia during PTCA [26]. The effect of calcium antagonists on restenosis was tested, but no advantage over placebo was found [27].

Several procedure-related factors have been tested. The balloon size to artery size ratio has been evaluated. Schmitz et al, in a small retrospective study, found significantly less restenosis when the balloon diameter was greater than the artery being dilated [28]. A prospective study at Emory University Hospital randomized the usually selected balloon size with the next-larger balloon size [29]. A continuation of that study indicated that there was more emergency bypass surgery required with the larger balloon size. The data are not yet complete, but no dramatic difference in restenosis rates has been seen. Higher balloon pressures have been associated with improved initial results [30], but higher restenosis rates have been seen with the use of high pressure [31,32]. It is difficult to make valid deductions from these retrospective studies, since harder lesions require higher pressures.

Prolonged balloon inflation [33] was suggested as one means of expressing more liquid from the plaque and hence improving results. Several methods for prolonging balloon inflation are being tried, including distal perfusion of oxygenated fluorocarbon or of blood, or the use of flow-through catheters. It is unclear, however, whether inflations longer than 45 seconds will reduce restenosis.

Analysis of Long-Term Results

Long-term follow-up results of PTCA patients are now becoming available. The 169 patients undergoing PTCA in Zurich before 1981 have been followed from five to eight years: cumulative survival for the 133 successfully treated patients is 93% at six years, and cardiac survival is 96% [19]. Of the initially successfully treated patients, 74% have exhibited maintained patency of the recanalized vessel without the need for coronary bypass surgery; 75% were asymptomatic at last follow-up. As all the Zurich patients were symptomatic and were considered candidates for bypass surgery prior to PTCA and as many as 40% of them had multi-vessel disease, these long-term follow-up results can be considered favorable. Follow-up of larger cohorts of patients is underway, and 468 patients treated at our hospital in 1981 show similar results [34]: excluding cases of repeat PTCA, 68% were free of myocardial infarction, death or coronary bypass surgery at 4.5 years, and cumulative survival was 96%.

PTCA in Conjunction with Thrombolysis for Acute Myocardial Infarction

PTCA has been used as a follow-up therapy to thrombolysis, and as primary therapy without thrombolysis, in the setting of evolving acute myocardial infarction. If neither intracoronary nor intravenous thrombolysis is successful in opening the vessel, then PTCA can be helpful in an additional percentage of patients.

An important question is whether PTCA should be used in the evolving phase of acute myocardial infarction, or as a follow-up therapy hours or days after thrombolysis. This point is being investigated at present in an addendum to the thrombolysis in myocardial infarction (TIMI) trial.

The case for urgent PTCA includes: a greater chance for reperfusion; more complete restoration of the coronary flow reserve; and avoidance of high levels of circulating thrombolytic agents. The case for trying thrombolysis first includes the ability to administer the agent and achieve potential reperfusion earlier and avoidance of the need for sophisticated catheterization equipment. Delaying PTCA may also allow more complete resolution of thrombus, thereby reducing acute reclosure of the artery and late restenosis following PTCA.

The best strategy must include very early reperfusion, in order to salvage significant amounts of myocardium. Therefore, early reperfusion administered by paramedics, followed within days by semielective PTCA, may become the treatment of the future. Current studies should shed additional light on the subject.

Future Developments

Many questions regarding PTCA technique and methods of obtaining the best initial outcome have been answered, and factors relating to acute closure and restenosis have been identified. New methods are now being developed to address the problems of opening chronic total occlusions and severe, tortuous and distal stenoses. Uninflated balloon dimensions have been reduced significantly. Balloons have now been placed on guidewires, so that almost any lesion that can be crossed with a wire can also be crossed with a balloon. Stronger balloon materials will allow adequate pressure to open these lesions. Methods for dealing with acute closure, of which intracoronary stents hold perhaps the most promise, are being developed. The bailout catheter and the newly developed flow-through catheters may also reduce the risk of acute closure. Potential yet speculative advances in the treatment of severe coronary atherosclerotic lesions include: a hot-tip catheter for crossing very tight or totally occluded vessels; vaporization by directly applied laser energy; and heating of the vessel wall by laser energy to weld layers back together.

The restenosis problem is being investigated, with more potent antiplatelet agents to attack thromboxane receptors in the vessel wall, and the use of antimitogenic agents. Other approaches, such as vascular stents and heat coagulation of the vessel wall, as well as mechanical atherectomy catheters and rotating high-speed plaque-destroying devices, are under investigation.

The future for interventional coronary work looks bright, but many questions remain to be resolved.

References

[1] Gruentzig A, Senning A, Siegenthaler W.
Non-operative dilatation of coronary artery stenosis: Percutaneous transluminal coronary angioplasty (PTCA).
N Engl J Med 1979; **301**: 61–8.

[2] Comparison of PTCA and CABG in patients with multivessel disease. National Heart, Lung and Blood Institute RO 1HL 33965-01A1; 1986.

[3] Bypass angioplasty reperfusion investigation (BARI).

[4] Dorros G, Cowley M, Janke L, Kelsey S, Mullin S, Van Raden M.
In-hospital mortality rate in the National Heart, Lung and Blood Institute Percutaneous Transluminal Coronary Angioplasty Registry.
Am J Cardiol 1984; **53**: 17C–21C.

[5] Cowley M, Dorros G, Kelsey S, Van Raden M, Detre K.
Acute coronary events associated with percutaneous transluminal coronary angioplasty.
Am J Cardiol 1984; **53**: 12C–16C.

[6] Detre K, Kelsey S.
NHLBI PTCA Registry. University of Pittsburgh Data Coordinating Center Publication, Nov. 1986.

[7] Bredlau C, Roubin G, Leimgruber P, Douglas J, King S, Gruentzig A.
In-hospital morbidity and mortality in patients undergoing elective coronary angioplasty.
Circulation 1985; **72**: 1044–52.

[8] Mabin T, Holmes D, Smith H *et al.*
Intracoronary thrombus: Role in coronary occlusion complicating percutaneous transluminal coronary angioplasty.
J Am Coll Cardiol 1985; **5**: 198–202.

[9] Anderson H, Roubin G, Leimgruber P, Douglas J, King S, Gruentzig A.
Primary angiographic success rates of percutaneous transluminal coronary angioplasty.
Am J Cardiol 1985; **56**: 712–7.

[10] Ellis S, Roubin G, Weintraub W, Cox W, Douglas J, King S.
Acute closure after elective native vessel PTCA: Risk factors and pre-procedural estimation of risk [Abstract].
Circulation 1986; **74**: II–194.

[11] Anderson H, Cox W, Roubin G, Weintraub W, Douglas J, King S.
Mortality of acute closure following coronary angioplasty (PTCA) [Abstract].
J Am Coll Cardiol 1987 (in press).

[12] Holmes DR, Vlietstra R, Smith H *et al.*
Restenosis after percutaneous transluminal coronary angioplasty (PTCA): A report from the PTCA Registry of the National Heart, Lung and Blood Institute.
Am J Cardiol 1984; **53**: 77C.

[13] Meier B, King S, Gruentzig A *et al.*
Repeat coronary angioplasty.
J Am Coll Cardiol 1984; **4**: 463–6.

[14] Kaltenbach M, Kober G, Scherer D, Vallbracht C.
Rezidivhäufigkeit nach erfolgreicher Ballondilatation von Kranzarterienstenosen.
Z Kardiol 1984; **73**: 161.

[15] David P, Renkin J, Morris A, Dagoisse V, Guiteras P, Bourassa M.
Can patient selection and optimization of technique reduce the rate of restenosis after percutaneous transluminal coronary angioplasty?
Am J Cardiol 1984; **3**: 470.

[16] Mabin T, Holmes D, Smith H *et al.*
Follow-up clinical results of patients undergoing percutaneous transluminal coronary angioplasty.
Circulation 1985; **71**: 754.

[17] Leimgruber P, Roubin G, Hollman J *et al.*
Restenosis after successful coronary angioplasty in patients with single vessel disease.
Circulation 1986; **73**: 710–7.

[18] Hollman J, Austin G, Gruentzig A, Douglas J, King S.
Coronary artery spasm at the site of angioplasty in the first two months after successful percutaneous transluminal coronary angioplasty.
J Am Coll Cardiol 1983; **2**: 1039–45.

[19] Gruentzig A, King S, Siegenthaler W, Schlumpf M.
Long-term follow-up of percutaneous transluminal coronary angioplasty.
Submitted for publication.

[20] Mabin T, Holmes D, Smith H *et al.*
Intracoronary thrombus: Role of coronary occlusion complication percutaneous transluminal coronary angioplasty.
J Am Coll Cardiol 1985; **5**: 198–202.

[21] Whitworth H, Pilcher G, Roubin G, Gruentzig A.
Do proximal lesions involving the origin of the left anterior descending artery have a higher restenosis rate after coronary angioplasty (PTCA)?
Circulation 1985; **72** (Suppl 3): III–398.

[22] Topol E, Ellis S, Fishman J et al.
Multicenter study of percutaneous transluminal angioplasty for right coronary artery ostial stenosis.
Submitted for publication.

[23] Douglas JR, Gruentzig AR, King SB et al.
Percutaneous transluminal coronary angioplasty in patients with prior coronary bypass surgery.
J Am Coll Cardiol 1983; 2: 745–54.

[24] Thornton M, Gruentzig A, Hollman J, King S, Douglas J.
Coumadin and aspirin in prevention of recurrence after transluminal coronary angioplasty: A randomized study.
Circulation 1984; 69: 721–7.

[25] Bredlau C, Hoffmeister J, Brown J, Douglas J, King S.
Is routine Dextran infusion during coronary angioplasty (PTCA) necessary?
Circulation 1985; 72: III–398.

[26] Serruys P, Van Den Brand M, Brower R.
Regional cardioplegic and protective effect of nifedipine during PTCA.
Circulation 1983; 68: III–142.

[27] Whitworth H, Gruentzig A, Hollman J, Galan K, Gershon L.
Effect of nifedipine on recurrent stenosis after percutaneous transluminal coronary angioplasty (PTCA).
J Am Coll Cardiol 1985; 5: 524.

[28] Schmitz H, Van Essen R, Meyer J, Effort S.
The role of balloon size for acute and late angiographic results in coronary angioplasty.
Circulation 1984; 70: II–295.

[29] Roubin G, Leimgruber P, Whitworth H et al.
Influence of balloon size on outcome after coronary angioplasty (PTCA).
Circulation 1985; 72: III–400.

[30] Meier B, Gruentzig A, King S et al.
Higher balloon dilatation pressure in coronary angioplasty.
Am Heart J 1984; 107: 619–22.

[31] Shaw R, Myler R, Fishman-Rosen J, Murphy M, Stertzer S, Topol E.
Clinical and morphologic factors in prediction of restenosis after multiple vessel angioplasty.
J Am Coll Cardiol 1986; 7: 63A.

[32] Marantz T, Williams D, Rhinehart S, Gewirtz H, Most A.
Predictors of restenosis after successful coronary angioplasty.
Circulation 1984; 70: 176.

[33] Kaltenbach M, Koberg G.
Can prolonged application of pressure improve the results of coronary angioplasty (PTCA)? [Abstract].
Circulation 1982; 66: II–123.

[34] Talley D, Hurst J, Weintraub W, Roubin G, Douglas J, King S.
Late clinical outcome of 428 consecutive patients who had percutaneous coronary angioplasty attempted in 1981 [Abstract].
Circulation 1986; 74: II–280.

LASER ANGIOPLASTY

[1] Percutaneous laser thermal angioplasty: initial clinical results with a laser probe in total peripheral artery occlusions.
Cumberland DC, Sanborn TA, Taylor DI et al, Northern Gen Hosp, Sheffield, UK.
Lancet 1986; i: 1457–9.

[2] Histopathology after Nd-YAG laser percutaneous transluminal angioplasty of peripheral arteries.
Geschwind H, Fabre M, Chaitman BR et al, St Louis Univ Med Sch, St Louis, MO, USA.
J Am Coll Cardiol 1986; 8: 1089–95.

[3] Experimental arteriosclerosis treated by argon ion and neodymium-YAG laser endarterectomy.
Eugene J, McColgan SJ, Pollock ME, Hammer-Wilson M, Moore-Jeffries EW, Berns MW, VA Med Cent, Long Beach, CA, USA.
Circulation 1985; 72 (Suppl II): 200–6.

[4] Factors contributing to perforations resulting from laser coronary angioplasty: observations in an intact human postmortem preparation of intraoperative laser coronary angioplasty.
Isner JM, Donaldson RF, Funai JR et al, Tufts-New England Med Cent, Boston, MA, USA.
Circulation 1985; 72 (Suppl II): 191–9.

[5] Coronary artery disobliteration by laser: a peroperative study (In French).
Fournial G, Choy D, Marco J et al, Hôp Purpan, Toulouse, France.
Arch Mal Coeur 1985; **78**: 1061–5.

[6] Vaporization of atherosclerotic plaques by spark erosion.
Slager CJ, Essed CE, Schuurbiers JCH, Bom N, Serruys PW, Meester GT, Erasmus Univ, Rotterdam, The Netherlands.
J Am Coll Cardiol 1985; **5**: 1382–6.

[7] Intraoperative coronary angioscopy. Technique and results in the initial 58 patients.
Chaux A, Lee ME, Blanche C et al, Cedars-Sinai Med Cent, Los Angeles, CA, USA.
J Thorac Cardiovasc Surg 1986; **92**: 972–6.

Comment. Laser angioplasty divides into two distinct types: the laser energy can either be used as a source of heat or it can be used directly to vaporize the constituents of an atheromatous plaque. The first has achieved some clinical success, but the second will remain a research technique until the problems of vessel perforation can be overcome. The successful application of laser thermal angioplasty has been described by Cumberland et al [1], who used a metal-tipped laser fiber during angioplasty of femoral/popliteal or iliac artery occclusions in 56 patients. Primary success was attained in 50 (89%) of the total occlusions, and thereby provided a channel for subsequent balloon dilatation. Prior to the procedure, 18 of the lesions treated had been adjudged untreatable using conventional angioplasty; four of the six failures occurred in this group of patients. One case of vessel perforation and two instances of entry into the vessel wall could be directly attributed to the use of the thermal laser probe; there were no sequelae to these complications. Distal thrombosis occurred in one non-heparinized patient and required therapy with local streptokinase, and there were two re-occlusions and one transient peripheral embolic episode within 24 hours of the procedure.

The effects of laser energy directly aimed at arterial walls is described by Geschwind et al [2], who performed laser recanalization of occluded femoral or popliteal arteries in 12 patients using a continuous wave neodymium yttrium aluminium garnet (Nd-YAG) laser with a specially designed catheter delivery system and cooling blood perfusate. They report on the histological findings in two of these patients. Specimens of the laser-irradiated arterial segments were obtained two and four weeks after the procedure. In the first patient, thermal injury to the inner quarter of the arterial wall was apparent; vacuolization was present and a rim of carbonization occupied 10% of the width of the arterial lumen. There was no thrombus formation. In the second patient, thermal injury was apparent at the crater site, and vacuolization was present in the intimal fibrous tissue. There were no fibrin deposits, atherosclerotic debris or thrombi at the intimal arterial edge. Samples investigated at four weeks showed new fibrous intimal tissue without endothelialization in some of the heavily calcified tissue sections. In areas where plaques were not calcified, re-endothelialization had occurred with only minimal damage to the surrounding tissue. No medial or elastic fibre disruption could be observed and no aneurysmal dilatation had occurred. Thus, histological findings at two and four weeks after laser irradiation showed there to be thermal injury of the inner quarter of the arterial vessel wall, but no evidence of thrombus formation.

Eugene et al [3] have shown that the argon laser is superior to the Nd-YAG laser in the aortae of 16 rabbits. Argon ion laser endarterectomy (8 rabbits) produced even depths of plaque removal and significantly better surfaces when compared with the

Nd-YAG laser (8 rabbits). Moreover, the argon ion energy was found to be readily absorbed by the atherosclerotic aortae whereas the Nd-YAG energy was transmitted to the surrounding tissues and produced thermal damage; perforation did not occur in any of the rabbits subjected to the argon ion laser, but 6 of 8 rabbits undergoing Nd-YAG laser endarterectomy suffered perforations.

The application of these techniques in coronary arteries is difficult. Isner *et al* [4] performed laser coronary angioplasty at 53 sites in 17 post-mortem hearts. Perforations were found to complicate laser angioplasty at 33 of the 53 sites; 29 of the 33 perforations were thermal. Perforation occurred at sites of extensive calcific deposits (21 of 33 instances) and at the origin of side branches (13 of 33 instances). In four cases, perforation was in part the result of excessive tortuosity of the artery. Fournial *et al* [5] report a preliminary study of the effects of an argon laser on the atheromatous coronary artery stenoses of 10 patients. The laser was used during coronary artery bypass grafting: 5 patients underwent laser therapy in association with coronary artery bypass grafting; 5 underwent laser therapy without distal bypass grafting. The immediate results showed a constant improvement (<25%) in the degree of stenosis. Angiography at 3 weeks revealed secondary occlusion in 88% of stenoses. Thus, although laser disobliteration of atheromatous plaques seems to be technically feasible *in vivo*, it is apparent that much clinical and experimental work remains to be done before this promising technique can be employed as a routine therapy in patients with coronary artery disease.

Two parallel developments that may help in the catheter treatment of arterial disease are spark erosion and fiberoptic angioscopy. Slager *et al* [6] describe a pulsed electrocardiogram R wave-triggered electrical spark erosion technique for the controlled vaporization of atherosclerotic plaques. The vaporization of fibrous and lipid plaques was achieved with minimal thermal side-effects in 30 aortic segments obtained from six human autopsy specimens. During preliminary trials *in vivo*, the method was found to be electrically safe in the coronary arteries of seven anesthetized pigs. The authors claim the advantages of this technique over laser irradiation are that it is simpler to perform and potentially easier to control.

Angioscopy enables the direct intraluminal visualization of coronary arteries, providing images with greater than 0.2 mm spatial resolution and excellent contrast resolution. Chaux *et al* [7] used ultrathin fiberoptic angioscopes (1.25–1.8 mm outer diameter) to visualize 81 native coronary arteries and 43 saphenous vein grafts in 58 patients during operation. The authors created a clear field of view by infusing crystalloid cardioplegic solution into the aortic root during cardiopulmonary bypass. To obtain high-quality images, sufficient cardioplegic solution must be perfused through the coronary circulation in order to displace all the blood, there must be adequate intraluminal illumination and the fiberoptic and lens system must be of a high quality. Angioscopic studies were incomplete in 14% of patients either because the aforementioned technical requisites were not fulfilled or because the scope lacked the necessary steerability. In 30% of patients, angioscopy revealed intimal flaps at vein-to-artery anastomoses, atheromatous plaques with adherent thrombi and hemorrhagic ulcerated plaques that had not been demonstrated on angiography. The procedure did not precipitate any serious complications in any of the patients, although in two patients a coronary intimal flap did develop proximal to the anastomosis during retrograde examination. Angioscopy was found to be safe in this group of patients and provided information potentially of clinical relevance. As the technique undergoes further development and refinement, it may prove valuable in conjunction with intraoperative balloon and laser angioplasty. In the future, it will be important to develop a light source that will enable the visualization of coronary arteries perfused with blood.

CURRENT ASPECTS OF CORONARY ARTERY SURGERY

Review: D. JOHN PARKER

The controversies raised by the publication of the Coronary Artery Surgery Study concerning the role of surgery in improving prognosis have diminished as careful comparative analysis with data from other trials has shown that the study fits into a particular part of the whole spectrum of clinical presentations of coronary artery disease, and does not necessarily contradict the European Coronary Artery Surgery Study. Other aspects of coronary artery disease have provoked increasing interest, including the relative roles of angioplasty and surgery, and thrombolysis and its implications for early follow-up revascularization, either by angioplasty or surgery. Also, the debate on the preferred conduit for coronary artery bypass grafting has been enlivened by the publication of several long-term follow-up reports of both vein grafts and the internal mammary artery.

The Trials: Effects of Surgery on Prognosis

The Coronary Artery Surgery Study (CASS) has continued to produce a large number of reports from the registry of 24 959 patients entered between July 1974 and May 1979. Many observational studies have been published, often using Cox proportional hazard analysis to try and evaluate complex situations. One such study examines the survival of patients undergoing surgery for severe angina pectoris [1]. The overall survival rate of surgical patients with class III and IV angina but with normal ventricular function was 92% at 5 years; among those electing to have medical treatment it was 74% ($P = 0.0001$). If ventricular function was abnormal, the respective figures were 82% and 52% at 5 years ($P = 0.0001$). These results contrast strongly with the much smaller but randomized CASS trial, emphasizing the importance of severity of angina in the assessment of management strategies.

Another important report from CASS looks at the effect of surgery and medical treatment on 1491 patients in the registry over the age of 65 [2]. Cox analysis suggested that surgery conferred an independent survival benefit ($P = 0.0001$); however, in a small group of patients with milder symptoms, similar to the CASS randomized subjects but older, no survival benefit was evident. These analyses emphasize the wide range of presentations of clinical coronary artery disease, and allow the randomized studies dealing with a limited aspect of this spectrum (mild to moderate angina in patients under 65 years of age) to be interpreted more usefully. This is highlighted by the eight-year survival of CASS randomized patients of 87% for the group assigned to surgery and 84% to medical treatment (not statistically different) [3].

Critical reviews have been provided by Kirklin *et al* [4], Rahimtoola [5] and Julian

[6]. All of the three major randomized studies, the Veterans Administration trial, the European Coronary Artery Surgery Study, and the CASS subset, have updated and extended their analyses.

The Veterans Administration trial has reported its long-term follow-up, averaging 11.5 years in 686 patients [7]. At seven years, survival was 70% in the medical and 77% in the surgical group ($P = 0.043$), but by 11 years survival was 57% and 58%, respectively ($P = 0.45$). Subgroup analysis, often criticized because of its prospective nature, revealed an angiographically high-risk group of three-vessel disease and impaired ventricular function, with a seven-year survival of 52% for medical and 76% for surgical assignment ($P = 0.002$); at 11 years, the figures were 38% and 50%, respectively ($P = 0.026$). A high-risk clinical subgroup showed similar differences. A low-risk clinical subgroup had better seven-year survival for medical than for surgical assignment, with 93% as against 82% ($P = 0.012$); furthermore, at 11 years, non-fatal myocardial infarction had occurred in 15% of surgical and 14% of medical patients ($P = 0.428$). However, the quality of surgery in this trial has been criticized in terms of operative mortality, the extent of revascularization undertaken and graft patency. These three factors compare very well now with surgical practice in the early 1970s. The loss after 11 years of an initial surgical benefit may not be relevant to patients who have undergone surgery more recently, particularly if an internal mammary artery graft has been used for bypassing obstruction in the left anterior descending coronary artery [8].

The European Coronary Artery Surgery Study has been updated as well, with survival statistics up to eight years [8]. This study, which was recruiting between 1973 and 1976, enrolled 768 patients (all men) under 65 years of age with an ejection fraction above 50%, but excluded single-vessel disease patients. Cross-over from medical to surgical treatment increased with time, and was more likely in patients with triple-vessel disease and class III angina (Canadian Cardiovascular Society). According to retrospective analysis, 42% of the patients were in class III angina, which makes this cohort considerably more symptomatic than the CASS subset and goes a long way towards explaining the different results of the two studies. The coronary angiography data have been reclassified, using a 75% as against 50% diameter reduction; this results in a significant change in distribution of one-, two- and three-vessel disease (to 27%, 47% and 26%, respectively).

Based on a criterion of 50% diameter reduction, survival was significantly better for the whole group and for three-vessel disease, but not for two-vessel disease. At eight years, survival in the surgical three-vessel disease group was 92%, as against 77% in the medical group ($P = 0.00015$), but in two-vessel disease the figures were 87% and 85%, respectively ($P = 0.20$).

From data based on the 75% stenosis classification criterion, the whole group had better survival at eight years ($P = 0.0022$), but single-vessel disease showed no benefit. Two-vessel disease had a surgical benefit at five years ($P = 0.045$) but had lost it by eight years ($P = 0.068$). However, if the two-vessel disease included a 75% proximal left anterior descending lesion there was definite benefit at both five years ($P = 0.005$) and ten years ($P = 0.013$). Thus, the earlier favorable results have been maintained with a benefit up to eight years. Non-fatal myocardial infarction at five years was 15% in the surgical as against 11% in the medical group ($P = 0.076$), and the difference is largely accounted for by an intraoperative infarction rate of 8%, included in the surgical figure.

110

The CASS randomized trial, including patients with mild angina or with no angina after a myocardial infarction, has been updated to an eight-year follow-up [3]. At eight years, this group of 780 patients, recruited between 1975 and 1979 inclusive, showed no benefit in terms of survival, with 87% for the surgical as against 84% for the medical group ($P = 0.14$). However, of the 160 patients who had an ejection fraction of between 35% and 50% (<35% was excluded from this trial), surgical patients had a seven-year survival of 88%, as against 65% in those undergoing medical treatment ($P = 0.009$).

Overall, the data suggest that most patients with severe angina – even those over the age of 65 and with poor ventricular function – will benefit prognostically from coronary artery bypass grafting. There is, however, no evidence to suggest that patients with single-vessel disease will derive any prognostic benefit.

For patients with mild (class I or II) angina, it seems that improvement is confined to patients with three-vessel disease or to those with two-vessel disease which includes proximal left anterior descending disease. This benefit is likely to be greater in cases where left-ventricular function is impaired. At present, there is no evidence of benefit in asymptomatic patients; however, specific groups, such as those with prior infarction or those with silent myocardial ischemia, will require prospective evaluation before conclusions can be drawn for asymptomatic patients in general.

The Choice of Conduit in Coronary Artery Surgery and its Management
Further information has recently become available about the long-term fate of different conduits used for coronary artery bypass surgery. Evidence favoring the use of the internal mammary artery, especially in the anterior descending position, is now more impressive, and at the same time more data have accumulated on the long-term complications of saphenous vein bypass grafting. Fuster and Chesebro have recently reviewed the subject of aortocoronary artery vein-graft disease [10], highlighting the initial thrombotic phase, which is followed by a phase of intimal hyperplasia lasting probably over the first year after surgery, and pointing to the later occlusions and narrowings due to atherosclerosis in the vein wall. The Montreal Heart Institute has updated its continuing review of the problems of graft atheroma [11]. This work confirms other reports that after the initial one-year period there appears to be a graft attrition rate of 1%–2% up to five years, which then more than doubles in the period 6–11 years. The Montreal group reports that by 11 years only 60% of the grafts are patent, and nearly half of these show evidence of some graft atheroma. Their sequential studies in a group of 278 patients, which included 40 with internal mammary artery grafts, confirmed the better patency of the internal mammary artery and its strong resistance to the development of atheroma. It is debatable whether current improved techniques for handling veins during harvesting and the use of preoperative antiplatelet therapy will affect these comparative results.

Data from the Cleveland Clinic, detailing a 10-year follow-up of nearly 6000 patients, approximately 40% of whom had internal mammary artery grafts to the left anterior descending artery, are of great interest [9]. It must be emphasized that this study was not randomized. Cox proportional hazard statistical analysis was used. The internal mammary artery was shown to be a superior conduit in terms of survival. In the group of patients (mean age, 52 years) with internal mammary artery grafts, 10-year survival was 86.6%, as against 75.9% for the saphenous vein group (mean age, 54 years)

111

($P = 0.0001$). This favorable effect was significant for the whole group and for one-, two- and three-vessel disease with varying degrees of left-ventricular dysfunction. Other important sequelae were influenced favorably by the use of internal mammary artery in the left anterior descending artery: less need for reoperation; reduced hospital admissions for cardiac causes; and a diminished incidence of late myocardial infarction. Several reviews have emphasized the importance of this artery [13,14]. Its extended use to sequential bypass grafting has been reported increasingly [15]. The 14-year experience with bilateral internal mammary artery grafting appears favorable [16].

Thus, at present, it seems appropriate to use the internal mammary artery as a preferred conduit, particularly for the left anterior descending coronary artery; provided the artery is of an acceptable size, its role can usefully be extended to sequential bypass grafting. In the younger patient, there is a good case for using both internal mammary arteries, and free internal mammary arteries appear to have satisfactory results.

In emergency situations, including post-angioplasty complications, it seems prudent to continue using the saphenous vein, as revascularization can be achieved more rapidly. There is as yet no evidence to suggest the internal mammary artery as a preferred conduit in older patients, and there is continuing concern as to the adequacy of flow it provides in the early postoperative period for large hypertrophied ventricles.

Care of the Saphenous Vein as a Conduit

It remains unknown whether the inevitable damage occurring to saphenous veins during harvesting and preparation for surgery is important in the short-term or long-term function of vein grafts, but this damage should be kept to a minimum. Unlimited pressure distension results in considerable intimal damage; there is interesting evidence to suggest that there is metabolic damage as well [17], although the significance of this is not established.

Fuster and Chesebro have reviewed the role of pharmacologic treatment with dipyridamole and aspirin, emphasizing its greater effect on the early thrombotic phase and the phase of intimal hyperplasia [10; see also p.379 this volume]. Whether aspirin, with or without persantine, can have any influence in diminishing the long-term development of graft atheroma or the progress of native coronary artery disease is not yet known.

References

[1] Kaiser GG, Davies KB, Fisher LD et al.
Survival following coronary artery bypass grafting in patients with severe angina pectoris (CASS). An observational study.
J Thorac Cardiovasc Surg 1985; **89**: 513–24.

[2] Gersh BJ, Krommal RA, Schaff HV et al.
Comparison of coronary artery bypass surgery and medical therapy in patients 65 years of age or older - A non-randomised study from the Coronary Artery Surgery Study (CASS) registry.
N Engl J Med 1985; **313**: 217–24.

[3] Killip T, Passamani E, Davis K et al.
Coronary Artery Surgery Study (CASS): A randomised trial of coronary bypass surgery - Eight years follow-up and survival in patients with reduced ejection fraction.
Circulation 1985; **72** (Suppl 5): V102–9.

[4] Kirklin JW, Blackstone EH, Roger WJ.
The plights of the invasive treatment of ischemic heart disease.
J Am Coll Cardiol 1985; **5**: 158–67.

[5] Rahimtoola SH.
     A perspective on the three large multicenter
     randomised clinical trials of coronary bypass
     surgery for chronic stable angina.
     Circulation 1985; **72** (Suppl 5): V123–35.
[6] Julian DG.
     The practical implications of the coronary
     artery surgery trials.
     Br Heart J 1985; **54**: 343–50.
[7] Detre KM, Takero T, Huttgren H *et al*
     Long term mortality and morbidity results of the
     Veterans Administration randomised trial of
     coronary artery bypass surgery.
     Circulation 1985; **72** (Suppl 5): V84–9.
[8] Varnauskas F, and the European Coronary
     Surgery Study Group.
     Survival, myocardial infarction and employ-
     ment status in a prospective randomised study
     of coronary bypass surgery.
     Circulation 1985; **72** (Suppl 5): V90–101.
[9] Loop FD, Lytle BW, Cosgrove DM *et al*.
     Influence of the internal mammary artery graft
     on 10-year survival and other cardiac events.
     N Engl J Med 1986; **314**: 1–6.
[10] Fuster V, Chesebro JH.
     Aortocoronary artery vein-graft disease: Ex-
     perimental and clinical approach for the under-
     standing of the role of platelets and platelet
     inhibitors.
     Circulation 1985; **72** (Suppl 5): V65.
[11] Bourassa MG, Fisher LD, Campeau L, Gillespie
     MJ, McConney M, Lesperance J.
     Long-term fate of bypass grafts: The Coronary
     Artery Surgery Study (CASS) and Montreal
     Heart Institute experiences.
     Circulation 1985; **72** (Suppl 5): V71.
[12] Grondin CM, Campeau L, Lesperance J, Enjal-
     bert M, Bourassa MG.
     Comparison of late changes in internal mam-
     mary artery and saphenous vein grafts in two
     consecutive series of patients 10 years after
     operation.
     Circulation 1984; **70** (Suppl 1): I208.
[13] Spencer FC.
     The internal mammary artery: The ideal coron-
     ary bypass graft?
     N Engl J Med 1986; **314**: 50–1.
[14] Tector AJ.
     Internal mammary artery – Its changing role in
     coronary artery bypass grafting procedures.
     Mayo Clin Proc 1986; **61**: 72–4.
[15] Orszulak TA, Schaff HV, Chesebro JH, Holmes
     DR.
     Initial experience with sequential internal mam-
     mary artery bypass grafts to the left anterior
     descending and left anterior descending di-
     agonal coronary arteries.
     Mayo Clin Proc 1986; **61**: 3–8.
[16] Lytle BW, Cosgrove DM, Loop FD, Borsh J,
     Goormaster M, Taylor PC.
     Peri-operative risk of bilateral internal mam-
     mary artery grafting. Analysis of 500 cases
     from 1971 to 1984.
     Circulation 1986; **74** (Suppl 3): III37–41.

SYNDROME X

Review: GRAHAM J DAVIES

Angina pectoris in patients with normal coronary arteries was reported by Osler in the Lumleian lectures on angina pectoris in 1910 [1]. The term Syndrome X has generally been accepted to describe those patients with chest pain of similar character to angina pectoris who have a positive exercise electrocardiogram for myocardial ischemia, but have normal coronary arteries when assessed by arteriography. The observed electro-cardiographic changes cannot be explained by other cardiovascular abnormalities, such as hypertension, cardiomyopathy and conduction disturbance, and the changes are independent of drug therapy. The syndrome has been reported frequently since the widespread application of coronary arteriography [2–6]. Its true incidence is unknown, but following a large arteriographic series it was reported to account for up to 10% of all patients investigated for chest pain [7]. However, the literature on this subject is misleading as the numerous series include non-diagnostic exercise test results for many patients who had presented with symptoms that only vaguely resembled angina pectoris. In series which do not include exercise stress tests, the incidence of normal coronary arteriograms may be as high as 25%, as in the case of the patients entered prospectively into the Coronary Artery Surgery Study (CASS) [8].

A further difficulty in classification relates to the definition of normality with respect to coronary arteriograms. It is conceivable that significant coronary lesions might have been missed in the older reports because of the limitations of the radiographic equipment of that era. Even with modern arteriography, the definition of normality is not consistent; some series include patients with minor (<50% of coronary diameter) lesions, but others confine normality to the complete absence of stenosis. This is an important consideration because it is known that factors which cause dynamic changes in coronary arterial flow can cause acute myocardial ischemia even in the presence of an atheromatous stenosis of moderate severity [9,10].

Myocardial Ischemia as the Cause of Syndrome X
There are conflicting reports regarding the pathogenetic basis of Syndrome X. Many reports suggest that it is related to acute myocardial ischemia. Indirect evidence for this has been obtained by the detection of transient abnormalities of left-ventricular function [11–13] including the detection of regional wall motion abnormality by two-dimensional echocardiography [13]. Other studies have found no abnormality of left-ventricular function by atrial pacing [14] or by pulmonary artery pressure monitoring during ambulatory recording [15]. Neither Arbogast and Bourassa [16] nor Boudoulas *et al* [17] could find an abnormality of left-ventricular function in their patients during atrial pacing, but there was regional lactate production in the presence of ST-segment depression suggesting that acute myocardial ischemia was the basis for the syndrome. As left-vent icular volume, and changes in stroke volume and wall motion are small during atrial pacing-induced ischemia, it is conceivable that regional hypokinesia may remain undetected.

There is reasonable, but not consistent, evidence to suggest a regional abnormality of myocardial perfusion in these patients. This evidence is based upon the results of xenon-133 imaging and washout [18], and on those of positron emission tomography [13]. However, continuous recording of coronary sinus oxygen saturation during atrial pacing shows a normal response, suggesting no abnormality of regional coronary flow [19]. Again, it should be remembered that the syndrome is defined by the presence of effort-induced ST-segment changes, not pacing-induced abnormalities.

The main body of evidence suggesting acute myocardial ischemia as the basis of Syndrome X has been obtained by measurement of regional myocardial lactate consumption or production [5,16,17,20,21].

Possible Mechanisms of Myocardial Ischemia in Syndrome X
Spasm of the epicardial coronary arteries is unusual in the complete absence of atheromatous lesions and has usually been excluded in these patients on the basis of provocative tests. In the absence of epicardial artery spasm and atheromatous stenosis, other mechanisms have been sought to explain the occurrence of myocardial ischemia. An abnormality of the oxygen dissociation curve of hemoglobin has been proposed and certain supporting evidence obtained [6,20,22]. However, this has not been confirmed

consistently. Structural alteration of small vessels has been found [23] but usually in those patients with skeletal muscle disorders in whom there is some suggestion of cardiomyopathy [24]. Currently, the most popular hypothesis is that of inadequency of the vasodilator capacity of the coronary circulation, imposing a restriction on coronary flow reserve [25].

Evidence for this consists of documentation of a reduced increment in coronary flow in response to atrial pacing, and a decrease in the flow increase observed in normal subjects in response to dipyridamole administration. The impaired flow response to atrial pacing can be exaggerated by the administration of ergometrine [26] without reduction in the caliber of the epicardial vessels. This indicates that a dynamic reduction in vasodilator capacity may occur at the level of the small vessels in this syndrome. The impaired vasodilator response may not be confined to the coronary circulation but may be part of a generalized smooth muscle disorder, affecting the whole of the systemic arterial system. The limited evidence for the hypothesis is based on the demonstration of a reduced hyperemic response to ischemia in the forearm of these patients [28]. Further evidence of a functional rather than an anatomic fixed restriction of coronary flow reserve is provided by the increased effort tolerance and increased coronary flow induced by verapamil [27].

The dynamic nature of coronary vascular resistance is also found during 24-hour ambulatory ST-segment monitoring in these patients. Thirty-three per cent of episodes of ST-segment depression are not preceded by an increase in heart rate. This indicates that, apart from restriction of flow increase as a mechanism of ischemia, an actual transient reduction in flow may be responsible for some episodes [13].

Relationship of Symptoms to Myocardial Ischemia

The occurrence, character and radiation of the pain is characteristic of angina pectoris, by definition, although the larger studies have often included patients with atypical chest pain, many of whom have had non-diagnostic exercise tests for myocardial ischemia. Myocardial ischemia may be effort related in Syndrome X, although the effort tolerance may vary greatly within individual patients from day to day and throughout the day. Spontaneous episodes are frequent and may be of long duration, but the typical pattern of nocturnal and early morning spontaneous angina, characteristic of variant angina, is not usually found.

The ischemic episodes may or may not be painful and it has been found that as many as 52% of episodes are not accompanied by symptoms on 24-hour ambulatory ST-segment monitoring [13]. This, however, is a lower incidence than that generally reported in unselected groups of patients with chronic stable angina [29]. Further investigation has revealed that patients with Syndrome X have a generalized enhancement in the perception of painful stimuli, indicated by a lower pain threshold and tolerance for forearm ischemia and electrical skin stimulation [30].

Natural History

The natural history of Syndrome X has not been established. It appears to be benign, but follow-up studies are inadequate because they are either based on populations with chest pain and normal coronary arteries without regard to the exercise test or of short duration. These patients with chest pain and normal coronary arteries generally have a good prognosis with a low mortality and an incidence of acute myocardial infarction not significantly greater than age- and sex-matched controls [7,21,31–34]. However, this incidence is higher than might be expected in a population with no coronary disease, because the control subjects were taken from an asymptomatic general population which undoubtedly contained a small incidence of coronary disease.

There is a tendency for symptoms to subside with time. Various figures are reported for persistence of unabated symptoms ranging from 20% to 80% at mean follow-up intervals of from two to four years. This great variability is to be expected because the results are based on ill-defined patient populations.

The relatively low incidence of morbid events is likely to be related to the small size of the populations studied and the short follow-up periods; in two of the larger studies, the morbid events tended to occur more than four years after initial cardiac catheterization [34,35]. Obviously, there is little value in continuing medication if there is no improvement in symptoms or objective tests for ischemia. Many patients obtain symptomatic relief with sublingual nitrates although the rapidity of the response is quite variable. It would seem reasonable in these cases to propose the continued use of nitrates. Generally, however, in view of the relatively benign prognosis, the tendency should be towards reassurance and minimization of drug therapy.

References

[1] Osler W.
The Lumleian lectures on angina pectoris.
Lancet 1910; **178**: 839–44.

[2] Likoff W, Kasparian H, Segal BL, Forman H, Novack P.
Coronary arteriography: correlation with electrocardiographic response to measured exercise.
Am J Cardiol 1966; **18**: 160–3.

[3] Proufit CC, Shirey EK, Sones FM Jr.
Selective cine coronary arteriography, correlation with clinical findings in 1000 patients.
Circulation 1966; **33**: 901–10.

[4] Likoff W, Segal BL, Kasparian H.
Paradox of normal selective coronary arteriograms in patients considered to have unmistakable coronary heart disease.
N Engl J Med 1967; **276**: 1063–6.

[5] Kemp HG, Elliot WG, Gorlin R.
The anginal syndrome with normal coronary arteriography.
Trans Assoc Am Physicians 1967; **80**: 59–70.

[6] Elliot RS, Bratt G.
The paradox of myocardial ischemia and necrosis in young women with normal coronary arteriograms.
Am J Cardiol 1969; **23**: 633–8.

[7] Ockene IS, Shay MJ, Alpert JS, Weiner BH, Dalen JE.
Unexplained chest pain in patients with normal coronary arteriograms. A follow-up study of functional status.
N Engl J Med 1980; **303**: 1249–52.

[8] CASS Principal Investigators.
Coronary Artery Surgery Study (CASS): a randomized trial of coronary artery bypass surgery.
J Am Coll Cardiol 1984; **3**: 114–28.

[9] Maseri A, Severi S, De Nes M et al.
"Variant angina" – one aspect of a continuous spectrum of vasospastic myocardial ischemia.
Am J Cardiol 1978; **42**: 10/9–35.

[10] Chierchia S, Brunelli C, Simonetti I, Lazzari M, Maseri A.
Sequence of events in angina at rest: primary reduction in coronary flow.
Circulation 1980; **61**: 759–68.

[11] Dwyer E, Wiener L, Cox J.
Angina pectoris in patients with normal and abnormal coronary arteriograms. Hemodynamic and clinical aspects.
Am J Cardiol 1969; **23**: 639–46.

[12] Cannon RO, Bonow RO, Bacharach SL et al.
Left ventricular dysfunction in patients with angina pectoris, normal epicardial coronary arteries, and abnormal vasodilatory reserve.
Circulation 1985; 71: 218–26.

[13] Kaski JC, Crea F, Nihoyannopoulos P, Hackett D, Maseri A.
Transient myocardial ischemia during daily life in Syndrome X.
Am J Cardiol 1986; 58: 1242–7.

[14] Mannohansingh P, Parker JO.
Angina pectoris with normal coronary arteriograms: hemodynamic and metabolic response to atrial pacing.
Am Heart J 1975; 90 (Suppl 5): 533–61.

[15] Levy RD, Shapiro LM, Wright C, Mockus L, Fox KM.
Syndrome X: the haemodynamic significance of ST segment depression.
Br Heart J 1986; 56: 353–7.

[16] Arbogast R, Bourassa MG.
Myocardial function during atrial pacing in patients with angina pectoris and normal coronary arteriograms. Comparison with patients having significant coronary artery disease.
Am J Cardiol 1973; 32: 257–63.

[17] Boudoulas H, Cobb TC, Leighton RF, Wilt SM.
Myocardial lactate production in patients with angina-like chest pain and angiographically normal coronary arteries and left ventricle.
Am J Cardiol 1974; 34: 501–5.

[18] Korhola O, Valle M, Frick M, Wiljasaalo M, Riihimaki E.
Regional myocardial perfusion abnormalities on Xenon-133 imaging in patients with angina and normal coronary arteries.
Am J Cardiol 1977; 39: 355–9.

[19] Crake T, Shapiro L, Crean P, Canepa-Anson RC, Poole-Wilson PA.
Continuous recording of coronary sinus oxygen saturation during atrial pacing in patients with coronary artery disease or Syndrome X.
Circulation 1986; 74 (Suppl II): 515.

[20] Neill WA, Kassebaum DG, Judkins MP.
Myocardial hypoxia as the basis for angina pectoris in a patient with normal coronary arteriograms.
N Engl J Med 1968; 279: 789–92.

[21] Bermiller C, Pepine C, Rogers A.
Long term observations in patients with angina and normal coronary arteriograms.
Circulation 1973; 47: 36–43.

[22] Eliot RS, Mizukani H.
Oxygen affinity of hemoglobin in persons with acute myocardial infarction and in smokers.
Circulation 1966; 34: 331–6.

[23] Mosseri M, Yarom R, Gotsman MS, Hasin Y.
Histological evidence for small vessel coronary artery disease in patients with angina pectoris and patent large coronary arteries.
Circulation 1986; 74: 964–72.

[24] James TN.
Angina without coronary disease.
Circulation 1970; 42: 189–91.

[25] Opherk D, Zebe H, Weihe E et al.
Reduced coronary dilatory capacity and ultrastructural changes of the myocardium in patients with angina pectoris but normal coronary arteriograms.
Circulation 1981; 63 (Suppl 4): 817–25.

[26] Cannon RO, Leon MB, Watson RM, Rosing DR, Epstein SE.
Chest pain in patients with normal coronary arteries - the role of small coronary arteries.
Am J Cardiol 1985; 55: 50B–60B.

[27] Bugiardini R, Ferrini D, Galvani M, Gridelli C, Pozzati A, Puddu P, Lenzi S.
Effects of vasodilators on exercise capacity and myocardial oxygen supply in patients with angina pectoris and normal coronary arteries.
Br Heart J 1985; 54: 610.

[28] Sax FL, Cannon RO, Epstein SE.
Forearm flow in patients with syndrome X: evidence of a generalised disorder of vascular tone?
Circulation 1986; 74 (Suppl II): 481.

[29] Deanfield JE, Maseri A, Selwyn AP, Ribeiro P, Chierchia S, Krikler S, Morgan M.
Myocardial ischaemia during daily life in patients with stable angina: its relation to symptoms and heart rate changes.
Lancet 1983; i: 753–8.

[30] Turiel M, Galassi AR, Glazier JJ, Kaski JC, Maseri A.
Generalized reduction in pain threshold and tolerance in patients with Syndrome X.
Am J Cardiol 1987 (in press).

[31] Waxler EB, Kimbiris D, Dreifus LS.
The fate of women with normal coronary arteriograms and chest pain resembling angina pectoris.
Am J Cardiol 1971; 28: 25–32.

[32] Neil WA, Judkins MP, Dkindsa DS, Metcalfe J, Kassebaum DG, Kloster FE.
Clinically suspect ischaemic heart disease not corroborated by demonstrable coronary artery disease.
Am J Cardiol 1972; **29**: 171–9.

[33] Kemp HG, Vokonas PS, Cohn PF, Gorlin R.
The anginal syndrome associated with normal coronary arteriograms. Reports of a six year experience.
Am J Med 1973; **54**: 735–42.

[34] Isner JM, Salem DH, Banas JS, Levine HJ.
Long term clinical course of patients with normal coronary arteriography: follow-up study of 121 patients with normal and nearly normal coronary arteriograms.
Am Heart J 1981; **102**: 645–53.

[35] Proudfit WL, Isrusckke AUG, Jones FM Jr.
Clinical course of patients with normal or slightly or moderately abnormal coronary arteriograms: 10 year follow-up of 521 patients.
Circulation 1980; **62**: 712–17.

MYOCARDIAL INFARCTION

THE PATHOLOGY OF ACUTE MYOCARDIAL INFARCTION AND SUDDEN ISCHEMIC DEATH

Review: MICHAEL J. DAVIES

Conceptual views on the pathology of both sudden ischemic death and acute myocardial infarction have undergone recent and radical alteration. The major change has come with the recognition that thrombosis is a dynamic process, the rate of change of which was previously underestimated: the pathologist, seeing the morphology of the coronary arteries at the moment of death (often many hours after the initiation of an acute event), was never well placed to be dogmatic about the cause of infarction.

However, the wide-scale use of coronary arteriography has allowed comparison of the angiographic morphology of the acute and chronic manifestations of ischemia, in particular of stable *versus* unstable angina [1]. Such a comparison shows the extent and degree of stenosis to be identical, but the former is associated with smooth-edged stenoses with a gradual transition to normal vessel (type I), the latter with abrupt, eccentric, ragged stenoses, often with overhanging edges (type II) – a fact recently confirmed by fiberoptic transmitted images during operations on the heart [2]. Intraluminal translucent defects thought to represent thrombi are associated with the ragged type of stenosis [3]. Morphologic analysis has been of major assistance in showing that type I lesions are stable 'chronic' plaques, while type II lesions are plaques over which thrombosis is developing in relation to the break-up and disintegration of an atheromatous plaque containing extracellular lipid [4]. The distinction between the different lesions can be made very accurately in high-resolution postmortem angiograms (Fig. 1).

Sudden Ischemic Death
When sudden ischemic death is the verdict in a patient who has died within six hours of the onset of pain in the last episode and who has coronary atheroma causing stenosis of more than 50% by diameter and no other cause of death discovered at necropsy, postmortem coronary angiography often demonstrates lesions which have a type II configuration, and histologic examination confirms these to be plaques which have undergone fissuring in relation to which thrombosis has developed [5,6]. A recent

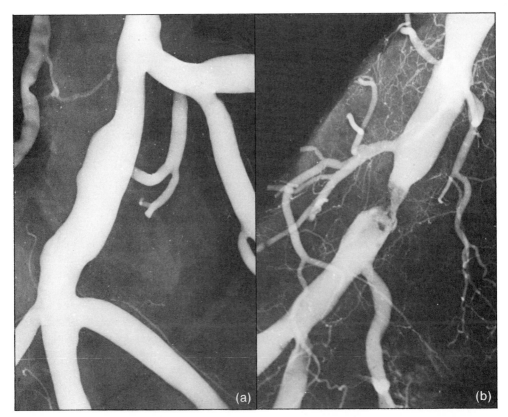

FIGURE 1: Postmortem angiograms, showing (a) typical smooth-edged, eccentric type I plaques; and (b) type II stenosis, with an abrupt transition from normal vessel to ragged stenosis associated with some intraluminal thrombus, shown as a translucent filling defect (taken from a patient with sudden death preceded by resting chest pain).

review of 90 cases of sudden ischemic death showed 86 (95%) to have such fissured plaques, while only four (5%) had no acute vascular lesion. The pathologic process in sudden ischemic death is therefore closer to that of unstable than to that of stable angina. In the 86 patients with plaque fissures, the overlying thrombosis had grown sufficiently to occlude the lumen and prevent filling of the distal vessel in 31 (36%), while in the other 55 patients (64%) there was mural thrombus over the plaque, with a patent vessel. Similar findings are reported from other centers in which postmortem angiography is used to study sudden ischemic death [7], while centers which use conventional dissection techniques at necropsy report a lower incidence [8].

A recent clinical study based on 310 survivors of out-of-hospital cardiac arrest has shown that only 19.4% develop acute myocardial infarction, as shown by the development of new Q waves [9]. Morphologic analysis also shows that the majority of victims of sudden ischemic death have a morphologically normal myocardium. In the study of 90 cases of sudden ischemic death, 45 (50%) had no demonstrable myocardial necrosis [6]. Two patterns of necrosis were identifiable in the remaining cases: regional coagulative necrosis was found in 22 (24.4%), while in the remaining 23 cases (25.6%) multiple microscopic foci of necrosis – particularly prevalent in the subepicardial zone – were found. Clinical and pathologic studies are therefore in accordance: approximately 20% of patients who die suddenly from ischemic heart disease have regional myocardial infarction.

The high incidence of mural thrombosis in a non-occluded coronary artery in victims of sudden ischemic death raises the possibility that microemboli invade the intramyocardial vessels, precipitating microscopic necrosis and thus ventricular fibrillation. A specific search for intramyocardial platelet emboli has shown that this mechanism exists [6,7]. Predominantly platelet thrombi are found in the intramyocardial vessels of up to 40% of sudden ischemic deaths, and are more common in patients who have had a prodrome of resting chest or arm pain in the two weeks prior to death. These microthrombi are specific for myocardial segments downstream of a fissured plaque, confirming that the platelet aggregates are emboli and not part of a widespread thrombotic tendency. Intramyocardial platelet emboli are associated with multiple microscopic foci of necrosis – particularly in the outer third of the myocardium.

The pathologic basis of sudden ischemic death has not always been so clear. Many autopsies in the field of sudden death are performed for primarily legal rather than scientific reasons, and techniques adopted in many previous series were never capable of sustaining the conclusion that thrombi had been absent when they were not found. A second cause of difficulty is in case selection and definition: if all sudden deaths in which there is no extra-cardiac cause and non-stenotic coronary atheroma is present are considered 'ischemic', the incidence of acute thrombotic lesions will fall.

The Pathologic Basis of Acute Myocardial Infarction
In strict terms, myocardial infarction means myocardial necrosis consequent upon reduction or cessation in the blood supply. At postmortem examination, such necrosis can be recognized to occur in a number of distinct patterns, which may have differing pathophysiologic bases. Large areas of necrosis can be visualized by the naked eye with the aid of techniques that demonstrate a loss of activity of such enzymes as succinic dehydrogenase. These large areas of necrosis can be classified as regional – that is, they involve one segment of the circumference of the left ventricle – or as more diffuse. Regional infarction can usually be seen to lie within the myocardial territory supplied by one major coronary artery or branch; it is further subdivided into transmural and subendocardial forms. Diffuse necrosis usually involves the subendocardial zone of the whole of the left ventricle. In addition to these forms of infarction (recognized macroscopically), there are cases in which no necrosis is identified until multiple tiny foci of necrosis are revealed under microscopic examination. Such microscopic foci may again be regional or diffuse. Any morphologic analysis of the pathogenesis of infarction, to be valid, must distinguish between these different forms.

Regional infarction induced by ligation of a coronary artery in an animal cannot be recognized by morphologic means unless there is survival for a minimum of six to eight hours. It seems unlikely that the human myocardium differs in this regard. Some pathologists in the past made what is now known to be an erroneous asssumption: that all sudden ischemic death is due to early myocardial infarction. Failure to make the distinctions between whether infarction was present or not and the different types led to hopeless confusion amongst pathologists over the role of thrombosis in causing myocardial necrosis. These matters have now been clarified by angiographic studies of patients with ECG-proven infarction (and therefore most likely to be regional in distribution).

The consensus among such studies is that within the first few hours of the onset of infarction there is a very high incidence of total occlusion in the subtending artery [10–12]. A proportion of these occluded vessels – perhaps as much as 40% – will spontaneously reopen with time. Use of intracoronary fibrinolysis will, however, re-establish flow in the majority of cases, and the time period within which this happens and the frequency with which intraluminal defects are present suggests that thrombosis rather than spasm is the major cause of occlusion. When blood flow is restored, a focal area of high-grade stenosis is revealed which has a typical type II configuration, suggesting an underlying plaque rupture [12].

Against this clinical background, pathologic studies that are specifically oriented to the study of demonstrable regional transmural infarction can be reassessed. Such studies, going back many years, are unanimous in describing that the subtending artery contains a large thrombus (Fig. 2) overlying a plaque which has broken down, thereby exposing free extracellular lipid to the blood [14–21]. The studies differ only in the name

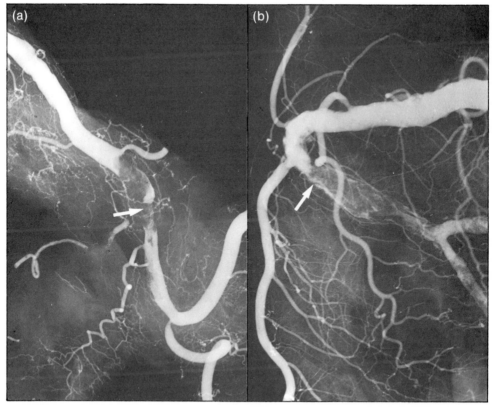

FIGURE 2: Postmortem angiograms from patients dying of regional myocardial infarction: (a) from the fissured plaque (arrow), thrombus has propagated both proximally and distally but, although there is a large intraluminal mass, there is filling of the distal vessel; (b) from the fissured plaque (arrow), thrombus has propagated downstream, and the distal vessel is only faintly outlined by contrast-media filling from the other coronary artery.

applied to this process, which is variously known as fissuring, cracking, rupture or ulceration. The high incidence of total occlusion in postmortems carried out in patients who survived 24–36 hours after the inception of infarction contrasts with the clinical angiograms showing a restoration of flow in up to 30% of patients who survive longer. This may imply that persistent occlusion is linked to a fatal outcome.

The microanatomy of the occlusive thrombi found in association with acute regional infarction has considerable relevance to the controversy over the timing of thrombosis in relation to the infarction [18–20]. Plaque fissuring or rupture allows blood to enter the intima from the lumen in a process aptly named by Fulton the 'dissecting hemorrhage' [22]: a platelet-rich thrombus forms within the intima, considerably enlarging the plaque. Immediately over this nidus, another platelet-rich thrombus forms in the lumen. The thrombus which occludes the lumen distal to this point is, however, formed by a far higher proportion of fibrin. Radiolabeled fibrinogen and platelets given to patients after the onset of infarction accumulated within this portion of the coronary thrombus, demonstrating its propagation [23,24]. In such studies, the head of the thrombus was not labeled [25], which demonstrated that it predated infarction. The distal propagation of thrombosis is more common in larger regional infarcts, again suggesting an association with higher mortality.

The pathogenesis of regional non-transmural infarction is less well established. Such pathologic studies as exist suggest a far lower incidence of persistent thrombotic occlusion than of regional transmural infarction [26]. Among the possibilities awaiting confirmation by clinical angiography are that pre-established collateral flow protects the sub-pericardial zone from necrosis, despite the occlusion of the subtending artery by thrombosis. More in keeping with the limited pathologic data available is that the artery has been occluded by thrombosis, but that flow was re-established by spontaneous lysis within the six-hour period that infarction takes to extend through the ventricular wall from endocardium to epicardium.

Focal microscopic necrosis, when regional in distribution and predominantly subpericardial, is associated with local platelet microemboli from a more proximal mural thrombus [6,7]. More widespread focal necrosis, predominantly subendocardial in distribution, is found in patients with left-ventricular hypertrophy – either in association with diffuse coronary artery stenosis or in isolation. Diffuse subendocardial necrosis (visible macroscopically) has no specific relationship to coronary thrombosis or even coronary atheroma, and reflects an overall fall in myocardial perfusion from a combination of increased left-ventricular wall thickness, increased left-ventricular volume, increased left-ventricular end-diastolic pressure and a fall in aortic root pressure. This pattern of necrosis is commonly seen in association with centrilobular liver necrosis in hypovolemic shock. When occurring in association with coronary atheroma, diffuse subendocardial necrosis may be superimposed on previous regional infarction as part of cardiogenic shock; it also occurs in the severe evenly distributed coronary stenosis with small-vessel extension typical of diabetes.

Relation of Arterial Spasm to Myocardial Infarction
Well-documented cases of regional infarction unrelated to coronary atheroma and ascribed to spasm are known [27], and spasm has itself been shown to elicit thrombosis [28]. Another documented cause is the myocardial bridging of an artery [29]. Even so,

the number of such cases is trifling compared with the number of patients documented who develop infarction on the basis of atheroma and plaque fissuring. Local spasm at the site of a plaque which fissures [30] and microvascular spasm within the myocardium itself, mediated through products released by platelet-rich thrombi, are both entirely feasible mechanisms, but they cannot be confirmed by morphologic analysis.

Morphologic analysis can do no more than describe the association between a fissured plaque and a thrombus occluding the lumen. The formation of thrombosis in the lumen is favored by any reduction in blood flow, caused: (i) by pre-existing high-grade stenosis; (ii) by local spasm; or (iii) by a reduction in distal run-off – all of which could be essential steps between plaque fissuring and the final occlusion of the arterial lumen by thrombus [30].

Central Role of Plaque Fissuring in Acute Ischemic Events

Epidemiologic and clinical studies have never been able to define risk factors which militate separately for the three acute symptoms – myocardial infarction, the crescendo form of unstable angina, and sudden ischemic death. Once plaque fissuring is seen to underlie all three, this fact becomes less surprising.

Plaque fissuring is a condition in which there is a potential space within the intima filled with cholesterol and cholesterol esters. There are some such plaques in the majority of patients with coronary atheroma; however, in a minority of (e.g. stable angina) cases, some have only plaques of this type while others have none. The mechanism by which a lipid pool develops involves necrosis ('atheronecrosis') of the basal layer of the intima, and occurs in natural human disease rather than experimental atheroma in animals. Current hypotheses attribute the process of 'atheronecrosis' to the lytic potential of macrophages that are activated by the ingestion and breakdown of lipid (with possible roles for elaboration of free radicals as a result). A number of plaques with such lipid pools undergo sudden fissuring: the cap breaks, allowing blood to enter the intima. The factors precipitating such rupture are unknown, but surges of blood pressure, local arterial spasm, mechanical fatigue of collagen or macrophage activity lysing collagen are all posssible.

The results of plaque fissuring are variable [30], and depend on the complex interplay of such factors as the magnitude of the break in the plaque cap, whether free lipid is extruded into the lumen, the degree of pre-existing stenosis at the site, blood flow and the thrombotic potential of the patient. Plaque fissuring asssociated with intraintimal thrombus – although not associated with the formation of mural intraluminal thrombus – still leads to an increase in plaque size, and is one mechanism by which a sudden increase in the degree of obstruction occurs [31]. When fissures are associated with superimposed mural thrombosis, sudden death and/or unstable angina can occur; if the thrombus lyses and the fissure reseals, the patient returns to normal; if the thrombus occludes, at least for a time, infarction may occur (Fig. 3). The prognosis of a patient who has recovered from unstable angina or an acute infarct depends in part on how many other plaques at risk of fissuring are present in that individual.

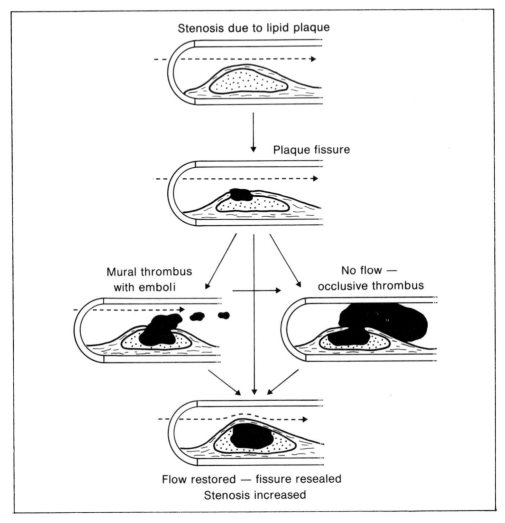

Stenosis due to lipid plaque

Plaque fissure

Mural thrombus with emboli

No flow — occlusive thrombus

Flow restored — fissure resealed
Stenosis increased

FIGURE 3: Diagrammatic representations of the possible progression of events after the formation of a plaque fissure in an atheromatous plaque with a lipid pool.

References

[1] Ambrose JA, Winters SL, Stern A *et al.* Angiographic morphology and the pathogenesis of unstable angina pectoris. *J Am Coll Cardiol* 1985; **5**: 609–16.

[2] Sherman CT, Litvack F, Grundfest ME *et al.* Fiberoptic coronary angioscopy identifies thrombus in all patients with unstable angina *Circulation* 1985; **72**: Abstract.

[3] Bresnahan DR, Davies JL, Holmes DR, High HC. Angiographic occurrence and clinical correlates of intraluminal coronary artery thrombus: Role of unstable angina. *J Am Coll Cardiol* 1985; **6**: 285–9.

[4] Levin DC, Fallon JT.
Significance of the angiographic morphology of localised coronary stenoses. Histopathological correlates.
Circulation 1982; **66**: 316–20.

[5] Davies MJ, Thomas AC.
Plaque fissuring - the cause of acute myocardial infarction, sudden ischaemic death and crescendo angina.
Br Heart J 1985; **53**: 363–73.

[6] Davies MJ, Thomas AC, Knapman PA, Hangartner JRW.
Intramyocardial platelet aggregation in unstable angina and sudden ischemic death.
Circulation 1986; **73**: 418–27.

[7] Falk E.
Unstable angina with fatal outcome: Dynamic coronary thrombosis leading to infarction and/or sudden death.
Circulation 1985; **71**: 699–708.

[8] Warnes C, Roberts WC.
Comparison at necropsy by age group of amount and distribution of narrowing by atherosclerotic plaque in 2995 five-mm-long segments of 240 major coronary arteries in 60 men aged 31–70 years with sudden coronary death.
Am Heart J 1984; **108**: 431–5.

[9] Hallstrom AP, Cobb LA, Ray R.
Smoking as a risk factor for recurrence of sudden cardiac arrest.
N Engl J Med 1986; **314**: 271–5.

[10] DeWood MA, Spores J, Notske R *et al.*
Prevalence of total coronary occlusion during the early hours of transmural myocardial infarction.
N Engl J Med 1980; **303**: 897–902.

[11] Stadius ML, Maynard C, Fritz JK *et al.*
Coronary anatomy and left ventricular function in the first twelve hours of acute myocardial infarction: The Western Washington randomized intracoronary streptokinase trial.
Circulation 1985; **72**: 292–301.

[12] Bertrand ME, Lefebvre JM, Laisne CL *et al.*
Coronary angiography in acute transmural myocardial infarction.
Am Heart J 1979; **97**: 61–9.

[13] Ambrose JA, Winters SL, Arora RR *et al.*
Coronary angiograph morphology in acute myocardial infarction: Link between the pathogenesis of unstable angina and myocardial infarction.
J Am Coll Cardiol 1985; **6**: 1233–8.

[14] Chapman I.
The cause-effect relationship between recent coronary artery occlusion and acute myocardial infarction.
Am Heart J 1984; **87**: 267–71.

[15] Davies MJ, Woolf N, Robertson WB.
Pathology of acute myocardial infarction with particular reference to occlusive coronary thrombi.
Br Heart J 1976; **38**: 659–64.

[16] Ridolfi RL, Hutchins GM.
The relationship between coronary artery lesions and myocardial infarcts: Ulceration of atherosclerotic plaques precipitating coronary thrombosis.
Am Heart J 1977; **93**: 468–86.

[17] Chandler AB.
Mechanisms and frequency of thrombosis in the coronary circulation.
Thromb Res 1974; **4**: 3–23.

[18] Davies MJ, Thomas A.
The pathological basis and microanatomy of occlusive thrombus formation in human coronary arteries.
Philos Trans R Soc Lond [Biol] 1981; **294**: 225–9.

[19] Horie T, Sekiguchi M, Hirosawa K.
Coronary thrombosis in pathogenesis of acute myocardial infarction. Histopathological study of coronary arteries in 108 necropsied cases.
Br Heart J 1978; **40**: 153–61.

[20] Falk E.
Plaque rupture with severe pre-existing stenosis precipitating coronary thrombosis. Characteristics of coronary atherosclerotic plaques underlying fatal occlusive thrombi.
Br Heart J 1983; **50**: 127–34.

[21] Constantinides P.
Plaque fissures in human coronary thrombosis.
J Atherosclerosis Res 1966; **6**: 1–17.

[22] Fulton WFM.
The coronary arteries: Arteriography, microanatomy and pathogenesis of obliterative coronary disease. Springfield, IL: Charles C. Thomas, 1965; pp. 230–96.

[23] Erhardt LR, Unge G, Boman G.
Formation of coronary arterial thrombi in relation to onset of necrosis in acute myocardial infarction in man.
Am Heart J 1976; **91**: 592–8.

[24] Henriksson P, Edhag O, Jansson B *et al.*
A role for platelets in the process of infarct extension.
N Engl J Med 1985; **313**: 1660–1.

[25] Davies MJ, Fulton WFM, Robertson WB.
The relation of coronary thrombosis to ischemic
myocardial necrosis.
J Pathol 1979; **127**: 99–110.

[26] Erhardt LR.
Clinical and pathological observations in different types of acute myocardial infarction: A
study of 84 patients deceased after treatment
in a coronary care unit.
Acta Med Scand 1974; **560** (Suppl): 1078–99.

[27] El-Maraghi NRH, Sely BJ.
Recurrent myocardial infarction in a young man
due to coronary arterial spasm demonstrated
at autopsy.
Circulation 1980; **61**: 199–207.

[28] Vincent MG, Anderson JL, Marshal HW.
Coronary spasm producing coronary thrombo-
sis and myocardial infarction.
N Engl J Med 1983; **309**: 220–3.

[29] Feldman AM, Baughman KL.
Myocardial infarction association with a
myocardial bridge.
Am Heart J 1986; **111**: 784–7.

[30] Maseri A, Chierchia S, Davies G.
Pathophysiology of coronary occlusion in
acute infarction.
Circulation 1986; **73**: 233–9.

[31] Willerson JT, Campbell WB, Winniford MD *et al*.
Conversion from chronic to acute coronary dis-
ease: Speculation regarding mechanisms.
Am J Cardiol 1984; **54**: 1349–55.

TECHNIQUES FOR USE IN THE DIAGNOSIS OF MYOCARDIAL INFARCTION

[1] Assessment of location and size of myocardial infarction with contrast-enhanced echocar-
diography.
Armstrong WF, West SR, Mueller TM, Dillon JC, Feigenbaum H, VA Hosp, Indianapolis, IN,
USA.
J Am Coll Cardiol 1983; **2**: 63–9.

[2] Nuclear magnetic resonance imaging of acute myocardial infarction in dogs: alterations in
magnetic relaxation times.
Higgins CB, Herfkens R, Lipton MJ *et al*, Univ California Med Cent, San Francisco, CA,
USA.
Am J Cardiol 1983; **52**: 184–8.

[3] Imaging and characterization of acute myocardial infarction in vivo by gated nuclear magne-
tic resonance.
Wesbey G, Higgins CB, Lanzer P, Botvinick E, Lipton MJ, Univ California San Francisco
Med Cent, San Francisco, CA, USA.
Circulation 1984; **69**: 125–30.

[4] Nuclear magnetic resonance analysis of acute myocardial infarction in dogs: the effect of
transient coronary ischemia of varying duration and reperfusion on spin lattice relaxation
times.
Brown JJ, Strich G, Higgins CB, Gerber KH, Slutsky RA, Univ California Med Cent, San
Diego, CA, USA.
Am Heart J 1985; **109**: 486–90.

Comment.   Echocardiography is now routinely used in the coronary care unit for the
examination of patients with acute myocardial infarction. Using contrast echocardiograms in a study in dogs, both the site and size of experimentally produced myocardial
infarctions could be accurately determined [1].

Nuclear magnetic resonance can also now be used for imaging in myocardial
infarction. This technique enables the accurate identification of acute myocardial
infarction in excised dog hearts as a positive image without contrast media [2,3], and it

may also be useful for monitoring the myocardial edema associated with reperfused myocardium [4].

RECIPROCAL ST-SEGMENT DEPRESSION DURING MYOCARDIAL INFARCTION

Review: ARSHED A. QUYYUMI

ST-segment depression in the 'remote' (anterior) electrocardiographic leads V_1 to V_3 during acute inferior myocardial infarction, and in the 'remote' (inferior) electrocardiographic leads during anterior myocardial infarction (with ST-segment elevation in leads V_1 to V_3), is often referred to as 'reciprocal' ST-segment depression. There is considerable debate as to the true significance of this 'reciprocal' change: some regard it as indicative of multi-vessel disease and ischemia in the myocardial wall which is remote from the site of infarction, whereas others believe that it is purely an 'electrical' electrocardiographic phenomenon. Several studies in recent years have invesigated patients with and without 'reciprocal' ST-segment depression at the time of myocardial infarction to determine the etiology of these changes. Although the results of these studies appear conflicting, important information can be obtained from the resting electrocardiograms recorded in the early phase after myocardial infarction.

Mechanisms of ST-Segment Change
Ischemic myocardium fails to depolarize fully and repolarizes incompletely, altering the magnitude and duration of the action potential. A potential difference exists at the boundary of ischemic and normal muscle throughout the cardiac cycle, which results in a shift of both the TQ and ST segments. The magnitude and polarity of the ST-segment change is dictated by the temporal and spatial relationships of the recording electrode to the ischemic myocardium [1]. The magnitude of ST-segment change is proportional, both to the distance the electrode is placed from the region of ischemia and to the intensity and duration of the ischemic insult. With epicardial or transmural myocardial infarction, a precordial electrode placed over the area will record ST-segment elevation; an electrode placed directionally opposite to the area of infarction will record ST-segment depression – a purely 'reciprocal' electrocardiographic phenomenon. Although most workers accept this explanation of why ST-segment depression occurs in leads remote from the region of infarction, there has been speculation that it may be due to islands of subendocardial ischemia interspersed within normal myocardium [2].

Incidence and Time Course of 'Reciprocal' ST-Segment Change
The incidence of ST-segment depression reported in leads remote from the site of infarction ranges in various studies between 34% and 100%. There is no doubt that this phenomenon is more likely to be observed if the electrocardiogram is performed early after infarction. In the series of Camara *et al*, in which electrocardiograms were obtained within a mean period of 3.7 hours from onset of chest pain, all patients with inferior myocardial infarction and 70% of those with anterior infarction had ≥ 0.5 mm ST-segment depression in leads remote from the area of infarction [3]. Shah *et al*

included patients admitted up to seven hours after the onset of symptoms, and reported a 45% incidence of ≥1 mm ST-segment depression [4].

It is also evident that 'reciprocal' ST-segment depression is often transient. Of 47 patients in the series reported by Croft *et al*, 83% had anterior ST-segment depression with inferior infarction [5]. Electrocardiograms in this group were recorded within a mean period of 7.3 hours from onset of symptoms. ST-segment depression lasted less than four hours in 11.5% of the patients, and had resolved in all but 12.8% of patients by 72 hours. Camara *et al* reported that 59% of their patients had no ST-segment depression within 24 hours of admission [3]. Furthermore, the magnitude of ST-segment depression was reduced in 91% of the remaining patients by that time.

Quyyumi *et al* measured ST-segment changes in inferior leads after balloon occlusion of the left anterior descending coronary artery during angioplasty [6], a maneuver which produces a situation analogous to the early stages of anteroseptal myocardial infarction. By measuring changes of 0.1 mm or greater, they were able to demonstrate ST-segment depression in one or more inferior leads in 90% of patients with isolated left anterior descending disease. The onset, the maximum change and the termination of ST-segment changes coincided in all leads where depression or elevation occurred, suggesting that these changes represented a truly reciprocal electrocardiographic phenomenon. We can conclude from these studies that ST-segment elevation during infarction is almost invariably accompanied by ST-segment depression in remote electrocardiographic leads. This change may nevertheless be transient and may be <1 mm in magnitude, which can be difficult to measure clinically, where a preinfarction baseline electrocardiogram is not always available for comparison.

The Magnitude of 'Reciprocal' ST-Segment Depression

A strong correlation has been reported between the magnitude of ST-segment elevation and the magnitude of ST-segment depression [3,5,7–10]. A significant correlation between the sum of ST-segment elevation and the sum of ST-segment depression has also been found [3]. Although this relationship holds true for both anterior and inferior myocardial infarction, the maximal size of ST-segment depression is significantly greater with inferior than with anterior infarcts [3]. Complex spatial and temporal factors determine the magnitude of ST-segment elevation during infarction [1], but the close relationship with ST-segment depression in remote electrocardiographic leads strongly suggests that the latter is a purely electrical phenomenon.

Infarct Size and 'Reciprocal' ST-Segment Depression

Direct and indirect estimates of infarct size have been made in several studies. In a study of 48 consecutive patients with inferior myocardial infarction, Gibson *et al* reported on 27 patients with ≥1 mm ST-segment depression in the precordial leads [7]. Compared to patients with <1 mm ST-segment depression in these leads, the patients had higher plasma peak creatine kinase levels, a higher prevalence of true posterior myocardial infarction by electrocardiographic criteria, a lower global ejection fraction and greater infarct-related asynergy. The authors attributed these findings to the presence of larger inferior or inferoapical infarcts. A higher QRS score, indicating a larger myocardial infarct, was also reported by Roubin *et al* in patients with ST-segment depression in remote leads [11]. A higher mean plasma creatine kinase level was also observed by

Gelman *et al* in patients who developed 'reciprocal' ST-segment changes [12]. The level was highest in the group of patients where the changes persisted for 48 hours or more, indicating that these patients had larger infarcts. Goldberg *et al* reported a higher plasma creatine kinase level and reduced ejection fraction in patients with anterior ST-segment depression during inferior myocardial infarction: 13 of the 14 patients had posterolateral wall dyskinesia in addition to inferior dyskinesia on radionuclide ventriculography; in contrast, patients with no ST-segment depression had inferior wall dyskinesia only [13]. These authors concluded that patients with anterior ST-segment depression during inferior wall myocardial infarction have more extensive areas of infarction, primarily involving the posterolateral region. By performing carbon-11 palmitate positron emission tomography, Billadello *et al* demonstrated that infarct-zone necrosis was greater in patients with $\geqslant 1$ mm ST-segment depression in remote electrocardiographic leads [10].

Thus, there is little doubt that the presence of significant ($\geqslant 1$ mm) ST-segment depression in remote electrocardiograpic leads during acute myocardial infartion indicates the presence of a more extensive infarct in the primary zone. From a solely electrocardiographic viewpoint, a larger area of necrosis leads to an ST-segment elevation which is greater in magnitude and longer in duration. This in turn would be expected to result in greater and more prolonged ST-segment depression in opposite electrocardiographic leads. Conversely, small areas of infarction will lead to smaller levels of ST-segment elevation persisting for shorter periods of time, and will result in less significant and more transient ST-segment depression in opposing leads. The results from several of the studies reviewed above clearly show that patients with more extensive infarcts were indeed the ones to develop ST-segment depression ($\geqslant 1$ mm in magnitude) in remote electrocardiographic leads, again suggesting that this is a purely 'reciprocal' electrical phenomenon.

'Reciprocal' ST-Segment Depression and Myocardial Ischemia

It has been hypothesized that during myocardial infarction, especially in the presence of multi-vessel disease, there is a net reduction of blood flow to the myocardium, so that ischemia often occurs even in areas of myocardium not directly supplied by the occluded coronary artery. These remote areas of ischemia are believed to be the cause of ST-segment depression. Clinical studies do not, however, support this hypothesis.

Cohen *et al* found angiographic wall motion abnormalities in the anterior and septal wall in fewer than 12% of their patients with acute inferior myocardial infarction and anterior ST-segment depression [14]. Goldberg *et al* performed radionuclide ventriculography early after inferior myocardial infarction, and demonstrated that a minority of their patients with ST-segment depression had anterior wall motion abnormalities [13]. Shah *et al* reported a 50% incidence of anteroseptal wall motion defects in patients with inferior infarction and anterior ST-segment depression, compared with 15% in patients without ST-segment depression [4]. Little *et al* and Ferguson *et al*, however, reported that none of their patients with 'reciprocal' ST-segment depression had wall motion abnormalities in the remote wall [8,9]. Billadello *et al* demonstrated isotope uptake in the anterior wall in three of nine patients with anterior ST-segment depression during inferior myocardial infarction, underscoring the difficulty in differentiating electrical reciprocity from ischemia at a remote site in the face of transmural inferior infarction using analysis of the electrocardiogram alone [10].

Several conclusions can thus be reached from these data. ST-segment depression in the 'remote' electrocardiographic leads during acute myocardial infarction does not invariably indicate the presence of ischemia in the 'distant' myocardium. Evidence of ischemia in the 'remote' myocardium was present in a minority of patients with ST-segment depression, and the lack of an adequate control group in most series reduces the specificity of this finding. In the majority of patients, ST-segment depression indeed appears to be a truly 'reciprocal' electrocardiographic phenomenon.

Does 'Reciprocal' ST-Segment Depression Indicate Presence of Multi-Vessel Disease?
Given the surgical option for the management of patients with multi-vessel disease, it is important to identify the presence of such disease in patients admitted with acute myocardial infarction. A number of studies have attempted, with conflicting results, to correlate the presence or absence of 'reciprocal' ST-segment depression with the severity of underlying coronary artery disease.

Salcedo *et al* reported on a group of 37 patients with inferior myocardial infarction and anterior ST-segment depression [15]: 95% of patients with ST-segment depression had concomitant left anterior descending coronary artery stenosis, whereas all of the eight patients with absence of ST-segment depression had single-vessel right coronary artery disease. Haraphongse *et al* reported a 31% incidence of left anterior descending coronary artery disease in patients with <1 mm ST-segment depression during inferior myocardial infarction, as opposed to a 68% incidence in patients with ≥1 mm ST-segment depression [16]. Similar findings were reported by Roubin *et al* [11]. Contrary to these results, four other studies failed to demonstrate an increased incidence of multi-vessel disease in patients with 'reciprocal' ST-segment depression [8–10,14].

It should be emphasized that the criteria for significant ST-segment depression, the time of recording of the first electrocardiogram from onset of symptoms and the criteria for significant disease varied between the different studies. For example, in the study of Salcedo *et al*, patients were included up to 24 hours after onset of symptoms [15]. This may have selected a population of patients with more extensive disease who still had persistent ST-segment depression. In the studies of Ferguson *et al* and Little *et al*, electrocardiograms were obtained relatively early (<4 hours and <9 hours, respectively) after onset of symptoms in groups with no manifest differences in coronary anatomy [8,9].

The size of myocardial infarction depends on the dominance of the vessel occluded, the state of collateral circulation and other hemodynamic factors. Patients with multi-vessel disease and reduced collateral flow are likely to suffer more extensive infarctions. This will result in greater ST-segment elevation and hence greater ST-segment depression in 'remote' leads due to the electrical reciprocal phenomenon. It is not surprising, therefore, that some studies have shown a greater incidence of multi-vessel disease in patients with 'reciprocal' ST-segment depression.

Overall, these findings suggest that patients with persistent ST-segment depression for several hours or days after the onset of symptoms tend to have more extensive infarcts and a greater likelihood of multi-vessel disease. Haraphongse *et al* were able to identify a group of patients with inferior myocardial infarction who had precordial ST-segment depression of ≥3 mm in magnitude [16]. All these patients had significant stenosis of the left anterior descending coronary artery. Such a severe degree of 'reciprocal' ST-segment depression probably indicates true subendocardial ischemia and the presence of significant disease in other vessels.

'Reciprocal' ST-Segment Depression as a Prognostic Indicator after Myocardial Infarction

Shah *et al* demonstrated that patients with anterior ST-segment depression during acute inferior myocardial infarction had a 50% incidence of developing heart failure and a 19% incidence of death in hospital, compared with the group without ST-segment depression in which no patient died [4]. Salcedo *et al* found that 92% of patients who developed complications after infarction had remote-wall ST-segment depression, whereas only 38% without ST-segment depression developed complications [15]. Nasmith *et al* reported that, during a 6-month follow-up, only 1 of 21 patients without 'reciprocal' ST-segment depression developed exertional angina pectoris [17]. In contrast, of the remaining 25 patients with ST-segment depression in the acute phase, 15 had exertional angina, 12 had rest pain, 2 had re-infarctions and 2 patients died. Other studies have confirmed the increased incidence of short-term and long-term complications in patients with 'reciprocal' ST-segment depression [7,16].

Thus, acute-phase 'reciprocal' ST-segment depression is a predictor of poor long-term and short-term prognosis. Outcome after myocardial infarction is closely related to the size of myocardial infarction: the greater the size of infarction, the greater the reduction in ejection fraction, the greater the magnitude and direction of ST-segment elevation and, as shown previously, the greater the likelihood of significant ST-segment depression in opposing electrocardiographic leads.

Conclusions

ST-segment depression in remote electrocardiographic leads, that is, in inferior leads during anterior myocardial infarction and anterior leads during inferior myocardial infarction, is virtually a consistent finding after acute myocardial infarction. Where absence is reported, this may be due to a failure to record an electrocardiogram early after the onset of symptoms, or more importantly due to the lower magnitude of change (<1 mm) which occurs with smaller infarcts.

The magnitude of ST-segment depression is directly related to the magnitude of ST-segment elevation. 'Significant' (≥1 mm) ST-segment depression occurs in patients with extensive myocardial infarction, and these patients tend to have a poor short-term and long-term prognosis.

As to the question of whether any conclusions can be drawn from the electrocardiogram after myocardial infarction: ST-segment depression in remote electrocardiographic leads on an electrocardiogram recorded early (<4 hours) after the onset of symptoms is an expected finding, and is not necessarily indicative of multi-vessel disease or remote-wall ischemia. However, a magnitude of ST-segment depression disproportionate to the magnitude of ST-segment elevation or greater than 3 mm in size is strongly suggestive of the presence of disease in other coronary arteries [16]. Persistence of ST-segment depression (for 24 hours or longer), especially with a reduction in the magnitude of ST-segment elevation, is strongly suggestive of the presence of multi-vessel disease and poor short-term and long-term outlook [12]. Critical analysis of serial electrocardiograms after infarction is likely to be helpful in identifying patients in whom a more aggressive diagnostic and therapeutic approach would be justified. Studies concentrating on the magnitude and duration of 'reciprocal' ST-segment depression after infarction, and correlating these with coronary anatomy, infarct size and prognosis, are required to clarify the picture further.

References

[1] Holland RP, Brooks H.
Precordial and epicardial surface potentials during myocardial ischemia in the pig: Theoretical and experimental analysis of the TQ and ST segments.
Circ Res 1975; 37: 471–80.

[2] Ekmekci A, Toyoshima H, Kwoczynski JK, Nagaya T, Prinzmetal M.
Angina pectoris IV. Clinical and experimental difference between ischemia with ST elevation and ischemia with ST depression.
Am J Cardiol 1961; 7: 412–26.

[3] Camara E Jr, Chandra N, Ouyang P, Gottlieb SH, Shapiro EP.
Reciprocal ST change in acute myocardial infarction: Assessment by electrocardiography and echocardiography.
J Am Coll Cardiol 1983; 2: 251–7.

[4] Shah PK, Pichler M, Berman DS et al.
Non-invasive identification of a high risk subset of patients with acute myocardial infarction.
Am J Cardiol 1980; 46: 915–21.

[5] Croft CH, Woodward W, Nicod P et al.
Clinical implications of anterior ST segment depression in patients with acute inferior myocardial infarction.
Am J Cardiol 1982; 50: 428–36.

[6] Quyyumi AA, Crake T, Rubens MB, Levy RD, Richards AF.
Importance of reciprocal electrocardiography changes during occlusion of left anterior descending coronary artery. Studies during percutaneous transluminal coronary angioplasty.
Lancet 1986; i: 347–50.

[7] Gibson RS, Crampton RS, Watson DD et al.
Precordial ST-segment depression during acute myocardial infarction: Clinical, scintigraphic and angiographic correlations.
Circulation 1982; 66: 732–41.

[8] Ferguson DW, Pandian N, Kio Schos JM, Marcus ML, White CW.
Angiographic evidence that reciprocal ST segment depression during acute myocardial infarction does not indicate remote ischemia: Analysis of 23 patients.
Am J Cardiol 1984; 53: 55–62.

[9] Little WC, Rogers EW, Sodums MT.
Mechanism of anterior ST segment depression during acute inferior myocardial infarction.
Ann Intern Med 1984; 100: 226–9.

[10] Billadello JJ, Smith JL, Ludbrook PA et al.
Implications of 'reciprocal' ST segment depression associated with acute myocardial infarction identified by positron tomography.
J Am Coll Cardiol 1983; 2: 616–24.

[11] Roubin GS, Shen WF, Nicholson M, Dunn RF, Kelly DT, Harris PJ.
Anterolateral ST segment depression in acute inferior myocardial infarction: Angiographic and clinical implications.
Am Heart J 1984; 107: 1177–82.

[12] Gelman JS, Saltups A.
Precordial ST segment depression in patients with inferior myocardial infarction: Clinical implications.
Br Heart J 1982; 48: 560–5.

[13] Goldberg HL, Borer JS, Jacobstein JG, Kluger J, Scheidt SS, Alonso DR.
Anterior ST segment depression in acute inferior myocardial infarction: Indicator of posterolateral infarction.
Am J Cardiol 1981; 48: 1009–15.

[14] Cohen M, Blanke H, Karsh KR, Holt J, Rentrop P.
Implications of precordial ST segment depression during acute inferior myocardial infarction. Arteriographic and ventriculographic correlations during the acute phase.
Br Heart J 1984; 52: 497–501.

[15] Salcedo JR, Baird MG, Chambers RJ, Bean-
lands DS.
Significance of precordial ST segment depression in anterior precordial leads in acute
inferior myocardial infarction: Concomitant left
anterior descending coronary artery disease?
Am J Cardiol 1981; **48**: 1003–8.

[16] Haraphongse M, Jugdutt BI, Rossall RE.
Significance of precordial ST segment de-
pression in acute transmural inferior infarction:
Coronary angiographic findings.
Cathet Cardiovasc Diagn 1983; **9**: 143–51.

[17] Nasmith J, Marpole D, Rahal D, Homan J, Stewart S, Sniderman A.
Clinical outcomes after inferior myocardial infarction.
Ann Intern Med 1982; **96**: 22–6.

NON-Q WAVE MYOCARDIAL INFARCTION

[1]   Coronary arteriographic findings soon after non-Q-wave myocardial infarction.
DeWood MA, Stifter WF, Simpton S *et al*, Deaconess Med Cent, Spokane, WA, USA.
N Engl J Med 1986; **315**: 417–23.

[2]   Diltiazem and reinfarction in patients with non-Q-wave myocardial infarction.
Gibson RS, Boden WE, Théroux P *et al*, and the Diltiazem Reinfarction Study Group, Med
Cent, Univ Virginia, Charlottesville, VA, USA.
N Engl J Med 1986; **315**: 423–9.

[3]   Non-Q-wave myocardial infarction (Editorial).
Kennedy JW, Univ Washington Sch Med, Seattle, WA, USA.
N Engl J Med 1986; **315**: 451–3.

[4]   Comparison of clinical features of non-Q wave myocardial infarction.
Ogawa H, Hiramori K, Haze K *et al*, Nat Cardiovasc Cent, Osaka, Japan.
Am Heart J 1986; **111**: 513–9.

Comment.   The correlation between the electrocardiographic changes and subsequent pathological findings in patients dying from a myocardial infarction is poor, particularly in relation to the presence or absence of Q waves; some patients without Q waves *do* have non-transmural infarction, whereas others have necrosis affecting the full thickness of the left ventricular wall, and the distinction cannot be made during life. Nevertheless, most clinical studies have shown that patients with non-Q wave infarction have, overall, a smaller release of cardiac enzymes and an initially lower mortality, but a higher incidence of re-infarction (or infarct extension), and a late mortality little different from those who develop Q waves. These observations suggest that there may be a different pathological process responsible for the two clinical types of infarction and, perhaps of even greater importance, that it may be possible to influence the late prognosis of the non-Q wave patients.

In a large series of patients who underwent coronary arteriography within one week of a non-Q wave infarction, DeWood *et al* [1] observed total occlusion of the responsible artery in only 26%, 37% and 42% of patients who were investigated within 24 hours, between 24 and 72 hours, and between 72 hours and one week, respectively, after the infarction. The frequency of a visible collateral circulation to the affected territory increased in parallel with that of coronary occlusion. These findings are in striking contrast with those after Q wave infarction, in which total coronary occlusion is observed almost universally in the early hours after infarction, with a tendency for patency to occur in subsequent weeks presumably as a result of spontaneous thrombolysis. Moreover, it is uncommon to observe collateral flow early after Q wave infarction. These observations suggest that non-Q wave infarction results from a severe reduction in coronary flow, whereas Q wave infarction results when flow is totally interrupted. Presumably, the residual flow is often precarious, for example in sub-total coronary occlusion or if collateral flow is compromised by disease in the feeding artery, and in these circumstances a further increase in ischemia results in extension of the infarct.

The possibility that treatment with the calcium antagonist, diltiazem, might prevent re-infarction in patients with non-Q wave infarction was investigated in a randomized controlled trial by Gibson *et al* [2]. Two hundred and eighty-seven patients were randomized to receive diltiazem 90 mg every 6 hours, and 289 to receive placebo; treatment was started 24–72 hours after the onset of infarction and continued for 14 days. Re-infarction occurred in 27 patients in the placebo group and in 15 in the diltiazem group; the 90% confidence interval of the reduction in re-infarction associated with active treatment was 7–67%. Active treatment also reduced the frequency of refractory unstable angina by 49.7% (confidence interval, 6–73%). However, mortality was similar in the two groups. In the editorial [3], Ward Kennedy argues that the most likely explanation for this apparently conclusive protection afforded by diltiazem is due to its platelet-inhibitor rather than its vasodilator actions.

Ogawa *et al* [4] studied the clinical spectrum and outcome of 119 patients with acute non-Q wave myocardial infarction and compared them with those of 354 patients with acute Q wave myocardial infarction. It was found that patients with non-Q wave myocardial infarction had a significantly higher incidence of pre-infarction angina (73% *vs* 63%), previous myocardial infarction (43% *vs* 22%), multivessel disease (73% *vs* 51%), post-infarction angina (55% *vs* 21%) and recurrent myocardial infarction during follow-up for an average of 25 months (17% *vs* 8%) when compared with patients with acute Q wave myocardial infarction. Patients with non-Q wave myocardial infarction also had a lower rate of complication of pump failure and smaller infarct size (as estimated by peak creatine phosphokinase levels) than those with Q wave myocardial infarction. There was no difference in in-hospital mortality between the two groups, although death due to cardiac rupture was observed only in the patients with Q wave myocardial infarction. The results of this study suggest that non-Q wave myocardial infarction has a more unstable clinical course than Q wave myocardial infarction.

RECENT ADVANCES IN CORONARY THROMBOLYSIS

Review: PHILIP A. LUDBROOK, BURTON E. SOBEL

History
With reduction of the hospital mortality attributable to ventricular fibrillation, heart failure has become the pre-eminent cause of death in patients hospitalized for acute myocardial infarction [1]. An inverse relationship between long-term prognosis and 'infarct size' has been established [2], but the limitation of infarct size by diminution of myocardial oxygen requirements has been only moderately successful [3]. Accordingly, the early restoration of myocardial oxygen supply by coronary thrombolysis, angioplasty, or both, has become a dominant focus of investigation and therapy.

Although 'coronary thrombosis' was first described by Herrick in 1912 [4], its role was controversial until recently, when DeWood *et al* demonstrated total coronary thrombotic occlusion in 87% of patients studied cinéangiographically within the first four hours of onset of infarction [5]. This observation lent credibility to the use of coronary thrombolysis as the primary approach in patients with acute myocardial infarction.

The phenomenon of fibrinolysis was recognized initially in 1769 by Morgagni [6]. Streptokinase was described by Tillet *et al* in 1933 [7]. Coronary thrombolysis with intravenous streptokinase was first attempted by Fletcher [8], but acceptance of this approach was limited because of potentially deleterious side-effects and difficulty in demonstrating clinical benefit. Ruegsegger *et al* in 1959 [9], and Kordenat and Kedzi in 1972 [10], demonstrated intracoronary thrombolysis with streptokinase in animals, with concomitant electrocardiographic and/or hemodynamic improvement. In 1976, Chazov *et al* documented successful thrombolysis in patients with intracoronary streptokinase [11]. In 1979, Rentrop *et al* elicited reperfusion in a patient with acute coronary thrombosis by guidewire fragmentation of the thrombus, followed by intracoronary streptokinase [12,13]. This study and a subsequent report of a pilot series of patients ignited the current burst of enthusiasm for coronary thrombolysis [13].

Plasminogen activator, the agent whose promise has recently stimulated multiple clinical trials, was first described in 1947 by Astrup [14]. The activator was isolated in 1969 by Kok [15]; it was purified initially from human uterine tissue by Rijken in 1979 [16], and subsequently in 1981 from the supernatant fraction of a human melanoma cell-line (mt-PA) by Rijken and Collen [17,18], in quantities sufficient for pharmacologic studies in animals [19] and pilot studies in man [20]. In 1983, the t-PA gene was cloned by Pennica *et al* [21], facilitating the production of pharmaceutical quantities of recombinant DNA-produced t-PA (rt-PA) and enabling the instigation of a pilot study [22] and large-scale clinical trials of rt-PA in patients with acute myocardial infarction [23–26].

Pharmacology

Thrombosis occurs through either intrinsic or extrinsic proteolytic pathways that ultimately generate thrombin, a protease that converts fibrinogen to fibrin. Physiologically, a counterbalancing fibrinolytic system precludes excessive or inappropriate intravascular thrombosis [27]. Fibrinolysis reflects the activation of plasminogen by tissue-type plasminogen activator (t-PA) to yield plasmin. Circulating plasmin can degrade not only fibrin but also fibrinogen, with consequent elaboration of fibrinogen degradation products (FDP), clotting factors V, VIII and XII, and other plasma proteins [28]. Physiologically, proteolysis by plasmin is restricted to fibrin in clots because of the high affinity of plasminogen, and plasminogen activator, for fibrin. Any excess plasmin released free into the circulation is promptly inactivated by inhibitors such as alpha$_2$-antiplasmin and alpha$_2$-macroglobulin. Conversely, fibrin-bound plasmin is protected from alpha$_2$-antiplasmin, as the lysine-binding sites of plasmin, which are involved in the binding between fibrin and plasmin, are also required for the interaction between alpha$_2$-antiplasmin and plasmin. In contrast to the 100-ms half-life of circulating free plasmin, the half-life of fibrin-bound plasmin is more than 10 seconds, which affords fibrinolysis and clot dissolution adequate time to commence – and to continue, provided that a continuous supply of plasminogen and activator is available at the eroding clot surface.

Plasminogen Activation

Physiologically, plasminogen is activated by endogenous t-PA elaborated by vascular endothelial cells in response to local intravascular thrombus. Release of t-PA can be stimulated also by epinephrine, ethanol, exercise, and nicotinic acid [29]. The circulating half-life of t-PA is 5–7 minutes. In contrast, the administration of streptokinase or urokinase induces massive activation of circulating plasminogen, resulting in the generation of sufficient plasmin to overwhelm the circulating plasmin inhibitors. Circulating plasminemia induces a prolonged 'systemic lytic state' characterized by fibrinogenolysis as well as fibrinolysis, depletion of alpha$_2$-antiplasmin and plasminogen; and accumulation of fibrin- and fibrinogen-degradation products ('split products'), which exert profound anticoagulant effects [30].

Free plasminogen is physiologically not activated in the circulation by dint of its low concentration and the low affinity of t-PA for non-fibrin-bound plasminogen. In the presence of intravascular thrombus, however, t-PA undergoes hydrophobic binding to fibrin, forming a binary complex with a very high affinity for plasminogen. Plasminogen binds via its lysine-binding sites to fibrin, producing a ternary complex of fibrin, plasminogen and t-PA. The close spatial orientation of t-PA, plasminogen and fibrin facilitates the activation of fibrin-bound plasminogen by fibrin-bound t-PA, producing plasmin juxtaposed to fibrin on the clot surface, where plasmin is protected from alpha$_2$-antiplasmin through the occupation of its lysine-binding sites in the process of fibrin-binding. Any excess plasmin released into the circulation is rapidly inactivated by alpha$_2$-antiplasmin [28–30].

Tissue-type plasminogen activator appears to be synthesized physiologically as a single-chain protein (MW 72 000 daltons). A two-chain form, with polypeptide components connected by a single disulfide bridge, results from limited proteolytic degradation. The functional properties of the two forms are similar [31], though their pharmacokinetics differ.

Listed below are several activators of the fibrinolytic system that are of pharmacologic interest.
(i) Tissue plasminogen activator (t-PA)
(ii) Streptokinase
(iii) Acylated (anisoylated) streptokinase/plasminogen
(iv) Urokinase
(v) Pro-urokinase
(vi) Streptokinase/fibrin-specific monoclonal antibody
(vii) Urokinase/fibrin-specific monoclonal antibody

Streptokinase, which is not a clot-selective activator, is synthesized by group C beta-hemolytic streptococci. It activates plasminogen indirectly by complexing with it, and unmasking an active proteolytic site on the plasminogen molecule, which in turn activates other plasminogen molecules. Streptokinase induces high concentrations of circulating plasmin and a systemic lytic state that predisposes to bleeding. As an antigenic foreign protein, streptokinase may commonly induce allergic reactions, including chills, fever and urticaria, although anaphylaxis is fortunately rare. Streptokinase may be partially inactivated by antibodies induced by prior exposure to streptococci. However, the extent of inactivation is generally modest, and can be overcome with the use of a loading dose to saturate the antibody-binding capacity [32,33].

In an effort to produce a more clot-selective plasminogen activator, streptokinase, modified by acylation, has been complexed with plasminogen to form an acylated streptokinase/plasminogen complex [34]. Prior to deacylation *in vivo*, this complex exerts no fibrinolytic activity; it can, however, bind to fibrin and resist inactivation by alpha$_2$-antiplasmin. After deacylation, the circulating complex is fibrinogenolytic. Two acylated agents have received the most attention in animal models and in clinical studies – the *p*-anisoyl derivative (BRL 26921) and the *p*-aminobenzoyl derivative (BRL 33575) [35]. In practice, however, deacylation entails a significant delay in activation of plasminogen on the clot surface, and hence delays thrombolysis [33]. Further, the considerable plasminemia, and consequent systemic fibrinogenolysis, encountered with this agent has been disappointing [36,37]. Nevertheless, in a controlled trial of anisoylated plasminogen streptokinase activator complex (APSAC) in 149 patients admitted with probable myocardial infarction, increased plasma activity of myocardial creatine kinase isoenzyme diagnostic of infarction was observed in 92% of control patients and 79% of APSAC-treated patients. The difference was more apparent in patients treated within 2.5 hours of onset of symptoms. Treated patients showed greater preservation of electrocardiographic R waves than control patients. More adverse effects were observed in the patients treated with APSAC (26%) than in the control population (3%) [38].

Urokinase is a human protein first isolated from urine; it has little antigenicity [33]. It activates plasminogen directly (without intermediate complexing with plasminogen), and elicits plasminemia. Despite reports of the efficacy of urokinase for the induction of thrombolysis in acute myocardial infarction patients [39] with slightly less systemic fibrinogenolysis than encountered with streptokinase, its acceptance and use have in general been limited by its relative expensiveness. Single-chain human urokinase-type plasminogen activator (scu-PA, or pro-urokinase) can be obtained from conditioned media of human cell culture, or synthesized by recombinant DNA technology. Because of plasma inhibitors of scu-PA-induced activation of plasminogen that are 'neutralized' by fibrin and fibrin breakdown products, it exhibits some clot selectivity, activating plasminogen only in the presence of fibrin. Studies in both experimental animals [40] and humans [41] have demonstrated coronary thrombolysis with only modest systemic fibrinogenolysis. In combination, t-PA and scu-PA (like t-PA and urokinase) appear to exhibit synergism, thrombolytic effects of the combination(s) in animal models being significantly greater than would be expected from the additive effects of each agent administered singly. Further, the systemic fibrinogenolysis observed after higher doses of urokinase was not observed with the t-PA/scu-PA combination given in equivalent thrombolytic doses. Although not yet confirmed clinically, these findings may presage the use of synergic thrombolytic combinations of t-PA and scu-PA in patients – it is to be hoped with diminished propensity to systemic fibrinogenolysis [42].

Recently, complexes of streptokinase or urokinase conjugated with monoclonal antibodies to human fibrin have been developed to provide clot selectivity through 'immunofibrinolytic' mechanisms [43,44].

Fibrin Specificity

Clot selectivity exhibited by t-PA reflects the high affinity of activator for fibrin-bound as opposed to circulating free plasminogen. However, clot selectivity is a relative rather than an absolute property. Tissue plasminogen activator does, in fact, possess some affinity for circulating plasminogen. Thus, inordinately high doses can induce plasminemia and ultimately a systemic lytic state [45,46]. Accordingly, carefully modulated dose regimens are necessary [45].

Physiologically based mathematical models simulating the multiple reactions participating in fibrinolysis demonstrate that inordinately high or prolonged dosages of t-PA may in fact result in the progressive depletion of fibrinogen and plasminogen, whereas judiciously chosen dose regimens generally result in only modest systemic fibrinolytic activation – much less than after streptokinase [47]. These findings have been confirmed in clinical studies. Such simulations provide information useful in developing dose regimens for t-PA suitable for the treatment of those diverse thrombotic entities in which preclusion of a systemic lytic state is desirable [45].

Results of Clinical Trials of Coronary Thrombolysis

Intracoronary Streptokinase

Initially, the intracoronary route was thought to be preferable for the administration of streptokinase to patients with myocardial infarction because of: (i) high concentrations of activator achievable at the clot surface; (ii) avoidance of a necessarily high systemic dose; and (iii) the need for angiographic documentation of lysis. However, intracoronary administration entails inherent delay and high costs, and is impractical for the majority of patients because of the relatively limited availability of catheterization facilities and skilled personnel [48]. Accordingly, it has largely been abandoned as the primary approach [49]. Nevertheless, several randomized and non-randomized trials of intracoronary streptokinase have established that thrombolysis can be achieved in 60%–94% of patients [50,51]. Pooled-data studies indicate an average incidence of thrombolysis of 72%–75% [52,53]. Incidences of thrombolysis after intracoronary streptokinase reported from the Registries of the Society for Cardiac Angiography (71.2%) [54] and the European Society of Cardiology (76%) are consistent with these results.

Improvement of regional perfusion [55] and myocardial metabolism [56] have been demonstrated after intracoronary streptokinase. However, improved left-ventricular function has been more difficult to document clinically, despite favorable reports from the Registry of the European Society of Cardiology [57], the Hoechst-Roussel Registry [58], and several small randomized [59] and non-randomized [32,60–64] studies. Because left-ventricular ejection fraction can improve spontaneously in some patients treated conservatively [65], prospective randomized placebo-controlled studies are necessary to determine the left-ventricular functional response to thrombolysis. A summary of results of five such studies [50] points out that ejection fraction improved in only one [59], and in this study the duration of ischemia was relatively brief (<3 hours). Reocclusion and reinfarction may have confounded the evaluation of left-ventricular function in certain studies [50]. Automated contrast ventriculographic analysis of regional left-ventricular wall motion [66] has demonstrated improvement of regional wall motion in 82% of patients exhibiting recanalization within two hours of onset of chest pain, but in only 46% of those in whom recanalization was induced later [67]. Clearly, myocardial salvage requires prompt reperfusion.

Furberg analyzed pooled data from nine relatively small randomized trials of intracoronary streptokinase (with fewer than 1000 patients in aggregate) [52]. No significant enhancement of survival by intracoronary streptokinase was evident. Likewise, no significant difference in six-month mortality was observed by Rentrop [68]. Nevertheless, results of several larger randomized trials have recently indicated that prompt administration of intracoronary streptokinase improves early survival. Thus, in the Western Washington trial, 30-day and 6-month mortality were significantly lower after streptokinase given within 24 hours after onset of symptoms than after placebo, particularly in patients with anterior infarction [69]. Survival, when statistically adjusted for disparities in infarct location and ejection fraction, was still improved 12 months after infarction in patients receiving intracoronary streptokinase [70]. Similarly, in the Netherlands Interuniversity Cardiology Institute study, which involved 533 patients studied within four hours of onset of infarction, intracoronary streptokinase lowered 14-day mortality significantly, with markedly improved survival evident also 12 months after infarction [71]. Infarct size measured and estimated enzymatically was significantly less, and left-ventricular ejection fraction significantly greater, in treated patients. Benefit was particularly striking in patients treated within two hours of onset of chest pain [72].

Intravenous Streptokinase
Although various protocols for the intravenous use of streptokinase have been suggested [73], most recent trials have employed a high-dose short-duration regimen (e.g. $1–1.5 \times 10^6$ IU given over 60 min) [74]. In studies that do not entail preintervention arteriography, the apparent recanalization rate has ranged from 73% to 96% [50]. In contrast, if the analysis is limited to patients in whom complete thrombotic occlusion of the infarct artery is confirmed angiographically prior to administration of streptokinase, the average incidence of recanalization is only 45% (range, 10%–62%) [50]. This discrepancy reflects: (i) the inclusion, in studies not requiring preintervention angiography, of patients with incomplete obstruction of the infarct-related vessel, observed in approximately 22% of patients; and (ii) the effects of spontaneous recanalization in a small percentage.

The NHLBI thrombolysis in myocardial infarction (TIMI) phase I study confirmed the relatively low incidence of coronary thrombolysis in patients given streptokinase intravenously [24]. Patients were randomized within the first six hours of onset of chest pain to receive intravenous streptokinase or rt-PA. Angiographically documented recanalization was observed in 35% of patients given streptokinase and 66% of those given t-PA.

The results of several large and recent clinical trials using intravenous streptokinase [75–77] have yielded promising conclusions.

In the largest study completed to date – the 'GISSI' trial, involving some 11 806 patients – intravenous streptokinase (1.5 million units over 1 hour) was administered within 12 hours of onset of chest pain [75]. Although no angiographic information was available to confirm thrombosis or thrombolysis, differences in early mortality were striking. Mortality at 21 days in the streptokinase group (10.7%) was 18% less than that in controls (13%). Benefit was highly dependent on the rapidity with which streptokinase was administered: a 51% reduction in mortality was observed in patients treated within one hour of onset of pain (8.2%); a 23% reduction was seen in patients treated within three hours. Significant reduction was not seen in patients treated six hours or more after onset of pain. Improved survival was seen only in patients with anterior infarction and whose age was less than 65 years.

Improved early survival was reported also by Simoons *et al* [71], who randomized 264 patients with acute myocardial infarction to conventional therapy, and 269 to thrombolytic therapy with either intracoronary streptokinase immediately after angiography (n=152) or intravenous streptokinase upon entry to hospital followed by intracoronary streptokinase after angiography (n=117). In addition, PTCA was performed in selected patients. Mortality 28 days after admission was significantly lower in patients treated with streptokinase (5.6%) than in those given placebo (11.7%). After one year, survival was 91% in treated patients compared with 84% in controls; the best results occurred in the subset in which intravenous preceded intracoronary streptokinase.

In the ISAM study, 1741 patients hospitalized within six hours of onset of acute myocardial infarction were randomized to treatment with either streptokinase (1.5 million IU intravenous over 1 hour) or placebo [76]. Global and regional ejection fractions were significantly higher in treated than in control patients with anterior or inferior infarction. Although mortality was statistically similar 21 days after hospitalization, a trend towards improved survival was observed in the treated group – particularly in patients receiving streptokinase within three hours of onset of symptoms.

In summary, thrombolysis can be induced in approximately 75% of patients by intracoronary and in 45% of patients by intravenous streptokinase. Intravenous administration is much more universally applicable than intracoronary therapy and can be implemented faster, thereby increasing the likelihood of achieving myocardial salvage, and thus improved ventricular performance and enhanced survival. Early- and medium-term survival may be improved in patients in whom thrombolysis is achieved promptly after onset of chest pain.

Tissue-Type Plasminogen Activator
Coronary thrombolysis with t-PA was demonstrated initially in dogs with coronary thrombosis which had been induced with thrombogenic copper coils inserted into the left anterior descending coronary artery. Intravenous t-PA elicited thrombolysis, accompanied by restoration of nutritive perfusion and intermediary metabolism and without induction of a systemic lytic state, within 15 minutes [19].

Studies in humans were undertaken soon afterwards. In an initial pilot study of t-PA, thrombolysis without significant fibrinogenolysis was demonstrated in six of seven patients with transmural infarction and angiographically documented coronary occlusions [22].

As soon as large quantities of t-PA became available via recombinant DNA technology (rt-PA), a multicenter dose-finding and efficacy trial was undertaken [23]. Recanalization of totally occluded infarct-related arteries was documented angiographically in 75% of 109 patients given intracoronary or intravenous rt-PA; it was accompanied by only modest fibrinogenolysis.

The first phase of the TIMI study involved an initial open-label, and a subsequent randomized, comparison between intravenous streptokinase (1.5×10^6 IU intravenous over 1 hour) and intravenous rt-PA (80 mg intravenous over 3 hours) [24]. These dosages were chosen on the basis of reported experience to represent the most efficacious regimens for each drug; drug equivalence was not implied. This study confirmed the superiority of rt-PA. Of 122 patients given intravenous streptokinase and 118 given intravenous rt-PA within seven hours of onset of chest pain, recanalization was demonstrated angiographically in 66% after rt-PA, and in 35% after streptokinase. Fibrinogen declined to less than 150 mg/dl in only 17% of patients given rt-PA, and to less than 100 mg/dl in only 3%. By contrast, in patients given streptokinase it declined to less than 150 mg/dl in 57%, and to less than 100 mg/dl in 27%.

In the European Cooperative Study, 129 patients with acute infarction were randomized to intravenous rt-PA (0.75 mg/kg over 90 min) or intravenous streptokinase (1.5×10^6 IU over 1 hour) [25]. In another arm of the study 124 patients were randomized to intravenous rt-PA or placebo [78]. Administration of agents was not preceded by coronary angiography, resulting in probable inclusion of some patients with incomplete coronary occlusion in the analyses. Consistent with results of other studies, thrombolysis occurred in 70% and 61%, respectively, of patients with only modest fibrinogenolysis given rt-PA and placebo. The patency rate after streptokinase was 55%.

Results of these trials corroborate those of earlier pilot studies, and indicate that thrombolysis can be induced with intravenous rt-PA in some 75% of patients with acute myocardial infarction, without induction of a systemic lytic state.

Pharmacodynamics and Pharmacokinetics of t-PA

Computer simulations [45,46,79] and laboratory results indicate that the pharmacodynamic effects of t-PA are dependent upon: (i) the initial concentration of circulating alpha$_2$-antiplasmin; (ii) the initial concentration, and the rate of synthesis, of plasminogen – particularly in the presence of prolonged infusions of t-PA; (iii) the dose and duration of infusion of t-PA; and (iv) circulating concentrations of alpha$_2$-macroglobulin, a slow-reacting inhibitor of plasmin whose effects become predominant after depletion of alpha$_2$-antiplasmin. After complete consumption of plasminogen, additional activator results paradoxically in no additional generation of plasmin and hence in no further fibrinolysis [79].

Augmentation of Myocardial Salvage

The major determinant of salvage appears to be the rapidity of reperfusion. Salvage is dependent also on the adequacy of restitution of nutritive flow and thus on the severity of the residual coronary artery stenosis [3]. Reocclusion is particularly frequent when the residual stenosis is severe (i.e. cross-sectional area <0.4 mm^2) [80]. Sheehan et al found that improvement in regional hypokinesis – and thus, presumably, the extent of myocardial salvage – was greater in patients in whom the residual minimal diameter of the infarct-related artery after thrombolysis was greater than 0.4 mm [81]. Among patients with more severe residual stenosis, significantly less improvement of regional dysfunction was evident. Others have demonstrated greater improvement in patients treated within two hours of onset of chest pain. Thus, in some patients, thrombolysis may restore angiographically demonstrable patency, but may restore insufficient nutritive coronary blood flow to induce salvage of jeopardized myocardium. Coronary angioplasty, by further reducing the severity of the residual stenosis, may be required to achieve adequate nutritive perfusion and thus effect salvage. Further, by reducing the severity of the residual coronary stenosis, angioplasty may reduce the incidence of reocclusion after pharmacologic thrombolysis.

In a randomized trial comparing intracoronary streptokinase and coronary angioplasty (PTCA) in 56 patients studied within 12 hours of onset of myocardial infarction, recanalization was accomplished in 24 of 29 patients by PTCA and in 23 of the 27 given streptokinase [82]. Although the incidence of recanalization was comparable, residual diameter stenosis was significantly less successful in patients subjected to PTCA (43% ±31%) than in those given intracoronary streptokinase (83% ±17%). While the time to reperfusion was comparable in the two groups, ventricular function prior to hospital discharge was significantly improved after PTCA but not after streptokinase. Residual ischemia with exercise was evident with thallium-201 scintigraphy in 47% of patients given streptokinase, but in only 14% of those treated with PTCA. Similarly, among 50 patients with acute infarction randomized 3:1 to placebo, intravenous rt-PA alone, or intravenous rt-PA followed by emergent PTCA, infarct-zone regional wall motion one week later was significantly improved in patients undergoing PTCA compared with those given rt-PA alone [83]. Thus, early PTCA may facilitate or augment myocardial salvage. From a practical point of view, a combined strategy may be best, entailing thrombolysis to 'buy time' until preparations for catheterization and angioplasty can be completed [84]. Obviously, public education emphasizing the need to reduce the time lag between onset of symptoms and treatment is of the utmost importance [3].

Several adjunctive pharmacologic approaches offer promise for augmenting protection of myocardium subjected to ischemia and reperfusion, and for prolonging the interval of ischemia after which jeopardized tissue can still be salvaged.

In dogs with experimentally induced coronary thrombosis, diltiazem given 30 minutes prior to streptokinase-implemented thrombolysis approximately doubled the extent of myocardial salvage, as delineated by positron emission tomography and by direct assay of myocardial creatine kinase activity, compared with salvage induced by thrombolysis alone [85].

Another pharmacologic approach employs scavengers of catabolic enzymes to limit accumulation of oxygen-derived free radicals and their metabolites, such as superoxide anion, hydrogen peroxide and the hydroxyl radical, that may mediate reperfusion injury [86]. Further, neutrophil depletion [87], and inhibitors of lipoxygenase and prostacyclin, may reduce infiltration of the neutrophils that adhere to vascular endothelium and stimulate release of oxygen free radicals in the infarcted region [86]. Despite their theoretical potential for protection against reperfusion injury, however, both benefit [88,89] and absence of benefit [90] have been reported after use of such agents in animal models, and their efficacy remains controversial.

Thrombolysis does not obviate the value of conventional management of acute myocardial infarction. Thus, for example, using adjunctive beta-adrenergic blocking agents to reduce myocardial oxygen requirements may potentiate salvage [91–93].

Reocclusion

Even when reperfusion is established early and adequately, reocclusion can obviate benefit.

After intravenous streptokinse, early reocclusion occurs with a frequency of 9%– 29% [73]. However, clinical manifestations of reinfarction occur only half as often; this may in part reflect the lack of salvage by the initial reperfusion. In the Netherlands Interuniversity Cardiology Institute study, clinical manifestations of recurrent ischemia were confined essentially to patients in whom thrombolysis of the infarct-related artery was initially successful: reinfarction occurred in 19% of patients in whom recanalization had occurred but in only 8% of those in whom recanalization failed [71]. In the GISSI trial, the incidence of reinfarction was 4.1% in patients given intravenous streptokinase, compared with 2.1% in controls [75]. Recently, 'ischemic double jeopardy' (i.e. infarction followed by recurrent ischemia) after thrombolysis has been emphasized [94]. The possibility has also been considered that small islands of surviving myocardium subject to recurrent ischemia may constitute foci of arrhythmogenesis, giving rise to sudden death.

Although the overall risk of reocclusion may be as high as 46% [95], reocclusion within 24 hours of thrombolysis is relatively infrequent [96], suggesting that interventions such as coronary angioplasty, intended to consolidate the benefit of thrombolysis and prevent reocclusion, can probably be delayed for at least 24 hours without inordinate risk of rethrombosis.

Although the short biologic half-life of t-PA in the circulation may be advantageous in permitting prompt offset in patients requiring surgery, it has been argued that it may set the stage for reocclusion. However, because the half-life of fibrin-bound t-PA is substantially longer, t-PA within the interstices of intravascular thrombi may continue to activate plasminogen locally, facilitating continued lysis and retarding reocclusion. In the same way, continued low-dose infusions may be protective against reocclusion. In experimental animals in which coronary thrombosis is induced by intracoronary placement of a thrombogenic copper coil, plasma concentrations of t-PA of as little as 10% of those required to induce lysis of established thrombi are sufficient to prevent reocclusion [97]. Prolonged infusions of subthrombolytic doses of t-PA can be given without induction of a systemic lytic state [97].

Gold *et al* have confirmed the efficacy of such prolonged low-dose infusions of rt-PA, for the prevention of early reocclusion in patients that have undergone successful thrombolysis [98]. Reperfused patients in whom the residual stenosis was less than 80% were found to be at low risk of reocclusion. Forty-six per cent of patients in whom residual stenosis was severe (greater than 80%) suffered reocclusion when treated with heparin alone. However, 86% of successfully reperfused patients with severe residual stenosis exhibited neither angiographic nor clinical evidence of reocclusion during hospitalization and follow-up for 10–14 days when treated with both heparin and a low-dose infusion of rt-PA. Only modest fibrinogen depletion was observed. Although the patient population was small, this suggests that prolonged low-dose infusions of rt-PA may constitute an effective alternative strategy for the prevention of early reocclusion.

Non-Invasive Markers of Reperfusion and Reocclusion

Two considerations dominate the management of patients treated initially with thrombolytic agents: (i) the presence or absence of reperfusion within a defined interval after the onset of ischemia; and (ii) the extent to which the magnitude of the mass of myocardium salvaged justifies invasive interventions designed to consolidate the gains [3]. Conventional non-invasive markers of reperfusion, such as 'early wash-out' of creatine kinase, are neither sensitive nor specific enough for these purposes [99]. Characterization of ratios of subforms of individual isoenzymes of creatine kinase in serial plasma samples may be useful. Because the tissue form of the MM creatine kinase isoenzyme (MM_A) undergoes sequential proteolytic conversion in plasma to the MM_B and MM_C subforms with consistent kinetics, the release of the MM creatine kinase isoenzyme from ischemic myocardium, and hence the time of onset of irreversible myocardial injury, can be estimated accurately [100]. Subform analysis offers promise for the detection of reperfusion, in view of the 10-fold or greater rate of rise of the MM_A/MM_C ratio in plasma over that seen during the evolution of acute myocardial infarction in the absence of reperfusion.

Note added at proof

Several important studies have recently been completed. Their results have clarified the role of early cardiac catheterization in the management of patients treated pharmacologically with fibrinolytic agents, the virtues and limitations of immediate, 'routine,' angioplasty for such patients, and the impact of coronary thrombolysis with tissue-type plasminogen activator on ventricular performance [101,102]. Diagnostic cardiac catheterization is needed immediately whenever deterioration compatible with early reocclusion or reinfarction is recognized. Should emergency, early coronary angiography following pharmacologic thrombolysis demonstrate severe stenoses with cross-sectional areas of 0.4 mm^2 or less, they should be dilated at once because of the high risk of early reocclusion. Many investigators believe that immediate angioplasty is the treatment of choice in this setting, although it is now recognized that angioplasty soon after pharmacologic induction of coronary thrombolysis is more prone to be associated with complications than angioplasty deferred until somewhat later. Results of three controlled trials clarify this important issue. Published data from the TAMI trial [101] as well as information presented from the European Cooperative trial and the TIMI IIA trial presented at the 1987 meeting of the American Heart Association are remarkably concordant. In all three trials, immediate cardiac catheterization and 'routine' angioplasty for amenable lesions not only failed to improve ventricular performance or early survival but also were associated with a two-fold higher incidence of adverse effects. Such effects include early recurrent infarction, bleeding requiring transfusions, coronary artery dissection requiring immediate surgery, and death. These persuasive results indicate that in the absence of complications mandating immediate invasive evaluation, angiography and possible angioplasty after coronary thrombolysis should be undertaken electively. These procedures may be reserved for patients with signs of ischemia at rest or signs of ischemia evoked by exercise testing performed prior to hospital discharge. The alternative view, namely that all patients with acute myocardial infarction treated with thrombolytic agents should undergo cardiac catheterization prior to hospital discharge, with angioplasty if anatomically suitable, has yet to be proven.

Results of several studies indicate that early coronary thrombolysis enhances ventricular performance. A recently published investigation of the effects of intravenous t-PA in this regard demonstrates conclusively that patients treated with intravenous t-PA within 3.2 $\pm$0.2 (SD) hours after the onset of symptoms indicative of acute transmural myocardial infarction exhibit a high patency rate of infarct-related arteries (66%) and that they manifest a higher mean ejection fraction than placebo-treated controls (53 $\pm$2 compared with 46 $\pm$2 [SE]) ten days after hospital admission and a diminution of the prevalence of congestive heart failure of 58%. Although angioplasty appears to increase exercise ejection fraction even further and reduce the incidence of postinfarction angina beyond the reduction associated with administration of t-PA alone, it does not appear to influence ejection fraction at rest[102]. It is likely that these results will be corroborated by a large Australian study from which some preliminary information has been presented informally and additional information is being compiled presently for formal scientific pub-lication.

Acknowledgments

Supported in part by National Heart, Lung and Blood Institute Grant RO1 HL25430, and Specialized Center of Research in Ischemic Heart Disease, Grant HL 17646, National Institutes of Health, Bethesda, Maryland, USA.

References

[1] Schwartz DE, Yamaga CC, for the Health and Public Policy Committee, American College of Physicians.
Thrombolysis for evolving myocardial infarction.
Ann Intern Med 1985; **103**: 463–9.

[2] Geltman EM, Ehsani AA, Campbell MK, Schechtman K, Roberts R, Sobel BE.
The influence of location and extent of myocardial infarction on long-term ventricular dysrhythmia and mortality.
Circulation 1979; **60**: 805–14.

[3] Sobel BE.
Coronary thrombolysis with tissue-type plasminogen activator (t-PA): Emerging strategies.
J Am Coll Cardiol 1986; **8**: 1220–5.

[4] Herrick JB.
Clinical features of sudden obstruction of the coronary arteries.
JAMA 1912; **41**: 2015–20.

[5] DeWood MA, Spores J, Notske MD *et al.*
Prevalence of total coronary occlusion during the early hours of transmural myocardial infarction.
N Engl J Med 1980; **303**: 897–902.

[6] Morgagni JB.
The Seats and Causes of Diseases Investigated by Anatomy. London: Johnson & Payne, 1769; **3**: 186.

[7] Tillet WS, Garner RL.
The fibrinolytic activity of hemolytic streptococci.
J Exp Med 1933; **58**: 485–502.

[8] Fletcher AP, Alkjaersig N, Smyrniotis FE, Sherry S.
The treatment of patients suffering from early myocardial infarction with massive and prolonged streptokinase therapy.
Trans Assoc Am Physicians 1958; **71**: 287–96.

[9] Ruegsegger P, Nydick I, Hutter RC *et al.*
Fibrinolytic (plasmin) therapy of experimental coronary thrombi with alteration of the evolution of myocardial infarction.
Circulation 1959; **19**: 7–13.

[10] Kordenat RK, Kedzi P.
Experimental intracoronary thrombosis and selective in situ lysis by catheter technique.
Am J Cardiol 1972; **30**: 640–5.

[11] Chazov EI, Mateeva LS, Mazaev AV, Sargin KE, Sadovshaya M, Ruda Y.
Intracoronary administration of fibrinolysin in acute myocardial infarction.
Ter Arkh 1976; **48**: 8–19.

[12] Rentrop KP, DeVivie ER, Karsch KR, Kreuzer H.
Acute coronary occlusion with impending infarction as angiographic complication relieved
by guide-wire recanalization.
Clin Cardiol 1978; **1**: 101–6.

[13] Rentrop KP, Blanke H, Karsch KR *et al.*
Acute myocardial infarction: Intracoronary ap-
plication of nitroglycerin and streptokinase.
Clin Cardiol 1979; **2**: 354–63.

[14] Astrup T, Permin PM.
Fibrinolysis in animal organism.
Nature 1947; **159**: 681–2.

[15] Kok P, Astrup T.
Isolation and purification of a tissue plasminogen activator and its comparison with urokinase.
Biochemistry 1969; **8**: 79–86.

[16] Rijken DC, Wijngaards G, Zaal-DeJong M, Wel-
bergen J.
Purification and partial characterization of plasminogen activator from human uterine tissue.
Biochim Biophys Acta 1979; **580**: 140–53.

[17] Rijken DC, Collen D.
Purification and characterization of the plasminogen activator secreted by human melanoma
cells in culture.
J Biol Chem 1981; **156**: 7035–41.

[18] Collen D, Rijken DC, VanDamme J, Billiau A.
Purification of human extrinsic (tissue type)
plasminogen activator in scintigram quantities
from a human melanoma cell culture fluid and
its conditioning for use in vivo.
Thromb Haemost 1982; **48**: 294–6.

[19] Bergmann SR, Fox KAA, Ter-Pogossian MM,
Sobel BE, Collen D.
Clot-selective coronary thrombolysis with
tissue-type plasminogen activator.
Science 1983; **220**: 1181–3.

[20] Weimar W, Strabbe J, vanSeyen AJ, Billiau A,
De Somer P, Collen D.
Specific lysis of an iliofemoral thrombus by
administration of extrinsic (tissue-type) plasmi-
nogen activator.
Lancet 1981; **ii**: 1018–20.

[21] Pennica D, Holmes WE, Kǿhr WJ *et al.*
Cloning and expression of human tissue-type
plasminogen activator cDNA in *E. coli.*
Nature 1983; **201**: 214–21.

[22] Van de Werf F, Ludbrook PA, Bergmann SR *et al.*
Coronary thrombolysis with tissue-type plasminogen activator in patients with evolving
myocardial infarction.
N Engl J Med 1984; **310**: 609–13.

[23] Collen D, Topol EJ, Tiefenbrunn AF *et al.*
Coronary thrombolysis with recombinant human tissue-type plasminogen activator: A
prospective, randomized, placebo-controlled
trial.
Circulation 1984; **70**: 1012–7.

[24] TIMI Study Group.
The thrombolysis in myocardial infarction
(TIMI) trial: Phase I findings.
N Engl J Med 1985; **312**: 932–6.

[25] Verstraete M, Bory M, Collen D *et al.*
Randomized trial of intravenous recombinant
tissue-type plasminogen activator versus intravenous streptokinase in acute myocardial
infarction.
Lancet 1985; **i**: 842–7.

[26] Collen D.
Human tissue-type plasminogen activator:
From the laboratory to the bedside.
Circulation 1985; **72**: 18–20.

[27] Tiefenbrunn AJ, Sobel BE.
Tissue-type plasminogen activator (t-PA): An
agent with promise for selective thrombolysis.
Int J Cardiol 1985; **7**: 82–6.

[28] Collen D.
On the regulation and control of fibrinolysis:
Edward Kowalski Memorial Lecture.
Thromb Haemost 1980; **43**: 77–89.

[29] Fox KAA, Bergmann SR, Sobel BE.
Coronary thrombolysis: Pharmacological considerations with emphasis on tissue-type plasminogen activator (t-PA).
Biochem Pharmacol 1984; **33**: 1831–8.

[30] Ludbrook PA.
Thrombolytic therapy with t-PA.
Cardiovasc Med 1986; **11**: 37–44.

[31] Rijken DC, Holyaerts M, Collen D.
Fibrinolytic properties of one-chain and two-
chain human extrinsic (tissue-type) plasminogen activator.
J Biol Chem 1982; **257**: 2920–5.

[32] Little WC.
Thrombolytic therapy of acute myocardial in-
farction.
Curr Probl Cardiol 1983; **8**: 1–47.

[33] Shafer KE, Santoro SA, Sobel BE, Jaffe AS.
Monitoring activity of fibrinolytic agents.
Am J Med 1984; **76**: 879–86.

[34] Smith RAG, Dupe RJ, English PD, Green J.
Fibrinolysis with acyl-enzymes: A new
approach to thrombolytic therapy.
Nature 1981; **290**: 505–8.

[35] Marder VJ, Rothbard RL, Fitzpatrick PG, Francis CW.
Rapid lysis of coronary artery thrombi with anisoylated plasminogen: Streptokinase activator complex.
Ann Intern Med 1986; **104**: 304–10.

[36] Walker ID, Davidson JF, Rae AP, Hutton I, Lawrie TDV.
Acylated streptokinase-plasminogen complex in patients with acute myocardial infarction.
Thromb Haemost 1984; **51**: 204–6.

[37] Green J, Harris GS, Smith RAG, Dupe RJ.
Acyl-enzymes: A novel class of thrombolytic agents. In: Collen D, Lijnen HR, Verstraete M, eds. Thrombolysis, Biological and Therapeutic Properties of New Thrombolytic Agents. Edinburgh: Churchill-Livingstone, 1985; pp. 124–67.

[38] Ikram S, Lewis S, Bucknall C et al.
Treatment of acute myocardial infarction with anisoylated plasminogen streptokinase activator complex.
Br Med J 1986; **293**: 786–9.

[39] Mathey DG, Schofer J, Sheehan F, Becher H, Tilsner V, Dodge HT.
Intravenous urokinase in acute myocardial infarction.
Am J Cardiol 1985; **55**: 878–82.

[40] Collen D, Stump D, Van de Werf F, Jang IK, Nobuhara H, Lijnen HR.
Coronary thrombolysis in dogs with intravenously administered human pro-urokinase.
Circulation 1985; **72**: 384–8.

[41] Van de Werf F, Nobuhara M, Collen D.
Coronary thrombolysis with human single-chain, urokinase-type plasminogen activator (pro-urokinase) in patients with acute myocardial infarction.
Ann Intern Med 1986; **104**: 345–8.

[42] Collen D, Stassen JM, Stump DC, Verstraete M.
Synergism of thrombolytic agents in vivo.
Circulation 1986; **74**: 838–42.

[43] Ito RK, Davis GL, Houranieh A, Yunis EJ, Statland BE.
Development of a thrombolytic agent using a human fibrin-specific monoclonal antibody as a conjugate-carrier for streptokinase.
Circulation 1985; **72** (Suppl 3): III–192.

[44] Bode C, Matsueda G, Haber E.
Targeted thrombolysis with a fibrin-specific antibody-urokinase conjugate.
Circulation 1985; **72** (Suppl 3): III–192.

[45] Sobel BE, Gross RW, Robison AK.
Thrombolysis, clot-selectivity, and kinetics.
Circulation 1984; **70**: 160–3.

[46] Tiefenbrunn AJ, Robison AK, Kurnik PB, Ludbrook PA, Sobel BE.
Clinical pharmacology in patients with evolving myocardial infarction of tissue-type plasminogen activator produced by recombinant DNA technology.
Circulation 1985; **71**: 110–6.

[47] Collen D, Bounameaux H, DeCock F, Lijnen HR, Verstraete M.
Analysis of coagulation and fibrinolysis during intravenous infusion of recombinant human tissue-type plasminogen activator in patients with acute myocardial infarction.
Circulation 1986; **73**: 511–7.

[48] Braunwald E.
The aggressive treatment of acute myocardial infarction.
Circulation 1985; **71**: 1087–92.

[49] Verstraete M.
Intravenous administration of a thrombolytic agent is the only realistic therapeutic approach in evolving myocardial infarction.
Eur Heart J 1985; **6**: 586–93.

[50] Rentrop KP.
Thrombolytic therapy in patients with acute myocardial infarction.
Circulation 1985; **71**: 627–31.

[51] Ludbrook PA, Rentrop KP.
Coronary thrombolysis with intracoronary streptokinase. In: Sobel B, ed. Cardiology Clinics. Philadelphia: WB Saunders, 1987.

[52] Furberg CD.
Clinical value of intracoronary streptokinase [Editorial].
Am J Cardiol 1984; **53**: 626–7.

[53] Lo YSA.
Intravenous versus intracoronary streptokinase in acute myocardial infarction.
Clin Cardiol 1985; **8**: 609–19.

[54] Kennedy JW, Gensini GG, Timmis GC, Maynard C.
Acute myocardial infarction treated with intracoronary streptokinase: A report of the Society for Cardiac Angiography.
Am J Cardiol 1985; **55**: 871–7.

[55] Markis JE, Malagold M, Parker JA et al.
Myocardial salvage after intracoronary thrombolysis with streptokinase in acute myocardial infarction: Assessment of intracoronary thallium-201.
N Engl J Med 1981; **305**: 777–82.

[56] Sobel BE, Geltman EM, Tiefenbrunn AJ et al.
Improvement of regional myocardial metabolism after coronary thrombolysis induced with tissue-type plasminogen activator (t-PA) or streptokinase.
Circulation 1984; **69**: 983–90.

[57] Rentrop P, Smith H, Painter L, Holt J.
Changes in left ventricular ejection fraction after intracoronary thrombolytic therapy. Results of the Registry of the European Society of Cardiology.
Circulation 1983; **68** (Suppl 1): I-55–60.

[58] Weinstein J.
Treatment of myocardial infarction with intracoronary streptokinase: Efficacy and safety data from 209 United States cases in the Hoechst-Roussel Registry.
Am Heart J 1982; **104**: 894–8.

[59] Anderson JL, Marshall HW, Bray BE et al.
A randomized trial of intracoronary streptokinase in the treatment of acute myocardial infarction.
N Engl J Med 1983; **308**: 1312–8.

[60] Ganz W, Buchbinder N, Marcus H et al.
Intracoronary thrombolysis in evolving myocardial infarction.
Am Heart J 1981; **101**: 4–13.

[61] Mathey DG, Kuck K-H, Tilsner V, Krebber H-J, Bleifeld W.
Nonsurgical coronary artery recanalization in acute transmural myocardial infarction.
Circulation 1981; **63**: 489–97.

[62] Smalling RW, Fuentes F, Matthews MW et al.
Sustained improvement in left ventricular function and mortality by intracoronary streptokinase administration during evolving myocardial infarction.
Circulation 1983; **68**: 131–8.

[63] Feit F, Rentrop KP.
Thrombolytic therapy in acute myocardial infarction.
Cardiovasc Rev Rep 1983; **4**: 426–44.

[64] Hugenholtz PG, Rentrop P.
Thrombolytic therapy for acute myocardial infarction: Quo Vadis?
Eur Heart J 1982; **3**: 395–403.

[65] Schwartz H, Leiboff RL, Katz RJ et al.
Arteriographic predictors of spontaneous improvement in left ventricular function after myocardial infarction.
Circulation 1985; **71**: 446–72.

[66] Sheehan FH, Mathey DG, Schofer J, Krebber H-J, Dodge HT.
Effect of interventions in salvaging left ventricular function acute myocardial infarction: A study of intracoronary streptokinase.
Am J Cardiol 1983; **52**: 431–8.

[67] Mathey DG, Sheehan FH, Schofer J, Dodge HT.
Time from onset of symptoms to thrombolytic therapy: A major determinant of myocardial salvage in patients with acute transmural infarction.
J Am Coll Cardiol 1985; **6**: 518–25.

[68] Rentrop KP, Feit F, Blanke H et al.
Effects of intracoronary streptokinase and intracoronary nitroglycerin infusion on coronary angiographic patterns and mortality in patients with acute myocardial infarction.
N Engl J Med 1984; **311**: 1457–63.

[69] Kennedy JW, Ritchie JL, Davis KB, Fritz JK.
Western Washington randomized trial of intracoronary streptokinase in acute myocardial infarction.
N Engl J Med 1983; **309**: 1477–82.

[70] Kennedy JW, Ritchie JL, Davis KB, Stadius ML, Maynard C, Fritz JK.
The Western Washington randomized trial of intracoronary streptokinase in acute myocardial infarction.
N Engl J Med 1985; **312**: 1073–8.

[71] Simoons ML, Serruys PW, van den Brand M et al.
Improved survival after early thrombolysis in acute myocardial infarction. A randomized trial by the Interuniversity Cardiology Institute in the Netherlands.
Lancet 1985; ii: 578–82.

[72] Vermeer F, Simoons ML, Frits WB et al.
Which patients benefit most from early thrombolytic therapy by intracoronary streptokinase?
Circulation 1986; **74**: 1379–89.

[73] Geltman EM.
Treatment of myocardial infarction with intravenous streptokinase. In: Sobel B, ed. *Cardiology Clinics*. Philadelphia: WB Saunders, 1987 (in press).

[74] Schroder R, Biamino G, von Leitner ER et al.
Intravenous short-term infusion of streptokinase in acute myocardial infarction.
Circulation 1983; **67**: 536–48.

[75] Gruppo Italiano per lo Studio della Streptochinasi nell'Infarto Miocardico (GISSI).
Effectiveness of intravenous thrombolytic treatment in acute myocardial infarction.
Lancet 1986; i: 397–401.

[76] ISAM Study Group.
A prospective trial of intravenous streptokinase in acute myocardial infarction (ISAM). Mortality, morbidity, and infarct size at 21 days.
N Engl J Med 1986; **314:** 1465–71.

[77] Simoons ML, Serruys PW, van den Brand M.
Randomized trial with intracoronary streptokinase. In: Effest S, Hugenholtz PG *et al*, eds. *Facts and Hopes in Thrombolysis*. Darmstadt: Steinkopff Verlag, 1986; pp. 61–6.

[78] Verstraete M, Brower RW, Collen D *et al*.
Double-blind randomized trial of intravenous tissue-type plasminogen activator versus placebo in acute myocardial infarction.
Lancet 1985; i: 965–9.

[79] Tiefenbrunn AJ, Graor RA, Robison AK, Lucas FV, Hotchkiss A, Sobel BE.
Pharmacodynamics of tissue-type plasminogen activator characterized by computer-assisted simulation.
Circulation 1986; **73:** 1291–9.

[80] Harrison BG, Ferguson DW, Collins SM *et al*.
Re-thrombosis after reperfusion with streptokinase: Importance of geometry of residual lesions.
Circulation 1984; **69:** 991–9.

[81] Sheehan FH, Mathey DG, Schofer J, Dodge HT, Bolson EL.
Factors that determine recovery of left ventricular function after thrombolysis in patients with acute myocardial infarction.
Circulation 1985; **71:** 1121–8.

[82] O'Neill W, Timmis GC, Bourdillon PD *et al*.
A prospective randomized clinical trial of intracoronary streptokinase versus coronary angioplasty for acute myocardial infarction.
N Engl J Med 1986; **314:** 812–8.

[83] Topol EJ, O'Neill WW, Langburd AB *et al*.
A randomized, placebo controlled trial of intravenous recombinant tissue-type plasminogen activator and emergency coronary angioplasty in acute myocardial infarction.
Circulation 1987; **75:** 420–8.

[84] Jaffe AS, Sobel BE.
Thrombolysis with tissue-type plasminogen activator in acute myocardial infarction.
JAMA 1986; **255:** 237–9.

[85] Knabb RM, Rosamond TL, Fox KAA, Sobel BE, Bergmann SR.
Enhancement of salvage of reperfused ischemic myocardium by diltiazem.
J Am Coll Cardiol 1986; **8:** 861–71.

[86] Werns SW, Shea MJ, Lucchesi BR.
Free-radicals and myocardial injury: Pharmacologic implications.
Circulation 1986; **74:** 1–5.

[87] Romson JL, Hook BG, Kunkel SL, Abrams GD, Schork A, Lucchesi BR.
Reduction of the extent of ischemic myocardial injury by neutrophil depletion in the dog.
Circulation 1983; **67:** 1016–23.

[88] Myers ML, Bolli R, Lekich RF, Hartley CJ, Roberts R.
Enhancement of recovery of myocardial function by oxygen free-radical scavengers after reversible regional ischemia.
Circulation 1985; **72:** 915–21.

[89] Werns SW, Shea MJ, Driscoll EM *et al*.
The independent effects of oxygen radical scavengers on canine infarct size: Reduction by superoxide dismutase but not catalase.
Circ Res 1985; **56:** 895–8.

[90] Gallagher KP, Buda AJ, Pace D, Gerren RA, Shlafer M.
Failure of superoxide dismutase and catalase to alter size of infarction in conscious dogs after 3 hours of occlusion followed by reperfusion.
Circulation 1986; **73:** 1065–76.

[91] Maroko PR, Braunwald E.
Modification of myocardial infarction size after coronary occlusion.
Ann Intern Med 1973; **79:** 720–33.

[92] Hammerman H, Kloner RA, Briggs LL, Braunwald E.
Enhancement of salvage of reperfused myocardium by early beta-adrenergic blockade (timolol).
J Am Coll Cardiol 1984; **3:** 1438–43.

[93] Beta-Blocker Heart Attack Trial Research Group.
A randomized trial of propranolol in patients with acute myocardial infarction: I. Mortality results.
JAMA 1982; **247:** 1707–14.

[94] Schaer DH, Katz RJ, Leiboff RH *et al*.
'Ischemic double jeopardy' following reperfusion for acute myocardial infarction.
Circulation 1985; **72** (Suppl 3): III–55.

[95] Leiboff RH, Katz RJ, Wasserman AG *et al*.
A randomized, angiographically controlled trial of intracoronary streptokinase in acute myocardial infarction.
Am J Cardiol 1984; **53:** 404–7.

[96] Chesebro JH, Smith HC, Holmes DR *et al*.
Re-occlusion and clot lysis between ninety minutes, one day, and ten days after thrombolytic therapy for myocardial infarction.
Circulation 1985; **72** (Suppl 3): III–5.

[97] Fox KAA, Robison AK, Knabb RM, Rosamond TL, Sobel BE, Bergmann SR.
Prevention of coronary thrombosis with sub-thrombolytic doses of tissue-type plasminogen activator.
Circulation 1985; **72**: 1346–54.

[98] Gold HK, Leinbach RC, Garabedian HD *et al*.
Acute coronary reocclusion after thrombolysis with recombinant tissue-type plasminogen activator: Prevention by maintenance infusion.
Circulation 1986; **73**: 347–52.

[99] Gore JM, Roberts R, Alfredo M *et al*.
Caution in the use of timing of peak creatine kinase (CK) as a marker for reperfusion.
Circulation 1985; **72** (Suppl 3): III–418.

[100] Hashimoto H, Abendschein DR, Sobel BE.
Early detection of myocardial infarction in conscious dogs by analysis of plasma MM creatinine kinase isoforms.
Circulation 1985; **71**: 363–9.

[101] Topol EJ, Califf RM, Kereiaks DJ, George BS.
Thrombolysis and Angioplasty in Myocardial Infarction (TAMI) trial.
J Am Coll Cardiol 1987; **10**: 65–74B.

[102] Guerci AD, Gersteinblith G, Brinker JA *et al*.
A randomized trial of intravenous tissue type plasminogen activator for acute myocardial infarction with subsequent randomization to elective coronary angioplasty.
N Engl J Med 1987; **317**: 1613–8.

PROGNOSIS OF ANGINA PECTORIS AND MYOCARDIAL INFARCTION

[1] Fifteen year survival study of patients with obstructive coronary artery disease.
Proudfit WJ, Bruschke AVG, MacMillan JP, Williams GW, Sones M Jr, Cleveland Clin Found, Cleveland, OH, USA.
Circulation 1983; **68**: 986–97.

[2] A life table and Cox regression analysis of patients with combined proximal left anterior descending and proximal left circumflex coronary artery disease: non-left main equivalent lesions (CASS).
Chaitman BR, Davis K, Fisher LD *et al*, St Louis Univ Med Cent, St Louis, MO, USA.
Circulation 1983; **68**: 1163–70.

[3] Natural history of coronary heart disease: a study of 586 men surviving an initial acute attack.
Graham I, Mulcahy R, Hickey N, O'Neill W, Daly L, St Vincent's Hosp, Dublin, Eire.
Am Heart J 1983; **105**: 249–57.

[4] Long-term prognosis after first Q-wave (transmural) or non-Q-wave (nontransmural) myocardial infarction: analysis of 593 patients.
Krone RJ, Friedman E, Thanavaro S, Miller JP, Kleiger RE, Oliver GC, Jewish Hosp, St Louis, MO, USA.
Am J Cardiol 1983; **52**: 234–9.

[5] Nontransmural versus transmural myocardial infarction. A morphologic study.
Freifeld AG, Schuster EH, Bulkley BH, Johns Hopkins Hosp, Baltimore, MD, USA.
Am J Med 1983; **75**: 423–32.

[6] Prognosis after extension of myocardial infarct: the role of Q wave or non-Q wave infarction.
Maisel AS, Ahnve S, Gilpin E *et al*, Univ California, San Diego Sch Med, La Jolla, CA, USA.
Circulation 1985; **71**: 211–7.

[7] Myocardial infarct extension: prevalence, clinical significance, and problems in diagnosis.
Buda AJ, Macdonald IL, Dubbin JD, Orr SA, Strauss HD, Toronto Western Hosp, Ontario, Canada.
Am Heart J 1983; **105**: 744–8.

[8] Relationship of specific coronary lesions and regional left ventricular dysfunction to prognosis in survivors of sudden cardiac death.
Vlay SC, Reid PR, Griffith LSC, Kallman CH, State Univ New York, Stony Brook, NY, USA.
Am Heart J 1984; **108**: 1212–20.

[9] Ventricular performance and prognosis after primary ventricular fibrillation complicating acute myocardial infarction.
Dewhurst NG, Hannan WJ, Muir AL, Royal Infirm, Edinburgh, UK.
Eur Heart J 1984; **5**: 275–81.

[10] Effect of ventricular fibrillation complicating acute myocardial infarction on long-term prognosis: importance of the site of infarction.
Schwartz PJ, Zaza A, Graz S *et al*, Univ Milano, Milano, Italy.
Am J Cardiol 1985; **56**: 384–9.

[11] Left bundle branch block: a predictor of poor left ventricular function in coronary artery disease.
Hamby RI, Weissman RH, Prakash MN, Hoffman I, State Univ New York, Stony Brook, NY, USA.
Am Heart J 1983; **106**: 471–7.

[12] Arteriographic predictors of spontaneous improvement in left ventricular function after myocardial infarction.
Schwartz H, Leiboff RL, Katz RJ *et al*, George Washington Univ Med Cent, Washington, DC, USA.
Circulation 1985; **71**: 466–72.

[13] Left ventricular aneurysm as a coronary risk factor independent of overall left ventricular function.
Cohen DE, Vogel RA, Univ Michigan, Ann Arbor, MI, USA.
Am Heart J 1986; **111**: 23–30.

[14] Variation in the size of jeopardized myocardium in patients with isolated left anterior descending coronary artery disease.
DePace NL, Iskandrian AS, Nadell R, Colby J, Hakki A-H, Hahnemann Univ, Philadelphia, PA, USA.
Circulation 1983; **67**: 988–94.

[15] Angiographic findings after myocardial infarction in patients with previous bypass surgery: explanations for smaller infarcts in this group compared with control patients.
Crean PA, Waters DD, Bosch X, Pelletier GB, Roy D, Theroux P, Montreal Heart Inst, Montreal, Quebec, Canada.
Circulation 1985; **71**: 693–8.

[16] Extent and severity of myocardial hypoperfusion as predictors of prognosis in patients with suspected coronary artery disease.
Ladenheim ML, Pollock BH, Rozanski A *et al*, Cedars-Sinai Med Cent, Los Angeles, CA, USA.
J Am Coll Cardiol 1986; **7**: 464–71.

[17] Incremental prognostic power of clinical history, exercise electrocardiography and myocardial perfusion scintigraphy in suspected coronary artery disease.
Ladenheim ML, Kotler TS, Pollock BH, Berman DS, Diamond GA, Cedars-Sinai Med Cent, Los Angeles, CA, USA.
Am J Cardiol 1987; **59**: 270–7.

[18] Mobile coronary care and community mortality from myocardial infarction.
Mathewson ZM, McCloskey BG, Evans AE, Russell CJ, Wilson C, Tyrone County Hosp, Omagh, UK.
Lancet 1985; i: 441–4.

[19] Five hundred patients with myocardial infarction monitored within one hour of symptoms.
O'Doherty M, Tayler DI, Quinn E, Vincent R, Chamberlain DA, Royal Sussex County Hosp, Brighton, UK.
Br Med J 1983; **286:** 1405–8.

[20] Self admission for myocardial infarction. Controlled trial.
Reynell PC, Bradford Royal Infirm, West Yorks, UK.
Br Heart J 1983; **49:** 364–7.

[21] Incidence and prognosis of unrecognized myocardial infarction. An update on the Framingham Study.
Kannel WB, Abbott RD, Boston Univ Sch Med, Boston, MA, USA.
N Engl J Med 1984; **311:** 1144–7.

[22] Cigar and pipe smoking related to four year survival of coronary patients.
Hickey N, Mulcahy R, Daly L, Graham I, O'Donoghue S, Kennedy C, St Vincent's Hosp, Dublin, Eire.
Br Heart J 1983; **49:** 423–6.

[23] Long term effect on mortality of stopping smoking after unstable angina and myocardial infarction.
Daly LE, Mulcahy R, Graham IM, Hickey N, St Vincent's Hosp, Dublin, Eire.
Br Med J 1983; **287:** 324–6.

[24] Cessation of smoking after myocardial infarction. Effects on mortality after ten years.
Aberg A, Bergstrand R, Johansson S *et al*, Ostra Hosp, Goteborg, Sweden.
Br Heart J 1983; **49:** 416–22.

[25] Smoking and myocardial infarction: secondary prevention.
Perkins J, Dick TBS, Leigh Infirm, Greater Manchester, UK.
Postgrad Med J 1985; **61:** 295–300.

[26] Effect of cigarette smoking on survival of patients with angiographically documented coronary artery disease. Report from the CASS Registry.
Vlietstra RE, Kronmal RA, Oberman A, Frye RL, Killip T III, Univ Washington, Seattle, WA, USA.
JAMA 1986; **255:** 1023–7.

[27] Smoking as a risk factor for recurrence of sudden cardiac arrest.
Hallstrom AP, Cobb LA, Ray R, Harbborview Med Cent, Seattle, WA, USA.
N Engl J Med 1986; **314:** 271–5.

[28] Psychosocial influences on mortality after myocardial infarction.
Ruberman W, Weinblatt E, Goldberg JD, Chaudhary BS, Health Insurance Plan Greater New York, NY, USA.
N Engl J Med 1984; **311:** 552–9.

[29] Type A behavior and survival after acute myocardial infarction.
Case RB, Heller SS, Case NB, Moss AJ and the Multicenter Post-Infarction Research Group, St Luke's-Roosevelt Hosp Cent, New York, NY, USA.
N Engl J Med 1985; **312:** 737–41.

[30] Alteration of type A behavior and reduction in cardiac recurrences in postmyocardial infarction patients.
Friedman M, Thoresen CE, Gill JJ *et al*, Mount Zion Hosp and Med Cent, San Francisco, CA, USA.
Am Heart J 1984; **108:** 237–48.

[31] Trial of relaxation in reducing coronary risk: four year follow up.
Patel C, Marmot MG, Terry DJ, Carruthers M, Hunt B, Patel M, London Sch Hygiene and Tropical Med, London, UK.
Br Med J 1985; **290:** 1103–6.

[32] The impact of marital status on survival after an acute myocardial infarction: a population-based study.
Chandra V, Szklo M, Goldberg R, Tonascia J, Johns Hopkins Univ Sch Hygiene and Public Health, Baltimore, MD, USA.
Am J Epidemiol 1983; **117**: 320–5.

Comment. The Cleveland Clinic have reported on 15-year survival in 598 patients with coronary artery disease [1]. Initially, patients were treated medically and were followed for 15 years. Death due to non-coronary causes was uncommon (5%) in the first five-year period but frequent (36%) in the third five-year period. Survival rates were 48%, 28%, 18% and 9% for patients with single-, double-, triple-vessel and left main stem disease, respectively. Abnormalities documented by ventriculography were related to survival. In 386 patients who would have been candidates for bypass surgery, survival rates were 58%, 55%, 26% and 11%, respectively, for those with single-, double-, triple-vessel and left main stem disease. Cardiac survival curves for single-, double- and triple-vessel disease in candidates for surgery and curves constructed on the basis of a 3% mortality per artery per year corresponded fairly closely. When an abnormal electrocardiogram was considered as a single variable in multivariate analysis, the five-year survival rates of candidates for surgery were influenced by the following, in order of importance: abnormal electrocardiogram; symptoms of at least five years' duration; triple-vessel disease; double-vessel disease; and arteriosclerosis obliterans. The survival rates for medically treated patients with 'left main equivalent' lesions were studied by Chaitman *et al* [2]. Patients with left main stem stenosis had a poorer prognosis than those with left main equivalent lesions. Proximal left anterior descending and proximal left circumflex disease indicated a high-risk subset of patients, but the risk was still not prognostically equivalent to left main stem stenosis.

The problem in accurately assessing prognosis following myocardial infarction and thereby devising the appropriate therapeutic strategy is emphasized by the conflicting data presented in terms of natural history. Grahame *et al* present a follow-up of 586 men who had survived an initial attack of either unstable angina (120 patients) or myocardial infarction (466 patients), and who were followed for up to 15 years [3]. A conservative approach to treatment was adopted (indeed, only two patients underwent surgery). Risk-factor advice was given and drugs were used only for symptoms. Survival at 5, 10 and 15 years was 80%, 61% and 43%, respectively.

However, a number of factors have been identified which will influence prognosis. A seven-year follow-up study of 593 patients following myocardial infarction grouped patients according to the presence or absence of Q waves on the electrocardiogram and also by level of cardiac enzymes [4]. Patients with Q-wave infarction together with markedly elevated enzyme levels had a high six-month mortality (11%). Patients with non-Q-wave infarction had excellent survival rates for two years (96.8%) [4]. An autopsy study of age-matched subjects comparing the features of 35 transmural with 35 non-transmural infarcts showed that non-transmural infarction had a greater tendency to be associated with evidence of prior infarction, more contraction-band (i.e. reflow) necrosis and fewer acute coronary thrombi than did transmural myocardial infarction, suggesting a different pathologic mechanism [5]. In a prospective study of 1253 patients with acute myocardial infarction, myocardial extension was found in 8% of non-Q-wave infarctions, 6% of Q-wave anterior and 6% of Q-wave inferior infarctions [6].

However, hospital mortality in patients with extension was 15% in those with Q-wave infarction *vs* 43% in those with non-Q-wave infarction; one-year survival rates for Q-wave infarction vs non-Q-wave infarction were 66% and 35%, respectively. Extension of myocardial infarction was found to be a predictor of poor prognosis in patients with Q-wave infarction, but it was the strongest predictor of one-year mortality in those with non-Q-wave infarction. In a further study of 103 hospitalized patients with acute myocardial infarction, secondary peaks of the creatine kinase MB isoenzyme were found in 31% of patients approximately six days after initial infarction [7]. In-hospital mortality was 16% for patients with infarct extension compared with 2.8% for those without extension, and no clinical variables, such as recurrent prolonged chest pain or ECG changes, singly or in combination were able to predict the risk of infarct extension in individual patients. This study emphasizes the need for improved diagnostic accuracy in the identification of infarct extension.

The importance of left-ventricular function in relation to prognosis is repeatedly being emphasized. One prospective study evaluated the relationship of specific coronary arterial and left-ventricular segments to the subsequent clinical outcome in 80 survivors of sudden cardiac death who were refractory to conventional antiarrhythmic therapy [8]. Survival outcome was inversely related to the degree of proximal left anterior descending coronary narrowing and the presence of severe left-ventricular dysfunction. In 22 survivors of acute myocardial infarction complicated by primary ventricular fibrillation, evidence from radionuclide ventriculograms suggested that primary ventricular fibrillation after anterior infarction is usually related to a large area of myocardial necrosis, whereas less extensive infarction may be accompanied by an arrhythmia when the inferior surface of the heart is affected [9]. As a result, patients with anterior infarction and primary ventricular fibrillation have a worse 5 year mortality (54%) than those without ventricular fibrillation (29%), whereas primary ventricular fibrillation does not influence mortality in inferior infarction [10]. The presence of left bundle branch block identified patients with severe left-ventricular dysfunction [11]. It is important to remember, particularly when investigating patients early in acute myocardial infarction and attempting to identify the appropriate therapeutic regimen according to the likely prognosis of patients, that spontaneous improvement in left-ventricular ejection fraction frequently occurs following acute myocardial infarction [12].

Cohen and Vogel [13] set out to determine whether left ventricular aneurysm is a risk factor independent of left ventricular function in patients with coronary artery disease by comparing retrospectively 39 patients with angiographically demonstrated segmental dyskinesis with 28 patients who had segmental akinesis and an ejection fraction of <60%. Follow-up was for a mean of 33 months after catheterization. The authors could not demonstrate any benefit from aneurysmectomy, and the patients with left ventricular aneurysm showed an insignificant trend towards more severe congestive heart failure and less angina. However, there was no significant difference in the re-infarction rate, and the incidence of ventricular tachycardia or embolism. The mortality rate was 38% in the patients with left ventricular aneurysm compared with 32% in the control subjects ($P=0.59$). Thus, Cohen and Vogel conclude that left ventricular aneurysm is not an independent risk factor for congestive heart failure, angina, ventricular tachycardia, re-infarction, embolism or death.

In one study of patients with isolated left anterior descending coronary artery stenosis the size of jeopardized myocardium was found to vary greatly [14]. In patients under the age of 50, moreover, more than 30% of the heart muscle could be put at risk. From another study [15], it would appear, however, that, although the incidence of occlusion of an infarcted artery in single-, double- and triple-vessel disease was similar in patients who either had or had not undergone previous coronary artery bypass graft surgery, the infarction in the surgically treated patient was more often caused by a distal arterial lesion and therefore it was smaller.

Another important determinant of prognosis in coronary artery disease is the amount of viable myocardium jeopardized by the disease. This can be assessed by exercise testing in combination with electrocardiography, radionuclide ventriculography or thallium scintigraphy. Exercise electrocardiography has already been discussed, but thallium scintigraphy provides a more viable indicator of the site and extent of ischaemia. In a study by Ladenheim *et al* [16], the value of exercise-induced myocardial hypoperfusion on thallium scintigraphy to predict coronary events was assessed in 1689 patients who had symptoms suggestive of coronary artery disease but no previous myocardial infarction or coronary artery bypass surgery. In the year after testing, 74 patients had a coronary event: 12 cardiac deaths, 20 non-fatal myocardial infarctions and 42 referrals for bypass surgery more than 60 days after testing. Only three independent predictors could be identified by stepwise logistic regression analysis: the number of myocardial regions with reversible hypoperfusion (which indicates the extent of hypoperfusion), the maximal magnitude of hypoperfusion (which indicates the severity of hypoperfusion) and the achieved heart rate (which indicates exercise performance). It was found that both extent and severity of hypoperfusion were exponentially correlated with event rate ($r > 0.97$), whereas achieved heart rate was linearly-correlated with event rate ($r = 0.79$). These results suggest that the extent and severity of myocardial hypoperfusion are important independent prognostic variables in patients with suspected coronary artery disease. In a subsequent study from the same group [17], the incremental prognostic power of clinical history, exercise ECG and myocardial perfusion scintigraphy was evaluated in order to define a strategy for prognostic testing, in 1659 patients who had symptoms suggesting coronary artery disease. Logistic analysis was used to derive a measure of prognostic power. In the year after testing, 74 patients suffered a coronary event. In 1451 patients who had a normal resting ECG, the clinical history alone had the greatest prognostic power (72%) which improved (by 5%) only when both tests were analysed. In 208 patients with abnormal findings on the resting ECG, the clinical history was a significant improvement in prognosis (an increment of 14% for each).

The value of the mobile coronary ambulance has been underlined by a recent study from Ireland. In two very similar Northern Irish communities [18], the mortality in the community with a mobile coronary care unit was found to be significantly lower than in the area without, and this difference was most marked in younger patients. Of the difference in mortality between the two areas, 48% occurred in the first two hours after onset of symptoms, despite the fact that only three patients had been resuscitated from cardiac arrest by the mobile team. These findings suggest that the benefits from the mobile coronary care unit may have been underestimated, and accrue not only from the unit's capacity to defibrillate patients in ventricular fibrillation, but also from the prompt treatment of pain, heart failure and arrhythmias. A group working in Brighton also claims improved survival from the prompt treatment of primary ventricular fibrillation [19]. Of 2886 patients monitored during acute myocardial infarction, 500 were seen within an hour of onset of symptoms. The following complications were more frequent in this group: pulmonary edema occurred in 26%, cardiogenic shock in 12%, death in 23%, and ventricular fibrillation in 20%. The authors conclude that prompt admission after myocardial infarction should improve survival by permitting the successful management of both ventricular fibrillation and other arrhythmias which may influence short-term and long-term prognosis. Several areas of the UK, Europe and the USA do not have the facilities for a mobile coronary care unit. In such circumstances, a potentially acceptable compromise is to improve access to the coronary care unit. In a randomized controlled trial of 511 men, half the patients were invited to readmit themselves to hospital if ischemic pain recurred [20]. The majority of the patients that were readmitted had taken advantage of this scheme. There is no evidence that they admitted themselves unnecessarily, and the time from onset of pain to admission was significantly reduced in those who made use of the scheme. All of the seven successful resuscitations among readmitted patients occurred in those who had bypassed their general practitioner and secured admission within 2.5 hours of onset of pain.

Unfortunately, many patients are unable to avail themselves of any means of admission to hospital because myocardial infarction may not be accompanied by the usual symptoms. More than 25% of 708 myocardial infarctions occurring among the 5127 participants in the Framingham Study were discovered only by the appearance of new diagnostic evidence during routine biennial ECG examinations [21]. Almost half of these infarctions were 'silent', and the remaining infarctions caused atypical symptoms. A high proportion of unrecognized infarctions occurred in women and in older men; unrecognized infarctions were uncommon in patients with angina. Unrecognized infarctions are as likely to cause death, heart failure or stroke as are recognized ones.

Several studies have reported on the effects of smoking on prognosis. Patients who survived an initial attack of unstable angina or myocardial infarction, and who continued to smoke cigarettes or cigars, had greater mortality than non-smokers, those who stopped smoking or cigarette smokers who changed to pipe smoking [22]. In a study of the same group, who had been followed for 15 years [23], mortality in those who had continued to smoke was significantly higher (82.1%) than in those who had stopped smoking (36.9%). These differences became more obvious with time, and were more marked in patients with unstable angina. The authors suggest that cessation of smoking appears to be the single most effective measure in reducing mortality from coronary artery disease. These findings were confirmed by a study from Sweden, in which 1023 smokers were followed for 10 years after their first myocardial infarction [24]. Those who stopped smoking had a considerably higher survival rate and a lower cumulative frequency of reinfarction. In a prospective study of 119 cigarette smokers who had survived their first myocardial infarction, the age-corrected mortality rate of men who continued to smoke cigarettes was found to be 2.2 times that of patients who stopped smoking after their infarction [25]. Women who continued to smoke were found to have 2.4 times the age-corrected mortality, and the age- and sex-corrected mortality rates for the combined group of men and women showed that those who stopped smoking after infarction had 55% of the mortality of those who continued to smoke.

156

Vlietstra *et al* [26] prospectively investigated the morbidity and mortality of 4165 patients with angiographically proven coronary artery disease in the Coronary Artery Surgery Study who were smokers; 2675 of those patients had continued to smoke, the remaining 1490 had stopped. After adjustment for baseline differences with Cox analysis, it was found that five-year mortality for those who continued smoking was 22%, and 15% for those who stopped; the relative risk of mortality for the smokers was found to be 1.55 times that of those who stopped smoking. Those who continued smoking were found to have a higher frequency of death associated with myocardial infarction and sudden death during follow-up than those who stopped smoking. Three hundred and ten survivors of out-of-hospital cardiac arrest who had been habitual smokers at the time of arrest were questioned about the cessation of smoking, and stratified according to mortality risk on the basis of recognized criteria [27]. The analysis of life-tables showed that at three years the reformed smokers had a lower incidence of recurrent arrest than patients who continued to smoke (19% *vs* 27%) in all the risk strata except the highest. The authors suggest that continued smoking led to an acceleration of atherosclerosis; the differences in early survival indicate that smoking may also act to enhance vulnerability to cardiac arrest in the short term.

Stress has often been suggested as an important factor in the quality of recovery following myocardial infarction, but there is little objective evidence for its relationship to prognosis. Psychosocial interviews with 2320 male survivors of acute myocardial infarction participating in the Beta-Blocker Heart Attack Trial identified those patients considered to be socially isolated and with a high degree of life stress as having more than four times the risk of death compared with men with low levels of both stress and isolation [28]. Surprisingly, high levels of stress and social isolation were most prevalent among the least-educated and least prevalent among the best-educated patients. In contrast, in a Multicenter Post-Infarction Research Group study, type A behavior measured within two weeks of acute myocardial infarction in 516 patients was found to have no relation to survival over 1–3 years [29]. In an attempt to try and clarify the importance of type A behavior, Friedman *et al* reported the results of a secondary prevention trial to determine whether type A behavior could be modified in patients who had survived an acute myocardial infarction and, if it could be altered, whether the individual so changed would have an improved prognosis [30]. Both group cardiologic counselling and type A behavior counselling were performed in 592 randomly selected patients, and 44% of this group showed evidence of a reduction in type A behavior; this was apparently associated with a highly significant reduction in 'cardiac recurrence rate' as compared with control patients (7.2% *vs* 13.2%). There was no difference in mortality, and the difference in recurrence rates was due to a reduction in non-fatal reinfarction.

In view of the conflicting data currently available, it would be premature to recommend a program of type A behavior counselling for the survivors of acute myocardial infarction. However, there is increasing evidence that alteration of stress may improve prognosis. Patel *et al* classified 192 subjects as having two or more coronary risk factors, and randomly assigned them to either a control group or a group to be subjected to behavior modification [31]. The treatment group had group sessions of one hour a week for eight weeks in which they were taught breathing exercises, relaxation, meditation and the management of stress. Follow-up at eight weeks and eight months showed a significantly greater reduction in systolic and diastolic blood pressure in the treatment group when compared with the control group; this difference had been maintained at the four-year follow-up. Plasma cholesterol concentrations and the number of cigarettes smoked were also lower in the treatment group at eight weeks and eight months, but not at four years. In addition, more subjects in the control group reported having had angina and treatment for hypertension and its complications. Moreover, the incidence of ischemic heart disease, fatal myocardial infarction and electrocardiographic evidence of ischemia was significantly greater in the control group.

Finally, a prospective study was carried out on the influence of marital status on the immediate and long-term survival of 1401 patients who had experienced an acute myocardial infarction [32]. The age-adjusted hospital mortality rate was 19.7% for married men and 23.3% for married women, whereas for unmarried men the mortality rate was 26.7% and for unmarried women it was 37.4%. Ten-year follow-up of 888 hospital survivors disclosed a highly significant difference in terms of mortality, in favor of married subjects of both sexes.

2. Congenital Heart Disease

SIMPLIFYING THE DESCRIPTION OF THE MORPHOLOGY OF CONGENITALLY MALFORMED HEARTS

Review: ROBERT H. ANDERSON

Polemics and controversy abound in all fields of science and medicine; cardiology is no exception. Those involved with any particular specialist area can usually cite examples of acrimonious disagreement; they perhaps imagine that such arguments are peculiar to their field. Certainly the area of congenital heart disease seems strewn with examples of unbecoming dissonance. Even the elder statesmen of the art have commented on the transatlantic 'war' which is perceived to be in progress concerning the philosophy and description of congenital cardiac malformations [1].

From the position of a protagonist (or antagonist, depending upon the stance of the observer) in this undeclared war, the conflict seems to be greatly exaggerated. There is a far greater understanding of the morphology of these malformations now than existed 10 years ago. In part this has to do with the great strides made in cross-sectional echocardiography, which puts cardiac anatomy at the fingertips of the clinician and places great significance upon an understanding and knowledge of the underlying cardiac structure. There is still room for improvement. If approached in a straightforward fashion, the structure of congenitally malformed hearts is easy to understand. It should be equally easy to describe, and there are steps we can all take to facilitate this description. There are also certain basic principles we can follow which will make the interchange of information such that the patient (or the parents) can understand the problems as readily as the diagnostician or the surgeon.

The Embryologic Approach

The conventional approach to the categorization of congenital heart disease is, in part, founded upon the belief that some lesions can be understood in terms of disordered cardiac development, and knowledge of the maldevelopment can lead to a means of eradicating the error and hence the disease. This may in the future prove to be the case. At present, this focus on embryology is diverting our attention and energy from the diagnosis and treatment of the lesions.

My interest in the subject of categorization grew out of embryologic investigations and interpretations [2,3], which in turn have led to much of the above-mentioned polemic and disagreement. The problem with the embryologic approach is that, at any given moment, one theory is as good as the next. My own treatment of the description of congenital cardiac malformations became more firmly based when I excluded embryologic assumptions from my descriptive vocabulary, categorizing cases exclusively on the basis of the observed anatomy [4]. Yet rare lesions are still described and interpreted in terms of armchair embryology [5]. It is difficult to see why authors who rarely display expertise in the field should see the need to add a gratuitous paragraph on development in papers devoted to congenital malformations – similarly, why editors should permit them this luxury in days when the pages of journals are full to bursting-point. Our first step towards the simplification of description and categorization of congenital cardiac anomalies, therefore, is to exclude considerations of development, while encouraging studies of cardiac embryology in their own right.

Terminology

We should then examine the very words we use to describe the lesions. Terminology is a touchy subject, and practitioners rightly object when the names seem to change so frequently. The conventional vocabulary of congenital heart disease is riddled with terms that are of obscure origin and not immediately understandable to the newcomer. As an example, consider 'situs solitus': this describes the usual arrangement of the organs of the body. Would it not be simpler to say 'usual organ arrangement'? I believe the time has come to anglicize (or to 'English') the vocabulary. English (or American English) is now the most popular international scientific language. We should accept this fact and describe congenital cardiac disease in English rather than Greco-Roman words. The Italians speak among themselves of 'il dotto', and not 'ductus arteriosus'. We should follow suit, and describe the 'arterial duct'. This has several advantages: it simplifies English style (the plural of duct is ducts and the adjective is ductal – how many know the correct Latin equivalents?), and concentrates the mind on the meaning of the term. I suddenly realized the role of the venous duct as opposed to the arterial duct when describing them in this fashion (previously I had simply learnt by rote the course of the 'ductus venosus'). Changes of this type also popularize and simplify the learning of cardiac anatomy. Pediatric cardiology should not be ruled by elitists who have their own jargon which all must learn before they are welcomed into the specialty.

The process of Englishing will certainly not be welcomed by all. There is much conservatism amongst the practitioners of pediatric cardiology. (I know that many of my close friends are less than convinced by my arguments.) It is also true that one can only go so far. English is an eclectic language, and multitudinous words of Greco-Roman origin are now fully incorporated into the Anglo-Saxon vocabulary. Certain words must remain. For example, it is most unlikely that 'tricuspid atresia' will ever pass from usage; at least, most are now aware that the atresia itself is usually produced by a complete absence of the right atrioventricular connection [6], rather than by an imperforate tricuspid valve. I submit, none the less, that 'common arterial trunk' is more readily understood than 'truncus arteriosus persistens', while 'caval veins' are more readily woven into the fabric of English style than are 'venae cava' (or whatever is the correct Latin for 'hollow veins').

Alpha-Numeric Cryptology

The third way we can improve description is by finding a practical replacement for alpha-numeric classification. Cryptology has its place in times of conflict, but I see no conflict in the attempt to simplify the description of congenitally malformed hearts. Perhaps the greatest philosophic difference between New World [7] and Old World [4] approaches has arisen in the matter of codification. The segmental approach originally introduced by Van Praagh [8] is generally accepted to have been the fundamental step forward in the logical analysis of congenital heart disease. Some of the value of this approach, however, has been removed by the use of formidable codes, such as '{I,L,D}'. In similar fashion, I see little benefit in describing 'tricuspid atresia type IIIC' or 'truncus arteriosus, Type IV'. Considerable prior knowledge is needed to interpret and understand these codes.

I favor the descriptive approach. Thus, I would describe 'transposition {I,L,D}' as 'mirror-image atrial arrangement, concordant atrioventricular and discordant ventriculo-arterial connections, with right-sided position of the discordantly connected aorta'. This description may be considerably longer; the listener also needs to know what is meant by concordant and discordant connections at the junctions of the cardiac segments. The approach, however – although basically the same as that of the Boston school, with added emphasis on junctional connections – is, I believe, more readily assimilated, and lends itself better to widespread communication.

Anatomy

My final suggestion for improvement of the description of congenital lesions relates to the role of normal cardiac anatomy. There has been a natural tendency over the years to consider defects within the heart in terms of the norm. Thus, atrial septal defects are related to the atrial septum and ventricular defects to the ventricular septum; problems with the left atrioventricular valve in 'endocardial cushion defects' have been considered in terms of 'mitral regurgitation'. To a point this is all well and good, but the approach is simplistic. All so-called atrial septal defects cannot exist within the setting of the normal atrial septum. The only true defects of the septum are those which exist within the confines of the oval fossa (egg-shaped depression?). Other holes are to be found which permit unequivocal interatrial communications: the sinus venosus, coronary sinus and ostium primum defects all fall within this category. None of these lesions, however, represents a deficiency of the atrial septum. The sinus venosus defect exists because either the caval or pulmonary veins (or both) have a connection to both atria, this bridging connection serving to provide the interatrial communication. The coronary sinus defect exists at the orifice of the sinus because of the unroofing of its course through the left atrioventricular groove. The ostium primum defect is due to a deficiency of the atrioventricular rather than the atrial septum [9]. I am not suggesting that these lesions should not be called 'atrial septal defects' – even though 'interatrial communications' would be a more accurate term – simply that their anatomy, particularly their cross-sectional echocardiographic appearance, can only be fully appreciated once their relationship to the limited extent of the atrial septum is known.

Similarly, the so-called 'supracristal' or doubly committed juxta-arterial ventricular septal defect cannot exist in the setting of the normal heart. This is because the larger part of the sub-pulmonary infundibulum of the normal heart is a free-standing rather than an interventricular structure. Knowing this, and also that the so-called 'inlet septum' of the normal heart separates the inlet of the right ventricle largely from the sub-aortic outlet component of the left ventricle, can lead to a better appreciation of the anatomy of interventricular communications. The anomaly of the 'endocardial cushion defect' can properly be understood only when it is known that the chamber communications take place primarily through a hole at the site of the atrioventricular septum of the normal heart [9]. This produces not only the potential for communication between atrial, ventricular, or atrial and ventricular chambers, it also results in a common atrioventricular junction guarded by a basically common valve, the left component of which bears no resemblance whatsoever to a mitral valve [10]. It is debatable how best to describe this valve, and many will probably continue to speak of a 'cleft mitral valve'. All that can be cited in support of this policy is tradition. For sheer accuracy, understanding and clinical significance, I should recommend the term 'trifoliate left valve' [11].

Summary

There has been much progress made in the past decade, which has resulted in widespread acceptance of some version or other of the logical segmental approach. We can go further in simplifying things, by using direct descriptors rather than interposing definitions. For example, we need no longer define a heart with double-inlet atrioventricular connection as 'single ventricle'. At one stroke, the description of a heart as having double-inlet left, right or solitary and indeterminate ventricle would cut through the extensive and non-productive disagreements which have surrounded the singularity of the ventricular mass in these anomalies. The relationship of this heart to those with the absent connection variant of atrioventricular valve atresia could then be recognized by acknowledging the univentricular nature of these atrioventricular connections [12]. No-one, however, should ever contemplate describing an individual heart in terms of its univentricular atrioventricular connection. It will always be possible to find a more apt and descriptive alternative.

We can do all a service first by avoiding concepts of embryology in deciding on categorizations, second by avoiding alpha-numeric cryptologies, and finally by using good Anglo-Saxon words for description.

Acknowledgment
Supported by the British Heart Foundation together with the Joseph Levy Foundation.

References

[1] Nadas AS.
Closing remarks. In: Doyle EF, Engle MA, Gersony WM, Rashkind WJ, Talner NS, eds. *Pediatric Cardiology*. Proceedings of the Second World Congress. New York: Springer-Verlag, 1986; 1323–6.

[2] Anderson RH, Wilkinson JL, Arnold R, Becker AE, Lubkiewicz K.
Morphogenesis of bulboventricular malformations, II. Observations on malformed hearts. *Br Heart J* 1974; **36**: 948–70.

[3] Anderson RH, Becker AE, Wilkinson JL, Gerlis LM.
Morphogenesis of univentricular hearts. *Br Heart J* 1976; **38**: 558–72.

[4] Tynan MJ, Becker AE, Macartney FJ, Quero-Jimenez M, Shinebourne EA, Anderson RH.
Nomenclature and classification of congenital heart disease. *Br Heart J* 1979; **41**: 544–53.

[5] Ekteish FMSA, Hajar R, Folger GM Jr.
Persistence of third aortic arch with fourth aortic arch agenesis. *Br Heart J* 1986; **55**: 607–10.

[6] Anderson RH, Wilkinson JL, Gerlis LM, Smith A, Becker AE.
Atresia of the right atrioventricular orifice. *Br Heart J* 1977; **39**: 414–28.

[7] Van Praagh R.
Diagnosis of complex congenital heart disease: Morphologic-anatomic method and terminology. *Cardiovasc Intervent Radiol* 1984; **7**: 115–20.

[8] Van Praagh R.
The segmental approach to diagnosis in congenital heart disease. In: *Birth Defects*. Original Article Series, Vol. 8. Baltimore: Williams & Wilkins, 1972; 4–23.

[9] Becker AE, Anderson RH.
Atrioventricular septal defects: What's in a name? *J Thorac Cardiovasc Surg* 1982; **83**: 461–9.

[10] Anderson RH, Zuberbuhler JR, Penkoske PA, Neches WH.
Of clefts, commissures and things.
J Thorac Cardiovasc Surg 1985; **90**: 605–10.

[11] Carpentier A.
Surgical anatomy and management of the mitral component of atrioventricular canal defects. In: Anderson RH, Shinebourne EA, eds. *Paediatric Cardiology 1977*. Edinburgh: Churchill-Livingstone, 1978; 477–86.

[12] Anderson RH, Becker AE, Tynan M, Macartney FJ, Rigby ML, Wilkinson JL.
The univentricular atrioventricular connection: Getting to the root of a thorny problem.
Am J Cardiol 1984; **54**: 822–8.

CATHETER TREATMENT IN CONGENITAL HEART DISEASE

Review: MICHAEL TYNAN, EDWARD J. BAKER

There are two broad types of treatment that can now be undertaken during cardiac catheterization - angioplasty and embolization. Although relatively new, these techniques have, in some conditions, already replaced surgery as the initial treatment of choice; in others their role is still being evaluated. Interventional catheterization has been used in congenital heart disease since the introduction of balloon atrial septostomy in 1966 by the late Dr William Rashkind [1]. This balloon catheter technique for the creation of an atrial septal defect in certain congenital heart malformations rapidly became and has remained the initial palliation of choice for transposition of the great arteries. It must be added that a report antedating Rashkind's proposed a catheter technique for the treatment of pulmonary and tricuspid stenosis [2], but this suggestion was not followed up for many years.

Progress in angioplasty had to await developments in plastics technology, which resulted in the production of catheter-mounted balloons that are in effect collapsible, non-distensible envelopes of predetermined size and geometry. When these 'balloons' are inflated, they exert force against any structures that deform them. This property allows them to inflict a limited injury on the deforming structure – for example, on stenosis in an artery. During the 1980s, results of experimental studies led to the application of these methods to congenital heart disease [3–7], and the first clinical reports of balloon valvoplasty and aortoplasty appeared in 1982 [8] and 1983 [9].

During this same period, embolization of vascular abnormalities emerged as a viable technique. A variety of devices and substances have been introduced, including plastic spheres [10], microspheres and gelfoam particles [11], tissue adhesives [12], metal coils [13] and detachable balloons [11,14]. Indications for these procedures are infrequent in patients with congenital heart disease, but attempts to widen them continue. As long ago as 1967, Porstmann *et al* reported a catheter method for the closure of persistence of the arterial duct [15]. Although successful, this technique was applicable only to adolescents and adults. It was Rashkind who developed a device and a technique for duct closure that could be used even in small children [16].

Valvoplasty and Angioplasty
Balloon angioplasty has been performed for pulmonary valve and pulmonary artery

stenosis, aortic valve stenosis, coarctation of the aorta, and postoperative coarctation restenosis. Attempts have been made to relieve venous stenosis, to treat subvalvar aortic stenosis and to palliate tetralogy of Fallot.

Pulmonary Valve Stenosis
The technique of balloon valvoplasty has been refined over the past four years. In its present use, cardiac catheterization is performed to confirm diagnosis and to establish the severity of the stenosis. A right-ventricular pressure in excess of 60 mmHg with a transvalvar gradient greater than 35 mmHg are the lower limits of hemodynamic disturbance at which to proceed with valvoplasty. In small infants, where the systemic arterial pressure may be in the region of 60–80 mmHg, these indications are modified, and a right-ventricular pressure of 60%–70% of the systemic arterial systolic pressure justifies valvoplasty. There is some debate about the precise hemodynamic indications, but at Guy's Hospital we have found these guidelines to be useful. There is no upper limit for right-ventricular pressure or pressure gradient. Prior to the valvoplasty a right-ventricular angiogram is performed in anterior and lateral projections, and the pulmonary valve 'ring' is measured in the lateral projection using the catheter's external diameter to correct for magnification. A balloon catheter of appropriate size is selected and introduced over a guidewire, which has been securely located with its tip in the periphery of the left pulmonary artery. The balloon is sited with its center portion at the level of the stenosed valve; it is then inflated with dilute contrast medium to the pressure recommended by the manufacturer. Inflation and deflation, which usually take less than 20 seconds, are carried out as rapidly as possible. With inflation the indentation of the valve on the balloon is seen to disappear. The inflation-deflation cycle is performed three or four times. The angioplasty catheter is removed, with the guidewire left in place; a cardiac catheter is reintroduced over the wire, which is then removed while withdrawal pressures are recorded. After removal of the guidewire, no further attempt should be made to cross the angioplasty site.

Using this technique, or one very similar, we [17] and several other groups have achieved considerable success in the relief of pulmonary valve stenosis, both in terms of immediate results and those obtained at review some months after the procedure [18–26]. Relief of the stenosis does not appear to be associated with significant pulmonary regurgitation, although in some an early diastolic murmur is heard, and in a number of patients there is suggestive evidence on Doppler echocardiography. However, there is no significant right-ventricular volume overload in any patients that we have studied [17].

No major complications have been reported as a result of the valvoplasty. We have had one fatality associated with a complex procedure: an infant with multiple hemangiomata, including a large hepatic arteriovenous malformation, who also had pulmonary valve stenosis, underwent combined balloon pulmonary valvoplasty and embolization of the hepatic artery. Death was due to hepatic failure, however, and was unrelated to the valvoplasty.

Our understanding of the mechanism of relief of pulmonary stenosis is sketchy, in part because the only valves observed after the procedure have been those referred for surgery, the one infant in our unit who died, and one patient in whom, at the start of our series, we performed the balloon valvoplasty intraoperatively. In our two cases the valve was split along the lines of commissural fusion; others have reported tearing or avulsion of a leaflet [22]. Whichever of these mechanisms is the more usual, it appears that relief is likely to be long lasting.

The first four years' experience have identified two reasons for failure. One is avoidable, namely the use of too small a balloon. Undue caution originally led to selection of balloons of the same diameter as, or a little smaller than, the pulmonary valve 'ring'. However, it was discovered, from work in lambs, that much larger balloons could be inflated in the outflow of the right ventricle without damage to the ventricle or pulmonary artery [27]. Analysis of our results shows that the probability of success increased from 58% when a balloon smaller than the valve ring was used, to 90% with a balloon 20% larger than the valve ring. The larger balloon has the advantage of maximizing the safe dilating force on the valve [28]. As yet no complications have occurred related to the use of larger balloons. On occasion it is impossible to attain the desired balloon size with one catheter. Two catheters can then be introduced side by side over separate guidewires, giving an effective diameter somewhat less than the combined diameter of the two balloons.

A second reason for failure can be the fact that not all pulmonary valves are suitable for balloon dilatation. A variant, known as the dysplastic valve, is grossly thickened with mucoid excrescences on the valve leaflets. This causes obstruction, as the bulk of the valve is a space-occupying lesion in the root of the pulmonary artery. This type of valve is not suitable for balloon valvoplasty, and should be treated by surgical excision or patch reconstruction of the pulmonary outflow. Such valves can be recognized angiographically by filling defects seen in the root of the pulmonary artery. We at Guy's Hospital no longer attempt to dilate them.

Age is not a limiting factor. The technique is applicable to newborn infants, children and adults [29].

In summary, balloon pulmonary valvoplasty is safe and effective. It is now the initial treatment of choice for most patients with pulmonary valve stenosis.

Aortic Valve Stenosis
The same basic principles apply to balloon valvoplasty in aortic as in pulmonary stenosis. There are, however, some differences in detail. Lababidi *et al* [30,31] described a modification that was designed to vent the left ventricle during the period of aortic orifice occlusion: in effect, the vascular lumen of the balloon catheter was connected to a venous catheter, which necessitated removal of the guidewire. Most workers now prefer the extra safety of having a guidewire in place, and make no attempt to vent the left ventricle. The presence of the guidewire, looped in the ventricle, assists in stabilizing the balloon in the outflow tract. This is important, as with inflation the balloon tends to be shot out of the ventricle like a bullet from a gun.

Another difference in technique is in balloon size. This should be no larger than the aortic orifice measured at the junction of the valve leaflets with the aortic sinuses [32]. Inflation and deflation should be performed rapidly, and in other respects the approach is similar to that in pulmonary stenosis.

Success has been reported in infants and children, and relief of stenosis has not been reported to be associated with significant aortic regurgitation [31,33–35]. However, deaths have occurred in infancy [36]. At present the literature is too sparse to give an accurate idea of the risks, but discussion at meetings suggests that in infants, especially neonates, there is a high incidence of fatal complications related to vascular or myocardial damage.

The indications for balloon aortic valvoplasty are less clear than for pulmonary stenosis. A transvalvar pressure gradient of 60 mmHg is a suitable level of hemodynamic disturbance at which to intervene in patients older than 1 year. In younger patients, left-ventricular dysfunction can result in relatively low left-ventricular pressures despite severe stenosis. Thus, relief is indicated in symptomatic infants when the stenosis appears severe on cross-sectional echocardiography or angiocardiography, and where no other anatomic cause for the cardiac decompensation can be found.

The major contraindication to the procedure is severe aortic regurgitation. Balloon valvoplasty is not ruled out by mild regurgitation [31], but to date we have rejected all patients when it has been detectable both clinically and angiocardiographically. This may be an excessively conservative approach, but the available literature on aortic valvoplasty is limited, and there are few large series with even intermediate-term follow-up.

There is little information available regarding the mechanism of relief of aortic stenosis. One case has been reported in which splitting of the commissures of a bicuspid valve occurred at autopsy, following operative transventricular balloon dilatation [38]. Other mechanisms will presumably be described.

The most obvious group of patients that may benefit from balloon aortic valvoplasty should be symptomatic neonates. Here, the natural history is very unfavourable and operative risk is high. It appears, however, that the risk of the balloon technique is also high, and it is a difficult procedure. Balloons of the appropriate size are mounted on large catheter shafts and may thus be impossible to introduce into the artery. Successes have been reported with small balloons [34], but this is contrary to the experience with pulmonary stenosis.

It has recently been shown that the balloon technique offers older people with calcific aortic stenosis at least palliative benefit [39].

In conclusion, aortic valve stenosis can be relieved by balloon valvoplasty. At present the indications and contraindications are still being worked out. Meanwhile, we perform this procedure only after full consultation on each case with our surgeons.

Coarctation of the Aorta and Coarctation Restenosis
Early studies in the dilatation of surgically excised [5,39] and experimental coarctation [6] showed that this approach was clinically feasible. An anatomic study, however, suggested that dilatation could carry a risk of aneurysm formation in approximately 30% of cases [40], and the experimental studies showed that the effect is achieved by inflicting intimal and medial damage. Clinical experience has given mixed results [9,22,41–44]. Good initial hemodynamic effects have been found to be only transient, or to be accompanied by no clinical improvement. The best results appear to be obtained with a balloon 1 or 2 mm smaller in diameter than the aorta proximal to the narrowed segment [45,46]. Deaths have been reported, one due to rupture of the aorta. Literature is sparse, but presentations and discussion at meetings have uncovered a significant incidence of late aneurysm formation [45]. Our group does not recommend balloon angioplasty for primary treatment but, despite potential complications [47], some centers continue to employ it in this role.

166

In contrast, balloon dilatation of coarctation re-stenosis has achieved a more secure place in interventional catheterization [9,47–49]. The balloon size recommended is the diameter of the aorta just proximal to the recoarcted segment. Results are less predictable than with pulmonary valvoplasty, but the technique appears to fulfill at least a palliative role.

Pulmonary Artery Stenosis
Experimental pulmonary artery stenosis can be ameliorated with balloons [4]. Dilatation of pulmonary artery stenosis is accomplished, however, only with concomitant extensive arterial damage [4,51]. Clinical experience has shown that relief is possible and can be maintained for at least an intermediate term [52–54]. However, the method unaccountably fails in approximately half of the patients. The reported complication rate is low, but perforation or rupture of a branch pulmonary artery has occurred, with one death [53,54]. Thrombosis of a pulmonary artery has also been reported when this procedure was performed after the Fontan operation [55]. Balloon angioplasty is not without risk in this setting and the results are not predictable, but it does offer an alternative treatment for unusually difficult lesions.

Balloon angioplasty has been used in other forms of congenital heart disease. A recent series has reported significant reduction in outflow tract gradients in discrete subaortic stenoses without serious aortic regurgitation [56]. Palliation of tetralogy has been undertaken successfully. Systemic venous stenoses – such as those which can complicate atrial correction of transposition – have been dilated [24,57], but congenital pulmonary vein stenoses have not [57,58].

Embolization
Until recently, embolization was reserved for the closure of major systemic to pulmonary artery collateral arteries [11,12,59,60], Blalock-Taussig shunts [11,61,62], and arteriovenous malformations in the lungs [11,14] or in the coronary system [11]. These procedures are safe and effective and can be performed in sick patients, even in those still needing postoperative intensive care. Detachable balloons offer the most controllable method, but coils or particle injection are effective in selected patients [11]. There are a small number of patients in whom these procedures are indicated. We have treated a total of nine in five years. However, since we have been involved in the trial of transcatheter occlusion of the arterial duct we have treated nine children in as many months.

The closure of the arterial duct is accomplished with the use of a double-umbrella device developed by Rashkind [16]. This device is introduced via the femoral vein using a long sheath and located in the duct, so that the distal umbrella is on the aortic aspect while the proximal umbrella is in the pulmonary artery. Over 100 implantations have been performed by Dr Charles Mullins. During the early part of his experience several problems were encountered, but in the last 70 or more patients closure has been achieved in almost all cases and without complications [63]. The accuracy of positioning the device remains, in our limited experience, the main problem during the learning phase. Devices of a similar type are under development for the closure of atrial septal defects [16], and with more experience their use will doubtless be extended to other types of congenital heart disease.

References

[1] Rashkind WJ, Miller WW.
Creation of an atrial septal defect without thoracotomy.
JAMA 1966; **196**: 991–2.

[2] Rubio-Alvarez V, Limon Lason R.
Treatment of pulmonary valvular stenosis and tricuspid stenosis with a modified cardiac catheter. In: *Proc 1st National Conference on Cardiovascular Disease*, Washington, DC, 1950.

[3] Abele JE.
Balloon catheters and transluminal dilatation: technical considerations.
Am J Roentgenol 1980; **135**: 901–6.

[4] Lock JE, Neimi BA, Enzig S, Amplatz K, Burke B, Bass JL.
Transvenous angioplasty of experimental branch pulmonary artery stenosis in newborn lambs.
Circulation 1981; **64**: 886–93.

[5] Lock JE, Castenada-Zuniga WR, Bass JL, Foker JE, Amplatz K, Anderson RW.
Balloon dilatation of excised aortic coarctation.
Radiology 1982; **143**: 698.

[6] Lock JE, Neimi BA, Burke B, Enzig S, Castenada-Zuniga WR.
Transcutaneous angioplasty of experimental aortic coarctation.
Circulation 1982; **66**: 1280.

[7] Kan JS, Anderson JH, White RI Jr.
Experimental basis for balloon valvoplasty of congenital pulmonary valvar stenosis. In: *Proc Sect Cardiol Am Acad Ped*, New York, Oct 1982; p.101A.

[8] Kan JS, White RI Jr, Mitchell SE, Gardener TJ.
Percutaneous balloon pulmonary valvoplasty: A new method for treating congenital pulmonary valve stenosis.
N Engl J Med 1982; **307**: 540.

[9] Singer M, Rowen M, Dorsey T. Transluminal aortic balloon angioplasty for coarctation of the aorta in the newborn.
Am Heart J 1982; **103**: 131–2.

[10] Luessenhop AJ, Kachman R, Shevlin W, Ferrero AA.
Clinical evaluation of artificial embolization in the management of large cerebral arteriovenous malformations.
J Neurosurg 1965; **23**: 400–17.

[11] Reidy JF, Jones ODH, Tynan MJ, Baker EJ, Joseph MC.
Embolization procedures in congenital heart disease.
Br Heart J 1985; **54**: 184–92.

[12] Zuberbuhler JR, Dakner E, Zoltun R, Burkholder J, Bahnson HT.
Tissue adhesive closure of aortic-pulmonary communications.
Am Heart J 1974; **88**: 41–6.

[13] Gianturco C, Anderson JH, Wallace S.
Mechanical devices for arterial occlusion.
Am J Roentgenol 1975; **124**: 428–35.

[14] White RI Jr, Ursic TA, Kaufman SL, Barth KH, Kin W, Gross GS.
Therapeutic embolization with detachable balloons.
Radiology 1978; **126**: 521–3.

[15] Postmann W, Wierny L, Warnke H.
Closure of persistent ductus arteriosus without thoracotomy.
Thoraxchirurgie 1967; **15**: 199–201.

[16] Rashkind WJ.
Interventional cardiac catheterization in congenital heart disease.
Int J Cardiol 1985; **7**: 1–11.

[17] Tynan M, Baker EJ, Rohmer J et al.
Percutaneous balloon pulmonary valvuloplasty.
Br Heart J 1985; **53**: 520–4.

[18] Lababidi Z, Wu J.
Percutaneous balloon pulmonary valvuloplasty.
Am J Cardiol 1983; **52**: 560–2.

[19] Kann JS, White RI Jr, Mitchell SE, Anderson JH, Gardener TJ.
Percutaneous transluminal balloon valvuloplasty for pulmonary valve stenosis.
Circulation 1984; **69**: 554–60.

[20] Rocchini AP, Kveselis DA, Crowley D, Dick M, Rosenthal A.
Percutaneous balloon valvuloplasty for the treatment of pulmonary valvular stenosis in children.
J Am Coll Cardiol 1984; **3**: 1005–12.

[21] Walls JT, Lababidi Z, Curtis JJ, Silver D.
Assessment of percutaneous balloon pulmonary and aortic valvuloplasty.
J Thorac Cardiovasc Surg 1984; **88**: 352–6.

[22] Brodsky SJ.
Percutaneous balloon angioplasty.
Am J Dis Child 1984; **138**: 851–4.

[23] Sullivan ID, Robinson PJ, Macartney FJ et al.
Percutaneous balloon valvuloplasty for pulmonary valve stenosis in infants and children.
Br Heart J 1985; **54**: 435–41.

[24] Miller GAH.
Balloon valvuloplasty, and angioplasty in congenital heart disease.
Br Heart J 1985; **54**: 285–9.

[25] Rey C, Marache P, Matina D, Mouly A.
Percutaneous transluminal valvuloplasty of pulmonary stenosis. Report of 24 cases.
Arch Mal Coeur 1985; **78**: 703–10.

[26] Fontes VF, Eduardo J, Sousa MR, Silva VD, Esteves CA, Pontes SC.
Percutaneous transluminal balloon valvuloplasty for pulmonic valve stenosis. In: Doyle EF, Engle MA, Gersony WM, Rashkind WJ, Talner NS, eds. *Pediatric Cardiology*. New York: Springer-Verlag, 1986; 326–30.

[27] Ring JC, Kulik TJ, Burke BA, Lock JE.
Morphologic changes induced by dilatation of the pulmonary valve annulus with overlarge balloons in normal newborn lambs.
Am J Cardiol 1984; **55**: 210–4.

[28] Abele JE.
Balloon catheters and transluminal dilation: Technical considerations.
Am J Roentgenol 1980; **135**: 901–6.

[29] Pepine CJ, Gessner IH, Feldman RL.
Percutaneous balloon valvuloplasty for pulmonic valve stenosis in an adult.
Am J Cardiol 1982; **50**: 1442–5.

[30] Lababidi Z.
Aortic balloon valvuloplasty.
Am Heart J 1983; **106**: 751–2.

[31] Lababidi Z, Wu J, Walls JT.
Percutaneous balloon aortic valvuloplasty: Results in 23 patients.
Am J Cardiol 1984; **53**: 194–7.

[32] Rupprath G.
Personal communication, 1986.

[33] Sanchez GR, Mehta AV, Ewing LL, Brickley SE, Anderson TM, Black IFS.
Successful percutaneous balloon valvuloplasty of the aortic valve in an infant.
Pediatr Cardiol 1985; **6**: 103–6.

[34] Rupprath G, Neuhaus KL.
Percutaneous balloon valvuloplasty for aortic valve stenosis in infancy.
Am J Cardiol 1985; **55**: 1655–6.

[35] Rickards AW, Somerville J.
Successful balloon aortic valvotomy in a child with a pulmonary hypertensive duct and aortic valve stenosis.
Br Heart J 1986; **56**: 185–6.

[36] Waller BF, Girod DA, Dillon JC.
Transverse aortic wall tears in infants after balloon angioplasty for aortic valve stenosis: Relation of aortic wall damage to diameter of inflated angioplasty balloon and aortic lumen in seven necropsy cases.
J Am Coll Cardiol 1984; **4**: 1235–41.

[37] Brown JW, Robison RJ, Waller BF.
Transventricular balloon catheter aortic valvotomy in neonates.
Ann Thorac Surg 1985; **39**: 376–8.

[38] Cribier A, Savin T, Saoudi N, Rocha P, Berland J, Letac B.
Percutaneous transluminal valvuloplasty of acquired aortic stenosis in elderly patients: An alternative to valve replacement?
Lancet 1986; i: 63–7.

[39] Sos T, Sniderman KW, Rettek-Sos B, Strupp A, Alonso DR.
Percutaneous transluminal dilatation of coarctation of the thoracic aorta post-mortem.
Lancet 1979; ii: 970.

[40] Pellegrino A, Deverall PB, Anderson RH *et al*.
Aortic coarctation in the first three months of life. An anatomopathological study with respect to treatment.
J Thorac Cardiovasc Surg 1985; **89**: 121–7.

[41] Lock JE, Bass JL, Amplatz K, Fuhrman B, Castenada-Zuniga WR.
Balloon dilation angioplasty of aortic coarctation in infants and children.
Circulation 1983; **68**: 109–16.

[42] Lababidi Z.
Neonatal transluminal balloon coarctation angioplasty.
Am Heart J 1983; **106**: 752–3.

[43] Sperling DE, Dorsey TJ, Rowen M, Gazzaniga AB.
Percutaneous transluminal angioplasty of congenital coarctation of the aorta.
Am J Cardiol 1983; **51**: 562–4.

[44] Finley JP, Beaulieu RG, Nanton MA, Roy DL.
Balloon catheter dilatation of coarctation of the aorta in young infants.
Br Heart J 1983; **50**: 411–5.

[45] Cooper RS, Ritter SB, Golinko RJ.
Balloon dilation angioplasty: Nonsurgical management of coarctation of the aorta.
Circulation 1984; **70**: 903–7.

[46] Lababidi ZA, Daskalopoulos DA, Stoeckle H Jr.
Transluminal balloon coarctation angioplasty: Experience with 27 patients.
Am J Cardiol 1984; **54**: 1288–91.

[47] Lock JE.
Now we can dilate, should we?
Am J Cardiol 1984; **54**: 1360.

[48] Kan JS, White RI Jr, Mitchell SE, Farmlet EJ, Donahoo JS, Gardener TJ.
Treatment of restenosis of coarctation by percutaneous transluminal angioplasty.
Circulation 1983; **68**: 1087–94.

[49] D'Souza VJ, Velasquez G, Weesner KM, Prabhu S.
Transluminal angioplasty of aortic coarctation with a two balloon technique.
Am J Cardiol 1984; **54**: 457–8.

[50] Lorber A, Ettedgui JA, Baker EJ, Jones ODH, Reidy J, Tynan M.
Balloon aortoplasty for recoarctation following the subclavian flap operation.
Int J Cardiol 1986; **10**: 57–63.

[51] Edwards BS, Lucus RV Jr, Lock JE, Edwards JE.
Morphological changes in the pulmonary arteries after percutaneous angioplasty for pulmonary artery stenosis.
Circulation 1985; **71**: 195–201.

[52] Lock JE, Castenada-Zuniga WR, Fuhrman B, Bass JL.
Balloon dilatation angioplasty of hypoplastic and stenotic pulmonary arteries.
Circulation 1983; **67**: 962–7.

[53] Rocchini AP, Kveselis D, MacDonald D, Crowly D, Snider AR, Rosenthal A.
Use of balloon angioplasty to treat peripheral pulmonary stenosis. *Am J Cardiol* 1984; **54**: 1069–73.

[54] Ring JC, Bass JL, Marvin W et al.
Management of congenital stenosis of a branch pulmonary artery with balloon dilation angioplasty.
J Thorac Cardiovasc Surg 1985; **90**: 35–44.

[55] Di Sessa TG, Yeatman LA, Williams RG, Lois JF, Friedman WF, Laks H.
Thrombosis complicating balloon angioplasty of left pulmonary artery after Fontan's procedure: Successful treatment with streptokinase.
Am J Cardiol 1985; **55**: 610–1.

[56] Suarez de Lezo J, Pan M, Sancho M et al.
Percutaneous transluminal balloon dilatation for discrete subaortic stenosis.
Am J Cardiol 1986; **88**: 619–21.

[57] Lock JE, Bass JL, Castenada-Zuniga WR, Fuhrman B, Rashkind WJ, Lucus RV Jr.
Dilatation angioplasty of congenital or operative narrowings of venous channels.
Circulation 1984; **70**: 457–64.

[58] Driscoll DJ, Hesslein PS, Mullins CE.
Congenital stenosis of individual pulmonary veins: Clinical spectrum and unsuccessful treatment by transvenous dilation.
Am J Cardiol 1982; **49**: 1767.

[59] Yamamoto S, Nozawa T, Aizawa T, Honda M, Mohri M.
Transcatheter embolization of bronchial collateral arteries prior to operation for tetralogy of Fallot.
J Thorac Cardiovasc Surg 1979; **78**: 739–43.

[60] Grinnel VS, Mehringer CM, Hielshima GB, Stanley P, Lurie PR.
Transaortic occlusion of collateral arteries to the lung by detachable balloons in a patient with tetralogy of Fallot.
Circulation 1982; **65**: 1276–8.

[61] Culham JAG, Izukawa T, Burns JE, Freedom RM.
Embolization of a Blalock-Taussig shunt in a child.
Am J Roentgenol 1981; **137**: 413–5.

[62] Florentine M, Wolfe RE, White RI.
Balloon embolization to occlude a Blalock-Taussig shunt.
J Am Coll Cardiol 1984; **3**: 200–2.

[63] Mullins C.
Personal communication, 1986.

TRANSPOSITION OF THE GREAT ARTERIES

Review: JOHN W. KIRKLIN, LIONEL M. BARGERON JR, EUGENE H. BLACKSTONE

Radical changes are occurring in the management of patients with transposition of the great arteries, although another 10–15 years of follow-up of patients now undergoing the *arterial* switch operation* will be required to determine whether the development of this relatively new operation will result not only in a higher proportion of surviving and

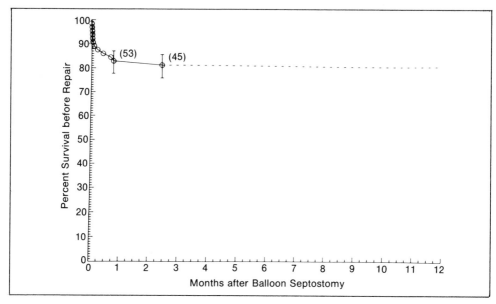

FIGURE 1: Actuarial survival after balloon septostomy but before repair with simple transposition of the great arteries (University of Alabama; 1970–1981; n = 65; deaths = 12). Patients were not censored when procedure other than repair was performed but were censored when an atrial switch repair was done (1 had repair three days after septostomy, 10 others had repair before 90 days of age). (Reproduced with permission from Kirklin *et al* [2].)

healthy patients, but also in simpler and less expensive management because of the need for only a single operation and the potentially simpler follow-up.

The setting in which this operation evolved reflects imperfections in management, despite remarkable progress since the advent of balloon atrial septostomy developed by Rashkind in 1966 [1]. Of babies born with transposition of the great arteries and intact ventricular septum, 5%–10% die prior to the possibility of balloon atrial septostomy [2], a situation that could be improved only by the earlier identification of the presence of a serious congenital cardiac anomaly, and by earlier referral to a facility equipped for balloon atrial septostomy. However, even with balloon atrial septostomy performed under optimal conditions, another 10% of babies with transposition of the great arteries and intact ventricular septum die before about three months of age unless an additional procedure is carried out (Fig. 1) [2,3]. Despite reports of the safety of an *atrial* switch operation* performed in the first month of life [4,5], most clinicians believe that the risk

* In the arterial switch operation, the repair of the transposition of the aorta to the right ventricle and of the pulmonary artery to the left ventricle (the anomaly in patients with transposition of the great arteries) is simply accomplished by dividing the great arteries and creating a neo-aorta by anastomosing the proximal end of the pulmonary artery to the distal aorta, and a neo-pulmonary artery by anastomosing the original proximal aortic end to the distal pulmonary artery. The coronary arteries are surgically transferred into the neo-aorta.

* The atrial switch operation can be performed using the Mustard or Senning technique. In both, the interiors of the atria are surgically rearranged so that caval blood drains through the mitral valve to the left ventricle and then out the aorta, and pulmonary venous blood drains through the tricuspid valve into the right ventricle and out the aorta.

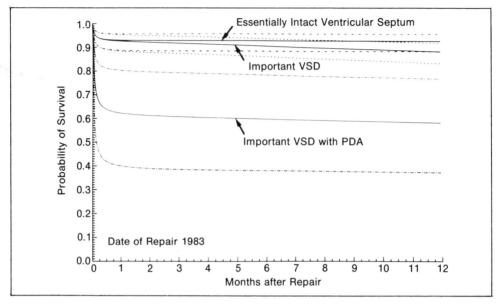

FIGURE 2: Parametric survival estimates for patients stratified with respect to status of hospital deaths, among those undergoing Senning atrial switch repair of all types of transposition of the great arteries (University of Alabama; 1977–1984; $n = 132$; 28 deaths including 22 hospital deaths). The dashed lines enclose the 70% confidence limits (CL). The estimated late survival figures for the group with essentially intact ventricular septum (simple transposition) at 5, 15 and 20 years are 89% (CL 85%–93%), 84% (CL 75%–90%) and 81% (CL 70%–88%), respectively. PDA = patent ductus arteriosus; VSD = ventricular septal defect. (Reproduced with permission from Kirklin *et al* [2].)

is higher in neonates than in infants 3–6 months old. Further, the 10- and 20-year survival after atrial switch operations is marred by a variable but continuing late mortality (Fig. 2) [6,7]. This, added to the initial hospital mortality from balloon atrial septostomy and atrial switch, results in 5- and 20-year survival of about 85% and 77%, respectively [8]. Most late deaths are associated with late degeneration of an initial sinus rhythm into a slow junctional rhythm, which may be followed by sudden death from a paroxysmal atrial tachyarrhythmia, ventricular tachycardia or fibrillation. Although pacemaker implantation at the point of development of slow junctional rhythm might prevent many such deaths, the overall results of this treatment protocol are not ideal.

Babies born with transposition of the great arteries and large ventricular septal defects, as well as those with large patent ductus arteriosus, often do not require balloon atrial septostomy, but the early development of congestive heart failure and signs of pulmonary vascular disease usually force surgical intervention before 3–6 months of age. The early risks of an *atrial* switch operation plus repair of the ventricular septal defects, whether done as a primary procedure or after a palliative pulmonary artery banding (with its intrinsic morbidity and mortality), are somewhat higher than when the ventricular septum is intact. Late arrhythmic problems in this setting are as prevalent as those in the setting of transposition of the great arteries with essentially intact ventricular septum. Additionally, impaired right-ventricular functional reserve with the high afterload imposed on it by systemic pressure combine to produce poor right-ventricular systolic function postoperatively and premature late death in 10%–30% of patients.

In contrast, in the hands of some surgeons, the *arterial* switch operation can be performed in neonates with transposition of the great arteries and intact ventricular septum with an early mortality approaching zero [9]. The arterial switch operation was conceptualized by many surgeons, but was never successfully accomplished until Jatene in Sao Paolo, Brazil, performed it in 1975. Although the operation was infrequently performed until a few years ago, more centers in developed countries are now using this procedure.

There appears to be no greater risk in performing the repair in infants of a few days of age than in those a few weeks of age. Prostaglandin infusion and balloon atrial septostomy are advisable in newborns with this condition when cyanosis is severe, if only for a few days prior to the *arterial* switch operation, as these bring the baby to operation in better condition. Further, no late deaths have followed the arterial switch operation over an eight-year follow-up period [8]. The results have been entirely similar in patients with transposition of the great arteries and large ventricular septal defects, although in these patients the arterial switch operation can often be deferred until 6–12 weeks of age.

A formal comparison of the results of the *arterial* switch operation with those of the *atrial* switch operation supports the superiority of the *arterial* switch repair [9]. The rapidity with which this procedure acquires general acceptance will be limited primarily by the time and effort required by cardiac surgeons treating congenital heart disease to acquire the proficiency now possessed by only a few, and by the tolerance of pediatric cardiologists of the inevitable initial complications that will accompany implementation of the procedure. Innovators in both medical and surgical specialties will be required for the development and definitive evaluation of these novel, beneficial approaches.

References

[1] Rashkind WJ, Miller WW.
Creation of an atrial septal defect without thoracotomy: A palliative approach to complete transposition of the great arteries.
JAMA 1966; **196**: 991–2.

[2] Kirklin JW, Barratt-Boyes B.
Cardiac Surgery. New York: John Wiley, 1986; 1182–3.

[3] Tynan M.
Survival of infants with transposition of great arteries after balloon atrial septostomy.
Lancet 1971; i: 621–3.

[4] Castaneda AR, Norwood WI, Jonas RA, Colan SD, Sanders P, Lang P.
Transposition of the great arteries and intact ventricular septum: Anatomical repair in the neonate.
Ann Thorac Surg 1984; **38**: 438–43.

[5] Matherne GP, Razook JD, Thompson WM Jr, Lane MM, Murray CK, Elkins RC.
Senning repair for transposition of the great arteries in the first week of life.
Circulation 1985; **72**: 840–5.

[6] Arciniegas E, Farooki ZQ, Hakimi M et al.
Results of the Mustard operation for dextro-transposition of the great arteries.
J Thorac Cardiovasc Surg 1981; **81**: 580–7.

[7] Trusler GA, Williams WG, Izukawa T, Olley PM.
Current results with the Mustard operation in isolated transposition of the great arteries.
J Thorac Cardiovasc Surg 1980; **80**: 381–9.

[8] Kirklin JK, Blackstone EH, Pacifico AD, Kirklin JW, Bargeron LM Jr.
Current comprehensive 5-year survival rates using a protocol of balloon septostomy and atrial switching in simple TGA.
Second World Congress of Pediatric Cardiology (June) 1985; Program 2: 157.

[9] Quaegebeur JM, Rohmer J, Ottenkamp J *et al*.
The arterial switch operation: An eight-year experience.
J Thorac Cardiovasc Surg (in press).

COMPLETE TRANSPOSITION

[1] Fate of infants with transposition of the great arteries in relation to balloon atrial septostomy.
Powell TG, Dewey M, West CR, Arnold R, Royal Children's Hosp, Liverpool, UK.
Br Heart J 1984; **51**: 371–6.

[2] Balloon atrial septostomy in the neonatal intensive care unit.
Baker EJ, Allan LD, Tynan MJ, Jones ODH, Joseph MC, Deverall PB, Guy's Hosp, London, UK.
Br Heart J 1984; **51**: 377–8.

[3] Fate of long-term survivors of Mustard procedure (inflow repair) for simple and complex transposition of the great arteries.
Ashraf MH, Cotroneo J, DiMarco D, Subramanian S, Children's Hosp, Buffalo, NY, USA.
Ann Thorac Surg 1986; **42**: 385–9.

[4] Late results of the Mustard procedure in transposition of the great arteries.
Stewart S, Alexson C, Manning J, Univ Rochester Med Cent, Rochester, NY, USA.
Ann Thorac Surg 1986; **42**: 419–24.

[5] Long-term results of the "palliative" Mustard operation.
Dhasmana JP, Stark J, de Leval M, Macartney FJ, Rees PG, Taylor JFN, Hosp for Sick Children, London, UK.
J Am Coll Cardiol 1985; **6**: 1138–41.

[6] Right and left ventricular function at rest and with exercise after the Mustard operation for transposition of the great arteries.
Ramsay JM, Venables AW, Kelly MJ, Kalff V, Royal Children's Hosp, Melbourne, Vic, Australia.
Br Heart J 1984; **51**: 364–70.

[7] Cardiac rhythm after the Mustard operation for complete transposition of the great arteries.
Flinn CJ, Wolfe GS, Dick M II *et al*, Univ Miami, Miami, FL, USA.
N Engl J Med 1984; **310**: 1635–8.

[8] The arterial switch operation. An eight-year experience.
Quaegebeur JM, Rohmer J, Ottenkamp J *et al*, Univ Hosp, Leiden, The Netherlands.
J Thorac Cardiovasc Surg 1986; **92**: 361–84.

[9] Up to 7 years of follow-up after two-stage anatomic correction of simple transposition of the great arteries.
Lange PE, Sievers HH, Onnasch DGW, Yacoub MH, Bernhard A, Heintzen PH, Univ Kiel, Kiel, FR Germany.
Circulation 1986; **74** (Suppl I): 1–47.

[10] Anatomic correction for complete transposition and double-outlet right ventricle.
Kanter KR, Anderson RH, Lincoln C, Rigby ML, Shinebourne EA, Brompton Hosp, London, UK.
J Thorac Cardiovasc Surg 1985; **90**: 690–9.

[11] Cognitive function and age at repair of transposition of the great arteries in children.
Newburger JW, Silbert AR, Buckley LP, Fyler DC, Children's Hosp Med Cent, Boston, MA, USA.
N Engl J Med 1984; **310**: 1495–9.

Comment. Complete transposition is the congenital lesion produced by the combination of a concordant atrioventricular with a discordant ventriculo-arterial connection. The physiologic effect of this anatomic arrangement is that the pulmonary and systemic circulations are in parallel rather than in series. The introduction of balloon atrial septostomy by Rashkind (who, sadly, died recently) and Miller revolutionized the prognosis of the lesion. Even now, however, the technique is not without its problems, a fact that must be borne in mind when considering the results of surgical correction (see below).

Powell *et al* [1] have analyzed their experience with balloon septostomy from January 1968 to January 1980. Their results are depressing in that, of the 124 infants studied, 38 (31%) died before they reached the age of 6 months. Surprisingly, nowhere in this paper do the authors give a detailed breakdown of the causes of death. They suggest that their results have been better in the period 1976–1979, but again give no details of deaths. It is of interest to study the literature they cite to indicate that results of septostomy are as poor elsewhere. The literature does not uphold their assertion. For example, the initial experience of the Pittsburgh group between June 1966 and April 1970 [reported by Baker *et al, Circulation* 1971; **43**(Suppl 1): 1–6] showed that only 6 of 43 patients died in the neonatal period (some of these as a result of palliative surgery), and only 1 patient died late unrelated to surgery. In the study of Gutgesell and colleagues (*Am J Cardiol* 1979; **44**: 96–100), covering more or less the same period as the Liverpool investigation [1], 34 of 112 patients died following septostomy. Detailed causes of death were given: 16 were related to surgery, and, of the rest, 2 were related to septostomy, 5 were medical deaths in the first year and 1 occurred in the second year. Such figures are lacking in the report of Powell *et al* [1], and in the study of Leanage and colleagues (*Br Heart J* 1981; **45**: 559–72), who simply report that, of all patients undergoing septostomy at Great Ormond Street, from 1976 to the end of the period of study only 86% survived to 6 months and 76.5% to 18 months. As indicated, these figures are highly relevant to the analysis of surgical results for the arterial 'switch' procedure.

Baker *et al* have performed balloon septostomy in the intensive care unit under cross-sectional echocardiographic control [2]. They argue that this approach permits the procedure to be performed in ideal conditions and with minimal delay. They further suggest that transfer to the catheterization laboratory, for a procedure they consider unnecessary, would have entailed delay, disturbance to the infant and also the infant's removal from a controlled thermal environment. They are convinced that the advantages of echo-controlled septostomy in the intensive care unit far outweigh the potential disadvantages.

In terms of surgical correction of the lesion, there is still no consensus concerning the ideal operation. The long-term results for the Mustard procedure have been encouraging. Ashraf *et al* [3] followed 106 patients who underwent this procedure. Arrhythmias developed in nearly one-third of the patients and six required a pacemaker. Obstructions of the newly constructed atrial pathways occurred in seven patients and a baffle leak in four. Actuarial survival at 18 years was 92% and event-free survival 83%. Most patients were in excellent health. Stewart *et al* [4] followed 35 patients who underwent this procedure. These patients developed fewer arrhythmias, although these were not searched for using 24-hour monitoring. There was no evidence of venous obstruction or baffle leaks and only one late death occurred, presumed to be due to an arrhythmia. All but three of the patients were judged to have had an excellent clinical result.

In the past (and presumably still on rare occasions) patients were first seen with irreversible pulmonary vascular disease, which usually occurs in the presence of a ventricular septal defect, but it can be found when the ventricular septum is intact. Lindesmith proposed that such patients could be palliated by performing an atrial redirection procedure while leaving open the ventricular septal defect. This approach was championed by the Great Ormond Street group, who extended its use to those with an intact ventricular septum by creating a defect [5]. This paper is a report of their experience with 41 patients who were operated on between 1973 and 1980. Three patients died in hospital and there were two late deaths. The survivors have now been followed from 3 to 10 years (mean follow-up of 74.7 $\pm$22.8 months). The results have been excellent: of the survivors, 33 were in NYHA class III prior to operation and the other four were in class IV; follow-up showed 18 to be in class I, 17 to be in class II and only one in class III. The pre-operative hemoglobin level was 19.43 $\pm$3.14 g/dl and arterial oxygen saturation was 63.44 $\pm$11.29%. Comparable levels at follow-up were 14.19 $\pm$2.3 g/dl and 89.12 $\pm$7.25%. Effective pulmonary blood flow had improved from 1.39 $\pm$0.39 to 2.6 $\pm$0.78 litres/minute/m^2, although there had been no change in pulmonary arterial pressure and resistance. Ideally, patients with complete transposition should be treated prior to the development of irreversible pulmonary vascular obstructive disease. This series, however, shows that excellent palliation can still be provided for those patients unfortunate enough to have developed vascular changes prior to operative correction.

Some of the 'complications' of atrial redirection procedures are investigated in subsequent papers [6,7]. Ramsay *et al* considered ventricular function in a group of patients that had undergone a Mustard operation in 1974 or earlier [6]. They observed not only right-ventricular dysfunction, well documented previously, but also left-ventricular dysfunction. As they say, this finding "points to a generalized problem with the myocardium which is not only related to the right ventricle's ability to cope with a systemic load". Their findings are of significance to present discussions concerning the roles of arterial or atrial switching operations for surgical treatment. The authors conclude, "the expected benefits from the [arterial] 'switch' may not be achieved", and add a note of caution by indicating that the full significance of their findings remains unclear.

Flinn *et al* undertook a collaborative venture to study the postoperative rhythm of 372 patients who had undergone Mustard's procedure [7]. During the year of operation, 76% were in sinus rhythm, but this decreased to 57% at the end of the eighth postoperative year. A significant number ($n=9$) of patients died suddenly, but no strong risk factor was identified. The investigators collected only 372 patients from eight centers. This is just under three times the number of patients reported by Ullal *et al (J*

Thorac Cardiovasc Surg 1979; **78**: 431–79) from a single center in London. Further-more, Ullal *et al* modified their surgical technique specifically to avoid the sinus node and its arterial supply. Following this approach, 109 of 113 patients discharged from hospital were in sinus rhythm as judged by the standard 12-lead ECG. This is surely more than the 'limited' success that the US team [7] attributes to modifications of the Mustard procedure that avoid the specialized conduction tissues. Other major pro-blems with the study are that no data were obtained from 24-hour recordings (generally accepted as the only accurate way of monitoring arrhythmias), no pre-operative tracings were studied and no information was given as to whether the same patients were followed over the postoperative period.

The arterial switch procedure was first achieved by Jatene in Sao Paulo just over ten years ago. Subsequently, the operation was championed by Yacoub, who persevered with the technique, despite a depressingly high mortality rate in his early experience. The dilemma now facing the surgeon is illustrated by four papers cited here. Quaegebeur *et al* [8] describe probably the largest recent experience with the arterial switch procedure. Brom was one of the first surgeons to follow the lead of Jatene and Yacoub, and his efforts have been extended by Quaegebeur. Since January 1977, all patients with complete transposition and ventricular septal defect along with those having double outlet right ventricle and sub-pulmonary ventricular septal defects were treated with the switch procedure. Since January 1983, all patients with essen-tially intact ventricular septum seen within the first month of life have also been recommended for this operation. The paper contains the results of treatment of 66 patients, but an addendum gives details of 43 additional patients treated between July 1985 and April 1, 1986. For the 66 patients, 11-month actuarial survival rate, including hospital and late deaths, was 81%, with 70% confidence limits of 75–86%. The hazard function (instantaneous risk of death in those who have not died) had a single phase of rapidly declining risk that overlapped that of the general population by 12 months after the operation. A low birth weight was an incremental risk factor for death, as was the presence of an arterial duct. The risk of death was less in those with an intact sep-tum and, most significantly, there was demonstration of a learning curve. Multivariate analysis predicted almost 100% survival rates in future unless there was a large ven-tricular septal defect or an arterial duct. This was borne out by analysis of the subse-quent 43 patients. Two patients with major associated lesions died but only one other death occurred. Analysis of the earlier experience had predicted three deaths. If the cases with severe lesions are excluded, the authors draw the inference that the improvement across time of the survival rate has continued. These excellent results show that in expert hands the arterial switch procedure can be performed with a mor-tality rate that matches or betters that obtained for atrial redirective procedures.

Lange *et al* [9] assess the follow-up (up to seven years) of 16 patients from Kiel who were corrected by Yacoub using a two-stage procedure. This involved preliminary banding of the pulmonary trunk to 'prepare' the left ventricle followed by subsequent arterial switch. In all the patients, bodyweight normalized 3–6 months after correction and was normal in most cases after one year. None had signs of coronary or myocar-dial insufficiency and no arrhythmias occurred. There was mild elevation of right ventricular pressure in 10 of 12 patients studied because of residual pulmonary stenosis at the site of banding, but right ventricular function was normal. The left ventricular volumes were increased but function was normal. The enlarged aortic root (initially the origin of the pulmonary trunk) did not dilate further. This study shows excellent intermediate results of follow-up of the arterial switch procedure.

Kanter *et al* have reported recent experience of the arterial switch operation at the Brompton Hospital, London [10]. Eight patients were operated upon who had an intact ventricular septum; all but one survived; these patients were significantly younger than the others (mean age 1.2 months). Fifteen patients had complete transposition and a ventricular septal defect; six of these cases died (40%). This figure is comparable with most reported series of repair of this combination of defects using atrial redirection. Seven patients had double-outlet right ventricle with subpulmonary defect (Taussig-Bing anomaly); in this group one patient died, giving results that are superior to any reported using atrial redirection. The pattern of coronary arteries did not cause any problems during surgery. When the arterial trunks were in front of one another, it proved possible to pass the aorta behind the pulmonary bifurcation during the repair (the Lecompte manoever) in all cases but one. This was not possible in any case with side-by-side arterial trunks. A major problem, identified in seven patients, was subvalvar outflow obstruction in the newly constructed pulmonary pathway (from the right ventricle), which was implicated as a cause of death in three of the eight patients who died. Furthemore, clinically unsuspected gradients were encountered across this outflow tract in 69% of patients at follow-up; they were thought to be related to the Lecompte procedure or the use of conduits, which is now avoided whenever possible at this center.

Thus, the long-term results show that the Mustard procedure has provided excellent clinical treatment of complete transposition so far; the predictions of the potential failure of the right ventricle have yet to become manifest. However, it has now been demonstrated unequivocally that the arterial switch procedure can be performed with results that match those obtained for atrial redirection. There is an obvious 'learning curve' for the arterial procedure but, once achieved successfully, it carries little or no risk of late death, which is not the case for atrial operations. The arterial switch procedure is becoming the treatment of choice for neonates with complete transposition.

The final paper in this section addresses an important topic on which there is little information at present available - namely, cognitive function after operation [11]. Although an important contribution, only one aspect of psychosocial function after operative repair was studied and only a limited number of tests performed. Nevertheless, highly significant results were obtained. The Boston group found that age at repair, when controlled for social index, was inversely associated with the results of the tests performed. Cognitive function, when tested similarly for patients with ventricular septal defect, bore no relation to age at repair. Surprisingly, the cognitive function of those who had ventricular septal defects was lower than that of a control group without congenital heart disease, a finding not discussed further. The results lead to the conclusion that delay in the repair of patients with complete transposition is associated with progressive impairment of cognitive function.

THE ROLE OF DOPPLER ECHOCARDIOGRAPHY IN CONGENITAL HEART DISEASE

Review: NEIL WILSON

Two-dimensional echocardiography has had a great influence on the diagnosis and management of the common and rarer forms of congenital heart disease [1–3]. Despite the ever-improving resolution of echocardiographic imaging, a fraction of pediatric patients persistently defy diagnosis because of limitations of the instrument, patient, or operator. Thus, some patients with structural heart abnormalities still require angiocardiography to delineate their cardiac anatomy. Nevertheless, and because of the ever-increasing demand for hemodynamic information by non-invasive means, the application of Doppler ultrasound to the detection and quantification of abnormalities of blood flow in the heart and great vessels has increased exponentially.

Qualitative Doppler

Suspected structural heart abnormalities can now be qualitatively confirmed [4–6] with pulsed Doppler echocardiography. Figure 1 demonstrates a typical use – the confirmation of a suspected ventricular septal defect in a child whose murmur was difficult to distinguish from that due to mitral regurgitation. Discrimination between murmurs due to mild semilunar valve stenosis and those which are innocent forms another extremely useful, if not well-publicized, role of Doppler in clinical pediatric cardiology.

Quantitative Doppler

Quantitative non-invasive hemodynamics, hitherto based on the secondary effects of chamber hypertrophy or dilatation detected by M-mode and two-dimensional echocardiography, as in the work of Blackwood [7], are now well established with delineation by Doppler echocardiography. The pioneering work of the Hatle [8] and Goldberg [9] teams has built a firm foundation for much of the state-of-the-art cardiac Doppler. The most recent applications to congenital heart disease have encompassed many desirable

(a)

(b)

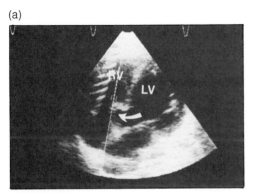
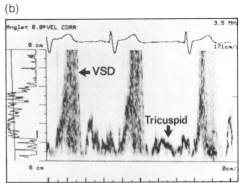

FIGURE 1: (a) Foreshortened apical four-chamber echocardiogram of a child with a ventricular septal defect. (b) The Doppler sample volume (short parallel lines) detects high-velocity turbulent blood flow from left to right across the ventricular septum. VSD = ventricular septal defect.

areas of hemodynamic quantification: semilunar and atrioventricular valve pressure gradient and orifice area calculation; pulmonary artery pressure measurement; volumetric blood flow for the quantification of intracardiac shunts; and semilunar valve regurgitation. Color flow mapping is on the horizon. It promises rapid qualitative diagnosis and perhaps quantitative virtues as well.

Stenotic Gradients

It has long been known that quantification of semilunar valve stenosis by applying the modified Bernouilli equation* to the peak blood flow velocity measured across the valve gives an accurate estimate of pressure gradient in terms of millimetres of mercury [10–12]. Recent work has extended these principles to deal with more complex ventricular outlet obstruction – with equally encouraging results [13], bearing in mind that, even at cardiac catheterization, outflow gradient measurement in complex congenital heart disease can be a time-consuming, difficult, and potentially hazardous procedure. Coarctation of the aorta, a stenotic lesion commonly encountered in pediatric cardiology, lends itself to quantification using the modified Bernouilli equation [14]. Figure 2 shows a typical time-velocity waveform across a coarctation in an older child, examined from the suprasternal notch. The hemodynamic assessment of this lesion is not so straightforward in the neonate, however, where ductal patency confounds conventional pressure gradient estimation [15].

Recently, much has been made of the temporal difference in gradients measured at cardiac catheterization (usually peak-to-peak gradient) and those measured in Doppler studies (instantaneous peak gradient). Zhang has tried to circumvent this problem by expressing aortic stenosis quantification by Doppler in terms of mean gradient [16], which is a reasonable compromise. The effort to convert an instantaneous Doppler

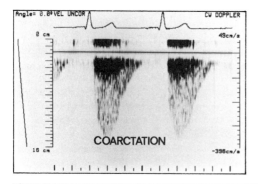

FIGURE 2: Time velocity waveform across a coarctation of the aorta in a 5-year-old boy. Note the typical, slurred slope of the deceleration limb. The peak velocity of 3.2 m/s corresponds to an instantaneous peak gradient of approximately 40 mmHg.

---

* The Bernouilli equation is a complex physical equation relating to fluid flow in cylinders. In practical terms, for clinical cardiology the equation may be shortened to:

$$P_1 - P_2 = 4 (V_2{}^2 - V_1{}^2)$$

where V_2 = velocity distal to the obstruction,
$\quad V_1$ = velocity proximal to obstruction,
$\quad P_1$ = pressure proximal to obstruction, and
$\quad P_2$ = pressure distal to obstruction.

When velocity is expressed in metres/second, the pressure difference ($P_1 - P_2$) is in mmHg. In most clinical situations the proximal velocity (V_1) is rarely significantly greater than 1 metre/second and is usually disregarded. The fully modified equation is thus:

$$\text{Pressure gradient} = 4 V_2{}^2.$$

gradient to a peak-to-peak measurement [17] is an interesting exercise, but is surely unphysiological.

Pulmonary Artery Pressure Estimation

Pulmonary artery pressure measurement is important in assessing congenital heart disease, and particularly the timing of palliative and corrective operations. Previous Doppler methods [18,19] have been simply extended and adapted observations of the work of Burstin [20]. Results with these methods, while they correlate well with measurements of invasive techniques in grouped studies, have wide confidence limits, which makes them unreliable predictors in the individual patient. The application of the modified Bernouilli equation to the peak blood velocity across a ventricular septal defect gives a reliable estimate of right-ventricular pressure and, in the absence of right-ventricular outflow tract obstruction, systolic pulmonary artery pressure in those children with a ventricular septal defect [21]. Children with an intact ventricular septum pose more of a problem. Applying the modified Bernouilli equation to a regurgitant jet across the tricuspid valve also gives an accurate measurement of right-ventricular pressure [22], but in practice quantitative estimation of this jet in children is difficult.

Volumetric Flow Calculation

Volumetric flow calculation is of considerable use in pediatric cardiology for the calculation of shunt magnitude in lesions causing left-to-right shunts. Using the product of the cross-sectional area and the mean velocity of blood at the site of the Doppler sample volume, an estimate can be made of blood flow at this site. Comparison of flow in a systemic artery with that in the pulmonary artery thus gives an estimate of shunt magnitude in terms of a Qp:Qs ratio [23]. While early studies validated the method at arterial sites, more recent work has demonstrated good correlation at intracardiac sites [24,25], extending the potential for shunt calculation in those cases where turbulent blood flow in the great arteries precludes accurate flow measurement.

The Doppler methods above rely on obtaining high-resolution imaging for area calculation and high-quality pulsed Doppler time-velocity waveforms for calculation of mean velocity. The studies quoted display good correlation but wide confidence limits, which again should provoke caution when applying the technique to the individual. Goldberg and Allen have applied volumetric flow calculation to the problem of quantifying semilunar valve regurgitation, with encouraging results [26]. This particular lesion usually defies all but the crudest quantification, even by invasive means. Teague et al [27] approach this problem in a different but simple way, using a half-time measurement method similar to that used in the calculation of pressure drop and valve orifice area in mitral stenosis. Both approaches are potentially useful.

Color Flow Mapping

The remarkable new extension of two-dimensional echocardiography to real-time blood-flow mapping is a form of pulsed Doppler which, within limits, gives an angiography-like image of cardiac blood flow. There is no doubt that, even in its infancy, this form of Doppler ultrasound affords rapid qualitative diagnosis. Particularly useful attributes, which put it ahead of more conventional Doppler, are those of speed and the ability to identify multiple or eccentrically placed stenotic jets, such as

181

those which occur in multiple ventricular septal defects [28], and in paraprosthetic valve leaks [29]. Although still very much a qualitative tool, the inevitable improvement in image resolution of color flow mapping seems set to pave the way for quantitative information, with some promise already of being able to quantify semilunar and atrioventricular valve regurgitation.

The Future

While Doppler echocardiography is in widespread use for confirmation of a clinical diagnosis, there are many quantitative questions still to be resolved. Now that the estimation of pulmonary artery pressure is feasible, what of diastolic pulmonary artery pressure? – and pulmonary vascular resistance? It seems likely that with the presence of pulmonary regurgitation – a common occurrence even in normal subjects [30] – application of the modified Bernouilli equation to the pulmonary regurgitant jet should result in a reasonably accurate estimate of pulmonary artery diastolic pressure. Figure 3 shows the Doppler waveform of a pulmonary regurgitant jet in a teenage girl with pulmonary hypertension. It is possible that the slope of the regurgitant waveform will also yield some information as to pulmonary vascular resistance in this patient.

Doppler ultrasound is now being applied to the heart of the developing fetus, and is already playing a small role in the antenatal diagnosis of congenital heart disease [31,32]. I anticipate that Doppler will play an even greater part in the delineation of changes that take place in the neonatal circulation with the adaptation to extrauterine life [33]. This information will be of practical value to those involved in the management of babies with persisting fetal circulation.

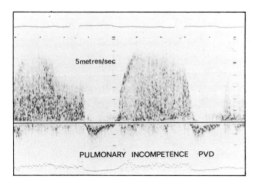

FIGURE 3: Time velocity waveform of the pulmonary regurgitant jet in a teenage girl with pulmonary vascular disease (PVD). The peak velocity in diastole is in excess of 5 m/s, indicating a diastolic pressure calculated by the modified Bernouilli equation greater than 100 mmHg.

References

[1] Sutherland GR, Godman MJ, Smallhorn JF, Guiterras P, Anderson RH, Hunter S.
Ventricular septal defect. Two dimensional echocardiographic and morphological correlations.
Br Heart J 1982; 47: 316–28.

[2] Huhta JC, Smallhorn JF, Macartney FJ.
Two dimensional echocardiographic diagnosis of situs.
Br Heart J 1982; 48: 97–108.

[3] Stark J, Smallhorn J, Huhta J et al.
Surgery for congenital heart defects diagnosed with real time echocardiography [Abstract].
Circulation 1982; 66 (Suppl 2): 30.

[4] Dickinson DF, Goldberg SJ, Wilson N.
A comparison of information obtained by ultrasound examination and cardiac catheterisation in paediatric patients with congenital heart disease.
Int J Cardiol 1985; 9: 275–85.

[5] Stevenson JG, Kawabori I, Stamm SJ et al.
Pulsed Doppler echocardiographic evaluation
of ventricular septal defect patches.
Circulation 1984; **70** (Suppl 1): 38–47.

[6] Minagoe S, Tei C, Kisanuki A et al.
Noninvasive pulsed Doppler echocardiographic detection of the direction of shunt flow in
patients with atrial septal defect: Usefulness of
the right parasternal approach.
Circulation 1985; **71**: 745–53.

[7] Blackwood RA, Bloom KR, Williams CM.
Aortic stenosis in children. Experience with
echocardiographic predictions of severity.
Circulation 1978; **57**: 263–8.

[8] Hatle L, Angelsen BA.
Doppler Ultrasound in Cardiology: Physical
Principles and Clinical Applications, 2nd edn.
Philadelphia: Lee & Febiger, 1985.

[9] Goldberg SJ, Allen HD, Marx GR, Flinn CJ.
Doppler Echocardiography. Philadelphia: Lee
& Febiger, 1985.

[10] Hatle L, Angelsen BA, Tromsdal A.
Noninvasive assessment of aortic stenosis by
Doppler ultrasound.
Br Heart J 1980; **43**: 284–92.

[11] Oliveira Lima C, Sahn DJ, Valdes Cruz LM et al.
Noninvasive prediction of transvalvular pressure gradient in patients with pulmonary stenosis by quantitative two dimensional echo Doppler studies.
Circulation 1983; **67**: 866–71.

[12] Stevenson JG, Kawabori I.
Noninvasive determination of pressure gradients in children: Two methods employing
pulsed Doppler echocardiography.
J Am Coll Cardiol 1984; **3**: 179–92.

[13] Reeder GS, Currie PJ, Fyfe DA, Hagler DJ,
Seward JB, Tajik AJ.
Extracardiac conduit obstruction: Initial experience in the use of Doppler echocardiography
for noninvasive estimation of pressure gradient.
J Am Coll Cardiol 1984; **4**: 1006–111.

[14] Wyse RKH, Robinson PJ, Deanfield JE,
Tunstall-Pedoe DS, Macartney FJ.
Use of continuous wave Doppler ultrasound
velocimetry to assess the severity of coarctation of the aorta by measurement of aortic flow
velocities.
Br Heart J 1984; **52**: 278–83.

[15] Sutherland GR, Wilson N.
Unpublished observations, 1986.

[16] Zhang Y, Nitter Hauge S.
Determination of the mean pressure gradient in
aortic stenosis by Doppler echocardiography.
Eur Heart J 1985; **6**: 999–1005.

[17] Zhang Y, Ihlen H, Nitter Hauge S.
Estimation of the peak to peak pressure gradient in aortic stenosis by Doppler echocardiography.
Int J Cardiol 1986; **10**: 197–212.

[18] Mahan G, Dabestani A, Gardin J, Allfie A, Burn
C, Henry W.
Estimation of pulmonary artery pressure by
pulsed Doppler echocardiography [Abstract].
Circulation 1983; **68** (Suppl 2): 367.

[19] Kosturakis D, Goldberg SJ, Allen HD, Loeber
C.
Doppler echocardiographic prediction of pul-
monary arterial hypertension in congenital
heart disease.
Am J Cardiol 1984; **53**: 1110–5.

[20] Burstin L.
Determination of pressure in the pulmonary
artery by external graphic recordings.
Br Heart J 1967; **29**: 396–404.

[21] Skjaerpe T, Hegrenaes L, Hatle L.
Noninvasive estimation of right ventricular
pressure by Doppler ultrasound in ventricular
septal defect [Abstract]. In: 5th Symp on Echo-
cardiology, Rotterdam 1983. Ultrasonar Bulle-
tin 92, 1983.

[22] Currie PJ, Seward JB, Chan KL et al.
Continuous wave Doppler determination of
right ventricular pressure: A simultaneous Doppler catheterization study in 127 patients.
J Am Coll Cardiol 1985; **6**: 750–6.

[23] Sanders SP, Yeager S, Williams R.
Measurement of systemic and pulmonary blood
flow and Qp:Qs ratio using Doppler and two
dimensional echocardiography.
Am J Cardiol 1983; **51**: 952–6.

[24] Goldberg SJ, Dickinson DF, Wilson N.
Evaluation of an elliptical area technique for the
calculation of mitral flow by Doppler echocardiography.
Br Heart J 1985; **54**: 68–75.

[25] Meijboom EJ, Horowitz S, Valdes Cruz LM,
Sahn DJ, Larson D, Oliveira Lima C.
A Doppler echocardiographic method for cal-
culating volume flow across the tricuspid valve:
Correlative laboratory and clinical studies.
Circulation 1985; **71**: 551–6.

[26] Goldberg SJ, Allen HD.
Quantitative measurement of semilunar insufficiency by Doppler echo with an internal
accuracy check [Abstract].
Circulation 1983; **68** (Suppl 3): 260.

[27] Teague SM, Heinsimer JA, Anderson JL, Olsen EG, Thadani U.
Accurate noninvasive assessment of aortic regurgitation utilising a Doppler half time index [Abstract].
J Am Coll Cardiol 1986; **7**: 101A.

[28] Ortiz E, Robinson PJ, Deanfield JE, Franklin R, Macartney FJ, Wyse RKH.
Localisation of ventricular septal defects by simultaneous display of superimposed colour Doppler and cross sectional echocardiographic images.
Br Heart J 1985; **54**: 53–60.

[29] Omoto R, Yokote Y, Takamoto S *et al*.
Diagnostic significance of real time two dimensional Doppler echocardiography (2D Doppler) in congenital heart diseases, acquired valvular diseases, and dissecting aortic aneurysms.
J Cardiography 1984; **14** (Suppl 5): 103–7.

[30] Yock PG, Naasz C, Schnittger I, Popp RL.
Doppler tricuspid and pulmonic regurgitation in normals: Is it real? [Abstract].
Circulation 1984; **70**: II–40.

[31] Huhta JC, Strasburger JF, Carpenter RJ, Reiter A.
Fetal echocardiography: Accuracy and limitations in the diagnosis of cardiac disease [Abstract].
J Am Coll Cardiol 1985; **5**: 387.

[32] Maulik D, Nanda N, Saini V.
Fetal Doppler echocardiography: Methods and characterisation of normal and abnormal hemodynamics.
Am J Cardiol 1984; **53**: 572–8.

[33] Wilson N, Reed KR, Allen HD, Marx GR, Goldberg SJ.
Doppler echocardiographic observations of pulmonary and transvalvular velocity changes after birth and during the early neonatal period.
Am Heart J 1987 (in press).

CROSS-SECTIONAL ECHOCARDIOGRAPHY AND DOPPLER TECHNIQUES

[1] Cross sectional echocardiographic diagnosis of congenital heart disease in infants [Editorial].
Macartney FJ, Hosp Sick Children, London, UK.
Br Heart J 1983; **50**: 501–5.

[2] Surgery without catheterization for congenital heart defects: management of 100 patients.
Huhta JC, Glasow P, Murphy DJ Jr *et al*, Texas Children's Hosp, Houston, TX, USA.
J Am Coll Cardiol 1987; **9**: 823–9.

[3] Cross-sectional echocardiographic features of "absent" pulmonary valve. Report of two cases.
Tenorio de Albuquerque AM, Ortiz J, Villela de Moraes A *et al*, Hosp Clin, Sao Paolo, Brazil.
Int J Cardiol 1984; **5**: 155–61.

[4] Anatomy of the echocardiographic crux cordis in the evaluation of the spectrum of atrioventricular valve atresia.
Magherini A, Azzolina G, Careri A, Tuscan Heart and Chest Cent, Florence, Italy.
Int J Cardiol 1984; **5**: 163–72.

[5] Complex congenital cardiac anomalies — morphological and echocardiographic correlations [Editorial].
Wilkinson JL, Royal Liverpool Children's Hosp, Liverpool, UK.
Int J Cardiol 1984; **5**: 174–7.

[6] Cor triatriatum sinistrum. Diagnostic features on cross sectional echocardiography.
Ostman-Smith I, Silverman NH, Oldershaw P, Lincoln C, Shinebourne EA, Brompton Hosp, London, UK.
Br Heart J 1984; **51**: 211–9.

[7] Prenatal screening for congenital heart disease.
Allan LD, Crawford DC, Chita SK, Tynan MJ, Guy's Hosp, London, UK.
Br Med J 1986; **292**: 1717–9.

[8] Evaluation of fetal arrhythmias by echocardiography.
Allan LD, Anderson RH, Sullivan ID, Campbell S, Holt DW, Tynan M, Guy's Hosp, London, UK.
Br Heart J 1983; **50**: 240–5.

[9] Fetal echocardiography. III. The diagnosis of cardiac arrhythmias using real-time-directed M-mode ultrasound.
DeVore GR, Siassi B, Platt LD, Women's Hosp, Los Angeles, CA, USA.
Am J Obstet Gynecol 1983; **146**: 792–9.

[10] Diagnosis of fetal abnormalities by echocardiography and its significance in obstetric and fetal management.
Pizzuto P, Colloridi V, Tulli A, Gallo P, Pachi I, Reale A, Univ 'La Sapienza', Rome, Italy.
Cardiologia 1985; **30**: 25–32.

[11] Noninvasive evaluation of the ratio of pulmonary to systemic flow in atrial septal defect by duplex Doppler echocardiography.
Kitabatake A, Inoue M, Asao M *et al*, Osaka Univ Med Sch, Osaka, Japan.
Circulation 1984; **69**: 73–9.

[12] A pulsed Doppler echocardiographic method for calculating pulmonary and systemic blood flow in atrial level shunts: validation studies in animals and initial human experience.
Valdes-Cruz LM, Horowitz S, Mesel E, Sahn DJ, Fisher DC, Larson D, Univ Arizona Health Sci Cent, Tucson, AZ, USA.
Circulation 1984; **69**: 80–6.

[13] Clinical utility of two-dimensional Doppler echocardiographic techniques for estimating pulmonary to systemic blood flow ratios in children with left to right shunting atrial septal defect, ventricular septal defect or patent ductus arteriosus.
Vargas Barron J, Sahn DJ, Valdes-Cruz LM *et al*, Univ Arizona Health Sci Cent, Tucson, AZ, USA.
J Am Coll Cardiol 1984; **3**: 169–78.

[14] Noninvasive determination of pressure gradients in children: two methods employing pulsed Doppler echocardiography.
Stevenson JG, Kawabori I, Univ Washington, Seattle, WA, USA.
J Am Coll Cardiol 1984; **3**: 179–92.

Comment. In an excellent editorial, Macartney [1] considers the expanding role of cross-sectional echocardiography in the diagnosis of congenital heart disease in infants. Its role in supplementing information provided by angiocardiography is discussed, as are those circumstances in which cardiac catheterization can be replaced. As the author states, there is now no variety of congenital heart disease which cannot be diagnosed with considerable accuracy by cross-sectional echocardiography; he adds: "sending a patient for operation without prior cardiac catheterization concentrates the mind wonderfully!". A review of the implications of the spread of cross-sectional echocardiography for the pattern of referral of neonates with congenital heart disease concludes the article. Macartney currently argues against a role for the pediatrician or cardiologist with particular experience of congenital heart disease in newborns and infants in the district general hospital, but sees a possible potential for the future. The final sentence is unarguably correct: "cross-sectional echocardiography has undoubtedly caused the biggest revolution in the management of congenital heart disease since the advent of open heart surgery".

Huhta *et al* analysed the effects of submitting patients to surgery without preoperative catheterization [2]. They compared the operative mortality in 100 patients managed without pre-operative catheterization with that of a group of 151 diagnosis-matched patients who did undergo catheterization. The majority of the patients studied had atrial septal defect, pulmonary stenosis/atresia, aortic stenosis, aortic coarctation or persistent patency of the arterial duct. When compared, mortality at operation was 18% in those who did not undergo catheterization but only 9% in those who did. Multiple logistic regression analysis demonstrated that these figures were not significantly different; rather, there was a trend toward lower mortality in the group who did not undergo catheterization. The investigators consider various factors related to the omission of catheterization, including financial savings. They conclude that accurate diagnosis can now be achieved without catheterization. When neonates and young infants are approached in this manner, the evidence from this study indicates a reduction in potential surgical mortality.

Several papers [3–6] illustrate the increasing value of cross-sectional echocardiography in the diagnosis of the most complex congenital cardiac lesions. They show that the correct answer can be obtained by anyone who has the appropriate echocardiographic machine and a reasonably sophisticated knowledge of cardiac morphology. The group from Brazil [3] show that, almost without exception, the so-called 'absent' pulmonary valve is represented by a ring of rudimentary leaflet tissue. They demonstrate how easy it is to see marked dilatation of the pulmonary arteries, and identify all the associated intracardiac lesions. The Italian workers [4] characterize fully the different anatomic substrates of atrioventricular valve atresia. They show the importance of the orientation of the ventricular septum in distinguishing between an imperforate valve membrane and an absent atrioventricular connection, also the value of anatomic knowledge in determining the extent of atrioventricular sulcus tissue and distinguishing it from a valve membrane. This is all put into perspective by Wilkinson's editorial [5], which emphasizes that "You diagnose what you know".

The paper from the Brompton Hospital [6] contains very good illustrations of the obstructing membrane in cases with a partitioned left atrium (cor triatriatum sinistrum). As the authors rightly conclude, cross-sectional echocardiography is vastly superior to angiocardiography as a means of distinguishing the different structures that can obstruct egress from the left atrium. They also show how a partitioned left atrium can readily be distinguished from totally anomalous pulmonary venous connection to the coronary sinus.

The Guy's Hospital Unit for fetal echocardiography probably has more experience in the field than any other unit. In an excellent review of fetal echocardiography [7], the authors emphasize how they have simplified the basic ultrasonic scan of the fetal heart so that most major defects can be detected by relatively unsophisticated ultrasonographers (in terms of cardiac malformation) from around the 16th week of gestation. The so-called 'four chamber' view of the heart, showing the connections of the atria and ventricles, can be achieved by experienced obstetric ultrasonographers and included in the routine scan. The normal appearance of this single scan effectively excludes most severe congenital heart lesions and, conversely, should detect abnormalities in over two pregnancies in each thousand studied. The number of lesions detected in the Guy's Hospital Unit has increased markedly since its inception in 1980. During the first nine months of 1985, 31 malformations were identified, of which the referring ultrasonographer suspected 22. Of the patients referred because of a lesion suspected in the four-chamber scan, four-fifths proved to have a cardiac malformation. This experience is important because it shows that recognition of abnormality in a solitary and easily performed scan is feasible, normality can be distinguished from abnormality in this way and fetal screening is already operating on a limited basis. In the authors' experience thus far, most mothers chose termination when learning of the fetal abnormality — for the remainder the fetus did not survive the malformation after birth. Earlier diagnosis of more lesions will offer greater options for counselling and also permit the fetus to be born in the optimal surroundings for treatment if this is the chosen course for pregnancy. The authors argue that extensions of their program and greater organization of teaching are now warranted, citing the development of such a program in France. Such a program has far-reaching implications, particularly in terms of social and ethical considerations.

Earlier experience of this group with fetal arrhythmias is described [8]; DeVore et al also discuss the topic [9]. Both groups report accurate diagnosis of a variety of fetal arrhythmias from the M-mode echocardiographic study of valvar, atrial and ventricular wall motion. The technique is of more than academic interest, because it permits prenatal treatment and may prevent unnecessary premature delivery after a mistaken diagnosis of fetal distress.

A further report [10] describes an experience of fetal echocardiography in keeping with that reported from Guy's Hospital and other centers. Pizzuto et al examined 294 high-risk pregnancies. Structural defects were predicted in nine fetuses, and these were confirmed at autopsy. The remaining 195 fetuses were considered to have normal hearts. Confirmation was obtained by clinical and echo studies after delivery. The authors point out the high risk of intrauterine death in fetuses with cardiac abnormalities, even in the absence of arrhythmias and/or fetal hydrops. Several psychologic, ethical and legal problems are raised, which have not yet been systematically addressed. It is likely that the solutions to such problems will differ according to the process of law within the society of each country.

The use of Doppler echocardiographic techniques is discussed fully elsewhere in this volume (see review by N. Wilson). The final papers in this section are representative of problems debated over the last few years. All four [11-14] are concerned with the pulsed Doppler technique, as opposed to the continuous wave format. The latter has been available for a longer period and evaluated in some detail by Hatle for the determination of pressure gradients.

Three of the studies are concerned with the estimation of pulmonary to systemic blood flow ratios [11-13], and the other is concerned with the determination of pressure gradients in children with arterial valve stenosis or pulmonary artery banding [14]. The work by Stevenson and Kawabori [14] is a good example of the scientific examination of a new technique. They give full credit to the pioneering studies of Hatle, and discuss frankly the problems involved in this technique, its limitations and the difficulties to be anticipated by newcomers. Despite the caveats pointed out, they achieved excellent prediction of pressure gradients. Stevenson and Kawabori argue that the pulsed Doppler format will probably be better for the evaluation of pressure gradients, since it has a cross-sectional format and will be easier for newcomers to use. It still seems likely that the continuous wave technique will provide more accurate measurements and will be less likely to underestimate pressure gradients, which is still a problem with the pulsed format.

THE ARTERIAL AND VENOUS DUCTS: CLOSURE, PERSISTENT PATENCY AND PHARMACOLOGIC MANIPULATION

[1] Autonomic mechanisms in the ductus venosus of the lamb.
Coceani F, Adeagbo ASO, Cutz E, Olley PM, Hosp Sick Children, Toronto, Ont, Canada.
Am J Physiol 1984; **247**: H17–24.
[2] Morphologic features of the ductus arteriosus after prostaglandin E₁ administration for ductus-dependent congenital heart defects.
Park I-S, Nihill MR, Titus JL, Texas Child Hosp, Houston, TX, USA.
J Am Coll Cardiol 1983; **1**: 471–5.
[3] Long-term prostaglandin E₁ therapy in congenital heart defects.
Teixeira OHP, Carpenter B, MacMurray SB, Vlad P, Children's Hosp Eastern Ontario, Ottawa, Ont, Canada.
J Am Coll Cardiol 1984; **3**: 838–43.
[4] Patent ductus arteriosus in neonates with severe respiratory disease.
Dudell GG, Gersony WM, Columbia Univ Babies Hosp, New York, NY, USA.
J Pediatr 1984; **104**: 915–20.
[5] Surgical closure of patent ductus arteriosus in 268 preterm infants.
Wagner HR, Ellison RC, Zierler S *et al*, for the National Collaborative Study on Patent Ductus Arteriosus in Premature Infants, Children's Hosp, Philadelphia, PA, USA.
J Thorac Cardiovasc Surg 1984; **87**: 870–5.
[6] Management of patent ductus arteriosus in the premature infant: indomethacin versus ligation.
Mavroudis C, Cook LN, Fleischaker JW *et al*, Univ Louisville Sch Med, Louisville, KY, USA.
Ann Thorac Surg 1983; **36**: 561–6.
[7] Indomethacin treatment for patent ductus arteriosus in very low birthweight infants: a double blind trial.
Rudd P, Montanez P, Hallidie-Smith K, Silverman M, Hammersmith Hospital, London, UK.
Arch Dis Child 1983; **58**: 267–70.
[8] Patent ductus arteriosus in adults — long-term follow-up nonsurgical versus surgical treatment.
Fisher RG, Moodie DS, Sterba R, Gill CC, Cleveland Clin Found, Cleveland, OH, USA.
J Am Coll Cardiol 1986; **8**: 280–4.

Comment. The mechanisms of closure of two of the vital components of the fetal circulation, namely, the venous and arterial ducts (ductus venosus and arteriosus, respectively), have become more fully understood in recent years. Much of this knowledge comes from the Toronto group led by Olley and Coceani. Their latest research has been concerned with autonomic mechanisms in the venous duct [1], and they have demonstrated a powerful potential role for adrenergic innervation in ductal closure — a mechanism which previously has often been doubted, in part because morphologists have not always agreed about the presence of adrenergic nerves within the muscular walls of the ducts. The pharmacologic evidence presented by Coceani *et al* [1] suggests that nervous regulation in life works in concert with priming by the prostaglandin system, the latter enhancing contractions initiated by the discharge from the neural elements. The important role of the prostaglandin system and its inhibition by aspirin or indomethacin was jointly elucidated by the Toronto group and Heymann and his colleagues from San Francisco in the late 1970s. Subsequent to these initial investigations, prostaglandins of the E series have been widely employed in centers dealing with neonatal heart disease to ensure patency of the arterial duct in lesions such as pulmonary atresia, where survival is dependent upon flow through the duct. Administration of the drugs, however, has not been without its problems.

In an early histologic study, Gittenberger-de Groot and her co-workers from Leiden suggested that prostaglandin administration produced significant changes in the wall of the arterial duct (*Br Heart J* 1978; **40**: 215). An extensive study by Silver and her colleagues from Ontario (*Hum Pathol* 1981; **12**: 1123) then questioned these conclusions, arguing instead that the changes observed were part of the normal closing process. Evidence to support this theory is now provided by Park *et al* [2] and Teixeira *et al* [3]. Park *et al* [2] studied arterial ducts from 12 neonates who died while receiving or within 4 days of administration of prostaglandin E_1, and compared these with similar material from 10 neonates who had not been treated with prostaglandins. Although the drug seemed to delay the natural maturational closing changes in the ductal wall, no deleterious histologic changes were seen and the duct seemed to close normally after prostaglandin was discontinued. Teixeira *et al* [4] used long-term intravenous prostaglandin E_1 in 17 neonates with various types of duct-dependent heart lesions. The average duration of drug administration was 39 days, with a range of 8–104 days. Although therapy was successful, they noted several significant side-effects, notably cortical hyperostosis of the long bones (which resolved when the drug was stopped) and refractory diarrhea. Histologic examination was possible in three cases, and all sections showed normal ductal closure only. The overall conclusion of the study is that long-term therapy with prostaglandin E_1 is both feasible and safe. Although the authors refer to the paper of Silove and his colleagues from Birmingham, UK (*Circulation* 1981; **63**: 682), they do not discuss it — a pity, because the UK team showed that a similar result could be achieved using oral therapy, with fewer side-effects.

Persistent patency of the arterial duct, although an advantageous feature in neonates with compromised pulmonary blood flow, is severely deleterious in premature infants or in those with respiratory distress. Dudell and Gersony studied 200 neonates with persistent patency of the arterial duct in association with respiratory distress [4], demonstrating clearly that patency beyond three days is a negative prognostic factor. Patency was investigated using the relatively non-invasive technique of contrast echocardiography via an umbilical catheter. None of the patients received treatment during the first three days. As the authors point out, the American

Collaborative Study (*J Pediatr* 1983; **102:** 895–906) established indomethacin as the treatment of choice for ductal closure, with surgery employed as a back-up. They are now concerned to establish whether such treatment given at diagnosis would prevent the mortality and morbidity which ensues if there is a delay.

The US Collaborative Study mentioned above has continued its investigations, and has now reported the results for surgical ductal closure in the premature infant [5]. Thirteen centers took part in the study, and 268 infants from a study population of 3559 patients underwent operation. No deaths occurred during operation, although 26% had intraoperative complications and 8 infants (3%) died within 36 hours of operation. Overall, 77% of the infants survived and were discharged from hospital at a mean age of 78 days. Some of the infants had received indomethacin previously; the only difference between them and those not receiving indomethacin was a later date of operation due to transient closure. The authors conclude that surgery is a safe and effective means of closing the duct in small premature infants.

Two further studies from individual units (as opposed to collaborative efforts) have also addressed the question of the most effective means of ductal closure. Mavroudis *et al* compared the use of indomethacin with surgical ligation [6]. This group previously reported the results of pharmacologic manipulation, and have now reported a sequential group of neonates treated surgically. The mean gestational age was 29.1 weeks and mean weight 1.1 kg. Overall mortality in the group treated pharmacologically was 40%, whereas the mortality following surgery was 17% — rising to 32% if preoperative pneumothorax was present. There were severe complications in both groups. Pharmacologic closure was the approach evaluated by Rudd *et al*, who treated 15 low-birthweight infants with indomethacin and compared the results with those from another 15 neonates of almost identical gestational age who received a placebo [7]. A response in terms of closure was achieved in 13 of the treated group, but permanent closure was achieved in only 7. In contrast, only three of the neonates receiving placebo closed their arterial duct, although this was a permanent effect in two of them. Indomethacin now seems established as the initial line of treatment for the persistently patent arterial duct, but surgery is still needed in a significant proportion of infants, particularly in those born prematurely.

One hundred and seventeen adult patients (age range 18–81 years, mean 36) with isolated patent ductus arteriosus (with or without pulmonary hypertension) have been seen at the Cleveland Clinic between 1951 and 1984; they have been followed for 1–37 years (mean 18) [8]. Forty-five patients were treated conservatively and 72 underwent surgical closure. After analysis, it was found that patients who were treated conservatively experienced significantly more cyanosis ($P=0.002$) and had fewer diastolic murmurs ($P>0.001$) than those patients who had been treated surgically. Among patients who had been treated conservatively, those who had cardiomegaly before treatment were more likely to die than those who did not ($P>0.001$). Among those treated surgically, patients who had cardiomegaly before operation had a poorer prognosis than those who did not ($P=0.09$). Of seven patients who presented with a pulmonary artery systolic pressure >100 mmHg, five were treated conservatively and two were treated surgically; two of those treated conservatively died, at four and 19 years follow-up, respectively. The authors conclude that adult patients with patent ductus arteriosus should be treated surgically, particularly if they have cardiomegaly at initial presentation.

190

DEFECTS OF THE ATRIAL, ATRIOVENTRICULAR OR VENTRICULAR SEPTAL STRUCTURES

[1] Is routine preoperative cardiac catheterization necessary before repair of secundum and sinus venosus atrial septal defects?
Freed MD, Nadas AS, Norwood WI, Castaneda AR, Children's Hosp, Boston, MA, USA.
J Am Coll Cardiol 1984; **4**: 333–6.

[2] Determinants and importance of atrial pressure morphology in atrial septal defect.
Parikh DN, Fisher J, Moses JW *et al*, New York Hosp-Cornell Med Cent, New York, NY, USA.
Br Heart J 1984; **51**: 473–9.

[3] Bidirectional shunt in uncomplicated atrial septal defect.
Galve E, Angel J, Evangelista A, Anivarro I, Permanyer-Miralda G, Soler-Soler J, Valle Hebron, Barcelona, Spain.
Br Heart J 1984; **51**: 480–4.

[4] Effect of age on pressure-flow dynamics in secundum atrial septal defect [Editorial].
Joffe HS, Bristol Royal Hosp Sick Children, Bristol, UK.
Br Heart J 1984; **51**: 469–72.

[5] Sinus node function and conduction system before and after surgery for secundum atrial septal defect: an electrophysiologic study.
Bolens M, Friedli B, Cantonal Univ Hosp, Geneva, Switzerland.
Am J Cardiol 1984; **53**: 1415–20.

[6] Electrophysiologic abnormalities of children with ostium secundum atrial septal defect.
Ruschhaupt DG, Khoury L, Thilenius OG, Replogle RL, Arcilla RA, Univ Chicago, Chicago, IL, USA.
Am J Cardiol 1984; **53**: 1643–7.

[7] Spontaneous closure of secundum atrial septal defect in infants and young children.
Cockerham JT, Martin TC, Gutierrez FR, Hartmann AF, Goldring D, Strauss AW, Washington Univ Sch Med/St Louis Children's Hosp, St Louis, MO, USA.
Am J Cardiol 1983; **52**: 1267–71.

[8] Atrioventricular septal defect with intact atrial and ventricular septal structures.
Silverman NH, Ho SY, Anderson RH, Smith A, Wilkinson JL, Cardiothoracic Inst, Brompton Hosp, London, UK.
Int J Cardiol 1984; **5**: 567–72.

[9] Atrioventricular septal defect with intact septal structures [Editorial].
Kirklin JW, Univ Alabama, Birmingham, AL, USA.
Int J Cardiol 1984; **5**: 573.

[10] Operative risk of correction of atrioventricular septal defects.
Rizzoli G, Mazzucco A, Brumana T *et al*, Univ Padua, Padua, Italy.
Br Heart J 1984; **52**: 258–65.

[11] Unequal cardiac care for children with Down's syndrome.
Sondheimer HM, Byrum CJ, Blackman MS, SUNY-Upstate Med Cent, Syracuse, NY, USA.
Am J Dis Child 1985; **139**: 68–70.

[12] Surgical and medical results of complete atrioventricular canal: a ten year review.
Clapp SK, Perry BL, Farooki ZQ *et al*, Children's Hosp Michigan, Detroit, MI, USA.
Am J Cardiol 1987; **59**: 454–8.

[13] Ventricular septal defect and subaortic stenosis: an analysis of 41 patients.
Vogel M, Freedom M, Brand A, Trusler A, Williams WG, Rowe RD, Sick Children's Hosp,
Toronto, Ont, Canada.
Am J Cardiol 1983; **52**: 1258–63.

Comment. Increased knowledge of septal morphology now dictates grouping of defects according to whether they involve the atrial, atrioventricular or ventricular septal structures. It should be noted then that the only true atrial septal defects are those within the confines of the oval fossa (fossa ovalis). The so-called sinus venosus, coronary sinus and ostium primum defects all unequivocally permit interatrial shunting of blood, but do so outside the confines of the true atrial septum. This is important not only in terms of diagnosis but also — in the case of the ostium primum defect — in terms of categorization. This latter septal deficiency, therefore, is correctly grouped with atrioventricular septal defects. The appropriate knowledge of septal morphology underscores the accuracy of diagnosis of the various septal defects using cross-sectional echocardiographic techniques. As reviewed in the section above devoted to echocardiography, the advent of cross-sectional echocardiography has made pediatric cardiologists re-examine the need for cardiac catheterization (Macartney, *Br Heart J* 1983; **50**: 501–5). It has been pointed out that many patients with relatively simple lesions could be referred for surgery on clinical examination alone.

This approach has been evaluated by analyzing the records of 161 patients from Boston Children's Hospital with atrial septal defects (excluding the 'ostium primum' variant of atrioventricular septal defect) [1]. Fifty-two patients (31%) underwent catheterization: 14 of these occurred early on in the study period and were routine, and the other 38 were performed because of atypical clinical and investigative findings. Of these, 50 were diagnosed as 'secundum' defects; this was a correct diagnosis in 46. The other 109 patients were not catheterized. Five underwent clinical studies only (no echo, etc.). The others had combinations of M-mode and cross-sectional echocardiography and radionuclide studies. The accuracy of diagnosis in this group was 84%. There was no operative mortality in either group, and there were no differences in complications between the groups. The authors conclude that patients with atrial septal defect could be referred for surgery without catheterization and experience no adverse effects, provided there were no atypical findings. Such atypical observations, to be expected in one-fifth of patients, would be an indication for invasive study. By following this strategy, a financial saving of 88% was made in the diagnosis and surgical referral of patients with uncomplicated atrial septal defect.

The hemodynamics of atrial septal defect were studied and discussed in an interesting series of papers in the *British Heart Journal* [2–4]. A right-atrial 'v' wave of greater amplitude than the 'a' wave ('v>a') is widely regarded as a classic feature of atrial septal defect. Parikh *et al* [2], however, observed this feature in only 20% of 15 adults and 63% of 80 children (aged <16 years) with isolated defects within the oval fossa (none of the patients had increased pulmonary vascular resistance or a predominant right-to-left shunt). This so-called 'left atrialization' of the right-atrial pressure wave was more frequent in younger adults, and occurred in those with higher right-atrial and right-ventricular end-diastolic pressures. In children, there were no age-related or hemodynamic determinants for the 'v>a' pattern. In addition, 67% of the adults, those who were older and had lower mean right-atrial, right-ventricular end-diastolic and

left-atrial pressures, had 'right atrialization' (i.e. 'a>v') in the left-atrial pressure contour. This observation was made in only 20% of the children, but in both groups there
seemed a tendency for it to be associated with larger left-to-right shunts. The authors
suggest that loss of left atrialization of the right atrium with increasing age might be a
consequence of declining systolic transatrial flow, which in turn is the result of a progressive alteration in compliance of the chronically dilated right ventricle.

Galve *et al* [3] reported on their study of bidirectional shunting in 40 patients with
uncomplicated atrial septal defects; 6 patients had a sizable step-down in oxygen
saturation between pulmonary vein and systemic artery. The only correlations found
with this right-to-left shunting were increasing age and lower left-to-right shunting
(none of the patients had raised pulmonary vascular resistance).

In an accompanying editorial, Joffe placed the above papers [2,3] in the context of
previous work, and attempted to explain these confusing and, in some respects,
paradoxical observations on the basis of the phasic gradients and flow between the
atria which must result from the complex interaction of left and right atrial and ventricular compliance [4]. He concluded that recognition (by the discovery of arterial
desaturation) of a 'sustained' right-to-left shunt, combined with a dominant right-
atrial 'a' wave (in contrast to the view of Parikh *et al* [2]), should be regarded as an
indication for closure of the defect, even if the left-to-right shunt is quite small,
because these occurrences may indicate decreasing compliance of the right-heart
chambers and herald the development of atrial arrhythmias and right-heart
failure.

The problem of postoperative arrhythmias was studied in two groups of children
with septal defects of the oval fossa. Bolens and Friedli [5] looked at a limited number
($n=18$) of older children (3–9 years, mean 10). The sinus node recovery time was prolonged in 14 before operation. It decreased in those who remained in sinus rhythm
after the operation, and an improvement was also noted in atrioventricular conduction. Abnormal rhythms, presumed to be a consequence of surgery, were produced in
five patients. Ruschhaupt *et al* investigated a larger group of much younger patients
(49 cases, aged 0.6–14 years, mean 4.3) [6]. They found preoperative abnormalities in
two-fifths of patients, but none in patients below the age of 2½. They found an
increase in abnormalities of atrioventricular conduction after operation (not significant). The important conclusion they reach is that the age of the subject is a crucial
factor in determining conduction-tissue abnormalities in patients with an atrial septal
defect in the oval fossa ('secundum' defect). This finding may favor early surgical
intervention for those with hemodynamically significant defects.

With ventricular septal defects, when determining the need for and timing of surgical closure, it is most important correctly to judge the chance for spontaneous closure
(or significant diminution in size) of the defect. Spontaneous closure of atrial septal
defects was the topic of another investigation [7]. Unfortunately, this paper raised as
many questions as it attempted to answer. The authors found that, of 87 patients
younger than age 4 years with a 'secundum' atrial septal defect undergoing cardiac
catheterization, 15 (17%) underwent spontaneous closure (still remarkably high when
set against Keith's experience, where only 15 of 445 underwent spontaneous closure
[reported in 1978 edition of Keith, Rowe and Vlad]). The 87 patients were from a total
load of 264. The authors compare their cases with what they term 'valve-incompetent

foramen ovale'. Since, in the discussion, they quote a deficiency in the rim of the oval fossa leading to a larger hole than the floor as the cause of a secundum defect, one wonders what the difference is between a small secundum defect and a valve-incompetent foramen ovale. Nine of the 15 patients had shown interatrial pressure ratios of <2. Again, one wonders whether these cases should not have been described as 'valve-incompetent foramen ovale'. In addition, why did they need to catheterize all these patients? The authors discuss their findings in relation to other papers reporting surgical repair in infancy with high mortality, although the subjects of these papers seem to be in quite a different category from those reported by the St Louis group, who lost 4 of 87 patients. A thought-provoking paper, but the discussion needs careful analysis and should not be taken at face value.

If an understanding of anatomy is important in the setting of interatrial communications, it is imperative in the context of deficiencies of the atrioventricular septum. The significance of this important septal component, formed in large part by the overlapping of the atrial and ventricular septal structures in the region of offsetting of the 'annular' septal attachments to the mitral and tricuspid valves, was clearly identified by the morphologic studies of Van Mierop and his colleagues (*Cardiovascular Clinics, Vol. 2.1*, Philadelphia: FA Davis, 1970) and the angiographic investigations of Brandt *et al (Australas Radiol* 1972; **16:** 367–76). It was Becker and Anderson, however, who promoted the concept of the atrioventricular septal defect (*J Thorac Cardiovasc Surg* 1982; **83:** 461–9), and their observations have recently been endorsed by detailed measurements by Penkoske and her colleagues (*J Thorac Cardiovasc Surg* 1985; **90:** 611–22). The keystone of this morphologic concept is the presence of a common atrioventricular junction, the left component of which is guarded by a three-leaflet valve, rather than by a deformed mitral valve, as had previously been assumed. It was the presence of this trifoliate left valve that permitted Silverman *et al* to recognize a heart with all the morphologic stigmata of an atrioventricular septal defect even when all the septal structures were intact, leaving no possibility of intracardiac shunting [8]. As discussed by the authors, the recognition of such a lesion in a heart without an atrioventricular septum, and its differentiation from hearts with isolated clefts of the mitral valve in the setting of normal atrioventricular septation, is highly significant for the group of anomalies otherwise described as 'endocardial cushion defects' or 'atrioventricular canal malformations'. As Kirklin says in an accompanying editorial [9], the recognition of the case with intact septal structures "emphasizes the nearly infinite variability of the spectrum".

The operative correction of this group of septal defects was the topic of a study by Rizzoli *et al* [10]. The paper provides an excellent analysis of seven years' experience (1976–1982) of surgical treatment at the University of Padua. Univariate and multivariate analyses were made of the influence of demographic, anatomic, clinical and operative variables in relation to operative mortality (death in hospital or within 30 days of operation). One hundred and eleven patients underwent surgery: 57 had separate right and left atrioventricular valves with no potential for interventricular shunting ('ostium primum defects'); 43 had common atrioventricular valves ('complete defects'); and 11 were considered to have intermediate forms of the lesion, that is, an ostium primum defect combined with a small interventricular communication.

Some of the findings of this study have previously been emphasized: the lower mortality for the simpler variants of the lesion (6% for ostium primum and 9% for inter-mediate forms) when compared with patients with common valve (37%); the high incidence of Down's syndrome in the overall group (46 of 111 patients); and the deleterious effect of either right- or left-ventricular dominance. The interesting and innovative aspect of this study is the detailed analysis of the mode of surgical repair of the left atrioventricular valve. Unlike those working in many other centers, the group from Padua have appreciated that, as discussed above, the left atrioventricular valve in all atrioventricular septal defects is *not* a cloven mitral valve, but a trifoliate struc-ture in its own right. Moreover, they show an improvement in the competence of this valve subsequent to their adoption of a repair based on the trifoliate concept emphasized by Alain Carpentier from Paris, as opposed to simple closure of the so-called 'cleft' to produce a bifoliate valve. They found that, "This approach resulted in a lower incidence of severe postoperative valvular dysfunction, although firm con-clusions cannot yet be drawn because of the broad confidence limits". The authors are convinced that "creating a two leaflet left atrioventricular valve [...] increases the risk of aggravating the original incompetence". Thus, the matter of an optimal repair of the left valve (not a mitral valve but a trifoliate left valve) is undecided as yet. This type of study is likely to provide the answer.

As shown by the results of Rizzoli *et al* [10], and from many other reports, atrioven-tricular septal defects can now be repaired with acceptably low mortality, whatever their type. An interesting paper from Sondheimer *et al* [11] examined the hypothesis that children with Down's syndrome and congenital cardiac malformations are at a disadvantage because they are referred to centers too late to benefit fully from such operative correction. The authors analyzed the referral patterns of patients with atrioventricular septal defect and common atrioventricular valve orifice ('complete atrioventricular canal defect') — a lesion known to be frequently associated with Down's syndrome: 18 had been referred prior to the age of one year, and surgery was possible in 17; half of the remainder, referred after the age of one year, were unsuitable for surgery. In contrast, all the patients without Down's syndrome had been referred before the age of one, and all were suitable for surgery. This finding certainly justifies the conclusion that children with Down's syndrome are being denied standard surgi-cal care because of late referral.

Clapp *et al* describe their surgical experience at the Children's Hospital, Michigan, between 1975 and 1984 for patients having atrioventricular septal defect with common valve orifice [12]. In all, 121 patients were seen. However, patients were excluded when they had significant pulmonary stenosis or associated tetralogy of Fallot. Corrective surgery was performed in 70 patients using the single-patch technique; 21 of these died (30%) in the peri-operative period. The mortality rate was reduced to 13% when significant risk factors were excluded. Of the patients not undergoing operation (51), 34 developed abnormal vascular obstructive disease. This had occurred within 12 months in 10 patients. A further eight patients died prior to planned surgery. The investigators conclude that, although the prognosis is good in those candidates without associated lesions, the overall prognosis must be guarded for this group of patients because of the frequently unfavorable anatomy and the known onset of early pulmonary vascular obstructive disease. On the basis of their experience, this group now performs catheterization at 4–6 months of age, following this with appropriate surgical intervention. Banding of the pulmonary trunk is recommended in selected patients. Success depends upon the prevention of pulmonary vascular disease.

The anatomy, cross-sectional echocardiographic and angiographic features of ventricular septal defects are, by now, well understood. Often, however, it is difficult to diagnose the association of sub-aortic stenosis in association with a ventricular septal defect. Vogel *et al* analyzed the findings from 41 patients with this combination [13]. Not surprisingly, the diagnosis was made clinically in only one case. There was a mean delay of 3.1 years between presentation and diagnosis of the stenosis, which was missed at catheterization in 17 patients. It was subsequently detected by further catheter studies in eight patients, surgery in five and autopsy in four. The stenosis was below the crest of the ventricular septum in 30. The authors anticipate that this combination of abnormalities will now be diagnosed both earlier and more accurately with cross-sectional echocardiographic techniques.

TETRALOGY OF FALLOT

[1] The first open heart corrections of tetralogy of Fallot.
Lillehei CW, Varco RL, Cohen M et al, Univ Minnesota Hosp, Minneapolis, MN, USA.
Ann Surg 1986; **204**: 490-502.
[2] Comparison of late clinical status between patients with different hemodynamic findings after repair of tetralogy of Fallot.
Chen D-G, Moller JH, Univ Minnesota Hosp, Minneapolis, MN, USA.
Am Heart J 1987; **113**: 767.
[3] The treatment of tetralogy of Fallot: early repair or palliation?
Sebening F, Laas J, Meisner H, Struck E, Buhlmeyer K, Zwingers Th, German Heart Cent, Munich, FRG.
Thorac Cardiovasc Surg 1984; **32**: 201-7.
[4] Risk factors for early and late failure after repair of tetralogy of Fallot, and their neutralization.
Kirklin JW, Blackstone EH, Pacifico AD, Kirklin JK, Bargeron LM Jr, Univ Alabama Sch Med, Birmingham, AL, USA.
Thorac Cardiovasc Surg 1984; **32**: 208-14.
[5] Surgical treatment of tetralogy of Fallot. Recent experience using a prospective protocol.
Villani M, Gamba A, Tiraboschi R, Crupi G, Parenzan L, Riuniti Hosp, Bergamo, Italy.
Thorac Cardiovasc Surg 1983; **31**: 151-5.
[6] Tetralogy of Fallot. Development of hypoplastic pulmonary arteries after palliation.
Laas J, Engeser U, Meisner H et al, German Heart Cent, Munich, FRG.
J Thorac Cardiovasc Surg 1984; **32**: 133-8.
[7] Surgical repair of tetralogy of Fallot. Long-term follow-up with particular emphasis on late death and reoperation.
Zhao H-X, Miller DC, Reitz BA, Shumway NE, Stanford Univ Med Cent, Stanford, CA, USA.
J Thorac Cardiovasc Surg 1985; **89**: 204-20.
[8] The correction of tetralogy of Fallot at age 40 years and older: long-term follow-up.
Hu DC, Seward JB, Puga FJ, Fuster V, Tajik AJ, Mayo Clin and Mayo Found, Rochester, MN, USA.
J Am Coll Cardiol 1985; **5**: 40-4.

[9] Ventricular arrhythmia in unrepaired and repaired tetralogy of Fallot. Relation to age, timing of repair, and haemodynamic status.
Deanfield JE, McKenna WJ, Presbitero P, England D, Graham GR, Hallidie-Smith K, Hammersmith Hosp, London, UK.
Br Heart J 1984; **52**: 77–81.

[10] Local abnormalities of right ventricular depolarization after repair of tetralogy of Fallot: a basis for ventricular arrhythmia.
Deanfield J, McKenna W, Rowland E, Hammersmith Hosp, London, UK.
Am J Cardiol 1985; **55**: 522–5.

[11] Ventricular arrhythmias and biventricular dysfunction after repair of tetralogy of Fallot.
Webb Kavey R-E, Deaver Thomas F, Byrum CJ, Blackman MS, Sondheimer HM, Bove EL, State Univ New York, Syracuse, NY, USA.
J Am Coll Cardiol 1984; **4**: 126–34.

[12] Analysis of adults with and without complex ventricular arrhythmias after repair of tetralogy of Fallot.
Burns RJ, Liu PP, Druck MN, Seawright SJ, Williams WG, McLaughlin PR, Toronto Gen Hosp, Toronto, Ont, Canada.
J Am Coll Cardiol 1984; **4**: 226–33.

[13] Hemodynamic effect of isoprenaline and dobutamine immediately after correction of tetralogy of Fallot. Relative importance of inotropic and chronotropic action in supporting cardiac output.
Jaccard C, Berner M, Rouge JC, Oberhansli I, Friedli B, Cantonal Univ Hosp, Geneva, Switzerland.
J Thorac Cardiovasc Surg 1984; **87**: 862–9.

[14] Tetralogy of Fallot with major aortopulmonary collateral arteries.
Ramsay JM, Macartney FJ, Haworth SG, Hosp for Sick Children, London, UK.
Br Heart J 1985; **53**: 167–72.

Comment. Open heart correction of congenital cardiac malformations started in two centers in the early 1950s: at the Mayo Clinic, Kirklin was developing the use of the heart-lung machine; Lillehei and his colleagues at the University of Minnesota in Twin Cities developed cross-circulation as the technique for bypass. Lillehei's efforts were unequivocally the first milestone in the development of surgery for major congenital malformations of the heart. In an important paper, Lillehei *et al* describe the follow-up of the first 106 patients operated on for tetralogy of Fallot between August 1954 and December 1960 [1]. The first six had their operation made possible by the use of cross-circulation. The follow-up of the patients is an encouraging account. (The paper also contains other important information relative to the development of cardiac pacemakers, another of Lillehei's innovations, and the performance of patch reconstruction of the pulmonary outflow tract.) Actuarial survival for the whole group was 77% at 30 years. Actuarial freedom from re-operation over the same period was 91%. Nearly one-third of the group (32%) completed college and 10 successfully passed through graduate school. As the authors conclude, many of the deaths from this early experience would not occur now.

The results of more recent surgery in Minneapolis have been reviewed by Chen and Moller [2]. The paper is a review of the long-term follow-up of 183 consecutive patients who underwent both continued clinical observation and cardiac catheterization after a reparative operation. The study included all patients undergoing repair up to the year 1981 in whom postoperative studies were available. They represent nearly half of the patients surviving the operation during this period. The patients were classified into one of three groups (excellent, satisfactory and unsatisfactory) according to the post-operative hemodynamic findings. Clinical status was similarly assessed and classified as ideal, fair or poor. Excellent hemodynamic results were found in 42 patients and almost all had ideal clinical status. Thirty patients had a satisfactory hemodynamic result and nearly all of these had either an ideal or a fair clinical result. Major abnormal hemodynamic findings were found in 72 cases. Perhaps surprisingly, nearly two-thirds of these still had ideal clinical results. Clinical results were poor in 20 patients. The authors analysed the reasons for poor results in detail and give a reasonable review of their findings in the light of the published literature; residual obstruction to the right ventricular outflow tract seems to have produced the worst late result. Taken overall, and considering the period in which the surgery was performed, this paper is extremely encouraging for those patients now undergoing surgical treatment for tetralogy of Fallot.

A paper from the Munich group [3] illustrates the overall excellence that can now be expected from the surgical treatment of tetralogy, but it does not address the major problem of optimal timing or the nature of treatment in great depth. Kirklin *et al* [4] identify 11 incremental risk factors for operative death, including such problems as old age, young age, high hematocrit, small pulmonary arteries, etc. They demonstrate how some of these factors are interrelated, for example a small pulmonary annulus, the use of a transannular patch and the postoperative persistence of high right-ventricular pressures. This is followed by a discussion of how all of these risk factors can best be neutralized. The problem of primary repair *versus* a two-stage approach is confronted, *viz*. "A rational protocol for patients with tetralogy of Fallot, based upon known risk factors, is primary repair down to the age where the hospital and interval risks of initial shunting and later repair are probably (non-overlapping 70% confidence limits) less than those of primary repair". Kirklin *et al* are of the opinion that if 1000 patients were operated on by primary repair, and they were compared with a similar group of 1000 undergoing two-stage correction, the results of initial palliation would be better.

The excellent results that can be obtained by others who follow the approach espoused by Kirklin are exemplified by the report of Villani *et al* [5]. They describe the results of surgical treatment of 218 consecutive patients with Fallot's tetralogy. No patient was refused surgery; 135 had total correction, with 5 hospital deaths. Incremental risk factors included young age, transannular patch and primary repair.

Initial palliation for young patients is a crucial step in the protocol recommended by Kirklin and his disciples [4,5]. Even those who espouse primary correction in infancy accept that a subset of patients with hypoplastic pulmonary arteries make unsuitable candidates. It is important to choose the palliative procedure that will best promote growth of the small pulmonary arteries. This is the topic addressed by Laas *et al* [6]. They palliated 31 patients, either with the Blalock-Taussig procedure ($n=9$), the Brock operation ($n=12$) or enlargement of the subpulmonary outflow tract with extracorporeal circulation ($n=10$). Measurements were done before and 24.8 ±20.9 months after palliation. The magnitude of growth was found to be inversely related to the initial size of the pulmonary arteries. With the shunt procedure, no growth of the pulmonary valve or trunk was observed. Both these structures enlarged with the other procedures.

A subsequent analysis of the results of operative correction of tetralogy of Fallot ranks alongside the study of Kirklin *et al* — the report by Zhao of the experience of Shumway and colleagues [7]. In 1963, Shumway presented an initial series of 25 consecutive cases operated on without mortality. Two years later, the series had expanded to 45 patients, still without mortality. Now the number of operated patients had reached 309; of these, 15 died in hospital or within 30 days of operation (4.9% ±1.3%). Seventeen patients died between 5 months and 16 years postoperatively. Of the 225 survivors who could be adequately followed, 97% were in NYHA functional class I; only one patient was judged to be in class III. Considering that 19 of the patients had pulmonary atresia in the setting of tetralogy, 1 had 'absent' pulmonary valve and several had other significant associated lesions, these are formidable results. Only young age, long cardiopulmonary bypass time and (probably) the extent of any right-ventricular outflow tract patch were found to be independent significant determinants of operative mortality. Based on these results, the Stanford group supports the conclusions of Kirklin *et al* that a two-stage approach (initial palliation followed by corrective operation) is probably safer in infants under 8 months of age with uncomplicated tetralogy (<12 months if a transannular patch is needed), and is definitely safer for infants under 6 and 8 months, respectively.

Although the papers discussed above show that the trend is to correct tetralogy of Fallot increasingly early in life, a number of patients, albeit small, reach adulthood before they come to correction. The Mayo Clinic group [8] have analyzed their experience with 30 patients aged 40–60 years who underwent total correction between 1960 and 1982. Only 11 of the patients had had palliative surgery 16–34 years before total correction. Preoperatively only four patients were in functional class I. Total correction was successful in all patients. Despite their age, the ratio of right-ventricular to left-ventricular pressure fell to 0.65 in 28 of the patients. Three patients died postoperatively. Follow-up at 5–244 months revealed seven late deaths. Of 22 survivors, 16 are in functional class I, 5 are in class II and 1 is in class III. From this series, it can be seen that age is not a contraindication for total correction of tetralogy of Fallot, even in patients with preoperative complications of shunting and polycythemia.

As discussed by the Stanford group, late deaths remain a problem after surgical correction of tetralogy of Fallot, and a good proportion may be related to ventricular arrhythmias. This topic has long fascinated Deanfield and co-workers, who have now reported two further aspects of their ongoing studies [9,10]. They placed the problem in perspective by examining first a preoperative group of patients ($n=60$) using 48-hour ambulatory ECG monitoring and comparing these with a group ($n=85$) that had undergone repair at various ages [9]. Of the unoperated group, 20% had ventricular arrhythmia, the prevalence increasing with age. The higher incidence of ventricular arrhythmia in the corrected group (44%) was associated with age at repair, but not with hemodynamic status, era of surgery or duration of follow-up.

Subsequently, Deanfield *et al* examined 22 patients in an attempt to correlate findings from ambulatory electrocardiographic monitoring and findings at intracardiac electrophysiologic study [10]. Intravenous conduction times and local endocardial electrograms were examined. Regional disordered local depolarization correlated with the severity and frequency of ventricular arrhythmia. There was no correlation between arrhythmia and disturbances of His-Purkinje conduction. The widespread nature of the myocardial repolarization abnormalities suggests that these are related to the disease process underlying tetralogy of Fallot rather than surgery. This supports the conclusion from the earlier study [9]: that earlier age at surgery might reduce long-term arrhythmia complications.

The presence of postoperative ventricular arrhythmias and their association with impaired ventricular function was the subject of two further studies [11,12]. Webb Kavey et al suggested that biventricular dysfunction was related to the presence of ventricular arrhythmia [11]. Of 38 postoperative patients evaluated, 18 were found to have ventricular arrhythmia of Lown grade 2 or greater on ambulatory monitoring and/or exercise testing. Ventricular function, as assessed by technetium radionuclide angiography, demonstrated a significantly lower left-ventricular ejection fraction ($P<0.05$) in the arrhythmia group, but no difference was found in right-ventricular function. The ratio between right and left end-diastolic dimension, as assessed by M-mode echocardiography, was also significantly elevated in the arrhythmia group ($P<0.005$). The authors suggest that evaluation of ventricular function allows selection of those patients at greatest risk of developing potentially lethal arrhythmias. They do not seem to have considered, however, that the arrhythmia may have produced the impaired ventricular function.

This association was investigated by Burns et al [12], who analyzed the clinical and hemodynamic features of 44 patients who had undergone surgical repair of tetralogy of Fallot, for features that correlated with complex ventricular arrhythmia observed during ambulatory monitoring or exercise testing. Those patients with arrhythmia (22) had a higher right-ventricular systolic blood pressure (46.9 ± 18.6 mmHg vs 33.1 ± 8.9 mmHg, $P=0.003$), a higher incidence of residual left-to-right intracardiac shunts (9 vs 0, $P<0.001$) and more frequently abnormal left-ventricular ejection fraction measured by radionuclide angiography at rest and on exercise than those patients without arrhythmia. The authors suggest that the patients with ventricular arrhythmia have subclinical left-ventricular dysfunction consequent on either a fibrotic process or right-ventricular pressure overload.

A different aspect of the postoperative course was analyzed by Jaccard et al [13], who gave isoproterenol and dobutamine immediately after correction to 12 randomly selected patients. Cardiac output was measured postoperatively by thermodilution before, during and after infusion of increasing doses of isoproterenol (0.05, 0.1 and 0.2 µg/kg/min) and dobutamine (2.5, 5 and 10 µg/kg/min) given successively in each patient. Central venous, left-atrial, pulmonary arterial and systemic arterial pressures were recorded simultaneously. Cardiac index increased significantly in response to all three doses of isoproterenol, whereas dobutamine produced only a small increase, which was not statistically significant. Stroke-volume index did not vary significantly with either drug. Therefore, cardiac index was found to be directly related to heart rate. Isoproterenol significantly reduced preload of the left ventricle as well as afterload ($P<0.01$ and $P<0.05$, respectively), but dobutamine did not. An increase in left-ventricular work index/min occurred with both drugs. Only isoproterenol, however, increased the work with an accompanying significant increase in cardiac index. The authors conclude that patients with tetralogy of Fallot usually have a small left ventricle, which responds to catecholamines immediately after correction with only an insignificant increase in stroke-volume index. Thus, the effect of catecholamines is one of chronotropy rather than increase in stroke-volume index. Isoproterenol is more effective than dobutamine in raising the cardiac index because of the increase in heart rate. Although this paper is important, the choice of two inotropes of such a dissimilar nature detracts somewhat from its impact. Moreover, the use of dobutamine in patients with tetralogy of Fallot is slightly unorthodox. It would have been useful if the authors had included dopamine in the trial: the extent of the observed differences might then not have been so large.

The final paper to be discussed concerning tetralogy of Fallot [14] addresses a feature of major diagnostic significance. Major aortopulmonary collateral arteries often provide the only source of pulmonary arterial supply in patients with pulmonary atresia and ventricular septal defect. They are usually multiple, producing a 'multifocal' blood supply, although occasionally a single collateral artery can supply the greater part of the intrapericardial pulmonary arterial network. Usually the presence of such systemic-pulmonary arteries in patients with pulmonary atresia excludes the possibility of the arterial duct persisting as an alternative source of pulmonary arterial supply. The commonest variant of pulmonary atresia with ventricular septal defect is tetralogy of Fallot, in which the outlet system is deviated to occlude the subpulmonary outlet completely rather than merely making it stenotic. It might be expected, therefore, that systemic-pulmonary collateral arteries coexist with tetralogy. This excellent study documents the coexistence of collateral supply in eight patients with tetralogy of Fallot. Most of the patients had two or more collateral arteries (which are not, and should not, be termed bronchial arteries); one had a single collateral artery. In all of the patients, all or the greater part of the pulmonary circulation was supplied by the intrapericardial 'central' pulmonary arteries, unlike the arrangement in pulmonary atresia. The authors also noted that two of the patients had 'mild' variants of tetralogy in the degree of subpulmonary stenosis. As in pulmonary atresia, however, selective injection into each collateral artery was recommended to determine the extent of its supply. The authors emphasize that investigation should concentrate on determining the presence of an alternative supply to the area fed by the collateral artery, and should exclude dual supply to any area of lung supplied by two or more collateral arteries in addition to the central supply. The criteria for surgical repair are based on the size of the central pulmonary arteries, and palliative surgery should aim at encouraging growth of these arteries if they are hypoplastic. The outlook is optimistic in most patients, because all or most of the bronchopulmonary segments are connected to the central pulmonary arteries.

COMMON ARTERIAL TRUNK ('TRUNCUS ARTERIOSUS')

[1] **Fifteen-year experience with surgical repair of truncus arteriosus.**
Di Donato RM, Fyfe DA, Puga F *et al*, Mayo Clin/Mayo Found, Rochester, MN, USA.
J Thorac Cardiovasc Surg 1985; **89**: 414–22.

[2] Surgical treatment of truncus arteriosus in the first 6 months of life.
Ebert PA, Turley K, Stanger P, Hoffman JE, Heymann MA, Rudolph AM, Univ California, San Francisco, CA, USA.
Ann Surg 1984; **200**: 451–5.

Comment. The Mayo Clinic group have now summarized their extensive experience of the operative repair of patients with a common arterial trunk [1]. The number of patients corrected at the clinic since October 1965 is 167, with 48 hospital deaths (28.7%). The authors identify several risk factors for operative death: age <2 years at operation; a post-repair ratio of pulmonary-arterial to left-ventricular pressure of >0.5 for patients with two pulmonary arteries and >0.6 for those with absence of one pulmonary artery; and a ratio of post-repair right-to-left ventricular pressure of >0.8. Di Donato *et al* [1] are aware that the influence of young age on death occurs because of the unique pattern of referral of cases to The Mayo Clinic. They accept that Ebert *et al* in San Francisco [2] have clearly demonstrated operation in infancy as the optimal treatment for this malformation. Despite this, the results of Di Donato *et al* are important. Reoperation was necessary in 36 patients (30%), mainly for replacement of the right-ventricular/pulmonary-arterial conduit and/or truncal valve. In this respect, the authors now recognize the potential benefit of using fresh antibiotic-restored aortic homografts, an option long promoted by Ross and Yacoub in the UK. In the series reported, insufficiency of the truncal valve produced major problems.

The extensive surgical experience of Ebert *et al* had been reported earlier. The Mayo Clinic group had shown that the Rastelli concept (using the common trunk as an outlet from the left ventricle and a conduit to connect the right ventricle to the pulmonary trunk) could be applied to older patients. Most patients, however, present in infancy, and the results of banding the pulmonary arteries at this stage are uniformly poor. From 1975 onwards, Ebert had achieved good results by performing immediate physiologic correction in the first year of life.

Ebert describes his experience in 106 infants in the first 6 months of life who were seen between 1974 and 1981 [2]. Six infants died prior to surgery while undergoing intensive medical treatment. Of the 100 patients submitted to surgery, 11 died at operation and 3 died later. Of the 86 long-term survivors, 55 returned to have their conduit replaced, because it had become obstructed either with natural growth or from pseudointimal proliferation; none of these patients died at or following the second operation. Several interesting points emerge from this study. Truncal valve incompetence is a very poor prognostic sign. All the infants dying prior to surgery had this problem, as did 8 of the 11 who died at operation. Ebert *et al* now suggest a more aggressive approach, with truncal valve replacement at the initial procedure. Moreover, none of the 11 patients receiving an allograft required replacement. Of those who had replacements, over half were given smaller, non-valved conduits at second operation. From these results it would appear that the best time to operate on patients with common arterial trunk is within the first six months of life.

PULMONARY AND AORTIC STENOSIS

[1] Percutaneous transluminal balloon valvuloplasty for pulmonary valve stenosis.
Kan JS, White RI Jr, Mitchell SE, Anderson JH, Gardner TJ, Johns Hopkins Univ Sch Med, Baltimore, MD, USA.
Circulation 1984; **69**: 554–60.

[2] Percutaneous balloon pulmonary vavuloplasty.
Tynan M, Baker EJ, Rohmer J *et al*, Guy's Hosp, London, UK.
Br Heart J 1985; **53**: 520–4.

[3] Balloon dilation angioplasty of hypoplastic and stenotic pulmonary arteries.
Lock JE, Casteneda-Zuniga WR, Fuhrman BP, Bass JL, Univ Minnesota Hosp, Minneapolis, MN, USA.
Circulation 1983; **67**: 962–7.

[4] Percutaneous balloon aortic valvuloplasty: results in 23 patients.
Lababidi Z, Wu J-R, Walls JT, Univ Missouri, Hosp and Clins, Columbia, MO, USA.
Am J Cardiol 1984; **53**: 194–7.

[5] Prognostic factors in valvotomy for critical aortic stenosis in infancy.
Gundry SR, Behrendt DM, Univ Michigan Hosps, Ann Arbor, MI, USA.
J Thorac Cardiovasc Surg 1986; **92**: 747–54.

Comment. The major interest in treatment of simple obstructions of the pulmonary and aortic outflow tracts has been in the development of balloon dilatation of valvar stenosis and more distal lesions of the pulmonary tree. The following papers describe the experience of pioneers in the various fields.

Kan *et al* were the instigators of non-invasive relief of valvar pulmonary stenosis. Their continuing experience is described, together with results from 20 patients [1]. Eighteen had 'typical' pulmonary valve stenosis, while a further two patients had, respectively, a dysplastic and a stenotic pulmonary atresia, the latter following an initial Brock procedure. Results were best for the 'typical' lesion. The right-ventricular pressure was halved after the procedure to levels of about 40 mmHg, and this reduction persisted during follow-up. As the authors state, this is still an elevated level, but it is below that which would be taken as an indication for surgery. Balloon size was increased during the series to the size of the pulmonary 'annulus' or slightly larger. It was also redesigned to permit more rapid inflation and to be shorter and stubbier. There were no untoward complications in the whole series.

It was the group from Guy's Hospital who introduced this technique to the UK. Their experience, together with the group at Leiden University, forms the basis of a collaborative study [2], which reports the results in 27 patients. Following valvoplasty, a significant fall in the transvalvar gradient was achieved in 22 patients, none of whom had a dysplastic valve. In contrast, dysplastic valves were present in three of the five patients in whom the technique was unsuccessful. Those patients in whom the technique was unsuccessful were operated upon early in the series, when the size of the balloon was inadequate. Subsequently, the authors used balloons 1–2 mm greater than the size of the pulmonary valve 'annulus', as judged by right-ventricular cineangiography, rather than 1–2 mm smaller, as had been their earlier policy. It was necessary to repeat the procedure in one patient. The second attempt was successful when a larger balloon was used. Follow-up has been conducted in six cases, with no evidence of restenosis. There were no important complications in any of the patients.

These studies justify the claim that valvoplasty should be the initial treatment for congenital pulmonary valve stenosis. Caveats concerning less satisfactory results in the presence of a dysplastic valve should, however, be borne in mind.

It was Lock and co-workers who promoted the use of balloons for dilatation of lesions of the pulmonary arteries, initially at the University of Minnesota [3]. The subjects were five children, with either stenosis or hypoplasia of both pulmonary arteries. Right-ventricular pressure fell from 104 ± 2 mmHg to 80 ± 30 mmHg ($P<0.05$). The gradient across the obstruction fell from 61 ± 51 mmHg to 32 ± 22 mmHg ($P<0.05$). The narrow segment diameter increased from 3.7 ± 1.2 mm to 6.8 ± 1.1 mm ($P=0.02$). Follow-up at 2–12 months in three patients showed persistence of the anatomic improvement.

In addition to aortic coarctation, the other lesion that has been attacked non-invasively by balloon dilatation is the stenotic aortic valve. Both these approaches were pioneered by Lababidi *et al* [4], who described their initial attempts at balloon dilatation of aortic valve stenosis in 23 consecutive patients aged between 2 and 17 years. Following the procedure there was a marked decrease in the pressure gradient across the valve, from 113 ± 48 mmHg to 32 ± 15 mmHg ($P<0.01$). Six of the 23 patients were restudied 3–9 months following dilatation, and none showed any evidence of restenosis.

Gundry and Behrendt present their results in the surgical treatment by valvotomy of critical aortic stenosis presenting in infancy [5]. They operated on 24 infants with a mean age of one month between January 1, 1978 and October 30, 1984 at the University of Michigan, Ann Arbor. Nearly two-fifths were operated on using cardiopulmonary bypass and the stenotic valve was approached through the ascending aorta. Their technique was to incise the fused valvar commissures to the periphery of their sinusal attachments. Two patients died in the operating room and three more died up to two weeks post-operatively. Only one of the last 11 patients undergoing surgery has died. There were two late deaths. When analysed for factors affecting survival, a low ejection fraction, a reduced left ventricular end-diastolic pressure and the presence of endocardial fibro-elastosis were all shown to be risk factors. Generally speaking, the results of operation for this lesion in infancy have been dismal. The results of Gundry and Behrendt and those of Messina *et al* (*J Thorac Cardiovasc Surg* 1984; **88:** 92–6) show that the lesion can be corrected in neonates with an acceptable operative mortality and good long-term results. Gundry and Behrendt conclude that a very young age and the presence of endocardial fibro-elastosis are unfavorable signs but they do not preclude operation. They recommend their open technique because it allows the performance of a precise repair.

HEARTS WITH A UNIVENTRICULAR ATRIOVENTRICULAR CONNECTION

[1] The univentricular atrioventricular connexion: getting to the root of a thorny problem.
Anderson RH, Becker AE, Tynan M *et al*, Cardiothoracic Inst, Univ London, UK.
Am J Cardiol 1984; **54:** 822–8.

[2] Early and intermediate-term (10-year) results of surgery for univentricular atrioventricular connection ("single ventricle").
Stefanelli G, Kirklin JW, Naftel DC *et al*, Univ Alabama, Birmingham, AL, USA.
Am J Cardiol 1984; **54**: 811–1.

[3] Subaortic stenosis, the univentricular heart, and banding of the pulmonary artery: an analysis of the courses of 43 patients with univentricular heart palliated by pulmonary artery banding.
Freedom R, Benson LN, Smallhorn JF, Williams WG, Trusler GA, Rowe RD, Hosp for Sick Children, Toronto, Ont, Canada.
Circulation 1986; **73**: 758–64.

[4] Surgical repair of univentricular heart (double inlet left ventricle) with obstructed anterior subaortic outlet chamber.
Barber G, Hagler DJ, Edwards WD *et al*, Mayo Clin, Rochester, MN, USA.
J Am Coll Cardiol 1984; **4**: 771–8.

[5] Extending the limits for modified Fontan procedures.
Mayer JE, Helgason H, Jonas RA *et al*, Children's Hosp, Boston, MA, USA.
J Thorac Cardiovasc Surg 1986; **92**: 1021–8.

[6] Fontan type operation for complex lesions. Surgical considerations to improve survival.
DeLeon SY, Ilbawi MN, Idriss FS *et al*, Children's Memorial Hosp, Chicago, IL, USA.
J Thorac Cardiovasc Surg 1986; **92**: 1029–37.

[7] Comparison of atriopulmonary versus atrioventricular connections for modified Fontan/Kreutzer repair of tricuspid valve atresia.
Lee C-N, Schaff HV, Danielson GK, Driscoll DJ, Mayo Clin, Rochester, MN, USA.
J Thorac Cardiovasc Surg 1986; **92**: 1038–43.

[8] The Fontan operation. Ventricular hypertrophy, age, and date of operation as risk factors.
Kirklin KJ, Blackstone EH, Kirklin JW, Pacifico AD, Bargeron LM Jr, Univ Alabama, Birmingham, AL, USA.
J Thorac Cardiovasc Surg 1986; **92**: 1049–64.

[9] Outcome of the Fontan procedure in patients with tricuspid atresia.
Mair DD, Rice MJ, Hagler DJ, Puga FJ, McGoon DC, Danielson GK, Mayo Clin and Mayo Found, Rochester, MN, USA.
Circulation 1985; **72**(Suppl II): 88–92.

[10] Relationship of pulmonary artery size to mortality in patients undergoing the Fontan operation.
Girod DA, Rice MJ, Mair DD, Julsrud PR, Puga FJ, Danielson GK, Indiana Univ Sch Med, Indianapolis, IN, USA.
Circulation 1985; **72**(Suppl II): 93–6.

[11] Exercise tolerance and cardiorespiratory response to exercise after the Fontan operation for tricuspid atresia or functional single ventricle.
Driscoll DJ, Danielson GK, Puga FJ, Schhaff HV, Heise CT, Staats BA, Mayo Clin, Rochester, MN, USA.
J Am Coll Cardiol 1986; **7**: 1087–94.

[12] Long-term results after Fontan procedure and its modification.
De Vivie E-R, Rupprath G, Univ Goettingen, Goettingen, FRG.
J Thorac Cardiovasc Surg 1986; **91**: 690–7.

[13] A new surgical technique for orthoterminal correction. Experimental development [In Spanish].
Fantidis P, Salvador JC, Fernandez Ruiz MA *et al*, Univ Autonoma, Madrid, Spain.
Rev Esp Cardiol 1984; **37**: 347–53.

[14] Modified Fontan procedure using a retroaortic atriopulmonary anastomosis.
Olert H, Borst HG, Hanover Med Sch, Hanover, GFR.
Thorac Cardiovasc Surg 1984; **32**: 392–4.

[15] Dynamics of right heart flow in patients after Fontan procedure.
Nakazawa M, Nakanishi T, Okuda H *et al*, Heart Inst Japan, Tokyo Women's Med Coll, Tokyo, Japan.
Circulation 1984; **69**: 306–2.

[16] Superior vena cava — pulmonary artery anastomosis [Editorial].
Glenn WWL, Yale Univ Sch Med, New Haven, CT, USA.
Ann Thorac Surg 1984; **37**: 9–11.

[17] Mechanical assistance of the pulmonary circulation after right ventricular exclusion.
De la Riviere AB, Haasler G, Bregman D, Columbia Univ, New York, NY, USA.
J Thorac Cardiovasc Surg 1983; **85**: 809–14.

[18] Radionuclide measurement of left ventricular ejection fraction in tricuspid atresia.
Baker EJ, Jones ODH, Joseph MC, Maisey MN, Tynan MJ, Guy's Hosp, London, UK.
Br Heart J 1984; **52**: 572–4.

[19] Pulmonary vascular structure in patients dying after a Fontan procedure. The lung as a risk factor.
Juaneda E, Haworth SG, Inst Child Health, London, UK.
Br Heart J 1984; **52**: 575–80.

[20] Effects of elevated coronary sinus pressure on left ventricular function after the Fontan operation. An experimental and clinical correlation.
Ilbawi MN, Idriss FS, Muster AJ *et al*, Children's Memorial Hosp, Chicago, IL, USA.
J Thorac Cardiovasc Surg 1986; **92**: 231–7.

Comment. Controversy has raged for years concerning hearts with an apparently single' ventricular chamber. It has long been appreciated that the majority of lesions designated 'single ventricle' possess two chambers within their ventricular mass, and arguments have revolved around the ventricular or non-ventricular status of the smaller chamber. These considerations have, in turn, led to disagreements about the relationship between classical tricuspid atresia and double-inlet left ventricle. There is still no agreement as to whether either, both or neither of these malformations should be called univentricular hearts.

The review by the 'European school' of nomenclaturists [1] points out that the feature held in common by all hearts with double-inlet ventricle and the majority with atrioventricular valve atresia is the connection of the atrial chambers to only one ventricle. A second chamber is present within the ventricular mass of most of these hearts, but it is incomplete and rudimentary because, of necessity, it has no connection with an atrial chamber. The authors posit that description of the hearts in terms of the atrioventricular connection (double-inlet, absent right connection, and so on) rather than the purported univentricular nature of the ventricular mass (which most do not have) resolves all the arguments. Adoption of this principle would mean that hearts can be described more accurately without resort to illogical conventions and that single ventricle' could be reserved for more appropriate use, namely to describe those hearts which truly do possess a solitary chamber within their ventricular mass. The anatomic principles underscoring this convention are vital both for diagnosis and determination of the appropriate surgical therapy, since it is the univentricular atrioventricular connection which underscores the options for 'correction'.

The above is emphasized by Stefanelli *et al* [2], who performed a thoughtful analysis of the results of surgical treatment in 116 patients with various forms of univentricular atrioventricular connection (mostly double-inlet). They compared them with a similar analysis of 89 patients undergoing operation for classic tricuspid atresia. As described by the European school [1], these hearts also have a univentricular atrioventricular connection, although most have considered them as separate entities until now, the true biventricular nature of the hearts being more obvious in patients with tricuspid atresia than in those with double-inlet left ventricle. The results of the Birmingham analysis [2] show that there is no scientific reason why this artificial division should continue. The overall actuarial survival of the 116 patients was 66% at 10 years — a significant improvement over the 'natural history' of such patients. The authors are appropriately optimistic about the results of palliative surgery. Only one hospital death occurred in 55 patients undergoing a shunt procedure. Actuarial survival of this subset at 10 years was 85%. Atrial septostomy was performed without operative death in 14 patients, actuarial survival being 76%. Banding was performed in a further 11 patients without hospital death (actuarial survival, 74%). Most of the mortality occurred following attempted 'corrective' procedures. Septation was attempted in 36 patients, with 13 hospital deaths. It is possible to extract an 'ideal group' of 13 patients with double-inlet left ventricle, left-sided rudimentary right ventricle, discordant ventriculo-arterial connection and no major associated lesion from this group of patients undergoing septation. There were no hospital deaths in this group, and 10 patients, all in NYHA class I or II, were still alive at the later follow-up (median, 1.96 years). The Fontan procedure was attempted in 73 patients, including 46 with classic tricuspid atresia. There were 16 hospital deaths. Risk factors identified were young age at operation, a diagnosis other than tricuspid atresia and the association of other complex lesions. Multivariate logistic analysis predicts an operative mortality of 4% at age 10 years and 11% at age 5 years for classic tricuspid atresia, with 16% at 10 years and 38% at 5 years for the other types of univentricular atrioventricular connection. These results are enviable.

Freedom *et al* continue their interest in the deleterious effects of banding of the pulmonary trunk in patients whose atrial chambers are connected only to the morphologically left ventricle with a rudimentary (incomplete) right ventricle and a discordant ventriculo-arterial connection [3]. The initial palliation for such patients with unobstructed pulmonary flow in infancy is to band the pulmonary trunk. Somerville *et al* (*Am J Cardiol* 1974; **34:** 206) first indicated the potential this procedure provided for ventricular hypertrophy and increasing restriction of the ventricular septal defect. As the interventricular communication provides the only route to the systemic circulation, the restriction produces effective sub-aortic obstruction. Freedom *et al* extended knowledge of this progression (*Am J Cardiol* 1977; **39:** 78), and the present investigation is the follow-up of their previous study. They point to the difficulties in nomenclature concerning univentricular hearts. They include in their analysis all patients with a dominant left and a rudimentary right ventricle, so that those with tricuspid atresia due to absent right atrioventricular connection and those with absent left atrioventricular connection are included in the analysis together with the more numerous patients who have double inlet left ventricle. It is difficult to understand, however, why they continue to describe the hearts as univentricular. The angiograms superbly illustrate the unbalanced nature of the ventricular mass, with a big left and a small right ventricle. The deleterious result of banding of the pulmonary trunk is restriction of the interventricular communication. How can a patient with only one ventricle have ventricular septal defect? There are other problems in the authors' selection of patients. They include those with a solitary right ventricle but exclude those with double inlet right ventricle and rudimentary left ventricle, and yet the rudimentary left ventricle in such cases is usually no more than a vestigial pouch. Its presence does not alter the clinical presentation and profile. Such patients should be included, as should those with double inlet right ventricle and concordant (or discordant) ventriculo-arterial connections. Although the Toronto group recognize some of the deficiencies of univentricular heart and expunge them, they continue to propagate equally deficient nosological concepts. In all, they studied 43 patients, having excluded patients who had sub-aortic stenosis prior to banding. Sub-aortic stenosis was seen in 31 (72%) patients, of whom only nine were still alive at writing. Surgical results of enlargement of a restrictive defect are poor (Penkaske *et al, J Thorac Cardivasc Surg* 1984 **87:** 767; Barber *et al, J Am Coll Cardiol* 1984; **4:** 771). The problem is mostly with patients who have a dominant left ventricle and discordant ventriculo-arterial connections. Such patients with unrestricted pulmonary flow must be banded early and tight to prevent pulmonary vascular disease (Juaneda and Haworth, *Br Heart J* 1985; **53:** 513). The experience of these authors suggests that most patients will then develop a restrictive ventricular septal defect. They are now pre-empting the need to enlarge the defect by constructing aorto-pulmonary shunts at the time of banding, in some instances going as far as to transect the pulmonary trunk and construct a systemic-pulmonary shunt to provide pulmonary blood flow. Whether such procedures will provide suitable ventricles and pulmonary vasculature is as yet unknown.

Another concept of 'univentricular hearts' is revealed in the analysis of the Mayo Clinic group of a cohort of patients with double-inlet left ventricle, a discordant atrioventricular connection and a restrictive ventricular septal defect [4]. Barber *et al* showed that obstruction at the ventricular septal defect in patients with double-inlet left ventricle and discordant ventriculo-arterial connection is an ominous development. Direct surgical relief of the obstruction, or bypass by construction of an aortopulmonary anastomosis, must be incorporated into the treatment of these patients. A detailed knowledge of the precise anatomy — particularly the abnormal course of the atrioventricular conduction axis — is necessary for successful surgery.

The major justification (other than the overwhelming anatomic evidence) for grouping together hearts with double-inlet ventricle and atrioventricular valve atresia is that the most successful and widely performed surgery for 'correction' of these lesions is the Fontan procedure or one of its modifications. It is now almost twenty years since Fontan first performed the procedure. Shortly after, Kreutzer carried out a very similar operation in Buenos Aires. Since then there have been many minor modifications in surgical technique. The simplest procedure remains a direct communication between the right atrium and the pulmonary arteries, thus excluding totally the ventricular mass from the pulmonary circulation. One major alternative is, when possible, to incorporate a rudimentary right ventricle into the circulation. These two options are described as atriopulmonary and atrioventricular connections, respectively. Initially performed in patients with tricuspid atresia (usual atrial arrangement, absent right atrioventricular connection with the left atrium connected to a dominant left ventricle in the presence of a right-sided rudimentary right ventricle), the procedure has subsequently been applied to diverse lesions, notably various forms of double inlet ventricle. Mayer *et al* [5] and Kirklin *et al* [8] describe their overall experience with the procedure in all types of lesion. The Boston group [5] describe 167 consecutive operations from 1973, whereas the Birmingham surgeons have performed the procedure 102 times since 1975 [8]. DeLeon *et al* [6] have selected 25 patients from their overall experience of 49 patients undergoing a Fontan-type operation. The selected patients had so-called complex lesions, although Fontan debated strongly against the inclusion within this category of those with tricuspid atresia and a discordant ventriculo-arterial connection ('transposition'). Lee *et al* [7] also selected a small subset of patients from their total of 421 patients undergoing this type of operation up to December 1985. They sought to compare the results of operation using direct atriopulmonary as opposed to an atrioventricular anastomosis; they chose 84 patients with classical tricuspid atresia for this purpose.

There are so many features of note in these important papers that they are required reading for all those with an interest in the treatment of congenital heart disease. Mayer *et al* [5] achieved 77% overall survival during the operative period. The best results were obtained in those with tricuspid atresia (85% operative survival). The indexed pulmonary arterial resistance was the most significant risk factor. Only 54% of those with an index >2 Wood units/metre^2 survived. Mayer *et al* also showed that several of the selection criteria established by Choussat *et al* (*Paediatric Cardiology* 1977, edited by Anderson RH and Shinebourne EA, Churchill Livingstone, Edingburgh, 1978, pp 559–66) could safely be exceeded. Nonetheless, success declined with each additional criterion exceeded, and no patient survived when more than three were broached (four patients). These results are in agreement with the updated experience of Fontan presented at the recent symposium on Pediatric Cardiology held in Vienna. Fontan would prefer to take 3 Wood units/metre^2 as his upper limit for pulmonary arterial resistance and not to contravene more than two of his selection criteria. As he indicates in his discussion of these papers (*J Thorac Cardiovasc Surg* 1986; **92:** 1044–8), his selection criteria were based on early experience and, in some cases, derived from theoretical rather than practical considerations. Despite this, it is salutary to note that survival is optimised by adhering strictly to all the 'commandments'. Mayer *et al* [5] also showed that young age (<4 years) was not a contraindication to surgery, a viewpoint endorsed by the results of Kirklin *et al* [8].

DeLeon *et al* [6] present excellent surgical results in their paper. They found it necessary to 'take-down' the procedure in four of their 25 patients, two of whom died. However, these were the only operative deaths. Significantly, three of the four had discordant ventriculo-arterial connections and a restrictive ventricular septal defect, giving sub-aortic stenosis in effect. All three had banding of the pulmonary trunk. This is recognized as a bad combination of features. In Vienna, Fontan suggested that immediate repair might be the best approach to this constellation of lesions irrespective of age. DeLeon *et al* [6] had three late deaths; 80% of their overall group, many of whom had a complex combination of lesions, were still alive at writing. It should be noted that at least one of their patients had sick sinus syndrome. Their demonstrated suture lines put the artery to the sinus node at high risk. This complication can be avoided by detailed attention to the atrial arteries as pointed out by Fontan in the discussion. DeLeon *et al* [6] also favour the construction of a Glenn shunt in certain patients, a viewpoint with which Fontan disagrees.

Lee *et al* [7] compared their patients with classical tricuspid atresia having atriopulmonary *versus* atrioventricular connections. Actuarial survival at 3.5 years post-operatively was virtually the same in the two groups (89 ±4% *vs* 88 ±7%). The only significant difference noted between the groups was an average right atrial pressure 2 mmHg higher in the atriopulmonary group. Lee *et al* conclude that the choice of procedure should be dictated by the patient's anatomy, particularly the size of the rudimentary right ventricle. Fontan, both in his discussion and at Vienna, stresses his desire to use the right ventricle whenever possible. He believes it is advantageous to use the native pulmonary valve. Nonetheless, he does exclude the apical trabecular component of this ventricle unless it is possible to insert a homograft between the right atrium and the right ventricle. If the ventricle is incorporated without such a homograft, it can enlarge and lead to significant complications.

Kirklin *et al* [8] show the major advantages conveyed by their use of sophisticated statistical analysis. All of the risks, their interrelations and their variance with time are demonstrated with exquisite detail. Their analysis showed a close correlation with an elevated right atrial pressure after repair and subsequent death. The operations with the best chance of success are those giving a low pressure immediately after operation. Kirklin *et al* demonstrated the deleterious effect of hypertrophy of the dominant ventricle. When this was taken into account, other apparent risk factors (such as double inlet atrioventricular connection) were shown not to be significant. Other factors exacerbated the effect of ventricular hypertrophy, notably a long aortic cross-clamp time. This is one factor that may be neutralized by more efficient myocardial protection. Kirklin *et al* also showed that young age is not a risk factor. They would now recommend this operation to be performed on patients between 2 and 3 years of age, even if shunting or banding are needed in earlier life.

Fontan's own report describing the results of his first hundred consecutive patients (*J Thorac Cardiovasc Surg* 1983; **85**: 647–58) revealed a mortality rate of 12 patients in 100, four of whom were in the first eight to be treated. Between 1973 and 1983 the Mayo Clinic group treated 90 patients with classical tricuspid atresia using the Fontan procedure [9]. The overall mortality was also 12%, which decreased to 7% during the second five-year period. Follow-up showed the majority of survivors (86%) to be in excellent condition; seven late deaths occurred. The interesting feature to emerge from this study is that, when the criteria outlined by Choussat for the selection of the ideal candidate for this procedure were fulfilled, there were no operative deaths. However, only 24 patients qualified as 'ideal' candidates; 30 patients did not fulfil one of the criteria, 25 did not meet two and 11 had three or more risk factors outside the 'ideal' criteria. The mortality rates of these three subgroups were 17, 16 and 18, respectively. Although it is advantageous for patients to fulfil all the criteria, 73% of them did not and more than four-fifths survived and, at follow-up, the great majority were found to have received significant benefit from the operation.

One of the criteria outlined by Choussat *et al* was normal size and distribution of the pulmonary arteries. A collaborative study by Girod *et al* [10] showed that the size of the pulmonary arteries was not a significant determinant of survival. The major feature identified as important in survival and benefit from the operation was good systolic and diastolic ventricular function. Consequently, the authors recommend that patients with tricuspid atresia should have the Fontan operation by the age of six years in order to protect ventricular function.

Driscoll *et al* describe the extensive experience of the Mayo Clinic group (a study of 81 consecutive patients with a functionally single ventricle seen between August 1981 and August 1984) [11], and De Vivie and Rupprath present their findings in a reasonably large group of patients (31) undergoing the Fontan procedure or its modifications between 1975 and 1984 at Göttingen, West Germany [12]. The Mayo Clinic team performed a maximal exercise study in their patients, studying all of them preoperatively and 29 after operation [11]. Seven patients were studied before and after the procedure. Only five patients were considered unsuitable for operation. The most significant findings were in the seven patients studied before and after operation. The patients increased significantly the total work performed ($P=0.019$), the duration of exercise ($P=0.019$) and the maximal oxygen uptake ($P=0.03$). A negative correlation overall was found with age and with age at operation. Exercise tolerance was also better in those receiving an atriopulmonary as compared with an atrioventricular connection, but this may have been related to age rather than the type of operation. Overall, the study demonstrated a significant increase in tolerance and an improvement in ventilatory response after the Fontan operation, together with reduction in exercise tolerance with increasing age. The authors cautiously conclude that the procedure is best considered during or before adolescence.

The Göttingen group give a broader view of their smaller group of patients [12]. Six of their 31 patients died in the early post-operative phase (17.1% mortality). Two of the patients with classical tricuspid atresia died (10.5%). All patients had pleural effusion or ascites in the post-operative period. Eleven required repeat thoracotomy and nine had temporary renal insufficiency. Follow-up of the 25 survivors showed excellent results in 17, good results in five and poor results in two. One patient had a residual shunt through a left atrial-coronary sinus window. The authors conclude that the Fontan procedure, with its modifications, must be seen as definitive palliation and they anticipate good long-term results when the criteria established by Fontan are strictly observed. The Mayo Clinic experience, however, suggests that re-appraisal of these criteria is now necessary.

Other modifications of the Fontan procedure have been described. In an experimental canine study [13], Fantidis *et al* carried out an ingenious technique which involved turning in the wall of the right atrial appendage and bringing the pulmonary venous return to the tricuspid valve. It is primarily applicable to patients with left atrioventricular valve atresia and not, as the authors suggest, to patients with tricuspid atresia. It also has the potential disadvantage of damaging the sinus node artery as it ascends through the interatrial groove. Another novel procedure is more innovative and exciting, and has been performed in one patient with tricuspid atresia [14]. Olert and Borst extended the atrial septal defect into the left atrium and then anastomosed the left atrium to the pulmonary trunk. This ingenious intra-atrial repair avoids all problems of conduit compression and should not damage the blood supply to the sinus node.

The final step in 'correction' of hypoplastic left heart syndrome — surgery which is increasingly being performed in the USA — involves a Fontan procedure. It is essential, therefore, that we understand how the pulmonary circulation works postoperatively in the various modifications of this procedure.

Nakazawa *et al* studied the performance of the right atrium after the variant of Fontan's procedure that produces an atriopulmonary connection [15]. They showed that right atrial contraction produced forward flow, and pulmonary regurgitation was not a problem even when they did not insert valves. Their conclusion, however, was that atrial contraction may not be a major determinant of cardiac output. The study shows that the end-result of the atriopulmonary connection is far from normal, which is why other centers strive to achieve an atrioventricular connection, hoping when possible to incorporate the rudimentary right ventricle as a functional part of the pulmonary circulation. Glenn's editorial [16] stresses that the original Fontan procedure was performed on a patient who had already undergone a Glenn procedure, and quotes support from Jane Somerville, who argues that long-term results for the Fontan procedure in tricuspid atresia will possibly be better when combined with a Glenn shunt, because this preserves the function of the left ventricle.

The experimental study from Columbia University [17] is also significant. Using dogs, the group studied the effect of counterpulsation on a valved right-atrial to pulmonary artery conduit distal to the implanted valve in a simulated 'Fontan' situation. There were no differences between 'direct' counterpulsation and that achieved through a graft sutured to the conduit. Counterpulsation increased cardiac output by 48% ($P<0.0001$) and right-atrial pressure fell by a mean of 4 mmHg ($P<0.003$). Left-atrial pressure was changed only by transfusion. Pulmonary vascular resistance fell by a mean of 35% ($P<0.002$). The authors suggest this as a feasible and effective method of assisting a failing right atrium.

Two of the most important criteria in surgery for tricuspid atresia and other varieties of univentricular connection are left-ventricular function and the state of the pulmonary vasculature. Baker *et al* [18] and Juaneda and Haworth [19] establish guidelines for determining these important parameters. The study of Baker *et al* [18] is a continuation of their investigation of radionuclide angiography's role in the evaluation of various congenital lesions. It is questionable whether the control group in this study is truly comparable, as there are fundamental differences in the geometry of the dominant left ventricle in tricuspid atresia and the left ventricle in hearts with biventricular atrioventricular connections, but the authors do recognize this. The ejection fraction in patients with tricuspid atresia was found to be significantly lower than in 'normals' ($P<0.001$). Furthermore, those who had undergone surgery for tricuspid atresia had a lower ejection fraction than those who had not ($P<0.05$), whereas those not undergoing surgery had a lower ejection fraction than controls ($P<0.01$). The authors are unable to ascribe this reduced functional capacity to any single factor. Although they consider the influence of hypoxia, they favor the effect of volume overload on an intrinsically abnormal left ventricle. This is because low ejection fractions were found in even the youngest patients and in those who had not undergone surgery. Once left-ventricular dysfunction has been identified, gated radionuclide angiography is a valuable technique for further investigation, as is echocardiography. It will be interesting to compare results of future investigations using both techniques.

Juaneda and Haworth [19] investigated the pulmonary vascular bed in 12 patients who died after a Fontan procedure. Of the patients studied, eight had classic tricuspid atresia, two had double-inlet left ventricle and two had hypoplastic right ventricle in a concordant atrioventricular connection. Eight had had low pulmonary blood flow during life; in seven of these patients, the pulmonary vascular structure was almost normal, and in the other, many intra-acinar arteries contained organized thrombus. Four patients had had increased pulmonary flow during life; in these, despite banding of the pulmonary trunk in three, significant pathologic changes were observed. It is clearly more difficult to fulfill the hemodynamic criteria for Fontan's procedure. Published results show that some patients can survive when they do not satisfy these criteria, but the lung can be a risk factor even in patients who do. As the authors indicate, preoperative lung biopsy will give a more accurate indication of the risk of operation. They recommend that the pulmonary trunk be banded more tightly when performing a palliative procedure in those patients in whom the right atrium must eventually propel blood to the lungs.

Using an ingenious experimental and clinical correlation, Ilbawi et al examined the effects of the elevation of coronary sinus pressure on left ventricular function after the Fontan procedure [20]. Left ventricular dysfuntion after the Fontan procedure is a serious complication. As abnormal left ventricular function is frequent in unoperated tricuspid atresia, anything that further limits it will worsen a patient's prognosis. In 13 dogs, the blood flow from the coronary sinus was diverted into a reservoir, and pressure within the sinus was increased markedly by elevating the reservoir in a stepwise fashion. A significant decrease in cardiac performance was found when coronary sinus pressure was elevated to 15 torr. These experimental results were then correlated with post-operative catheterization findings in 24 patients who had been corrected using the Fontan procedure. Again, a significant difference in ventricular performance was found between patients with a mean right atrial pressure <15 torr and those who had a higher pressure ($P<0.001$). The authors conclude that elevation of coronary sinus pressure impairs ventricular function after the Fontan procedure. Any action that would alleviate this, such as leaving the coronary sinus in communication with the left atrium or using a rudimentary right ventricle in the Fontan circulation, might decrease coronary sinus hypertension and improve the long-term results of surgery.

COARCTATION OF THE AORTA

[1] Aortic coarctation in the first 3 months of life: an anatomico-pathological study with respect to treatment.
Pellegrino A, Deverall PB, Anderson RH et al, Cardiothoracic Inst, London, UK.
J Thorac Cardiovasc Surg 1985; 89: 121-7.

[2] Should elective repair of coarctation of the aorta be done in infancy?
Campbell DB, Waldhausen JA, Pierce WS, Fripp R, Whitman V, Milton S Hershey Med Cent, Hershey, PA, USA.
J Thorac Cardiovasc Surg 1984; 88: 929-38.

[3] Prosthetic repair of coarctation of the aorta with particular reference to Dacron onlay patch grafts and late aneurysm formation.
Clarkson PM, Brandt PWT, Barratt-Boyes BG, Rutherford JD, Kerr AR, Neutze JM, Green Lane Hosp, Auckland, New Zealand.
Am J Cardiol 1985; **56**: 342-6.

[4] Transluminal balloon coarctation angioplasty: experience with 27 patients.
Lababidi ZA, Daskalopoulos DA, Stoeckle H Jr, Univ Missouri Hosps and Clins, Columbia, MO, USA.
Am J Cardiol 1984; **54**: 1288-91.

[5] Cystic medial necrosis in coarctation of the aorta: a potential factor contributing to adverse consequences observed after percutaneous balloon angioplasty of coarctation sites.
Isner JM, Donaldson RF, Fulton D, Bhan I, Payne DD, Cleveland RJ, Tufts-New England Med Cent, Boston, MA, USA.
Circulation 1987; **75**: 689-95.

[6] Coarctation in the first year of life. Patterns of postoperative effect.
Waldman JD, Lamberti JJ, Goodman AH *et al*, Child Hosp, San Diego, CA, USA.
J Thorac Cardiovasc Surg 1983; **86**: 9-17.

[7] Therapeutic effect of propranolol on paradoxical hypertension after repair of coarctation of the aorta.
Gidding SS, Rocchini AP, Beckman R *et al*, CS Mott Children's Hosp, Ann Arbor, MI, USA.
N Engl J Med 1985; **312**: 1224-8.

[8] Persistent ventricular adaptations in postoperative coarctation of the aorta.
Kimball BP, Shurvell BL, Houle S, Fulop JC, Rakowski H, McLaughlin PR, Toronto Gen Hosp, Toronto, Ont, Canada.
J Am Coll Cardiol 1986; **8**: 172-8.

[9] Coarctation of the aorta and tetralogy of Fallot: two cases.
Rey C, Coeurderoy A, Dupuis C.
Arch Mal Coeur 1984; **77**: 526-33.

[10] Coarctation of the aorta of unusual morphology.
Poulias GE, Polemis L, Skoutas B, Doundoulakis N, Papaioannou K, Red Cross Gen Hosp, Athens, Greece.
J Cardiovasc Surg 1984; **25**: 211-5.

[11] Interruption of the aortic arch and coarctation of the aorta: pathogenetic relations.
Van Mierop LHS, Kutsche LM, Univ Florida Sch Med, Gainesville, FL, USA.
Am J Cardiol 1984; **54**: 829-34.

Comment. The optimal surgical procedure for repair of aortic coarctation remains to be established. In recent years, there have been attempts to relieve the obstructive lesion in the aortic pathway using balloon dilatation techniques. The collaborative anatomic study of Pellegrino *et al* [1], which examines the obstructive lesions present in a series of infants dying within the first three months of life, is pertinent to both these matters. The authors observed wide variations in morphology, characterizing the three major patterns as shelf lesions, waisting of the aortic wall and tubular hypoplasia of a segment of the arch. They also noted marked variability in the proximity of origin of the left subclavian artery to the obstructing lesion. Their observations prompt them to suggest that no single surgical procedure is likely to be suitable for all cases — rather, each case should be treated on its own merits. They also point out that very few obstructive lesions seen in early life seem amenable on morphologic grounds to balloon dilatation. Relief of the obstruction would, in most cases, be achieved at the expense of ripping the medial wall of the aorta.

When surgical results are considered worldwide, it is clear that many centers now use the subclavian flap procedure for repair even in infants. It is therefore illuminating to read the report of the accumulated 10-year experience of Waldhausen and co-workers at Hershey Medical Center, Pennsylvania [2]. Along with Hahrwold, it was Waldhausen who first described this procedure in 1966. This paper [2] is concerned with 53 infants — 6 with isolated coarctation and 18 with major intracardiac lesions. The other cases had either patent arterial duct or ventricular septal defect. Only two infants died — one with arterial duct and one with hypoplastic left ventricle. Banding of the pulmonary trunk was performed in five cases: one with a 'simple' ventricular septal defect and the others with complex lesions. Further surgery was required in eight cases: four had isolated ventricular septal defects, and one died. The simple defect of the ventricular septum identified in 11 further cases regressed spontaneously and did not require further surgery. Of the complex cases, seven died, including all four (with double-outlet right ventricle) who underwent further surgery after coarctation repair. These results show that the coarctation lesion can be dealt with effectively using the subclavian flap approach and it produces excellent results in 'simple' cases. The problems remain in patients with complicated major lesions. The discussion reflects the division of opinion existing over the relative merits of the subclavian flap approach and those of resection followed by end-to-end anastomosis. This issue is by no means resolved.

Other groups have advocated a third procedure in repair, namely the use of prosthetic grafts to enlarge the site of narrowing. One paper is of the utmost significance to those who support the use of this alternative [3]. The authors present long-term follow-up in 72 patients in whom either onlay patches or tube grafts of Dacron were used to repair coarctation of the aorta at the Green Lane Hospital, Auckland, between 1958 and 1976. Follow-up was complete in all but one patient, and ranged from 8 months to 24 years after operation. Late aneurysm formation was noted in 3 of 20 patients who had a Dacron tube graft. An onlay patch was used in 34 patients; either true or false late aneurysms were found in five of these patients. Actuarial follow-up showed only a 3% probablility of aneurysm formation at 10 years ($\pm3\%$), but a very large increase to 38% probability ($\pm16\%$) was observed at 14 years after operation. The recommendations of the Green Lane Hospital team are clear-cut and difficult to dispute — synthetic-only patches should not be used for the repair of coarctation of the aorta in infancy. It is worth noting that those who continue to espouse the technique (*Ann Thorac Surg* 1984; **38**: 21–5) have yet to follow their patients beyond the critical 10-year point.

In the section on pulmonary and aortic stenosis, the pioneering efforts of Lababidi and co-workers were discussed relative to balloon dilatation of aortic stenosis (p. 203). They have also attempted dilatation of coarctation lesions [4], and present their experience of balloon angioplasty in 27 patients: 7 within the first year of life, 7 with restenosis following previous surgical repair and 13 (including one 27-year-old adult) with 'native' coarctation. All the infants had associated lesions. No deaths occurred and no aneurysms were found in a follow-up period extending to 24 months. Following the procedure, all patients had a significant decrease in the gradient across the lesion and an increase in diameter of the site of obstruction. The excellent studies of Lock *et al* (*Circulation* 1982; **66:** 1280– 6; *Circulation* 1983; **68:** 109–16) showed that relief is achieved by rupturing the aortic wall; the autopsy study of Pellegrino *et al* discussed above [1] confirmed these observations, showing that the wall was the only tissue (in most cases) which could be dilated. Lababidi *et al* [4] have shown that relief can be achieved without mortality or morbidity. It will be interesting to see if these results can be matched by other workers, and whether balloon angioplasty for coarctation becomes accepted as widely and rapidly as it has been for pulmonary stenosis. Despite this excellent initial experience, more caution would seem indicated when dilating 'native' lesions of the aortic isthmus.

Several investigators have noted the development of aneurysms following balloon dilatation. Marvin *et al* (*J Am Coll Cardiol* 1986; **7:** 117a) were the first to report this; more recently, Cooper *et al* have observed similar findings (*Circulation* 1987; **75:** 600–4). To a certain extent, some aneurysm formation is to be expected, because the procedure is known to work by splitting the aortic medial coat. Isner *et al* suggest that the aortic wall at the site of coarctation is particularly vulnerable to disruption [5]. They have studied the coarcted site removed at surgery ($n=31$) or obtained at autopsy ($n=2$) from 33 patients. They observed depletion and disarray of elastic tissue in all cases. These changes were dubbed 'cystic medial necrosis' by Erdheim, and they are thought to be precursors to the development of aortic aneurysms with increasing age. Isner *et al* graded the extent of these changes and found two-thirds of them to have severe alterations in aortic histology. Their thorough dissection puts these changes into perspective, and their claim that the weakened wall provides a basis for aneurysm formation is well reasoned. Clinical experience, however, with longer follow-up will be the final arbiter of the success and use of balloon angioplasty for native coarctation. ˙

Waldman *et al* [6] report the late results of operation in 31 infants with isolated coarctation operated on within the first year of life: 30 children survived. No differences were observed hemodynamically between those with end-to-end anastomosis ($n=14$), subclavian flap aortoplasty ($n=6$), patch aortoplasty ($n=5$), or other procedures ($n=6$). Sixty-nine per cent had postoperative residual arm-to-leg gradients that spontaneously resolved, 13% had persistent gradients and 13% progressive gradients. Stress-testing frequently unmasked gradients that were latent at rest.

Apart from residual coarctation, the other feared complications after repair are persistence of hypertension or the occurrence of paradoxical hypertension. Gidding *et al* reported results of a controlled trial of treatment with propranolol before repair relative to the latter complication [7]. Seven children were randomly assigned to receive propranolol for two weeks prior to surgery and for one week after surgery, and seven children received standard postoperative care. Both groups were found to have a similar significant increase in plasma norepinephrine in response to surgery, although the propranolol-treated group had a reduced rise in both systolic and diastolic blood pressure in comparison with the standard-care group ($P=0.004$ and $P=0.003$, respectively). The postoperative increase in plasma renin activity was also reduced in the propranolol-treated group ($P<0.01$). The authors conclude that prophylactic propranolol can prevent paradoxical hypertension following repair of coarctation of the aorta. As such, it should become standard perioperative care for patients undergoing this procedure.

In an important study from Toronto General Hospital, left ventricular function following repair of coarctation was studied in 25 subjects [8]. Their mean age at time of study was 26.1 years (range 18–41), and they had undergone operative correction at a mean of 10.6 years (range 2–25 years) before the study. Various techniques had been used for correction, including interposition grafting, synthetic patch aortoplasty, end-to-end anastomosis and subclavian flap aortoplasty. In all patients, ventricular performance and myocardial contractility were studied at rest and exercise using radionuclide ventriculography together with quantitative cross-sectional echocardiography. The results were compared with values obtained from an age- and sex-matched normal population. Clinical evaluation showed all the patients to be asymptomatic, with only two receiving treatment for persistent hypertension. The measured arterial pressures, both systolic and diastolic, were considered to be indistinguishable from those of the control groups. The presence of fundamental abnormalities in ventricular performance and intrinsic contractility was a highly significant finding. The ventricular performance was enhanced relative to the control values, with accentuation of both global left ventricular ejection fraction and maximal ejection velocity. The investigators argue that this relative ventricular over-compensation is a persistence of the changes induced in early life during the imposition of congenital pressure overload with residuary characteristics, suggesting incomplete resolution after surgical correction. It will be very interesting to see whether similar abnormalities in ventricular function are found in patients corrected in the first year of life, a trend that is developing in many centers at which this lesion is seen.

In recent years, it has become fashionable to argue that coarctation of the aorta is a result of abnormal fetal flow patterns. In the process of establishing this concept, its advocates have dismissed highly significant anatomic studies pointing to some role for ductal tissue in the production of coarctation (Wielenga and Dankmeijer, *J Path Bact* 1968; **95**: 265–74), which have also predicted that coarctation is an impossibility in association with lesions which have increased aortic flow, such as tetralogy of Fallot. Rey, Coeurderoy and Dupuis [9] describe two cases of tetralogy of Fallot coexisting with coarctation. Interestingly, both cases also had a right aortic arch. Poulias *et al* [10] describe coarctation occurring in three unusual sites along the arch. The first case had two obstructions, one at the anticipated site and the other proximal to the left subclavian artery. The second had obstructive lesions between the carotid arteries, while in the final case the lesion was in the thoracic aorta in a supradiaphragmatic position. All cases were successfully repaired at surgery. It is difficult to account for any of these lesions on the basis of abnormal fetal flow.

The final paper in this section is also concerned with the pathogenesis of coarctation, together with what can be considered an extreme form of coarctation: namely, interruption of the aortic arch. In an excellent example of anatomic 'detective work', Van Mierop and Kutsche [11] studied cases from their own collection (9 hearts with interruption at the isthmus and 21 with interruption between the left common carotid and left subclavian arteries) and then found an additional 54 cases with isthmal interruption and 124 with carotid-subclavian segment interruption in the literature. They compared the anatomic findings with 57 cases from their material, which had come from children less than 2 years old with aortic coarctation. They showed that ventricular septal defect was more commonly associated with interruption at the carotid-subclavian segment, and was characteristically of the malalignment type which obstructs the subaortic left-ventricular outlet. Anomalous origin of the right subclavian artery and DiGeorge syndrome were also commonly associated with this type of interruption, but they were rare in the other study groups. Abnormal intracardiac connections or presence of an aortopulmonary window, however, were more commonly found with interruption at the isthmus. On the basis of their findings, the authors postulated that interruption at the carotid-subclavian segment is a developmental error involving the neural crest, as is the DiGeorge syndrome. In contrast, aortic coarctation and interruption at the isthmus could be lesions acquired prenatally and pathogenetically distinct from the other group. These inferences are vital for those concerned with genetic counselling because when risks of recurrences are calculated it would be misleading to group these lesions together as 'coarctation and interruption'. The concept as advanced is convincing. The note of caution expressed by Van Mierop and Kutsche is also realistic: those who are inductive in their approach would see a single case of anomalous subclavian artery with interruption at the isthmus as significant.

PULMONARY VASCULAR DISEASE

[1] Left ventricular function in persistent pulmonary hypertension of the newborn.
St John Sutton MG, Meyer RA, Children's Hosp Med Cent, Cincinnati, OH, USA.
Br Heart J 1983; **50**: 540–9.

[2] Pulmonary vascular disease in different types of congenital heart disease. Implications for interpretation of lung biopsy findings in early childhood.
Haworth SG, Inst Child Health, London, UK.
Br Heart J 1984; **52**: 557–71.

[3] Reversibility of plexogenic pulmonary arteriopathy following banding of the pulmonary artery.
Wagenvoort CA, Wagenvoort N, Draulans-Noe Y, Univ Amsterdam, Amsterdam, The Netherlands.
J Thorac Cardiovasc Surg 1984; **87**: 876–86.

Comment. Persistent fetal circulation (persistent pulmonary hypertension of the newborn) is a major problem for the pediatric cardiologist. As discussed by Sutton and Meyer [1], it has previously been considered primarily a problem of the pulmonary vasculature. Left-ventricular echocardiograms in 23 neonates with this disorder were analyzed, and showed significant abnormalities of both systolic and diastolic left-ventricular function. There was an inordinately high mortality rate in this series in that almost one-quarter of the neonates died, but only those infants with the most severe pulmonary hypertension had been selected. Four possible factors are suggested to explain the left-ventricular dysfunction: the pulmonary hypertension itself, the alteration in left-ventricular geometry by the pressure-overloaded right ventricle, hypoxemia producing generalized myocardial ischemia and metabolic acidemia. What is fascinating is that, of the three neonates coming to autopsy, all had left-ventricular hypertrophy. Two of the three had subendocardial hemorrhage and papillary muscle necrosis in both left and right ventricles.

Recent improvements in surgical techniques have reduced but not abolished operative mortality in the management of most of the congenital lesions. One factor underscoring these deaths is the morphologic state of the pulmonary vascular bed. The importance of pulmonary vascular disease as an incremental risk factor has been recognized since the categorization of its severity by Heath and Edwards (*Circulation* 1958; **18**: 533–47). Reid extended the work of Heath and Edwards, initially at the Brompton Hospital and subsequently at Boston. Haworth continued this work; in collaboration with the Boston group, she was instrumental in showing the value of lung biopsy in clinical decision-making (Rabinovitch *et al*, *Circulation* 1978; **58**: 1107–22). One reservation about lung biopsy is whether it is representative. Haworth [2] studied serial reconstructions of the pulmonary vascular tree in 3 normal subjects and 16 patients with congenital heart disease (ventricular septal defect, 3; complete transposition and ventricular septal defect, 7; atrioventricular septal defect, 4; and atrial septal defect, 2). Precise findings along the pathways which varied from lesion to lesion are described. The reconstructed segments were compared with random sections taken from elsewhere in the lung and shown to be representative. This study confirms the value of a lung biopsy in providing an indication of the state of the pulmonary vasculature, and should be studied in depth by all those interested in the surgical treatment of congenital heart disease.

One of the pioneers of the histologic study of pulmonary vascular disease who, like Donald Heath, studied with Jesse Edwards while he was at the Mayo Clinic, is Cees Wagenvoort, recently retired as Professor of Pathology at the University of Amsterdam. He and his colleagues studied 28 patients with congenital lesions in whom lung biopsies were taken during the placement of a pulmonary band for excessive pulmonary flow [3]. Additional biopsies were obtained at the time of complete repair 2.5–10 years later. Histologic investigation showed regression of some features, such as medial hypertrophy or intimal fibrosis and thickening; however, other features, such as fibrinoid necrosis and plexiform lesions, showed a tendency to progress. The discussion of the findings is of considerable interest, because it is supplemented by a commentary from the manuscript reviewer, Marlene Rabinovitch of Toronto, and a reply from Wagenvoort and co-workers. This paper and the addenda are of significance to the whole area of vascular changes in pulmonary hypertension, and should be read by all those interested in the surgical treatment of congenital heart disease. As Rabinovitch states, it "answers many questions and dispels many myths".

MISCELLANEOUS CONDITIONS AND OTHER TOPICS

[1] Congenital heart disease: prevalence at livebirth. The Baltimore-Washington Infant Study.
Ferencz C, Rubin JD, McCarthy RJ *et al*, Univ Maryland Sch Med, Baltimore, MD, USA.
Am J Epidemiol 1985; **121**: 31–6.

[2] The presentation of symptomatic heart disease in infancy based on 10 years' experience (1973–82). Implications for the provision of services.
Scott DJ, Rigby ML, Miller GAH, Shinebourne EA, Brompton Hosp, London, UK.
Br Heart J 1984; **52**: 248–57.

[3] A possible increase in the incidence of congenital heart defects among the offspring of affected parents.
Rose V, Gold RJM, Lindsay G, Allen M, Univ Toronto, Toronto, Ont, Canada.
J Am Coll Cardiol 1985; **6**: 376–82.

[4] Primary preventive health care in children with heart disease.
Uzark K, Collins J, Meisenhelder K, Dick M, Rosenthal A, CS Mott Children's Hosp, Univ Michigan, Ann Arbor, MI, USA.
Pediatr Cardiol 1983; **4**: 259–4.

[5] Costs and results of cardiac operations in infants less than 4 months old. Are they worthwhile?
Watson DC Jr, Bradley LM, Midgley FM, Scott LP, Univ Tennessee Cent Hlth Sci, Memphis, TN, USA.
J Thorac Cardiovasc Surg 1986; **91**: 667–73.

[6] Magnetic resonance imaging in patients with congenital heart disease.
Higgins CB, Byrd BF III, Farmer DW, Osaki L, Silverman NH, Cheitlin MD, Univ California Med Cent, San Francisco, CA, USA.
Circulation 1984; **70**: 851–60.

[7] Autoantibodies to SS-A/Ro in infants with congenital heart block.
Reed BR, Lee LA, Harmon C *et al*, Univ Colorado Sch Med, Denver, CO, USA.
J Pediatr 1983; **103**: 889–91.

[8] Complete heart block in HLA B27 associated disease. Electrophysiological and clinical characteristics.
Bergfeldt L, Vallin H, Edhag O, Huddinge Univ Hosp, Huddinge, Sweden.
Br Heart J 1984; **51**: 184–8.

[9] Superiority of radionuclide over oximetric measurement of left to right shunts.
Baker EJ, Ellam SV, Lorber A, Jones ODH, Tynan MJ, Maisey MN, Guy's Hosp, London, UK.
Br Heart J 1985; **53**: 535–40.

[10] Amiodarone treatment of critical arrhythmias in children and young adults.
Garson A Jr, Gillette PC, McVey P *et al*, Texas Children's Hosp, Houston, TX, USA.
J Am Coll Cardiol 1984; **4**: 749–55.

[11] Congenital pulmonary vein stenosis.
Bini RM, Cleveland DC, Ceballos R, Bargeron LM Jr, Pacifico AD, Kirklin JW, Univ Alabama, Birmingham, AL, USA.
Am J Cardiol 1984; **54**: 369–75.

[12] Mitral atresia. Morphological details.
Gittenberger-de Groot AC, Wenink ACG, State Univ, Leiden, The Netherlands.
Br Heart J 1984; **51**: 252–8.

[13] Innominate artery compression of the trachea in infancy and childhood: is surgical therapy justified?
Welz A, Reichert B, Weinhold Ch *et al*, Univ Munich, Munich, FRG.
Thorac Cardiovasc Surg 1984; **32**: 85–8.

[14] Left ventricular false tendons in children: prevalence as detected by 2-dimensional echocardiography and clinical significance.
Perry LW, Ruckman RN, Shapiro SR, Kuehl KS, Galiato FM Jr, Scott LP, Children's Hosp Nat Med Cent, Washington, DC, USA.
Am J Cardiol 1983; **52**: 1264–6.

Comment. The first paper in our miscellaneous section is the report from the Baltimore-Washington Infant Study [1]. Eligible infants were enrolled on diagnosis at the study centers, and searches were made in the records of 52 community hospitals so as not to exclude infants with cardiac malformation who died outside the centers. Cases were coded according to the system of the International Society of Cardiology (1970), which is not optimal but did provide a diagnosis for all the cases encountered. Over the two-year period covered, 179 697 livebirths occurred within the study area. Of these, 664 infants were found to have a congenital cardiac malformation within the first year of life (prevalence, 3.7/1000). The results were compared with those of eight other studies, which gave figures remarkably close to 0.4 as the percentage of infants with confirmed congenital heart disease. The total prevalence of congenital malformation in these earlier studies varied from 5.51 to 8.56/1000 livebirths. The authors indicate that the study will be continued to establish the prevalence of congenital heart disease by school entry. This study demonstrates the need for similar collaborative efforts elsewhere, and for a generally agreed classification system so that results can be directly compared.

Scott *et al* analyzed their 10-year experience of admission of 1665 symptomatic infants with congenital cardiac malformations to the Brompton Hospital, London, during the period 1973–1982 [2]. They studied congenital heart disease, rather than cardiac illnesses of the infant period, and their criterion for selection was "a gross structural abnormality of the heart or intrathoracic great vessels that is actually or potentially of functional significance" (Mitchell *et al, Circulation* 1971; **43**: 323–32). An arterial duct was included when it occurred as the only abnormality in a symptomatic infant presenting within the first 14 days of life. It was not possible to determine the overall incidence of this disease here, but it was estimated at 2.6 infants in every 1000 livebirths from the New England Regional Infant Cardiac Program (NERICP). The authors used this figure to calculate that the Brompton Hospital provides emergency pediatric cardiologic care for 11% of the total population of England and Wales. They provide a detailed analysis of the types of individual lesions seen, together with combinations of lesions, and make sensible recommendations for the 'grading' of severity of given lesions, so that each constellation is represented only by its most significant individual malformation. A remarkably close correlation was found between the distribution of lesions within the Brompton study and NERICP data. The authors conclude that there has probably been a change between the two series in terms of the 'prevalence' of complete transposition (concordant atrioventricular and discordant ventriculo-arterial connections — defined incorrectly in Table 2), which is declining, and right-ventricular outflow tract obstruction, which is increasing. Although the title of the paper promises a discussion of the "Implications for the provision of services", this is disappointingly brief and superficial.

All those concerned with the diagnosis and treatment of congenital heart disease are eager to have reliable data on the recurrence rate of given anomalies; therefore studies such as that of Rose *et al* [3] are welcome. Moreover, they are necessary to confirm the validity of the polygenic or multifactorial concept of the inheritance of congenital cardiac defects, which states that congenital heart disease may be caused by the interaction of a large number of genes with or without some contribution from environmental factors. If this is the case, then the expected incidence of disease in first degree relatives of affected subjects would approximate to the square root of p, where p is the frequency of the given lesion in the general population. Given the known population incidence rates, early findings of recurrence risks of between 1% and 5% were consistent with the polygenic concept. However, subsequent investigations began to cast doubt over these figures.

The Toronto workers have investigated four defects: atrial septal defect, aortic coarctation, aortic valve stenosis and 'complex dextrocardia'. The choice of atrial septal defect is somewhat surprising, but that of 'complex dextrocardia' is much more so; neither is a 'pure' defect, and the authors give no information concerning the specific diagnosis of the cases chosen. They examined the records of the Hospital for Sick Children, Toronto, for all subjects born prior to 1959 who had one of the selected defects; 921 probands were identified initially, 219 of whom participated in the investigation. There were 462 pregnancies in this group, which resulted in 385 live-births. Congenital heart disease was found in 40 of these live-births (10.4%). When 'minor' lesions were excluded, such as ventricular pre-excitation or mitral valve prolapse, the recurrence risk was 8.8%. This is considerably higher than the figures found to support the polygenic model (3%, see *Tetralogy* 1970; **3:** 325–30). It is interesting that none of the five patients with 'complex dextrocardia' had offspring with congenital heart disease. Only 16 of the 40 offspring had the same lesion as their affected parent. The authors postulate that their results favor an environmental mechanism for the causation of congenital heart disease. Their conclusion concerning counselling is that each unit should produce its own figures, or at least quote figures relative to their own environment. When this is not possible, the authors point out that advice concerning the risk of recurrence of congenital heart disease should be moderated by an awareness of the higher recurrence risks found in recent studies. This important paper deserves to be studied in depth by all who counsel patients on the risk of recurrence of congenital heart disease.

In an important paper, Uzark *et al* address a much-neglected aspect of care of patients with congenital heart disease [4]. They studied the preventive health care offered to 215 children with heart disease and compared it with that offered to 284 control children without known chronic illness. Immunizations were incomplete in a surprising 32.7% of the heart disease group, compared with only 2.5% of the control group ($P<0.0001$). Also, 29% of children over 3 years with heart disease had not received routine dental care within the past year, compared with 23.4% of controls (this difference was not statistically significant). It is also surprising that parents of the children with heart disease paid less 'out-of-pocket' money for health care than did parents of the control group. It is concluded that important aspects of primary health care are neglected — at least in Michigan — in a large group of children with heart disease. All those who treat such children elsewhere should study the proposed educational program suggested for improving care by both professionals and parents.

In China and Russia at present it is tacitly understood that neonates will not consume national resources for correction of congenital heart disease. Should a degree of 'selection' also take place in the West and, if so, how is the selection to be made? Watson *et al* [5] provide some of the data that must be debated in the determination of these issues. The group at the Children's Hospital National Medical Center, Washington, DC analysed a cohort of 220 infants undergoing first operation below the age of 4 months from January 1979 to December 1983. In total, 256 operations were performed, which comprised 19% of all cardiac surgical procedures during the study period. Operations were considered primary (229) or non-primary (36); 97 were open procedures. Forty-three patients died, 18 after open procedures. Complete follow-up was obtained for 142 long-term survivors, and status was found to be normal in only 29%. The average difference in cost for a survivor (80 000 1984 US dollars) was not significantly different from a non-survivor (57 000 1984 US dollars). Although still not statistically significant, the cost of a survivor with abnormal function was almost 50% higher than that for a 'normal' survivor. The only pre-operative variable found to correlate with higher total cost was the length of pre-operative hospitalization. When cost of non-survivors was distributed across the group, the effective hospital cost per survivor was 110 000 1984 US dollars. The authors provide a thoughtful analysis that should be studied in detail by all concerned with Pediatric Cardiology. They falter only when they fail to address their own provocative question — are such operations worthwhile?

Several recent studies have demonstrated the role of gated magnetic resonance imaging in defining intracardiac anatomy. This technique should be ideal for distinguishing the abnormal anatomy found in congenitally malformed hearts. The San Francisco group [6] studied 22 patients, aged from 2 months to 75 years, with congenital cardiac lesions, aged from 2 months to 75 years, and 16 adult control volunteers. The images produced are convincing, but their value is dissipated by the use of confusing terminology. For example, Fig. 2 illustrates the aorta to be anterior and to the left of the pulmonary trunk; it also shows a right-sided right ventricle. The patient is said to have 'uncorrected L-transposition': does this mean surgically or congenitally uncorrected? Confusion is compounded by the table, where the only patient with 'L-transposition' is said to have a single ventricle with a rudimentary right ventricle (another contradiction in terms) and a small pulmonary trunk; this is not the patient shown in Fig. 2. This article underlines the need for the use of sensible terminology in congenital heart disease, although deficiencies in description should not detract from the potential of this technique for demonstrating cardiac anatomy. The illustrations in this paper are superb and have been oriented in a way that is easy to understand.

The problem of autoimmunity in the pathogenesis of congenitally complete heart block is assessed by two groups of workers [7,8]. Reed *et al* demonstrated the strong correlation between the presence of SS-A/Ro autoantibodies and congenitally complete heart block [7]. It is becoming increasingly clear that the commonest type of congenitally complete heart block is indeed related to transplacental passage of maternal SS-A/Ro antibodies. Bergfeldt *et al* [8] conducted an electrophysiologic study of 12 patients with complete heart block and HLA B27 associated disease. This study shows that the atrioventricular block seems to be located preferentially in the atrioventricular node, although the conduction system could be widely affected.

Baker *et al* used oximetry along with a first-pass radionuclide technique to measure the ratio of pulmonary to systemic flow in 100 children with suspected left-to-right shunts [9]. A good overall correlation between the two methods was observed, but it was found to be stronger for shunts at the ventricular than at the atrial level. These findings imply that, in patients with atrial shunts, the inaccuracy lies in the oximetric method — presumably a consequence of estimating mixed venous oxygen saturation under these circumstances.

Garson *et al* used amiodarone to treat 39 young patients with a variety of arrhythmias, most of which were associated with organic heart disease [10]. Patients' ages ranged from 6 weeks to 30 years; nine were under 2 years. The mean daily dose was 8.2 mg/kg (range, 2.5–21.6). Arrhythmia was abolished in 15 of 16 patients with atrial flutter, 11 of 14 with ventricular tachycardia, and 5 of 9 with supraventricular tachycardia. No side-effects occurred in patients under 10 years of age. Of the older patients, seven had symptomatic side-effects: rash ($n=3$), headache ($n=2$), nausea ($n=1$), and neuropathy ($n=1$). As has been noted previously, corneal microdeposits seem to be a less frequent occurrence in children; these developed in seven, but disappeared after the drug had been discontinued. Three patients who developed bradycardia required pacemaker implantation. Serum thyroxine and reverse tri-iodothyronine were increased. Amiodarone was judged to be highly effective in this resistant group, but although the side-effects observed were comparatively mild, the long-term effects of the drug are not known.

Congenital stenosis of all the pulmonary veins is a rare condition. Bini *et al* [11] found 38 cases in the literature and 10 patients with the lesion in the experience of the University of Alabama — the largest reported series to date. There was a striking similarity in the history of all but one of the patients: failure to thrive and increasingly severe dyspnea and subcostal retraction to a point where medical advice was sought. The diagnosis was suspected clinically in 6, and discovered at autopsy in two. In the outstanding case, the lesion was discovered unexpectedly at catheterization. At catheterization, all patients had an abnormal pulmonary wedge pressure, although specific details varied. Surgery was attempted in the eight patients in whom the diagnosis was made in life, and five survived the operation. These cases underwent rapid and progressive restenosis over several months and all died eventually, three after a second operation. In all cases, the stenosis afflicted all four of the pulmonary veins, mainly at their junction with the left atrium. Obstruction of one or two veins is compatible with life and may go undetected, but stenosis of all four veins seems fatal. There is no medical treatment. Balloon dilatation has been attempted with some success, but this has always been followed by restenosis (*Am J Cardiol* 1981; **48**: 585–9; *Am J Cardiol* 1982; **49**: 1767–70). Various surgical techniques were tried, but none had long-term success. The only reports of successful surgery have been in older patients and, in the authors' opinion, when only one or two veins have been involved. The elegant pathologic studies performed hold out little hope for any improvement in treatment.

Much has been learnt recently concerning the nature of atrioventricular valve atresia. This lesion can be produced either because there is a formed but imperforate valve membrane between the afflicted atrium and an underlying ventricle, or because the connection between atrium and ventricular mass is completely lacking. In the latter case there is no macroscopic evidence of the existence of the atrioventricular connection. The study by the Leiden workers [12] has enlarged our knowledge of the development of valve atresia by studying mitral atresia in 30 hearts using the light microscope. The authors were able to show a fibrous connection between atrial floor and ventricular roof with the light microscope, even when there was no gross evidence of a connection between the left atrium and the underlying left ventricle. In other words, the connection was present during early development but subsequently regressed. As the authors state, these latter cases, with only microscopic evidence of a connection, can be classified practically as absence of the left atrioventricular connection.

There were some workers sceptical of the incidence of tracheal compression due to an anomalous origin of the brachiocephalic (innominate) artery when the condition was highlighted by Rowe and co-workers at Johns Hopkins. The paper from the Munich group [13] attests to the problems the condition can produce and to the excellent results produced by surgically suspending the artery from the sternum ('innominate arteriopexy'). Compression of the trachea was seen in 18 patients. Six patients who underwent surgery all had apneic attacks and severe tracheal stenosis, as revealed by tracheoscopy. Arteriopexy relieved symptoms in all those undergoing operation.

The final paper in this section [14] demonstrates the increasing sensitivity of cross-sectional echocardiographic machines and also the fact that you see what you are looking for. The authors observed 'false tendons' spanning the left ventricle in 0.8% of 3847 consecutive cross-sectional echocardiograms. What is interesting is that they observed 9 in 1981, 16 in 1982, and 5 in the first quarter of 1983. These 'false tendons' have previously been observed by pathologists, and are known as 'telegraph wires'. In this echo series, all except one extended from a papillary muscle to the ventricular septum. They are almost certainly comparable with the false tendons seen in animal hearts with considerable frequency, which are known to be ramifications of the left bundle branch. Another interesting observation here is the association between these tendons and a Still's murmur. These structures are probably even more common than the authors suggest; however, as far as is known, they are of no functional significance.

3. Valve Disease

MITRAL VALVE PROLAPSE

[1] Mitral valve prolapse. Disease or illness?
Retchin SM, Fletcher RH, Earp JA, Lamson N, Waugh RA, Univ North Carolina, Chapel Hill, NC, USA.
Arch Intern Med 1986; **146**: 1081–4.
[2] Relation between clinical features of the mitral prolapse syndrome and echocardiographically documented mitral valve prolapse.
Devereux RB, Kramer-Fox R, Brown WT, New York Hosp-Cornell Med Cent, New York, NY, USA.
J Am Coll Cardiol 1986; **6**: 763–72.
[3] Echocardiographically documented mitral-valve prolapse. Long-term follow-up of 237 patients.
Nishimura RA, McGoon Md, Shub C, Miller FA, Ilstrup DM, Tajik AJ, Mayo Clin and Mayo Found, Rochester, MN, USA.
N Engl J Med 1985; **313**: 1305–9.
[4] Mitral valve prolapse and cerebral ischemic events in young patients.
Jackson AC, Boughner DR, Barnett HJM, Univ Hosp, London, Ont, Canada.
Neurology (Cleveland) 1984; **34**: 784–7.

Comment. Many of the symptoms ascribed to mitral-valve prolapse are common in the general population, and there is a strong suspicion that attribution of these symptoms to the valvular abnormality is a result of the assessment of highly selected patients without a comparable control group. In a study by Retchin *et al* [1], symptoms and functional impairment were assessed in 274 patients; all had been referred for echocardiography with the suspicion of mitral-valve prolapse, and they were grouped according to whether or not the diagnosis was sustained. After 14–36 months, 158 patients were re-assessed and although they were not very well there was no correlation between the presence or absence of mitral valve prolapse with disability, health-care utilization or symptoms.

Devereux *et al* [2] describe an ingenious attempt to establish what clinical features can correctly be ascribed to mitral valve prolapse. Eighty-eight patients with echocardiographically documented prolapse were compared with 81 first-degree relatives with prolapse and 172 first-degree relatives and 60 spouses without prolapse. (The point being that symptoms wrongly thought to be attributable to mitral valve prolapse could result in clinical suspicion of the diagnosis and, therefore, in its detection even though it is not responsible for the symptoms.) Comparison of the relatives with and without prolapse demonstrated true associations between the prolapse and clicks, murmurs or both, thoracic bony abnormalities, low systolic blood pressure and bodyweight, and palpitation, whereas a comparison of those with prolapse with normal relatives and spouses showed no association with chest pain, dyspnea, panic attacks, anxiety or repolarization abnormalities on the electrocardiogram.

Nishimura *et al* [3] determined the long-term prognosis of patients with mitral-valve prolapse that had been documented by echocardiography: 237 minimally symptomatic or asymptomatic patients were followed for a mean of 6.2 years. It was found that the actuarial probability of survival at eight years for these patients was not significantly different to that of a matched control population. The best echocardiographic predictor of subsequent need for mitral-valve replacement was an initial left ventricular diastolic dimension >60 mm. Most patients had a benign course, but a subset of patients with redundant mitral-valve leaflets was identified who are at high risk of the development of progressive mitral regurgitation, sudden death, cerebral embolic events or infective endocarditis.

The association between mitral valve prolapse and cerebral ischemic events in patients under the age of 45 years is well known, but the prognosis subsequent to such an occurrence is not. Thirty-two patients (19 men and 13 women) were followed up by Jackson *et al* [4] for an average of eight years after the initial ischemic attack which, for 75% of them, was a stroke. Average follow-up from the time of diagnosis of mitral prolapse-associated ischemia was four years; during this period, only 16% of patients suffered recurrences, and in none of them did the recurrence result in a new permanent neurologic deficit; 63% of patients were taking either 'antiplatelet' or anticoagulant therapy at the time of follow-up. Thus, the prognosis appears to be favorable, although whether it is influenced by treatment cannot be determined.

AORTIC VALVULOPLASTY

[1] Balloon dilatation of calcific aortic stenosis in elderly patients: postmortem, intraoperative, and percutaneous valvuloplasty studies.
Mckay RG, Safian RD, Lock JE *et al*, Beth Israel Hosp, Boston, MA, USA.
Circulation 1986; **74**: 119–25.

[2] Treatment of calcific aortic stenosis by balloon valvuloplasty.
Isner JM, Salem DN, Desnoyers MR *et al*, Tufts-New England Med Cent, Boston, MA, USA.
Am J Cardiol 1987; **59**: 313–7.

[3] Transluminal balloon catheter aortic valvuloplasty: a new therapeutic option in aortic stenosis in the elderly patient.
Cribier A, Savin T, Saoudi N *et al*, Hop Charles Nicolle, Rouen, France.
Arch Mal Coeur 1986; **79**: 1678–86.

[4] Inoperable aortic stenosis in the elderly: benefit from percutaneous transluminal valvuloplasty.
Jackson G, Thomas S, Monaghan M, Forsyth A, Jewitt D, King's Coll Hosp, London, UK.
Br Med J 1987; **294**: 83–6.

[5] Assessment of left ventricular and aortic valve function after aortic balloon valvuloplasty in adult patients with critical aortic stenosis.
McKay RG, Safian RD, Lock JE *et al*, Beth Israel Hosp, Boston, MA, USA.
Circulation 1987; **75**: 192–203.

Comment. Several centers have reported their experience of aortic balloon valvuloplasty, but, despite the excellent results in some patients, most groups emphasize the palliative nature of the procedure and suggest that the overall results cannot compete with those obtained following valve replacement in any but the most frail and elderly patients.

A study by McKay and colleagues [1] is of considerable interest to those familiar with the morbid anatomy of calcific aortic stenosis and who may have greeted the first reports of successful balloon dilatation with some incredulity. Dilatation was carried out on five valves at post-mortem, preliminary to aortic valve replacement on a further five, and percutaneously in two elderly patients. In all the valves that could be inspected, the procedure resulted in increased mobility of the leaflets. Partial or complete separation of the leaflets occurred in the three valves with pre-operative commissural fusion, and fracture of calcified leaflets was seen in two cases with heavy nodular calcification. In no instances were the valve leaflets torn, the annulus disrupted or valvular debris released.

In two separate reports of balloon valvuloplasty for calcific aortic stenosis in elderly patients [2,3], the results obtained were similar to those achieved by other groups. Isner *et al* [2] operated on nine patients, in whom the mean aortic valve area was increased from 0.42 ± 0.04 to $0.81 \pm 0.06 \, cm^2$. The procedure was totally unsuccessful in only one patient. Valvuloplasty did not create significant aortic regurgitation in any of the nine patients, but it was complicated by one cerebral embolism. In a large series of 44 patients [3] whose average age was 77 years, valve area increased from 0.5 ± 0.18 to $1.0 \pm 0.42 \, cm^2$, and the mean gradient after dilatation was <40 mmHg in 37 cases. In-hospital mortality was 4.6% (two patients), and all but four survivors experienced useful symptomatic improvement.

In a further report, by Jackson and colleagues [4], elderly patients with severe calcific aortic stenosis, who were considered to be unsuitable for valve replacement, were treated by percutaneous transluminal valvuloplasty. One patient died 4 hours after the procedure. All four who presented with heart failure improved immediately and remained well 6 months later, the patient who presented with angina was symptom free at 9 months, and two of the three patients who presented in cardiogenic shock showed an immediate improvement which was maintained over 3 and 9 months of follow-up. Although the authors were very cautious in their claims for the new technique, the paper provoked letters from cardiac surgeons pointing out that the quoted figures for operative mortality were misleading and emphasizing the incomparably better hemodynamic results after valve replacement (*Br Med J* 1987; **94**: 510). Another letter described treatment by valvuloplasty in a District General Hospital (*Br Med J* 1987; **294**: 510). It is clear that, at present, the technique should be applied only to patients in whom the risk of valve replacement would be extremely high.

McKay *et al* [5] report on their detailed hemodynamic study of 32 patients (mean age 79 years) undergoing balloon dilatation for severe calcific aortic stenosis. The mean peak-to-peak aortic valve gradient was reduced from 77 ± 27 to 39 ± 15 mmHg, cardiac output increased from 4.6 ± 1.4 to 5.2 ± 1.8 litres/minute and mean calculated valve are increased from 0.6 ± 0.2 to $0.9 \pm 0.3 \, cm^2$. Patients with depressed left ventricular ejection fraction showed a slight improvement, and there was an overall decrease in left ventricular end-diastolic volume index. However, these mean values reflect a wide range of response, from that of little change to dramatic improvement. There were no embolic complications, and valvular regurgitation increased only slightly.

MITRAL VALVULOPLASTY

[1] In vitro analysis of mechanisms of balloon valvuloplasty of stenotic mitral valves.
Kaplan JD, Isner JM, Karas RH et al, Tufts-New England Med Cent, Boston, MA, USA.
Am J Cardiol 1987; 59: 318–23.
[2] Percutaneous catheter commissurotomy in rheumatic mitral stenosis.
Lock JE, Khalilullah M, Shrivastava S, Bahl V, Keane JF, Children's Hosp, Boston, MA, USA.
N Engl J Med 1985; 313: 1515–8.
[3] Percutaneous double-balloon mitral valvotomy for rheumatic mitral-valve stenosis.
Al Zaibag M, Ribeiro P, Al Kassab S, Al Fagih MR, Riyadh Military Hosp, Riyadh, Kingdom of Saudi Arabia.
Lancet 1986, i: 757–61.

Comment. The mechanism by which balloon valvuloplasty can relieve mitral stenosis was examined by dilatation of 15 valves, which had been excised intact at the time of mitral valve replacement from patients who had at most grade 2–4 mitral regurgitation [1]. Balloon inflation caused a mean increase in valve area of 185% (range 34–407%) and the valves split through their commissures, even in the presence of heavy calcification. There was no gross evidence of detachment of tissue fragments. These findings indicate that balloon valvuloplasty operates by a similar mechanism to standard surgical valvotomy, and suggest that indications for the technique could be expanded to include relatively immobile, and even calcified, stenotic mitral valves in adult patients.

Lock and colleagues report the results of percutaneous balloon mitral commissurotomy carried out in 8 children and young adults with rheumatic mitral stenosis [2]. The valvuloplasty balloon was positioned across the mitral orifice over a guidewire, which had previously been inserted transseptally by means of a balloon flotation catheter into the aorta. An immediate fall in the pressure gradient occurred, with an increase in cardiac output and an increase in mitral-valve area from a mean value of 0.73–1.34 cm^2/m^2. Minimal mitral regurgitation was produced in one child, and at follow-up catheterization between 2 and 8 weeks later the hemodynamic benefit was found to have persisted, although partial restenosis had occurred in one patient.

Al Zaibag et al describe a development of the technique of percutaneous balloon mitral valvotomy, in which two balloons are used instead of one [3]. The balloons are positioned across the mitral orifice through two separate septal punctures, thus avoiding the need to create a rather large atrial septal defect to accommodate the bigger single balloon catheter. A further advantage over the single-balloon technique is that when the two balloons are inflated side by side, the resulting 'figure of eight' section should not totally occlude the valve, thus avoiding complete circulatory obstruction. Nine young patients (average age 25) with severely stenotic, mobile valves were treated. The technique failed in the first two because the balloons were too small, but excellent results were achieved in the others with virtual abolition of the mitral-valve gradient, both acutely and at six-week follow-up.

NUTRITIONAL STATUS

Should nutritional status be assessed routinely prior to cardiac operation?
Abel RM, Fisch D, Horowitz J, van Gelder HM, Grossman ML, Newark Beth Israel Med Cent, NJ, USA.
J Thorac Cardiovasc Surg 1983; **85**: 752-7.

Comment. There is increasing evidence that structural and functional impairment of the myocardium may result from protein-calorie malnutrition. However, in a well-conducted study on 100 consecutive patients undergoing cardiac operations, Abel *et al* failed to produce any specific markers of nutritional status that correlated significantly with the morbidity and mortality in the population. This is in marked contrast to similar studies performed (mainly) in Great Britain. Much of this discrepancy is explained by the different populations investigated, those in the USA being principally ischemic whereas those in the UK are mainly valvar. Reports from the UK still found a relationship in ischemic patients, but this was less pronounced than in valvar patients.

MECHANICAL VALVES

[1] Performance characteristics of the Starr-Edwards Model 1260 aortic valve prosthesis beyond ten years.
Miller DC, Oyer PE, Mitchell RS *et al*, Stanford Univ Sch Med, Stanford, CA, USA.
J Thorac Cardiovasc Surg 1984; **88**: 193-207.
[2] Late results after mitral valve replacement with Bjork-Shiley and porcine prostheses.
Marshall WG, Kouchoukos NT, Karp RB, Williams JB, Univ Alabama Med Cent, Birmingham, AL, USA.
J Thorac Cardiovasc Surg 1983; **85**: 902-10.
[3] Thrombotic obstruction of the Bjork-Shiley valve: the Glasgow experience.
Ryder SJ, Bradley H, Brannan JJ, Turner MA, Bain WH, Western Infirm, Glasgow, UK.
Thorax 1984; **39**: 487-92.
[4] A prospective evaluation of the Bjork-Shiley, Hancock, and Carpentier-Edwards heart valve prostheses.
Bloomfield P, Kitchin AH, Wheatley PR, Lutz W, Miller HC, Royal Infirm, Edinburgh, UK.
Circulation 1986; **73**: 1213-22.
[5] Long-term follow-up of the Ionescu-Shiley mitral pericardial xenograft.
Gabbay S, Bortolotti U, Wasserman F, Tindel N, Factor SM, Frater RWM, Albert Einstein Coll Med, Bronx, NY, USA.
J Thorac Cardiovasc Surg 1984; **88**: 758-63.

Comment. The results of the valve with the longest life-history are reported by Miller *et al* [1], who outline the performance characteristics of the Starr-Edwards non-cloth-covered silicone ball (Model 1260) aortic-valve prosthesis in a large sequential series of 449 patients. The long-term function of this valve was analyzed over a total of 2896 patient-years of follow-up, which extended beyond 13 years. Valve-related complications expressed in actuarial [%($\pm$SEM) free at 10 years] and linearized (%/

patient-year) terms, respectively, were found to have occurred at the following rates: thromboembolism, 76 ±3 and 2.7; anticoagulant-related hemorrhage, 74 ±3 and 3.1; prosthetic-valve endocarditis, 92 ±2 and 0.9; reoperation, 90 ±2 and 1.1; valve failure, 82 ±2 and 2.2; all valve-related morbidity and mortality, 51 ±3 and 6.0; and valve-related death, 88 ±2 and 1.3. Thirteen per cent of hospital and 18% of late deaths were due to valve-related causes; 12% ±2% of patients had died of valve-related complications by 10 years, and fully 49% ±3% had had some form of serious valve-related complication. No case of structural failure was documented. Thus, the prosthesis has been shown to have a good structural durability record up to 13 years, and its long-term performance is satisfactory. This study will undoubtedly become the standard against which the performance characteristics of the newer valves will be measured.

In a retrospective evaluation of isolated mitral-valve replacement in 357 patients receiving Bjork-Shiley disc prostheses and 96 receiving xenografts (Vascor or Carpentier-Edwards) between 1973 and 1978 in Birmingham, Alabama [2], the groups were comparable in all respects except for follow-up, which was a median of 46 months in the former group and 32 months in the latter. Five-year patient survival was 70% and 68%, respectively; 77% of the disc-valve patients and 78% of the xenograft patients were free of thromboembolism. All of the disc-valve patients and 14 of the 96 xenograft patients received long-term anticoagulation; 56% of disc-valve patients and 49% of xenograft patients were alive and free of thromboembolism, complications related to anticoagulant therapy or other valve-related complications at the time of the report. The claims of xenograft superiority therefore have not been substantiated in this series. However, Ryder et al [3] report on the incidence of thrombotic obstruction of the Bjork-Shiley valve in a series of 900 patients in whom 1186 valves were implanted between 1971 and 1982. Ninety-three of the patients died in hospital; the remaining 807 were considered at risk of developing thrombotic complications and were followed for 4146 patient-years. The authors calculated the incidence of thrombotic complications at 0.46 per 100 patient-years for all valve positions, 0.79 for single mitral-valve replacement and 0.18 for aortic-valve replacement. The maximum possible incidence of the complication in this population was calculated to be 1.4 per 100 patient-years. The authors identified the following risk factors: inadequate anticoagulation control, poor preoperative exercise capacity and the implantation of an inappropriately small prosthesis. As this series covers the period 1971–1982, it does not encompass the recent design and fracture problems seen in Bjork-Shiley valves. The results are chiefly those of one surgeon, and they are superior to many other reports on mechanical-valve embolizations. It is possible that this group of patients was more compliant with anticoagulant control.

In a similar study from Edinburgh [4], 540 patients who underwent valve replacement between 1975 and 1979 were entered into a randomised trail to receive either a Bjork-Shiley valve ($n = 273$) or a porcine heterograft prosthesis (Hancock valve in 107 patients and a Carpentier-Edwards in 160). Two hundred and sixty-two patients underwent mitral-valve replacement, 210 aortic-valve replacement and 60 mitral and aortic-valve replacement. Eight patients underwent associated tricuspid-valve replacement. Hospital mortality was not found to be significantly different among patients receiving the three prostheses for aortic-valve replacement (7.6% overall), and mitral and aortic-valve replacement (10% overall); however, patients undergoing mitral-valve replacement with the Carpentier-Edwards bioprosthesis had a higher hospital mortality (15.5 *vs* 8.8% overall, $P=0.03$). This difference could not be explained by any of the 34 pre-operative and operative variables analysed. Median follow-up was 5.6 (range 2.8–8.3) years. At seven years, actuarial survival for patients undergoing mitral-valve replacement was 56.7 ±7.0%, for those undergoing aortic-valve replacement it was 69.6 ±9.6% and for those undergoing combined mitral and aortic-valve replacement it was 62.5 ±20.0% (not significant). Reoperation for valve failure was undertaken in 37 patients; no significant difference was found among the three different valves. Eleven patients died at reoperation, giving an overall reoperative mortality of 29.7%. Up to seven years following surgery, no significant difference could be found in the incidence of thrombo-embolism between patients with different prostheses undergoing mitral or aortic-valve replacement. Moreover, the authors were unable to demonstrate a significant beneficial effect of anticoagulant therapy in patients undergoing mitral or aortic-valve replacement with porcine prostheses, but patients had not been randomly allocated to such treatment. All patients who received a mechanical valve were given anticoagulant therapy. After multivariate analysis of the factors associated with embolism, atrial fibrillation was found to be linked with mitral-valve replacement ($P<0.001$) and an age of <65 years and a rheumatic cause of valvular disease were found to be linked with aortic-valve replacement (both $P<0.01$). The risks of anticoagulant therapy were found to be low, with an overall incidence of complications of about one for every 100 years of treatment. Further follow-up will be conducted because important differences may yet emerge among the three valves.

The report by Gabbay *et al* [5], on the second-generation Ionescu-Shiley valve implanted in the mitral position, is disturbing. The results are at variance with those previously reported from series in the UK. Of 40 patients who underwent mitral-valve replacement with an Ionescu-Shiley pericardial xenograft from 1977 to 1980, seven experienced valve failure. This degree of dysfunction prompted the authors to follow-up the remaining patients. At six years postoperatively, there was an actuarial survival rate of 72%, an actuarial probability of being free of embolism of only 62%, and a freedom from prosthetic failure of 60%. Explanted valves showed a complete absence of the neo–endothelial lining of the Dacron-covered frame and lesions which resembled those observed when the xenografts were placed in the fatigue tester after a mean of $29 \pm 17 \times 10^{6}$ cycles. The discrepancies between this series and those from the UK are difficult to explain. However, this paper should alert physicians caring for patients with implanted pericardial valves to some potential problems.

MISCELLANEOUS

[1] Factors influencing postoperative survival in aortic regurgitation. Analysis by Cox regression model.
Louagie Y, Brohet C, Robert A *et al*, Univ Louvain, Brussels, Belgium.
J Thorac Cardiovasc Surg 1984; 88: 225-33.

[2] The risk of thromboembolism and hemorrhage following mitral valve replacement. A comparative analysis between the porcine xenograft valve and Ionescu-Shiley bovine pericardial valve.
Gonzalez-Lavin L, Tandon AP, Chi S *et al*, Palo Alto Med Clin, Palo Alto, CA, USA.
J Thorac Cardiovasc Surg 1984; **87**: 340–51.

[3] The place of repair procedures for rheumatic mitral valve disease.
Girinath MR, Southern Railway Headquarters Hosp, Madras, India.
Indian Heart J 1983; **35**: 147–8.

[4] Closed mitral valvotomy: early results and long-term follow-up of 3724 consecutive patients.
John S, Bashi VV, Jairaj PS *et al*, Christian Med Coll Hosp, Vellore, India.
Circulation 1983; **68**: 891–6.

Comment. The preoperative catheterization data obtained from 103 of 114 patients who underwent aortic-valve replacement for severe aortic regurgitation at the University of Louvain from 1965 to 1981 were analyzed [1]. The authors were able to follow 98% of the survivors. They found long-term survival to be significantly different between patients in preoperative functional class I-II and those in class III-IV ($P<0.03$); those with a preoperative cardiothoracic ratio <0.64 *vs* >0.64 ($P<0.001$); and those with a preoperative ejection fraction >0.50 *vs* <0.50 ($P<0.03$). The authors performed a multifactorial analysis to identify the dominant preoperative prognostic variables affecting survival. Three of the 13 parameters examined simultaneously were found to influence survival rates independently: cardiothoracic ratio ($P = 0.001$), strain pattern on the electrocardiogram ($P = 0.072$) and left-ventricular end-systolic pressure ($P = 0.127$). After stratification of the population into two groups according to preoperative functional class, the predictive variables were found to be cardiothoracic ratio ($P = 0.014$), strain pattern ($P = 0.05$) and acute/chronic form of aortic regurgitation ($P = 0.034$).

The authors then used this statistical analysis to derive a mathematical equation for predicting a patient's probability of survival, and found a close fit between the predicted and the observed survival rates. It is the generation of this mathematical model, which appears very accurate in predicting the postoperative survival of individual patients with severe aortic regurgitation, that makes this paper so important. It should be read by all cardiologists.

Two major causes of morbidity and mortality after successful mitral-valve replacement are thromboembolism and anticoagulant-related hemorrhage. Gonzalez-Lavin *et al* [2] performed a retrospective analysis of two groups of patients who had undergone mitral-valve replacement with a bioprosthesis in order to ascertain the risk of thromboembolism and anticoagulant-related hemorrhage. Two hundred and six patients underwent replacement with porcine xenograft valves. They were followed for 524.3 patient-years (mean, 30.5 months) and received long-term oral anticoagulation therapy (>8 weeks, mean 6 months). Three hundred and twenty-two patients underwent replacement with bovine pericardial valves. They were followed for 1106 patient-years (mean, 46.4 months) and received short-term anticoagulation therapy (6 weeks). There were thromboembolic events in the porcine bioprosthesis group of 4.6% per patient-year, and 0.63% in the bovine bioprosthesis group. There were bleeding episodes of 2.5% per patient-year in the porcine bioprosthesis group and 0.63% in the bovine bioprosthesis group. There were six deaths in the porcine bioprosthesis group (four as a result of thromboembolic events and two as a result of bleeding episodes) and none in the bovine group. The authors conclude that the low risk of thromboembolism with the bovine pericardial valve is due to its superior hydraulic characteristics. The use of this valve does not require long-term oral anticoagulation therapy, which reduces the risk of anticoagulant-related hemorrhage. If these results are substantiated, they will have far-reaching consequences.

It is easy for those living and working in Western industrialized societies to forget that in much of the world the ravages of rheumatic fever eclipse other forms of heart disease and can easily overwhelm the often-limited cardiologic services. An epidemiologic study from Taiwan (*Indian Heart J* 1983; **35**: 139–46) suggests that mortality from acute rheumatic fever and rheumatic heart disease is declining in parallel with socioeconomic development. For those already affected, conservative surgery of the mitral valve, even when dominantly regurgitant, can provide valuable palliation [3]. A report from Vellore, India [4], gives the results of closed mitral valvotomy in 3724 patients. This large series of operations was carried out between 1956 and 1980. Preoperative cardiac catheterization was carried out in only a minority. Nearly all of the patients were severely disabled (41.5% in class IV), and many were in an advanced state of malnutrition; most remarkably, the valve area estimated at operation was 0.5 cm^2 or less in over 80%. During the last 5 years the hospital mortality was 1.5%. Only 11 patients (0.3%) developed severe mitral regurgitation requiring valve replacement; postoperative systemic embolism, which occurred in less than 1%, was more frequent in patients with sinus rhythm who were not anticoagulated than in those with atrial fibrillation who were. Actuarial survival at 24 years was 84.2%, and 86% of the 15-year survivors had persisting symptomatic benefit from the operation. These excellent results attest to the value of closed valvotomy when carried out by experienced surgeons in correctly selected patients.

4. Endocardial, Myocardial and Pericardial Disease

HYPERTROPHIC CARDIOMYOPATHY

PATHOPHYSIOLOGY

[1] Intramural ("small vessel") coronary artery disease in hypertrophic cardiomyopathy.
Maron BJ, Wolfson JK, Epstein SE, Roberts WC, NHLBI, NIH, Bethesda, MD, USA.
J Am Coll Cardiol 1986; **8**: 545–57.

[2] Relation between left ventricular gradient and relative stroke volume ejected in early and late systole in hypertrophic cardiomyopathy. Assessment with radionuclide cineangiography.
Sugrue DD, McKenna WJ, Dickie S *et al*, Royal Postgrad Med Sch, London, UK.
Br Heart J 1984; **52**: 602–9.

[3] Septal myomectomy and mitral valve replacement for idiopathic hypertrophic subaortic stenosis: Short- and long-term follow-up.
Fighali S, Krajcer Z, Leachman RD, St Luke's Episcopal Hosp, Houston, TX, USA.
J Am Coll Cardiol 1984; **3**: 1127–34.

Comment. Patients with hypertrophic cardiomyopathy have a variety of clinical and morphological features, including angina pectoris or atypical chest pain, ECG abnormalities, myocardial fibrosis and abnormalities of coronary blood flow and lactate production during stress. In one study, Maron *et al* investigated the hypothesis that structural alterations in the intramural coronary arteries could be involved in the myocardial ischemia observed in many patients with hypertrophic cardiomyopathy [1]. Histological examination of left ventricular myocardium obtained at necropsy was undertaken in 48 patients with hypertrophic cardiomyopathy (who did not have atherosclerosis of the extramural coronary arteries) and in 68 subjects who had either a normal heart or acquired heart disease (control subjects). It was found that abnormal intramural coronary arteries were characterized by thickening of the vessel wall, due to the proliferation of medial or intimal components or both, and a decrease in the size of the lumen in the patients with hypertrophic cardiomyopathy; 40 (83%) had these abnormalities in the ventricular septum ($n=33$), the anterior left ventricular free wall ($n=20$) or the posterior free wall ($n=9$). Also, tissue sections with considerable myocardial fibrosis more frequently contained abnormal intramural coronary arteries than those with little or no fibrosis ($P<0.001$). The authors also discovered abnormal intramural coronary arteries in three of eight infants who died of hypertrophic cardiomyopathy before the age of one year. However, abnormal intramural coronary arteries could be identified in only six (9 %) of 68 controls; in comparison to those seen in the patients with hypertrophic cardiomyopathy, these arteries exhibited only mild thickening of the wall and minimal narrowing of the lumen. Also, abnormal arteries were found to be 20 times more frequent in patients with hypertrophic cardiomyopathy. These abnormal intramural coronary arteries, present in increased numbers in patients with hypertrophic cardiomyopathy, may represent a congenital component of the underlying pathophysiological process and may cause the myocardial ischemia observed, as suggested by their presence in areas of substantial myocardial fibrosis.

The significance of the pressure difference between the body and the outflow tract of the left ventricle in many patients with hypertrophic cardiomyopathy has been a source of controversy ever since the disease was first described. In a study from the Royal Postgraduate Medical School [2], left-ventricular time-activity curves (technetium-99m) were analyzed in 57 patients with hypertrophic cardiomyopathy, of whom 8 had a resting pressure difference of 30 mmHg or more, 18 a provokable gradient, and 31 neither. The results were compared with similar analyses in a control group of 18 normal subjects. The time-to-peak left-ventricular ejection was shorter, and the proportion of the stroke volume ejected in the first third, the first 50%, and the first 80% of systole was higher in patients than in controls, but there was no difference between the three patient groups, and the total duration of systole in patients and controls was similar.

These data do not support the hypothesis that gradients reflect obstruction to left-ventricular ejection (although it must be acknowledged that studies of the flow pattern in the aortic root have led to a different conclusion). Moreover, they can be used as a theoretical objection to the practice of left-ventricular myomectomy, which nevertheless does appear to alleviate symptoms in many patients [3]. The findings are also consistent with observations of no difference in clinical features or prognosis between patients with and without intraventricular pressure gradients.

ARRHYTHMIAS

[1] Amiodarone for long-term management of patients with hypertrophic cardiomyopathy.
McKenna WJ, Harris L, Rowland E et al, Royal Postgrad Med Sch, London, UK.
Am J Cardiol 1984; 54: 802–10.

[2] Improved survival with amiodarone in patients with hypertrophic cardiomyopathy and ventricular tachycardia.
McKenna WJ, Oakley CM, Krikler DM, Goodwin JF, Royal Postgrad Med Sch, London, UK.
Br Heart J 1985; 53: 412–6.

[3] Potentially lethal arrhythmias and their management in hypertrophic cardiomyopathy.
Frank MJ, Watkins LO, Prisant LM et al, Section of Cardiology, Med Coll Georgia, Augusta, GA, USA.
Am J Cardiol 1984; 53: 160–13.

Comment. The demonstration, by workers at the Royal Postgraduate Medical School and the National Institutes of Health[1,2] that patients with hypertrophic cardiomyopathy who have episodes of ventricular tachycardia on ambulatory electrocardiography are at high risk of dying suddenly, marked an important advance in our knowledge of the natural history of the disease. Three recent papers have addressed two important secondary questions: can survival be improved by antiarrhythmic therapy which suppresses the ventricular tachycardia? If so, how often should ambulatory electrocardiography be repeated for patients without ventricular tachycardia at initial assessment?

The most promising agent to investigate for effectiveness as prophylaxis against sudden death is undoubtedly amiodarone. Fifty-three patients with hypertrophic cardiomyopathy and a variety of tachyarrhythmias received amiodarone for a median period of 18 months [1]. Ventricular tachycardia was suppressed in 24 patients (92% of those with this arrhythmia) by a relatively modest dose of 100–400 mg/day, and none of the patients in this group died suddenly over a mean follow-up period of 27 months. (Moreover, amiodarone proved highly effective in suppressing symptomatic supraventricular tachycardias.) In a subsequent paper from the Royal Postgraduate Medical School, the results of amiodarone treatment in 21 out of 82 consecutive patients with hypertrophic cardiomyopathy in whom ventricular tachycardia was detected by 48-hour ambulatory monitoring (three or more consecutive ventricular extrasystoles at a rate of 120 beats/min or greater) were reported [2]. The three-year survival of these patients was compared with that in a retrospective control group comprising 86 patients, of whom 24 had had ventricular tachycardia and had received conventional antiarrhythmic drugs. The arrhythmia was suppressed in all the amiodarone-treated patients, and none died during follow-up, although there were two sudden deaths among the untreated patients whose ambulatory electrocardiograms had not shown ventricular tachycardia. In the control group, ventricular tachycardia had been suppressed in only 5 of the 24 patients, and 5 had died suddenly; 3 patients without the arrhythmia had also died.

These data provide compelling evidence of a protective influence of amiodarone for patients with ventricular tachycardia; unfortunately, they fall short of the proof which could be obtained only from a prospective, randomized, controlled trial.

The recommendation by Frank *et al* [3], that patients with hypertrophic cardiomyopathy should undergo annual Holter monitoring, seems to be justified by the results of their study of 50 patients who were followed up for 2–14 years. The incidence of conductive system disease (sick sinus syndrome or His-Purkinje disease) in 47 patients free of the condition at entry was 5% at 5 years and 33% at 10 years; for ventricular couplets or ventricular tachycardia, the corresponding incidences were 26% and 75%, and, for ventricular tachycardia only, 18% and 40%. Few of these arrhythmias, for the most part justifiably regarded by the authors as 'potentially lethal', were accompanied by new symptoms. All the patients were receiving large doses of beta-blocking drugs.

[1]McKenna WJ, England D, Doi YL *et al.*
Arrhythmias in hypertrophic cardiomyopathy. 1. Influence on prognosis.
Br Heart J 1981; **46:** 129–36.
[2] Maron BJ, Savage DD, Wolfson JK *et al.*
Prognostic significance of 24 hour ambulatory electrocardiographic monitoring of patients with hypertrophic cardiomyopathy: A prospective study.
Am J Cardiol 1981; **48:** 252–7.

DRUG THERAPY

[1] Effects of verapamil on haemodynamic function and myocardial metabolism in patients with hypertrophic cardiomyopathy
Wilmshurst PT, Thompson DS, Juul SM, Jenkins BS, Webb-Peploe MM, St Thomas' Hosp, London, UK.
Br Heart J 1986; **56**: 544–53.
[2] Does verapamil improve left ventricular relaxation in patients with myocardial hypertrophy?
Hess OM, Murakami T, Krayenbuehl HP, Univ Hosp, Zurich, Switzerland.
Circulation 1986; **74**: 530–43.
[3] Effects of long-term treatment with amiodarone on exercise hemodynamics and left ventricular relaxation in patients with hypertrophic cardiomyopathy.
Paulus WJ, Nellens P, Heyndrickx GR, Ziekenhus, Aalst, Belgium.
Circulation 1986; **74**: 544–54.

Comment. Although verapamil has been recommended for the treatment of patients with hypertrophic cardiomyopathy, the rationale for such a treatment regimen is not clear. This recommendation was based on results obtained in animal models of cardiomyopathy which have no proven relation to the human condition. Moreover, the earlier results showing that verapamil could have the potential to reverse left ventricular hypertrophy are in dispute. Verapamil has been claimed to improve symptoms and exercise tolerance in patients with hypertrophic cardiomyopathy despite results showing it does not improve systolic or diastolic left ventricular function, and a lack of information on the metabolic effects of this agent in this condition. Wilmshurst *et al* [1] studied the effects of an intravenous dose of verapamil (20 mg) over a range of heart rates in 12 patients with hypertrophic cardiomyopathy, six of whom had an appreciable left ventricular outflow tract gradient and six of whom did not. Verapamil was found to reduce myocardial oxygen consumption in proportion to a reduction in left ventricular pressure. However, verapamil's negative inotropic effect was found to be counteracted by its non-specific vasodilator activity, therefore cardiac index was not altered at any heart rate and consequently verapamil did not affect myocardial efficiency. Although some patients underwent an improvement in anaerobic myocardial metabolism after verapamil, an equal number had their lactate metabolism impaired. On the basis of clinical features, echocardiographic findings or hemodynamic variables measured before therapy with verapamil, the authors were unable to predict which patients would experience hemodynamic or metabolic improvement on treatment with verapamil.

In another study, by Hess *et al* [2], intravenous verapamil (1 mg/kg) was administered to 10 patients with hypertrophic cardiomyopathy and 13 with aortic stenosis; M-mode echocardiography and left ventricular measurements were performed simultaneously at rest and 10–15 minutes after drug administration. It was found that verapamil improved left ventricular relaxation in the patients with hypertrophic cardiomyopathy but it was decreased in the patients with aortic stenosis. As no changes were observed in the hemodynamic determinants of left ventricular relaxation, this indicates there was an intrinsic but opposite effect of verapamil on the myocardium of patients with primary and patients with secondary myocardial hypertrophy. It was thought that this beneficial effect of verapamil in the patients with hypertrophic cardiomyopathy was related to an improvement in relaxation and diastolic filling, as evidenced by the increase in cycle efficiency that occurred with a decrease in left ventricular asynchrony.

Amiodarone is commonly used in patients with hypertrophic cardiomyopathy and dysrhythmias. Paulus *et al* [3] administered oral amiodarone (600 mg daily for the first week, 400 mg daily second week, 200 mg daily afterwards) to patients with hypertrophic cardiomyopathy for five weeks. Measurements of rest-exercise hemodynamics ($n=9$) and echocardiographic relaxation indices ($n=11$) were made under control conditions and after treatment. In patients at rest, amiodarone caused a significant drop in heart rate ($P<0.05$) and a rise in mean pulmonary artery pressure and mean pulmonary capillary wedge pressure. Systemic arterial pressure, cardiac output and systemic vascular resistance were found to be unaltered by treatment with amiodarone. On serial supine bicycle stress testing, exercise tolerance was reduced in six of the nine patients. Both pulmonary capillary wedge pressure and mean pulmonary artery pressure rose at both the highest identical workloads and maximal symptom-limited workloads with amiodarone treatment, but at maximal exercise no significant differences were observed in heart rate, systemic arterial pressure, cardiac output and exercise factor. Echocardiography did not reveal any change in isovolumic relaxation time, end-diastolic posterior wall thickness and peak posterior wall thining rate after treatment. The authors postulate a negative inotropic action for amiodarone to explain the worsened rest and exercise hemodynamics observed in these patients. As relaxation indices did not alter despite an elevation in left ventricular filling pressure, it is possible that amiodarone has a deleterious effect on myocardial inactivation, whose mechanism of action may be similar to that seen in depressed myocardial inactivation in patients with hypothyroidism.

INHERITANCE

[1] Asymmetric septal hypertrophy and hypertrophic cardiomyopathy.
Emanuel R, Marcomichelakis J, Withers R, O'Brien K, Natl Heart Hosp, London, UK.
Br Heart J 1983; **49**: 309–16.

[2] Patterns of inheritance in hypertropic cardiomyopathy: Assessment by M-mode and two-dimensional echocardiography.
Maron BJ, Nichols PF III, Pickle LW, Wesley YE, Mulvihill JJ, NHLBI, NIH, Bethesda, MD, USA.
Am J Cardiol 1984; **53**: 1087–94.

Comment. Hypertrophic cardiomyopathy frequently affects more than one member of a family, and it is of considerable importance to determine the mode of inheritance so that genetic counselling can be given to patients with the disease.

Emanuel *et al* [1] studied the families of 19 patients with fully developed hypertrophic cardiomyopathy in which the disease was manifest in at least two successive generations and for whom first-degree relatives were available for investigation. In this familial form of the disease, isolated asymmetric septal hypertrophy — in which the echocardiographic ratio of septal to posterior left-ventricular wall thickness was equal to or greater than 1.3:1, in the absence of any other clinical, radiologic or elec-trocardiographic evidence of heart disease — had the same genetic implications as hypertrophic cardiomyopathy itself: a parent with hypertrophic cardiomyopathy could produce an offspring with either isolated asymmetric septal hypertrophy or clinical hypertrophic cardiomyopathy. The pattern of affected individuals was most consistent with inheritance through a dominant gene with variable penetrance.

In a study from the National Institutes of Health, Maron et al [2] examined 367 relatives in 70 families of patients with hypertrophic cardiomyopathy using M-mode and two-dimensional echocardiography. The disease appeared to be genetically transmitted in 39 and sporadic in 31, so that the study differs in an important way from that from the National Heart Hospital [1], in which only the familial form was studied. In 30 affected families, occurrence of the disease suggested autosomal-dominant inheritance, but overall analysis was not consistent with single-gene Mendelian transmission. As in the British study, the manifestations of the disease varied among affected members of the same family.

HYPERTROPHIC CARDIOMYOPATHY IN CHILDHOOD

[1] Development and progression of left ventricular hypertrophy in children with hyper-trophic cardiomyopathy.
Maron BJ, Spirito P, Wesley Y, Arce J, NHLBI, NIH, Bethesda, MD, USA.
N Engl J Med 1986; 315: 610–4.
[2] Hypertrophic cardiomyopathy: An important cause of sudden death.
McKenna WJ, Deanfield JE, Royal Postrgrad Med Sch, London, UK.
Arch Dis Child 1984; 59: 971–5.

Comment. Maron et al have continued their series of investigations into hypertrophic cardiomyopathy [1]. It is not known whether the magnitude and distribution of the left ventricular hypertrophy in patients with hypertrophic cardiomyopathy are established at birth, or whether they evolve during the first years of life. In some patients, marked left ventricular hypertrophy is present at or shortly after birth, whereas in others these changes have been detected during intra-uterine life. The results of this careful study show that the findings of hypertrophic cardiomyopathy are not always present and can appear or increase markedly during childhood and adolescence. Thirty-nine patients who met the criteria for hypertrophic car-diomyopathy were studied using cross-sectional echocardiography between 1979 and 1985. All patients were below the age of 15 years at initial echocardiographic evalua-tion and had been followed for at least two years. Seventeen of the patients were found to have substantial increases in the magnitude and overall distribution of left ven-tricular hypertrophy. In addition, five children who initially had morphologically normal hearts were found to develop hypertrophy over a period of 2–6 years. The latter findings are particularly significant; gross anatomical features of hypertrophic car-diomyopathy are not always present at birth. Therefore, a normal echocardiographic study in a young child genetically predisposed to hypertrophic cardiomyopathy does not absolutely exclude the diagnosis. The authors discuss the implications for genetic counselling: they recommend that, if hypertrophic cardiomyopathy is suspect in asymptomatic young children with a family history of the disease, subsequent echocardiograms should be obtained about every three years until the patients reach adulthood and have a mature body size.

McKenna and Deanfield describe a retrospective study of 37 patients in whom the diagnosis of hypertrophic cardiomyopathy was made during childhood (up to the age of 14 years) [2]. At the time of diagnosis, 19 patients were asymptomatic; the remaining 18 had the characteristic symptoms of chest pain, dyspnea or disturbance of consciousness. An additional 17 patients were excluded: they were diagnosed during the same period as a result of family screening of probands dying from the disease, and such individuals are known to have a poor prognosis. The average length of follow-up was nine years. During this period 18 patients died — 11 suddenly, of whom 4 had been asymptomatic.

A history of syncope and electrocardiographic evidence of right-ventricular hypertrophy were found to be significant markers of sudden death, although these data-derived associations should be accepted with some reservation because the use of standard statistical tests of significance for multiple subgroup analysis (18 variables were examined for their prognostic associations) is scientifically questionable, particularly in a retrospective study involving relatively small numbers. As ambulatory electrocardiographic monitoring was not carried out, it was not possible to ascertain whether serious ventricular arrhythmias reflect a poor prognosis — as is the case for adults. However, it is clear that the diagnosis of hypertrophic cardiomyopathy in childhood is accompanied by a high mortality.

INFECTIVE ENDOCARDITIS

INCIDENCE AND ETIOLOGY

[1] The teeth and infective endocarditis.
     Bayliss R, Clarke C, Oakley CM et al, BCS, MSSG, London, UK.
     Br Heart J 1983; **50**: 506–12.
[2] The microbiology and pathogenesis of infective endocarditis.
     Bayliss R, Clarke C, Oakley CM et al, MSSG, BCS, CDSC, London, UK.
     Br Heart J 1983; **50**: 513–9.
[3] The bowel, the genitourinary tract, and infective endocarditis.
     Bayliss R, Clarke C, Oakley CM et al, RCP Research Unit, BCS, CDSC, London, UK.
     Br Heart J 1984; **1**: 339–45.

Comment. The British Cardiac Society, the Medical Services Study Group of the Royal College of Physicians and the Communicable Diseases Surveillance Center attempted to obtain information on all cases of infective endocarditis occurring in the UK over a two-year period, by asking physicians to complete a simple questionnaire. Although it is apparent that reporting was incomplete, there is no reason to believe that it was unrepresentative in any way that might have distorted the conclusions.

Reports were obtained on 544 cases in 541 patients [1,2], indicating that there had been no major fall in the incidence of the disease since before the introduction of penicillin. This is explained by the disclosures that in over 40% of cases heart disease had not been suspected before the development of infection (32% had probably had normal hearts), and that while the mouth and pharynx were the most likely source of the commonest organism — *Streptococcus viridans* — only 13% had undergone any form of dental procedure within three months of the onset of infection. In 60% of cases, the portal of entry could not be ascertained. In other words, prophylaxis is being administered to only a small proportion of those at risk.

The aortic valve was the commonest site of infection; 17% of patients had undergone previous cardiac surgery, and 6% had had a previous episode of infective endocarditis. Mortality was 14% overall, and 30% for patients with staphylococcal infection. The authors recommend that antibiotic prophylaxis should still be given before dental procedures, but that more emphasis should be placed on the maintenance of good dental hygiene.

In a subsequent paper, the same authors give details of the 87 patients (out of 582) in whom the infecting agent was thought to have gained entry through the alimentary or genitourinary tracts [3]. In 75 cases, the organisms were normal bowel residents (most were *Streptococcus* spp.), and in 12 others the endocarditis was associated with disease, or with a wide variety of operations or investigations of the alimentary or genitourinary tracts. The average age of the patients was higher than that of the study group as a whole, and in 41% of them there was no knowledge or evidence of a pre-existing cardiac abnormality. In 40 of the 75 cases infected with bowel organisms, there was no apparent initiating event.

These findings emphasize the importance of giving antibiotic prophylaxis to patients with susceptible heart lesions scheduled for gastrointestinal or genitourinary surgery or instrumentation, although it is conceded that this does not provide infallible protection. A case could be made for this provision in older patients, even when the heart is thought to be normal (see also below).

ANTIBIOTIC PROPHYLAXIS

[1] Apparent failures of endocarditis prophylaxis. Analysis of 52 cases submitted to a national registry.
Durack DT, Kaplan EL, Bisno AL, Duke Univ Med Cent, Durham, NC, USA.
J Am Med Assoc 1983; **250**: 2318–22.

[2] Endocarditis prophylaxis for patients with mitral valve prolapse. A quantitative analysis.
Bor DH, Hummelstein DU, Harvard Med Sch, Boston, MA, USA.
Am J Med 1984; **76**: 711–7.

[3] Mitral valve prolapse and bacterial endocarditis: When is antibiotic prophylaxis necessary?
Hickey AJ, MacMahon SW, Wilcken DEL, Prince Henry Hosp, Sydney, Australia.
Am Heart J 1985; **109**: 431–4.

Comment. There has never been a clinical trial on the value of antibiotic prophylaxis for patients with endocarditis-susceptible cardiac lesions, so that its overall effectiveness, quite apart from its effectiveness in specific clinical circumstances, is unknown.

Even when prophylaxis is administered, it can fail. Durack and colleagues [1] published data, from a registry established by the American Heart Association, on 52 cases of endocarditis which occurred despite prophylactic treatment. Mitral valve prolapse was the most frequent underlying lesion (33% of cases); 19% of infections occurred on prosthetic valves; 48 cases (92%) occurred after dental procedures — a reflection presumably of the large number of patients undergoing dental treatment and the universal belief in its importance in the etiology of endocarditis; 39 cases (75%) were caused by *Streptococcus viridans*, and 7 (14%) by *Staphylococcus aureus*. Most of the patients received oral penicillin, but only six (12%) were on regimens recommended by the American Heart Association; 63% of patients for whom antibiotic sensitivities were available were infected with an organism susceptible to the prophylactic agent.

The value of prophylactic treatment for low-risk patients must be questioned. Bor and Hummelstein [2] attempted a risk-benefit analysis for patients with mitral valve prolapse, based on published data of the prevalence (of 6%-10%) of the condition, the projected incidence of fatal and non-fatal endocarditis if unprotected and the risk of fatal reactions to penicillin or erythromycin. They estimated that both no prophylaxis and penicillin prophylaxis might be expected to result in a similar number of deaths, whereas the equation of risk and benefit for erythromycin was in favor of prophylactic treatment.

In a slightly less speculative investigation from Australia, Hickey *et al* [3] conducted a case-control study of the association between mitral valve prolapse and infective endocarditis in 56 patients with endocarditis and 168 sex- and age-matched controls who had undergone echocardiography: 20% of patients and 4% of controls had evidence of mitral valve prolapse on echocardiogram, but an increased risk of endocarditis was confined to those who had had a pre-existing systolic murmur, which was present in 9 of 11 cases. The data indicate a relative risk of endocarditis of 5 for patients with mitral valve prolapse, although the attributable risk is very small — 11 cases/100 000 patients with mitral valve prolapse/year.

Overall, findings support the usual clinical practice, which is to recommend prophylactic treatment only for patients with a murmur of mitral regurgitation; they incidentally cast further doubt on the significance of 'echo-only' prolapse as anything more than a variation of normality in many subjects.

5. Heart Failure

CURRENT CONCEPTS IN CARDIAC FAILURE

Review: HENRY J. DARGIE

Clinical interest in heart failure has never been greater. No single reason for this can be identified but there is little doubt that a deeper understanding of the pathophysiology, a clearer definition of the structural pathology during life and the development of new therapeutic interventions have all contributed to the resuscitation of a previously falling interest in the failing heart.

In the 1970s, appreciation of the potential value of vasodilatation in improving cardiac function led to the adoption of a new philosophy of 'unloading' the heart. This was facilitated, if not stimulated, by the development of flow-directed cardiac catheters that allowed the measurement of right-heart and indirect left-heart pressures not only in the cardiac catheterization laboratory but also in the clinical laboratory and at the bedside. This development enabled the acute and chronic effects of vasodilators and other interventions to be described and quantified, and led to what might be termed the 'invasive period' in the approach to heart failure.

The next milestone was the recognition of the role played by neuroendocrine factors, leading to the tentative use of beta-blockers to obviate the harmful effects of excess adrenergic activity [1]. The angiotensin converting enzyme inhibitors then arrived, concentrating further interest on the neuroendocrine response, and redirecting attention to the kidney and its role in heart failure.

Although the chronic effects of treatment can be assessed by repeat cardiac catheterizations, the recent availability of an array of non-invasive techniques has facilitated both the definition of the underlying cause of heart failure and the long-term evaluation of its response to treatment. This might be termed the current 'non invasive' period. Moreover, long-term studies of medical treatment have led to speculation about the possibility that the poor survival [2] in patients with heart failure might be improved.

What is Heart Failure?

Heart failure is among the commonest of clinical diagnoses, yet it is a term that eludes precise definition. Sir Thomas Lewis deemed the heart to be failing when it could not supply sufficient oxygen for the needs of the metabolizing tissues [3]. However, most clinicians diagnose heart failure from a constellation of clinical factors that includes the typical symptoms of dyspnea and fatigue and the characteristic signs of fluid retention in the context of an acceptable history of heart disease. Modern diuretics have allowed the emergence of a large class of patients with 'heart failure' who may be edema free, have normal venous pressure and clear lung fields. This is analogous to, but not identical with, the situation preceding fluid retention in less advanced cardiac disease, when symptoms occur only during moderate or severe exercise when the cardiac output, which may be normal at rest, fails to rise appropriately.

A broad functional classification, such as that of the New York Heart Association which divides patients according to symptoms and activity, has been of some clinical value in assessing the severity of heart failure, especially when the classification has been made on the basis of exercise capacity measured objectively. However, the same apparent degree of intrinsic cardiac dysfunction may allow a patient to be in any of the classes from I to IV; apart from treatment, several factors including previous physical fitness, obesity and personality significantly affect symptoms and can add to uncertainty concerning the severity of the heart disease. A symptom-based functional classification is most useful when accompanied by information about the nature and degree of the underlying cardiac structural abnormality.

The causes of heart failure are well known but diverse. Anemia, thyrotoxicosis, Paget's disease and arteriovenous fistulae may all cause heart failure despite a high cardiac output. Nevertheless, these conditions, however interesting, are numerically insignificant compared with heart failure that is due to a low cardiac output associated with left-ventricular dysfunction secondary to ischemic heart disease, right-ventricular dysfunction secondary to lung disease or pressure or volume overload from valvar dysfunction.

Thus, heart failure is not a diagnosis in itself. An acceptable modern clinical description would be that situation when the heart is unable to deliver sufficient oxygen for the needs of the metabolizing tissues causing fatigue and/or dyspnea, possibly at rest but commonly on effort. This may be due to a cardiac pathology that should be identified and quantified either non-invasively or invasively. In the later stages it is associated with activation of a number of so-called 'compensatory' mechanisms directed at the maintenance of an adequate blood pressure and an effective blood volume. The main clinical consequences of this are tachycardia, fluid retention and peripheral vasoconstriction. This review will concentrate on those aspects of heart failure concerning physiologic mechanisms as applied to medical treatment in which most progress has been made recently; most attention will be focused on heart failure secondary to left-ventricular functional impairment.

Hemodynamic Considerations
Hemodynamically, cardiac function can be described in terms of the preload, afterload, myocardial contractility and the heart rate [4]. Preload, the extent of fibre stretch in diastole, is represented in the clinical setting by the end-diastolic volume which is determined by venous tone, the intravascular volume, ventricular compliance and the extent of ventricular systolic emptying. Although end-diastolic pressure and volume are not linearly related (pressure rising more steeply for any given increase in volume), the left-ventricular end-diastolic pressure or filling pressure nonetheless provides a useful clinical assessment of preload. In the absence of mitral valve disease, the left-ventricular end-diastolic pressure correlates well with the pulmonary capillary wedge pressure and usually with the pulmonary artery end-diastolic pressure. In simple clinical terms, an increase in left-ventricular preload may lead to pulmonary congestion and to the symptom of dyspnea.

Afterload, the left-ventricular wall stress that must be overcome for the contents to be ejected, is determined by a number of factors including the radius of the ventricle, its thickness and its pressure, and the arteriolar tone. Since preload affects the volume and, therefore, the radius of the ventricle, it also influences the afterload. For practical clinical purposes, systemic vascular resistance is the main contributor to the afterload and is used as an approximation for it. Systemic vascular resistance is calculated simply from a knowledge of the cardiac output (usually measured by thermodilution) and the systemic arterial and cardiac filling pressures. In heart failure, systemic vascular resistance increases in response to a number of vasoconstrictor stimuli that form part of the neuroendocrine response. In a ventricle with impaired contractility, this depresses the stroke volume much more than in a normal ventricle, emphasizing the importance of afterload not only in determining stroke volume but also as a mechanism worth modulating in efforts to increase it.

When myocardial contractility is impaired, stroke volume is maintained by an adaptive increase in end-diastolic volume which has been regarded, historically but probably simplistically, as the recruitment of the Frank–Starling mechanism. Sodium and water retention by the kidney facilitates this by increasing intravascular volume as does increased venous tone mediated mainly through the sympathetic nervous system. Both factors may be modulated by neuroendocrine mechanisms and the interaction of these and other factors have been well reviewed recently [5,6].

Non-Invasive Techniques
The wider availability of non-invasive cardiological techniques has led to increased diagnostic accuracy and has provided new ways not only of investigating the nature and severity of cardiac functional impairment but also of assessing its response to treatment.

Echocardiography, the least invasive of the non-invasive imaging techniques, is of immense value diagnostically. All three echocardiographic techniques, M-mode, cross-sectional or real-time and, more recently, Doppler are relevant to heart failure. M-mode echocardiography provides information on chamber dimensions and wall thickness from which echocardiographic ejection-phase indices, such as fractional shortening, may be calculated and left-ventricular mass determined. Using digitizing techniques, it is possible to derive information on rate of change of dimensions, which is particularly useful for defining abnormalities of diastolic function. Abnormalities of relaxation or diastolic function often coexist with systolic dysfunction, reminding us that cardiac output is as dependent on ventricular filling as on emptying [7]. Poor ventricular filling is typified by the restrictive and hypertrophic cardiomyopathies, but is also a prominent feature of acute myocardial ischemia [8]. How important these abnormalities of diastolic function are in determining cardiac output in the enlarged, poorly contracting ventricle that results from chronic coronary heart disease and is characteristic of dilated (congestive) cardiomyopathy is unknown at present, but the contractile or inotropic abnormalities seem dominant.

Ventricular volumes are more easily calculated and regional wall-motion abnormalities more readily identified from the cross-sectional echocardiogram which is also useful in standardizing the point at which end-diastolic and end-systolic dimensions are measured. In addition to assessing valvar stenosis or incompetence, Doppler provides information on the velocity of blood flow from which cardiac output may be estimated with reasonable accuracy, but it remains to be established conclusively whether these techniques can be used for quantitative, meaningful measurements.

From radionuclide ventriculography, data concerning ventricular shape and volume may be acquired more accurately and cardiac output estimated. But the most important information gained is the left-ventricular ejection fraction which has powerful prognostic significance [9], even though it reflects an average of several parameters.

Treadmill exercise remains a simple and safe method of determining the nature and severity of the limiting symptom in a given patient. Many protocols are available both for the assessment of ischemic heart disease and to determine exercise capacity [10].

Direct measurement of oxygen consumption provides objective data about oxygen delivery to the exercising muscles and, by inference, of the cardiac output during exercise. This technique brings the clinician closer to the physiology of heart failure, which is defined as an inadequate delivery of oxygen for the needs of the body. Oxygen consumption may be predicted from the heart -rate response but this is subject to considerable error. By simultaneously measuring CO_2 production, ventilation and oxygen consumption, the onset of anerobic respiration or the anerobic threshold can be determined with reasonable accuracy [11]; at this point the patient is exercising maximally. Quite clearly, this technique is very valuable in the initial assessment of the patient and in evaluating the response to treatment because exercise time, oxygen consumption and anerobic threshold are end-points that may have some bearing on the symptoms of tiredness and breathlessness. Moreover, functional limitation can be accurately determined leading to better patient classification [12].

Whether the limiting symptom in patients with poor left-ventricular function is fatigue or breathlessness may depend on the type of test. A 'fast' test may result in a higher value for oxygen consumption but a shorter exercise time than a 'slow' test when the patient usually stops because of leg or general fatigue [13].

Exercise testing is of particular importance in patients with ischemic heart disease because, in the absence of digoxin, significant ST-segment depression with or without chest pain might imply that an important component of left-ventricular dysfunction is due to ischemia and, therefore, reversible.

Ambulatory electrocardiographic monitoring is another method of objective assessment in patients with heart failure due to left-ventricular dysfunction. Survival of such patients is poor [3,14] and many die suddenly, presumably from a ventricular tachyarrhythmia [15,16]. Studies in such patients have shown a high frequency of ventricular ectopic activity and this has been found to be closely related to survival. Knowledge of the frequency of such arrhythmias is also important from the functional point of view because poorly compliant ventricles tolerate such arrhythmias badly when the atrial component of ventricular filling is lost. There is no evidence to date that the use of antiarrhythmic drugs in patients with heart failure prolongs life.

Especially in those patients with underlying coronary heart disease, who are the majority, a further application of ambulatory monitoring will be in the detection of silent ischemia since a proportion of patients presenting with heart failure from this cause will have been unaware of any pain. The extent of silent ischemia in this group is as yet completely unknown, but clearly could be a factor not only of prognostic but also of therapeutic importance.

Thus, non-invasive techniques provide a different spectrum of information on cardiac function than hemodynamic variables, facilitating rapid and frequent assessment of patients on a long-term basis. These two approaches are not mutually exclusive; rather they should be regarded as complementary, providing a broader base for the management of the patient with heart failure.

Neuroendocrine Mechanisms in Heart Failure

Increased sympathetic nervous activity as reflected by high plasma and urinary catecholamines could be considered compensatory for the decrease in cardiac output associated with heart failure [17,18].

Indeed, the chronotropic and inotropic effects seem appropriate but the adrenergically mediated peripheral vasoconstriction could potentially depress left-ventricular ejection fraction and stroke volume further. Activation of the renin–angiotensin–aldosterone axis, which occurs in many but not all patients with heart failure, could also be considered compensatory as an attempt to maintain blood pressure and an effective blood volume in the presence of a falling cardiac output. Angiotensin II–mediated vasoconstriction and its effects on the kidney, both directly and indirectly via aldosterone, may be appropriate following blood loss or other causes of hypotension, but are disadvantageous in heart failure. Increased vasopressin secretion may also lead to vasoconstriction and fluid retention so that the collective effects of neuroendocrine stimulation, potentially, are unfavorable to cardiac function and could be responsible, at least in part, for the edema that typifies the clinical syndrome of heart failure; these aspects have been the subject of several recent reviews [5,6,19,20].

Neuroendocrine mechanisms may be stimulated by heart failure treatment, especially by diuretics but also by conventional vasodilators such as hydralazine and prasozin, and therefore may be a factor in the observed decreased long-term efficacy of these agents [21]. Thus, there has been considerable interest in the development of antagonists of the renin–angiotensin system at a variety of sites. The most interesting group of compounds available so far are the angiotensin converting enzyme (ACE) inhibitors. Captopril was the first orally acting ACE inhibitor and has been followed by enalapril. Of considerable experimental interest is a new group of compounds, the renin inhibitors. These drugs block the formation of angiotensin I by antagonizing the action of renin on its substrate [22].

It would be unusual if all the hormonal responses to heart failure were deleterious, and the exciting discovery recently of atrial natriuretic peptide secreted from granules in the right atrium is an example of a beneficial compensatory response. Plasma levels of this hormone which cause natriuresis and vasodilatation are often considerably elevated in many patients with heart failure and indeed a fairly close correlation has been found between the right atrial pressure, pulmonary artery end-diastolic pressure, left-ventricular and end-diastolic pressure and the level of atrial natriuretic peptide [23,24]. The therapeutic potential of this and related synthetic compounds remains to be realized.

Effects of Drug Therapy

The assessment of drug therapy in patients with heart failure was greatly facilitated by the development of flow-directed catheters for accurate documentation of cardiac hemodynamics [25].

Although arteriolar vasodilators significantly increase cardiac output, this may change little with a venodilator and under some circumstances it may fall. A simplistic view of the situation based on the observations of Starling [26,27] would be that the lowering of the filling pressure by a venodilator would reduce pulmonary congestion and therefore breathlessness, whereas an increase in cardiac output with a drug having

248

positive inotropic effects or an arteriolar vasodilator would improve tiredness. This would certainly be the hope of the clinician. Hemodynamic studies can classify a new agent as a drug having inotropic effects or being a venodilator or an arterial vasodilator, but reports of the same drug being classified as a drug having inotropic effects, a vasodilator and possessing both properties reflect the difficulty in establishing such basic data in man [28,30]. In general, acute studies do help to define the mechanism of action of a drug but, unfortunately, beneficial acute effects are not necessarily predictive of long-term hemodynamic effects of some older vasodilators and some newer drugs with inotropic effects; unfortunately, the promises of the cardiac catheterization laboratory are not always fulfilled in clinical practice.

Moreover, it is inconvenient to carry out invasive procedures that carry some risk and which are difficult to repeat sequentially to define the chronic effect of a drug. Therefore, there is considerable interest in non-invasive methods of describing drug action and in the design of studies to ascertain long-term efficacy.

There is obvious interest in the interrelationships among these functional variables and the biochemical markers of the heart failure state, such as renin, angiotensin II, arginine, vasopressin, aldosterone and, more recently, atrial natriuretic peptide. It has been suggested, for example, that stimulation of neuroendocrine mechanisms by vasodilators might compromise their therapeutic potential [21]. In contrast, the potentially favorable therapeutic profile of ACE inhibitors in heart failure includes vasodilatation mediated not only by reduced angiotensin II levels, but also by decreased sympathetic activity and vasopressin secretion. Whether increased levels of bradykinin (occurring as a result of inhibition of its degradation by converting enzyme) contribute to the effects of ACE inhibitors is unknown at present. Moreover, since the renin-angiotensin system may already be activated by the heart-failure state and further stimulated by diuretic therapy [31,32], treatment with ACE inhibitors seems logical and indeed has been associated with improvement in body potassium status [33] presumably because of the reduction in aldosterone levels.

The development of the ACE inhibitors has focused attention once more on the kidney, not only in the production of the heart failure state but also on the effects of therapeutic agents on renal function. Although the effects of the ACE inhibitors on renal function are being investigated, and to some extent have been described [33,34], there is very little information on the long-term effects of other new therapeutic interventions. In future, these aspects are likely to be important in the overall assessment of anti-heart-failure treatment. There will be a greater need for standardization in clinical methodology as non-invasive techniques continue to proliferate so that we may properly evaluate the increasing number of new chemical entities presenting for clinical assessment. These include new drugs with inotropic effects, such as milrinone and enoximone, and their congeners, which, by inhibiting phosphodiesterase, lead to increased levels of cyclic AMP, which in turn cause both an inotropic and a peripheral arteriolar vasodilating effect. New partial $beta_1$-agonists like xamoterol, together with full $beta_1$-agonists such as dopexamine, are also dependent for their inotropic effect on enhancement of cyclic AMP levels by $beta_1$-adrenoceptor-mediated stimulation of adenyl cyclase. New arteriolar vasodilators such as the more vascular selective dihydropyridine 'vascular' calcium antagonists including felodipine, nicardipine and nisoldipine may also have a role in the future [35,36]. It remains to be seen whether new generation ACE inhibitors will have substantially different hemodynamic, renal or metabolic effects from their forerunners captopril and enalapril.

It is becoming clear that patients with lesser degrees of cardiac functional impairment will be targeted for study with several of these new agents and, as hemodynamic assessments will be inappropriate in these patients, even greater reliance will be placed on non-invasive methods with its attendant problems for quantitation. In addition, it will be important to develop and standardize methods of assessing symptomatic improvement in response to treatment. Although preliminary attempts with visual analog scales have been moderately successful [33], there is considerable interest in the application of quality of life analysis to the assessment of heart failure.

Prognosis in Heart Failure
Patients with severe and irreparable myocardial dysfunction cannot be expected to have a normal or near normal survival and indeed once an in-hospital diagnosis of heart failure secondary to left-ventricular dysfunction has been made, survival is short; most patients in functional classes III and IV will be dead within two years [14,37]. Interestingly, a significant proportion of these deaths is sudden and unheralded by acute deterioration in cardiac function, suggesting that they may be due to ventricular tachyarrhythmia. It is now apparent that poor left-ventricular function is associated with a high frequency of ventricular arrhythmias although opinion is divided concerning the prognostic significance of these in patients with heart failure [33,38,39]. A number of factors have been identified as being predictive of a poor prognosis in heart failure; these include ventricular arrhythmias, low blood pressure, poor exercise capacity, hyponatremia and plasma norepinephrine concentration. These variables seem interrelated [16,37] and to be determined ultimately by the extent of left-ventricular dysfunction.

Despite uncertainty surrounding the continued efficacy of nitrates and hydralazine on cardiac function, the combination of these two agents has recently been shown to improve prognosis in patients with heart failure secondary to left-ventricular dysfunction [40], thus reopening the question of the place of conventional vasodilators especially in comparison with the ACE inhibitors. These aspects have gained new importance with the very recent demonstration of improved survival in patients with very severe heart failure in NYHA Grade IV when ACE inhibition was added to conventional therapy [41]. Although one would expect that the careful application of modern medical treatment to patients with very severe heart failure would improve their short-term prognosis, the nitrate/hydralazine study [40] demonstrated that vasodilator therapy prolonged life in less severely affected patients in the longer term. Other mechanisms, however, might also be important and, as several studies have demonstrated the presence of frequent ventricular arrhythmias to be a strong predictor of long-term mortality, it may be that efforts to improve survival of patients with heart failure should not only be aimed at improving cardiac function, but also specifically targeted against the accompanying ventricular arrhythmias. Only properly controlled randomized studies will answer these questions. It should not be forgotten that cardiac transplantation in selected patients with very severe heart failure must now be considered as a realistic option when the very poor prognosis is considered. Whether it will ever be possible, or indeed desirable, to compare such treatment with the very best available medical therapy remains to be seen.

Conclusions

The scene in heart failure is changing rapidly. The relative ease and accuracy of modern clinical investigation mean that symptoms alone form an inadequate basis for a therapeutic strategy that is likely to be lifelong. New therapeutic strategies are challenging older concepts and a host of new chemical entities are presenting their own new problems of assessment. Such diversity in mechanisms of action is both interesting and potentially valuable to the heart-failure patient but each must be considered carefully; hopefully, our newly acquired diagnostic precision will enable us to match the treatment to the pathology. However, only time and much more clinical investigation will provide the answer.

References

[1] Alderman J, Grossman W.
Are beta adrenergic blocking drugs useful in the treatment of dilated cardiomyopathy?
Circulation 1985; 71: 854–7.

[2] Kannel WB, Savage D, Casteli WP.
Cardiac failure in the Framingham Study: 20 year follow-up.
Am J Cardiol 1985; 55: 15A–30A.

[3] Lewis, Sir Thomas.
Diseases of the Heart. London: MacMillan, 1933.

[4] Sonnenblock EH, Ross J Jr, Braunwald E.
Oxygen consumption of the heart. New concepts of its multifactorial determination.
Am J Cardiol 1968; 22: 328–36.

[5] Parmley WW.
Pathophysiology of congestive heart failure.
Am J Cardiol 1985; 55: 9A–14A.

[6] McCall D, O'Rourke RA.
Congestive heart failure 1. Biochemistry, pathophysiology and neurohumoral mechanisms.
Mod Conc Cardiovasc Dis 1985; 54: 55–9.

[7] Soufer R, Wohlgelernter D, Vita NA *et al.*
Intact systolic left ventricular function in clinical congestive heart failure.
Am J Cardiol 1985; 55: 1032–6.

[8] Kumada R, Karliner GS, Pouleur H *et al.*
Effects of coronary occlusion on early ventricular diastolic events in conscious dogs.
Am J Physiol 1979; 237: 8542–9.

[9] Greenberg H, McMaster P, Dwyer EF and the Multicenter Post Infarction Research Group.
Left ventricular dysfunction after acute myocardial infarction: results of a prospective multicenter study.
J Am Coll Cardiol 1984; 4: 867.

[10] Sheffield LT.
Exercise stress testing in heart disease.
In: Braunwald E, ed. *A Textbook of Cardiovascular Medicine.* Philadelphia: WB Saunders, 1980; 253.

[11] Weber KT *et al.*
Oxygen utilization and ventilation during exercise in patients with chronic cardiac failure.
Circulation 1982; 65: 1213–23.

[12] Weber KT, Janicki JS.
Cardiopulmonary exercise testing for evaluation of chronic cardiac failure.
Am J Cardiol 1985; 55: 22A–31A.

[13] Lipkin DP, Canepa-Anson R, Stephens MR, Poole-Wilson P.
Factors determining symptoms in heart failure: comparison of fast and slow exercise tests.
Br Heart J 1986; 55: 439–45.

[14] Franciosa JA, Wilen LPN, Ziesche RN, Cohn JN.
Survival in men with severe chronic left ventricular failure due to either coronary heart disease or idiopathic dilated cardiomyopathy.
Am J Cardiol 1983; 51: 831–6.

[15] Packer M.
Sudden unexpected death in patients with congestive heart failure: a second frontier.
Circulation 1985; 72: 681–5.

[16] Dargie HJ, Cleland JGF, Leckie B, Ingles C, Ford I.
Electrolytes, arrhythmias and survival in patients with heart failure.
Circulation 1987; 75: 89–107.

[17] Chidsey CA, Braunwald E, Morrow AG.
Catecholamine excretion and cardiac stores of norephinephrine in congestive heart failure.
Am J Med 1965; 39: 442.

[18] Chidsey CA, Harrison BC, Braunwald E.
Augmentation of plasma norephinephrine response to exercise in patients with congestive heart failure.
N Engl J Med 1982; **267**: 650.

[19] Francis GS.
Neurohumoral mechanisms involved in congestive heart failure.
Am J Cardiol 1985; **55**: 15A–21A.

[20] Lee WH, Packer M.
Prognostic importance of serum sodium concentration and its modification by converting enzyme inhibition in patients with severe chronic heart failure.
Circulation 1986; **73**: 257–67.

[21] Bayliss J, Norell MS, Canepa-Anson R, Reid C, Wilson P, Sutton G.
Importance of the renin angiotensin system in chronic heart failure: double blind comparison of captopril and prazosin.
Br Med J 1985; **290**: 1861–5.

[22] Haber E.
Renin inhibitors.
N Engl J Med 1984; **311**: 1631–3.

[23] Palluk R, Gaida W, Hofke W.
Atrial natriuretic factor.
Life Sci 1985; **36**: 1415–25.

[24] Richards AM, Cleland JGF, Tonolo G et al.
Atrial natriuretic peptide in heart failure.
Br Med J 1986; **293**: 409–12.

[25] Forrester JS, Ganz W, Diamond G et al.
Thermodilution cardiac output determination with a single flow-directed catheter.
Am Heart J 1972; **83**: 306–11.

[26] Starling F.
The Linacre lecture on the law of the heart. London: Longmans Green: 1918; 1.

[27] Ross J Jr et al.
Left ventricular performance during muscular exercise in patients with and without cardiac dysfunction.
Circulation 1966; **34**: 597–608.

[28] Benotti JR, Grossman W, Braunwald E, Donolos DD, Alonsi AA.
The hemodynamic assessment of amrinone.
N Engl J Med 1978; **299**: 1373–7.

[29] Wilmshurst PT et al.
Haemodynamic effects of amrinone in patients with impaired left ventricular function.
Br Heart J 1983; **49**: 77–82.

[30] Konstam MA, Cohen SR, Weiland DS et al.
Relative contribution of inotropic and vasodilator effects to amrinone induced hemodynamic improvement in congestive cardiac failure.
Am J Cardiol 1986; **57**: 242–8.

[31] Davies JO, Freeman SH.
Mechanisms regulating renin release.
Physiol Res 1976; **56**: 1.

[32] Zanchetti A, Stella A.
Neural control of renin release.
Clin Sci Molec Med 1975; **48**: 215.

[33] Cleland JGF, Dargie HJ, Hodsman GP et al.
Captopril in heart failure: a double blind control study.
Br Heart J 1984; **52**: 530.

[34] Cleland JGF, Dargie HJ.
ACE inhibition in renal function.
Kidney Int 1987 (in press).

[35] Dargie HJ.
New therapeutic strategies in heart failure.
In: Brown MJ, ed. *Recent Advances in Medicine.* Edinburgh: Churchill Livingstone, 1986; 243–58.

[36] Hamer J.
Therapeutic aspects of heart failure.
Curr Opinion Cardiol 1986; **1**: 354.

[37] Cohn JN, Levine TB, Olivari MT.
Plasma norepinephrine as a guide to prognosis in patients with chronic congestive heart failure.
N Engl J Med 1984; **311**: 819–23.

[38] Unverfert DV, Magorian RD, Moeschberger ML, Baker PB, Fetters JK.
Factors influencing the one year mortality of dilated cardiomyopathy.
Am J Cardiol 1984; **54**: 147.

[39] Meinertz T, Hoffman T, Kasper W et al.
The significance of ventricular arrhythmias in idiopathic dilated cardiomyopathy.
Am J Cardiol 1984; **53**: 902.

[40] Cohn JN et al.
Effect of vasodilator therapy on mortality in chronic congestive heart failure: results of a Veterans Administration Co-operative Study.
N Engl J Med 1986; **314**: 1547.

[41] The Consensus Trail Study Group.
The effects of enalapril on mortality in severe congestive heart failure: results of the co-operative North Scandinavian enalapril survival study.
N Engl J Med 1987; **316**: 1429–34.

THE NEUROENDOCRINE AXIS IN HEART FAILURE

[1] Untreated heart failure: clinical and neuroendocrine effects of introducing diuretics.
Bayliss J, Norell M, Canepa-Anson R, Sutton G, Poole-Wilson P, Cardiothoracic Inst, London, UK.
Br Heart J 1987; **7**: 17–22.

[2] Acute vasoconstrictor response to intravenous furosemide in patients with chronic congestive heart failure. Activation of the neurohumoral axis.
Francis GS, Siegel RM, Goldsmith SR, Olivari MT, Levine TB, Cohn JN, Univ Minnesota Med Sch, MN, USA.
Ann Intern Med 1985; **103**: 1–6.

[3] Neurohumoral activation during exercise in congestive heart failure.
Kirlin PC, Grekin R, Das S, Ballor E, Johnson T, Pitt B, Univ Michigan, Ann Arbor, MI, USA.
Am J Med 1986; **81**: 623–9.

Comment. Despite their widespread use in the treatment of chronic heart failure, the initial effects of diuretic agents have seldom been studied. Recently, attention has been focused on the importance of the neuroendocrine response to heart failure and several trials of drugs that oppose the activation of the renin-angiotensin system and the sympathetic system have been conducted. Although angiotensin converting enzyme inhibitors have been shown to have a beneficial effect in patients with moderate to severe heart failure already being treated with diuretics, it is possible that this is partly because they offset the activation of the renin-angiotensin system caused by the diuretics. In a study of 12 previously untreated patients with heart failure, all of whom were limited by breathlessness on exercise and one of whom was edematous, Bayliss *et al* [1] assessed the clinical and neuroendocrine response to one month's treatment with furosemide (40 mg) and amiloride (5 mg) at rest and during exercise. It was found that there was a significant change in the patients' weight and their exercise capacity doubled. Levels of plasma noradrenaline were normal at rest but abnormally high on exercise. There were significant increases in plasma renin activity and plasma aldosterone at rest and on exercise. Although diuretics cause a marked clinical improvement with chronic heart failure, they stimulate the renin-angiotensin system. Bayliss *et al* conclude that the activation of the renin-angiotensin system is a response to diuretic therapy and not a response to the disease process.

Similar conclusions were drawn in an acute study of 15 patients with severe chronic heart failure who were given furosemide intravenously (1.3 ±0.6 [SD] mg/kg body wieght) [2]. By 20 minutes, it was found that left ventricular pump function had deteriorated and left ventricular filling pressure had increased. The following variables were also found to increase: heart rate, mean arterial pressure, systemic vascular resistance, plasma renin activity, plasma noradrenaline and plasma arginine vasopressin levels. During the following three and a half hours, all patients experienced diuresis and the expected fall in filling pressure; the neurohumoral indicators also returned towards control levels. The authors conclude that in patients with severe chronic heart failure, intravenous furosemide is associated with acute pump dysfunction which is temporally related to activation of the neurohumoral axis.

The response of the neurohumoral axis to exercise has been studied by Kirlin *et al*

[3], who investigated the activation of the renin-angiotensin-aldosterone system and the release of hormone during exercise in 14 patients with chronic heart failure (NYHA functional class II or III) and 9 age-matched normal subjects. Plasma renin activity, plasma antidiuretic hormone, plasma noradrenaline and plasma adrenaline concentrations were measured at rest and during moderate (50 W) or strenuous (100 W) bicycle exercise. Patients with heart failure were found to have elevated plasma renin activity and plasma antidiuretic hormone concentration at rest. During strenuous exercise, plasma renin activity almost doubled in the subjects with heart failure but underwent only minimal change in the control subjects; the concentration of plasma antidiuretic hormone did not change with exercise in patients with heart failure, but in the control subjects undertaking strenuous exercise it rose to levels similar to those in patients with heart failure. Plasma noradrenaline concentrations were not significantly elevated either at rest or during exercise in patients with heart failure; plasma adrenaline concentrations were found to be similar. From these results, it would appear that independent neurohumoral activation occurs during exercise in patients with heart failure, and activation of the renin-angiotensin-aldosterone system is predominant.

ACE INHIBITORS IN HEART FAILURE

[1] Arginine vasopressin and the renal response to water loading in congestive heart failure.
Goldsmith SR, Francis GS, Cowley AW Jr, Hennepin Country Med Cent, Minneapolis, MN, USA.
Am J Cardiol 1986; **58**: 295–9.

[2] Vasopressin, renin and norepinephrine levels before and after captopril administration in patients with congestive heart failure due to idiopathic dilated cardiomyopathy.
Riegger GAJ, Kochsiek K, Med Univ, Wurzburg, FRG.
Am J Cardiol 1986; **58**: 300–3.

[3] Effects of captopril and a combination of hydralazine and isosorbide dinitrate on myocardial sympathetic tone in patients with severe congestive heart failure.
Daly P, Rouleau J-L, Cousineau D, Montreal Gen Hosp, Montreal, Canada.
Br Heart J 1986; **56**: 152–7.

[4] Neurohumoral consequences of vasodilator therapy with hydralazine and nifedipine in severe congestive heart failure.
Elkayam U, Roth A, Hsueh W, Weber L, Freidenberger L, Rahimtoola SH, Univ Southern California Sch Med, Los Angeles, CA, USA.
Am Heart J 1986; **111**: 1130–5.

[5] The renal response to neuroendocrine inhibition in chronic heart failure: double-blind comparison of captopril and prazosin.
Bayliss J, Canepa-Anson R, Norell M, Poole-Wilson P, Sutton G, Hillingdon Hosp, Uxbridge, UK.
Eur Heart J 1986; **7**: 877–84.

[6] Preservation of glomerular filtration rate in human heart failure by activation of the renin-angiotensin system.
Packer M, Lee WH, Kessler PD, Mount Sinai Med Cent, New York, NY, USA.
Circulation 1986; **74**: 766–74.

[7] Comparison of captopril and enalapril in patients with severe chronic heart failure.
Packer M, Lee WH, Yushak M, Medina N, Mount Sinai Med Cent, New York, NY, USA.
N Engl J Med 1986; **315**: 847–53.

Comment. The neurohumoral consequences of cardiac failure and their response to treatment are of great interest because changes in catecholamines, activation of the renin-angiotensin system, and vasopressin might account for phenomena that cannot be easily explained in purely hemodynamic terms.

Goldsmith *et al* [1] examined the relation between plasma arginine vasopressin and serum and urinary osmolality in 26 patients with severe heart failure and 14 control subjects. The patients with heart failure had a higher resting arginine vasopressin level than the control subjects but they had a proportionately lesser degree of suppression in response to a water load, despite a similar fall in serum osmolality. Overall urinary dilution in response to the water load was less in the patients than in the control subjects, but the patients appeared to fall into two groups: those with an appropriate fall in urine osmolality and those in whom the decrease was very small. These differences could not be explained solely in terms of the responses of arginine vasopressin.

Riegger and Kochsiek [2] studied 10 patients with heart failure before and after 4 weeks of captopril treatment. Baseline vasopressin levels were elevated relative to the decreased plasma osmolality, and although there was no immediate effect from the captopril, long-term therapy, which was accompanied by a sustained improvement in cardiac function, restored the vasopressin-osmolality relation to normal. As in previous studies, captopril caused an elevation of plasma renin concentration and a decrease in plasma noradrenaline. Thus, despite evidence from the use of specific antagonists that in some patients with heart failure elevated vasopressin levels contribute to the inappropriate vasoconstriction, the acute hemodynamic effects of captopril are not a result of a reduced plasma vasopressin concentration.

A probable explanation for the sustained benefit from angiotensin converting enzyme inhibitors in patients with severe heart failure is that these agents reduce sympathetic stimulation, whereas 'conventional' vasodilators, such as prazosin, with which the benefits tend to be transient, cause an increase in plasma adrenaline and noradrenaline concentrations. The authors of two recent papers have further explored this aspect of treatment. Daly *et al* [3] compared changes in circulating catecholamines and transmyocardial catecholamine balance in patients with heart failure after treatment with captopril ($n = 10$) and the combination of hydralazine with isosorbide dinitrate ($n = 8$). Both regimens resulted in qualitatively comparable hemodynamic changes, but catecholamine concentrations were unchanged with captopril and increased after hydralazine-isosorbide dinitrate.

Elkayam *et al* [4] compared the neurohumoral effects of vasodilator therapy with hydralazine and nifedipine in 18 patients with severe heart failure. Baseline noradrenaline concentrations were elevated, and unaffected by either drug but, whereas the high baseline adrenaline concentration was also unaffected by nifedipine, its concentration was increased after hydralazine. The two agents also differed in their effects on the renin-angiotensin system. There was no change either in plasma renin concentration or in aldosterone level after hydralazine. Nifedipine increased plasma renin, but there was no resulting increase in aldosterone level after hydralazine. The different responses to the two agents can be explained by the known effects of calcium blockade on the secretory cells of the adrenal gland; their clinical significance, if there is any, is unknown.

The consequences for renal function of converting enzyme inhibition in patients with severe heart failure can be unpredictable. In the eperimental animal with a reduced renal perfusion pressure, glomerular filtration is maintained by angiotensin II-mediated constriction of the efferent arterioles. It is not known whether this mechanism operates in man or whether the deterioration in renal function that sometimes results from captopril or enalapril therapy is merely a consequence of reduced perfusion pressure. In a study by Bayliss *et al* [5], in which the effects of captopril were compared with those of prazosin, both agents produced a sustained fall in systemic vascular resistance, but they had opposite effects on the renal vascular resistance. A fall in renal vascular resistance with captopril was accompanied by an increase in cardiac output, an increase in the proportion of the cardiac output distributed to the kidneys and a reduction in bodyweight, whereas renal blood flow and the percentage of cardiac output distributed to the kidneys fell with prazosin, and there was an increase in weight.

Packer *et al* [6] studied systemic and renal hemodynamics in 56 patients with severe heart failure three months after initiation of converting enzyme inhibition. In the patients who had pre-treatment renal perfusion pressures of <70 mmHg, those with preserved renal function (creatinine clearance >50 ml/minute/1.73 m^2) had high pre-treatment plasma renin activities, and creatinine clearance declined after treatment with captopril or enalapril. By contrast, those with low perfusion pressures accompanied by low pre-treatment creatinine clearances had low plasma renin activities, and converting enzyme inhibition had no influence on renal function, despite a similar fall in systemic blood pressure. In patients with renal perfusion pressures >70 mm Hg, there was no correlation between creatinine clearance and plasma renin activity, and renal function was not influenced by therapy. These findings indicate that the renin-angiotensin system is important in the maintenance of glomerular filtration in patients with reduced renal perfusion, and the effect is independent of its action on systemic blood pressure.

Both captopril and enalapril are effective when added to diuretic therapy in patients with severe heart failure, but it has been suggested that enalapril, with its prolonged inhibition of converting enzyme, might have advantages over captopril, which requires more frequent dosing if 24-hour suppression of the renin-angiotensin system is to be achieved. In a study by Packer *et al* [7] 42 patients were randomly assigned to a fixed dosage regimen of either captopril or enalapril. Although both agents resulted in comparable hemodynamic and clinical improvement, serious symptomatic hypotension occurred mainly in the patients taking enalapril, and an overall decline in glomerular filtration rate (creatinine clearance) and evidence of potassium retention occurred only in the patients treated with enalapril. These results do not necessarily indicate that captopril is 'better' than enalapril for the treatment of heart failure because both agents were used in high fixed dosage (captopril 150 mg and enalapril 40 mg daily); it is possible that the problems with enalapril could have been overcome by a reduction in dose without compromising the beneficial effects. Nevertheless, other workers have drawn attention to the occurrence of the more prolonged (and, therefore, more dangerous) hypotension that occurs with enalapril than with captopril in patients who react badly to the first dose of an angiotensin converting enzyme inhibitor.

6. Electrophysiology, Heart Rate and Rhythm

ELECTROPHYSIOLOGIC STIMULATION PROTOCOLS FOR THE EVALUATION AND MANAGEMENT OF VENTRICULAR ARRHYTHMIAS

Review: ANTHONY W. NATHAN

Ventricular arrhythmias are the commonest cause of sudden cardiac death. Many of these arrhythmias are not associated with an acute myocardial infarction, although most patients have organic heart disease – usually atherosclerotic coronary artery disease or cardiomyopathy. Ambulatory monitors attached fortuitously during episodes of sudden cardiac death have demonstrated that many cases of ventricular fibrillation are preceded by ventricular tachycardia, although ventricular fibrillation may occur *de novo*. Many forms of therapy are available to treat ventricular arrhythmias: these include drugs, pacemakers, non-specific and specific surgical techniques and, most recently, the automatic implantable cardioverter/defibrillator.

Once a diagnosis is established, the type of therapy to be used should be tailored to each individual case, as no single therapy is either effective or ideal for all cases. Selection may be made empirically (in the case of drug therapy with or without the use of drug plasma levels), using non-invasive methods such as ambulatory monitoring and exercise stress testing, or using invasive electrophysiologic studies with programmed electrical stimulation [1,2].

It is worth emphasizing that when treating potentially lethal arrhythmias some sort of testing is necessary: empiric therapy alone is very often unsuccessful and carries a high mortality. Myerburg *et al* have shown an improvement in survival by ensuring adequate plasma levels of a given drug [3], but this approach is still associated with a significant mortality. Lown's group have encouraged the use of non-invasive testing [4], but the value of this may be highly dependent on the patient group studied: Gradman *et al* favorably compared ambulatory monitoring with exercise testing, but 58% of their patients had ventricular tachycardia on their ambulatory monitoring recordings, an unusually high prevalence [5]. Davies has pointed out [6] that programmed electrical stimulation, first reported for the induction of ventricular arrhythmias in 1972 [7], has become the 'gold standard' for the assessment of therapy for ventricular arrhythmias.

Aims of Electrophysiologic Studies

The commonest reason for performing an electrophysiologic study is to assess the value of drug therapy, either in patients with recurrent monomorphic or multiple monomorphic (also known as pleomorphic) ventricular tachycardia or in those who have been resuscitated from ventricular fibrillation. Most patients have some kind of structural heart disease, although others have apparently normal hearts. However, as shown in Table I, electrophysiologic studies may be performed for other reasons in patients with

Table I. Potential reasons for performing electrophysiologic studies in patients with suspected ventricular arrhythmias

---

Establishing that a tachycardia is ventricular
Prognosis in patients with frequent ventricular premature beats
Prognosis in patients following myocardial infarction
Assessing the value of drug treatment in patients with recurrent ventricular arrhythmias
Establishing suitability or otherwise for antitachycardia pacemaker
Establishing inducibility prior to arrhythmic surgery
Catheter mapping prior to antiarrhythmic surgery
Establishing inducibility prior to use of automatic implantable cardioverter/defibrillator
Establishing efficacy of prior surgical treatment, automatic implantable cardioverter/defibrillator
    or pacemaker
Investigating syncope of unknown cause

---

ventricular arrhythmias, whether previously suspected or proven. The North American Society of Pacing Electrophysiology (NASPE) policy statement on the minimally appropriate electrophysiologic study for the initial assessment of patients with documented sustained monomorphic ventricular tachycardia is worth studying [8,9]. This defines the various ventricular arrhythmias and recommends the appropriate baseline status of the patient, measurements, recording leads, characteristics of the stimulator and other pieces of equipment, as well as personnel requirements. Recommendations for initiating and terminating protocols are also included.

End-points
Before discussing the various protocols it must be recognized that different authors have used different definitions of successful end-points. For example, Livelli *et al* defined sustained ventricular tachycardia as a run of ventricular complexes requiring intervention to stop it [10]. Richards *et al* defined sustained ventricular tachycardia as a run of ventricular complexes lasting at least 10 seconds [11], and Morady *et al* as a ventricular tachycardia lasting at least 30 seconds or requiring emergency measures to terminate it in less than 30 seconds [12]. This variety of definitions can make comparison of different protocols difficult; it is to be hoped that the NASPE guidelines will be universally accepted in the future.

Very limited end-points, such as the repetitive ventricular response, have been studied by several authors. Green *et al* considered the repetitive ventricular response (two or more ventricular premature beats provoked by a single ventricular premature stimulus during atrial drive pacing) to be a useful prognostic indicator in patients with recurrent ventricular tachycardia [13], although others, such as Naccarelli *et al* [14], Breithardt *et al* [15] and Mason [16], have refuted this. End-points such as ventricular fibrillation must be viewed cautiously: as discussed later, aggressive protocols may induce ventricular fibrillation in nearly normal subjects [17]. Even in patients being investigated prognostically during recovery from acute myocardial infarction, induced ventricular fibrillation seems to be of limited clinical significance – certainly in comparison with induced sustained ventricular tachycardia [18].

259

The Effect of Different Factors on the Electrophysiologic Study

Wellens *et al* have listed a number of factors that can or cannot be controlled by the investigator during stimulation studies [19]. These, with some additions and modifications, are listed in Tables II and III. There is no doubt that more aggressive protocols will induce more arrhythmias, but an optimal protocol in terms of predictive value (specificity and sensitivity) has yet to be fully defined. The practising physician requires the most effective, the safest and the least time-consuming protocol in relation to any given problem.

The Stimulus

The current employed for stimulation is usually direct current, from a fully isolated source, of the constant-current type [20]. Mower *et al* have suggested the use of alternating current [21], but all patients in their study were being considered for the automatic implantable defibrillator, and specificity was sacrificed for the sake of sensitivity. This may be a rapid method of inducing a known arrhythmia, but as well as being

Table II. Factors controllable by the investigator during electrophysiologic studies

Stimulus
    type of current
    duration
    strength
    number of basic stimuli
    rate of basic stimuli
    number of premature stimuli
    interval/s of premature stimulus/stimuli
    pause between each stimulation attempt

Site of Stimulation
    basic stimuli
    premature stimuli

Mode of Stimulation
    unipolar
    bipolar

Interelectrode Distance

Patient Medication
    sedation
    local anesthetic
    antiarrhythmic drugs
    isoprenaline (isoproterenol)
    other drugs (including anti-ischemics)

Prevailing Psychologic Stress (partially controllable)

Patient Posture

Table III. Factors not controllable by the investigator during electrophysiologic studies

Type of spontaneous arrhythmia
Etiology of spontaneous arrhythmia
Resting heart rate
Resting autonomic tone
Electrophysiologic properties of arrhythmia substrate
Autonomic response to pacing or drug administration
Hemodynamic consequences of pacing or drug administration
Ischemic consequences of pacing or drug administration

non-specific it may carry a considerable risk of inducing unwanted ventricular fibrillation.

A stimulus duration of 1 or 2 ms is used in most laboratories – usually the latter, because of its suitable stimulation characteristics when assessed during strength–duration curves [22]. To obtain consistent capture most investigators use a stimulus strength of twice the diastolic threshold. Higher current strengths will result in a larger area of simultaneous depolarization, and may also allow ventricular capture at closer coupling intervals than might otherwise be obtained. Morady *et al* have examined the effect of increasing current strength on the induction of ventricular tachycardia in 41 patients, 30 of whom had documented ventricular tachycardias and 11 syncope [23]. Irrespective of the result of the standard protocol at twice the diastolic threshold (0.6–1.5 mA), they increased the current to 10 mA. Of the patients non-inducible at twice diastolic threshold, 16 were rendered inducible by the higher current, although some became non-inducible. Whether or not this is merely a problem of reproducibility remains a point for speculation. Some of the patients who became inducible (although not all) had the arrhythmia induced at closer coupling intervals that were previously possible. Richards *et al* investigated 111 patients who had no history of ventricular arrhythmias and 27 patients with documented ventricular arrhythmias [11]. They compared the use of stimulation at twice diastolic threshold and at 20 mA, achieving a higher sensitivity in the patients with previous ventricular arrhythmias without affecting specificity. Their suggestion that 20 mA might become a new standard for stimulation, however, could not be fully supported by Morady's results. A factor often ignored in drug studies is the effect of some drugs on stimulation thresholds. Flecainide, for example, has a major effect on thresholds, which may markedly affect results [24].

Stimuli may be delivered during the spontaneous rhythm, which is usually sinus rhythm. Interestingly, Somberg *et al* have shown that vulnerability may be increased during atrial fibrillation [25]. Stimuli may also be delivered following a drive train of stimuli at a fixed rate (or even at a variable rate). The number of stimuli given in a train is usually eight, with the NASPE recommendation that at least six of these capture the stimulated chamber [8,9]. The cycle length of the drive may vary from 600 ms to 300 ms (100–200 beats/min). Sensitivity certainly increases when drive pacing is used or when its rate is increased [26], but the effect on specificity is less well documented in the literature.

When considering the number of premature stimuli to be chosen there is no doubt that increasing the number of extrastimuli increases sensitivity, but it does so at the expense of specificity – both in terms of non-clinical tachyarrhythmias in those patients who do have previously documented arrhythmias and in terms of arrhythmia induction in those patients with no history of serious arrhythmias [27]. The order of the stimulation protocol may also be important. Whether to use a single extrastimulus in the basic rhythm followed by two and then three extrastimuli in that rhythm followed by drive-pacing routines, or to use one extrastimulus in basic rhythm followed by one extrastimulus in slow-drive rhythm and one extrastimulus in fast-drive rhythm and so on, is still a point of contention.

The coupling intervals of the extrastimuli are usually critical. Coupling intervals are usually decremented in steps of 5–20 ms until they are effective in inducing tachycardia or until refractoriness is reached. Most investigators add a second stimulus, with the first set at 5–20 ms longer than the refractory period, but some prefer using a relatively long coupling interval for the first extrastimulus when the second is introduced. The starting point of the decrementing sequence also varies from laboratory to laboratory, but is usually 20–50 ms shorter than the spontaneous or drive rate. If extrastimuli are ineffective some investigators use bursts of pacing, either at a constant rate or with the rate increasing, decreasing, or both within the same burst; this kind of maneuver, however, lacks specificity and reproducibility [27]. Finally, the pause between each stimulation attempt should be long enough to allow hemodynamic stabilization without wasting too much time: usually 3 to 5 seconds will suffice.

Site of Stimulation
The site of stimulation is a highly important variable. Ventricular arrhythmias can sometimes be induced (i) with an atrial extrastimulus alone [28]; (ii) with an atrial extrastimulus following atrial drive pacing; (iii) with a ventricular extrastimulus alone; (iv) with a ventricular extrastimulus following atrial drive pacing; and (v) most commonly with a ventricular extrastimulus following ventricular drive pacing. In addition, different ventricular sites can be used for stimulation; the most frequently used are: the right-ventricular apex, right-ventricular outflow tract [29,30], and left-ventricular apex [31]. In my experience, using atrial extrastimuli or atrial drive pacing for the induction of ventricular arrhythmias is time-consuming and rarely effective.

The most commonly used ventricular site is the right-ventricular apex; this site allows a conventional pacing catheter to be left in a stable position for days or even weeks during serial drug testing. The right-ventricular outflow tract is rarely stable in an ambulatory patient, and the serial use of this site may necessitate reinsertion of the pacing electrode for each test. Left-ventricular stimulation obviously requires fresh arterial catheterization on each occasion unless left-ventricular capture can be achieved from the distal coronary sinus. Although left-ventricular stimulation seemed fashionable in the early 1980s, the use of multiple extrastimuli, rapid-drive cycle lengths, increased stimulation energies and multiple right-ventricular sites have obviated the need for it in most patients.

The optimum site of stimulation is theoretically that closest to the arrhythmic focus; in practice, however, this is not always so.

Mode of Stimulation and Interelectrode Distance
Stimulation is usually bipolar, in order to localize the area of depolarization. Very little work has been performed on assessing unipolar stimulation for electrophysiologic

studies. It is of interest to note, however, that electrophysiologic studies have been performed in a significant number of patients using implantable pulse generators [32]. These are usually specially adapted devices, or at least devices with special programmers, and until very recently most of these pacemakers were unipolar. Results from these studies seem to vary little from test results on temporary pacing catheters of the bipolar variety. In the electrophysiology laboratory interelectrode distances used for stimulation generally vary from 5 mm to 10 mm.

Patient Factors
It has been suggested that patients suffering from arrhythmias associated with different types of heart disease may differ in their response to programmed electrical stimulation. Certainly the response of those with the long QT syndrome and torsade de pointes differs considerably from others, and patients with congestive cardiomyopathy and ischemic heart disease may also differ in their response to stimulation [33,34].

Some work has been performed in so-called normals [17,35], examining the induction of ventricular arrhythmias. In fact, these normals are usually patients undergoing electrophysiologic study for documented supraventricular arrhythmias with no evidence of underlying heart disease. Sustained monomorphic ventricular tachycardia is very rarely induced in such patients; polymorphic ventricular tachycardia or ventricular fibrillation can occasionally be induced, but this is thought to be of no clinical significance. True normals have rarely been studied – for obvious ethical reasons.

Most patients are studied in the non-sedated state, although light sedation/premedication may be used. Lignocaine (lidocaine) is normally used for local anesthesia, but the quantity and strength should be minimized in order to keep circulating levels as low as possible [36]. Antiarrhythmic drugs may be given deliberately during electrophysiologic testing in order to assess their efficacy, but if a baseline study is being performed administration should be stopped for at least three to five half-lives prior to testing. Termination of a sustained arrhythmia by an intravenous dose of a drug may sometimes predict its efficacy in terms of prevention; conversion from the inducible to the non-inducible state with a drug, intravenously and then later orally, is an even better predictor [37]. If full prevention cannot be achieved, the fact that induction is more difficult after administration of a drug may imply a partial cure [38]. Where the patient has been receiving other medications, such as anti-ischemic drugs, these should be continued during testing. Isoprenaline (isoproterenol) may be needed in some instances [30] either actually to induce arrhythmias or to facilitate the induction of an arrhythmia during programmed stimulation – particularly if the clinical arrhythmia is effort-related. Some have used deliberate psychologic stress, and some investigators, for example Cassagneau *et al*, have usefully employed alterations in patient posture, using a tilt table [39].

Termination Regimens
It is obviously crucial that the arrhythmias be terminated after electrophysiologic study. This is also usually achieved by programmed stimulation. If the arrhythmia is well tolerated, single or double extrastimuli can be systematically scanned through the tachycardia cycle. If the arrhythmia is not well tolerated, rapid bursts are usually the most effective [40], but these may degenerate the arrhythmia. Facilities for direct-

current cardioversion and defibrillation, as well as other resuscitative facilities, must be available at all times. An alternative to pacing worthy of mention is low-energy endocardial cardioversion [41,42], using a special high-surface-area transvenous electrode. Although not always effective (perhaps even in situations where pacing is effective) and sometimes painful, the technique is useful and may, in some patients, avoid the necessity for anesthesia in external transthoracic cardioversion.

Table IV. Suggested stimulation protocols for patients with suspected or documented ventricular arrhythmias

---

A. Constant current, 2-ms impulses, at twice diastolic threshold (re-measured after drug administration), using bipolar pacing electrodes with 5-mm electrode spacing; 3-s pauses used between stimulation cycles.
  1. 1 VPS during basic rhythm, from RVA.
  2. 2 VPS during basic rhythm, from RVA.
  3. 1 VPS during VP (8 beats) at 600 ms (or 40–50 ms faster than the basic rhythm if cycle length of basic rhythm less than 60 ms), from RVA.
  4. 2 VPS during VP at '600' ms, from RVA.
  5. 1 VPS during VP at 400 ms, from RVA.
  6. 2 VPS during VP at 400 ms, from RVA.
  7. 3 VPS during basic rhythm, from RVA.
  8. 3 VPS during VP at '600' ms, from RVA.
  9. 3 VPS during VP at 400 ms, from RVA.

B. Repeat all of above from RVO.

C. Repeat A and then B at 20 mA.

D. Burst pacing from RVA, either at constant rate or at increasing or decreasing rates. Adjust rates up to exit block if necessary.

E. Repeat D from RVO.

F. Repeat A from the LVA.

G. Repeat F at 20 mA.

H. Repeat D from the LVA.

I. Infuse isoprenaline (isoproterenol)
  Then repeat A1, A2, A5, A6, A7 and A9;
         B1, B2, B5, B6, B7 and B9;
         D, E;
         F1, F2, F5, F6, F7 and F9.

J. Use alternating current from RVA.

Abbreviations: LVA = left-ventricular apex; RVA = right-ventricular apex; RVO = right-ventricular outflow tract; VP = ventricular drive pacing; VPS = ventricular premature stimulus/stimuli.

Approaches for Different Patient Groups

When assessing the response to tachycardia reversion pacing or to an implantable defibrillator, or when mapping prior to arrhythmia surgery, the mode of tachycardia initiation is relatively unimportant. If 12-lead ECGs of the presenting arrhythmias are available, any method of inducing the clinical tachycardia quickly and safely will suffice – for example, rapid-drive pacing with multiple extrastimuli, burst pacing, or even alternating current. When assessing potential risk in an 'asymptomatic' patient following myocardial infarction, or assessing the results of drug therapy or previous arrhythmia surgery, a more stratified approach is necessary.

The strategy currently used in my clinical practice is shown in Table IV. Prior to electrophysiologic study the underlying heart disease is usually fully investigated, and most patients with suspected ventricular arrhythmias undergo coronary angiography before electrophysiologic study is considered. In general, patients with absolutely critical coronary artery disease are excluded from electrophysiologic study, as they may not survive induced ventricular fibrillation. Once a decision has been made to undertake stimulation, a strategy is used which has been compiled in accordance with a consensus of published data. The extent of stimulation depends on the presenting problem: for example, in a patient with no documented arrhythmia but presenting with syncope of unknown origin, steps A1–A6 and B1–B6 would be performed; in patients with documented monomorphic ventricular tachycardia causing a previous cardiac arrest, the entire protocol may be undertaken. Note has to be made of the patient's tolerance to the procedure, and any protocol may require modification accordingly.

Recently, some attention has been paid to the reproducibility of inducing arrhythmias [43]. In a series of 77 patients, McPherson *et al* reported that, of 66 who had inducible ventricular tachycardia at first study, only 53 (80%) were inducible at a second study performed under similar conditions within 72 hours [44]. Kudenchuk *et al* studied 114 patients with documented sustained ventricular arrhythmias, performing two baseline electrophysiologic studies within 24 hours [45]. Non-reproducibility increased as the number of extrastimuli increased from one (7%) to four (27%), although non-reproducibility with three and four extrastimuli was not significantly greater than when two were used. Although this study had a lower inducibility rate than many other studies, these findings certainly have some implications for patients subjected to multiple drug trials.

References

[1] Mason JW, Winkle RA.
Electrode-catheter arrhythmia induction in the selection and assessment of antiarrhythmic drug therapy for recurrent ventricular tachycardia.
Circulation 1978; **58**: 971–85.

[2] Breithardt G, Seipel L, Abendroth RR, Loogen F.
Serial electrophysiological testing of antiarrhythmic drug efficacy in patients with recurrent ventricular tachycardia.
Eur Heart J 1980; **1**: 11–24.

[3] Myerburg RJ, Zaman L, Kessler KM, Castellanos A.
Evolving concepts of management of stable and potentially lethal arrhythmias.
Am Heart J 1982; **103**: 615–25.

[4] Graboys TB, Lown B, Podrid PJ, DeSilva R.
Long-term survival of patients with malignant ventricular arrhythmia treated with antiarrhythmic drugs.
Am J Cardiol 1982; **50**: 437–43.

[5] Gradman AH, Batsford WP, Rieur EC, Leon L, Van Zetta AM.
Ambulatory electrocardiographic correlates of ventricular inducibility during programmed electrical stimulation.
J Am Coll Cardiol 1985; **5**: 1087–93.

[6] Davies DW.
The electrophysiological investigation of patients with ventricular tachyarrhythmias and resuscitated sudden death.
Curr Opin Cardiol 1986; **1**: 22–8.

[7] Wellens HJ, Schuilenburg RM, Durrer D.
Electrical stimulation of the heart in patients with ventricular tachycardia.
Circulation 1972; **46**: 216–26.

[8] Waldo AL, Akhtar M, Brugada P *et al.*
The minimally appropriate electrophysiologic study for the initial assessment of patients with documented sustained monomorphic ventricular tachycardia.
J Am Coll Cardiol 1985; **6**: 1174–7.

[9] Waldo AL, Akhtar M, Brugada P *et al.*
The minimally appropriate electrophysiologic study for the initial assessment of patients with documented sustained monomorphic ventricular tachycardia.
PACE 1985; **8**: 918–22.

[10] Livelli FD, Bigger JT, Reiffel JA *et al.*
Response to programmed ventricular stimulation: Sensitivity, specificity and relation to heart disease.
Am J Cardiol 1982; **50**: 452–8.

[11] Richards DA, Cody DV, Denniss AR, Russell PA, Young AA, Uther JB.
A new protocol of programmed stimulation for assessment of predisposition to spontaneous ventricular arrhythmias.
Eur Heart J 1983; **4**: 376–82.

[12] Morady F, Scheinman MM, Hess DS, Sung RJ, Shen E, Shapiro W.
Electrophysiologic testing in the management of survivors of out-of-hospital cardiac arrest.
Am J Cardiol 1983; **51**: 85–9.

[13] Greene HL, Reid PR, Schaeffer AH.
The repetitive ventricular response in man: A predictor of sudden death.
N Engl J Med 1978; **299**: 729–34.

[14] Naccarelli GV, Prystowsky EN, Jackman WM, Heger JJ, Rinkenberger RL, Zipes DP.
Repetitive ventricular response: Prevalence and prognostic significance.
Br Heart J 1981; **46**: 152–8.

[15] Breithardt G, Abendroth RR, Borggrefe M, Yeh HL, Haerten K, Seipel L.
Prevalence and clinical significance of the repetitive ventricular response during sinus rhythm in coronary disease patients.
Am Heart J 1984; **107**: 229–36.

[16] Mason JW.
Repetitive beating after single ventricular extrastimuli: Incidence and prognostic significance in patients with recurrent ventricular tachycardia.
Am J Cardiol 1980; **45**: 1126–31.

[17] Morady F, Shapiro W, Shen E, Sung RJ, Scheinman MM.
Programmed ventricular stimulation in patients without spontaneous ventricular tachycardia.
Am Heart J 1984; **107**: 875–82.

[18] Holley LK, Denniss AR, Cody DV *et al.*
Comparison of clinical significance of programmed stimulation induced ventricular tachycardia and fibrillation in survivors of acute MI.
PACE 1983; **6**: A73.

[19] Wellens HJJ, Brugada P, Stevenson WG.
Programmed electrical stimulation of the heart in patients with life-threatening ventricular arrhythmias: What is the significance of induced arrhythmias and what is the correct stimulation protocol?
Circulation 1985; **72**: 1–7.

[20] Morady F, Hess D, Scheinman MM.
Electrophysiologic drug testing in patients with malignant ventricular arrhythmias: Importance of stimulation at more than one ventricular site.
Am J Cardiol 1982; **50**: 1055–60.

[21] Mower MM, Reid PR, Watkins L, Mirowski M.
Use of alternating current during diagnostic electrophysiologic studies.
Circulation 1983; **67**: 69–72.

[22] Brugada P, Wellens HJJ.
Standard diagnostic programmed electrical stimulation protocols in patients with paroxysmal recurrent tachycardia.
PACE 1984; **7**: 1121–8.

[23] Morady F, DiCarlo LA Jr, Liem LB, Krol RB, Baerman JM.
Effects of high stimulation current on the induction of ventricular tachycardia.
Am J Cardiol 1985; **56**: 73–8.

[24] Hellestrand KJ, Burnett PJ, Milne JR, Bexton RS, Nathan AW, Camm AJ.
Effect of the antiarrhythmic agent flecainide acetate on acute and chronic pacing thresholds.
PACE 1983; **6**: 892–9.

[25] Somberg JC, Torres V, Gotlieb S, Butler B, Levitt B, Miura DS.
The enhancement of myocardial vulnerability by atrial fibrillation.
Circulation 1983; **68:** III56.

[26] Estes NAM, Garan H, McGovern B, Ruskin J.
Use of multiple decremental drive cycle length protocol increases sensitivity of programmed ventricular stimulation.
Circulation 1984; **70:** II398.

[27] Mann DE, Luck JC, Griffin JC *et al.*
Induction of clinical ventricular tachycardia using programmed stimulation: Value of third and fourth extrastimuli.
Am J Cardiol 1983; **52:** 501–6.

[28] Wellens HJJ, Bar FW, Farre J, Ross DL, Wiener I, Vanagt EJ.
Initiation and termination of ventricular tachycardia by supraventricular stimuli: Incidence and electrophysiologic determinants as observed during programmed stimulation of the heart.
Am J Cardiol 1980; **46:** 576–82.

[29] Doherty JU, Kienzle MG, Waxman HL, Buxton AE, Marchlinski FE, Josephson ME.
Programmed ventricular stimulation at a second right ventricular site: An analysis of 100 patients with special reference to sensitivity, specificity and characteristics of patients with induced ventricular tachycardia.
Am J Cardiol 1983; **52:** 1184–9.

[30] Brugada P, Wellens HJJ.
Comparison in the same patient of two programmed ventricular stimulation protocols to induce ventricular tachycardia.
Am J Cardiol 1985; **55:** 380–3.

[31] Michelson EL, Spielman SR, Greenspan AM, Farshidi A, Horowitz LN, Josephson ME.
Electrophysiologic study of the left ventricle: Indications and safety.
Chest 1979; **75:** 592–6.

[32] Menozzi C, Brignole M, Monducci I, Lolli G.
Noninvasive serial electrophysiological testing using an implanted pacemaker for management of recurrent ventricular tachycardia.
PACE 1986; **9:** 589–93.

[33] Poll DS, Marchlinski FE, Buxton AE, Doherty JU, Waxman HL, Josephson ME.
Sustained ventricular tachycardia in patients with idiopathic dilated cardiomyopathy: Electrophysiologic testing and lack of response to antiarrhythmic drug therapy.
Circulation 1984; **70:** 451–6.

[34] Naccarelli GV, Prystowsky EN, Jackman WM, Heger JJ, Rahilly GT, Zipes DP.
Role of electrophysiologic testing in managing patients who have ventricular tachycardia unrelated to coronary artery disease.
Am J Cardiol 1982; **50:** 165–71.

[35] Vandepol CJ, Farshidi A, Spielman SR, Greenspan AM, Horowitz LN, Josephson ME.
Incidence and clinical significance of induced ventricular tachycardia.
Am J Cardiol 1980; **45:** 725–31.

[36] Nattel S, Rinkenberger RL, Lehrman LL, Zipes DP.
Therapeutic blood lidocaine concentrations after local anesthesia for cardiac electrophysiologic studies.
N Engl J Med 1979; **301:** 418–20.

[37] Mason JW, Winkle RA.
Accuracy of the ventricular tachycardia-induction study for predicting long-term efficacy and inefficacy of antiarrhythmic drugs.
N Engl J Med 1980; **303:** 1073–7.

[38] Fisher JD, Fink D, Matos JA, Kim SG, Waspe L.
Programmed stimulation and ventricular tachycardia therapy: Benefits of partial as well as complete "cures".
PACE 1983; **6:** 313.

[39] Cassagneau B, Puel J, Fauvel JM, Bounhoure JP, Rangueil CMU.
Interest of tilt-test during electrophysiologic provocative studies for antiarrhythmic drug selection in recurrent tachycardias.
Eur Heart J 1984; **5** (Suppl 1): 194.

[40] Fisher JD, Mehra R, Furman S.
Termination of ventricular tachycardia with bursts of rapid ventricular pacing.
Am J Cardiol 1978; **41:** 94–102.

[41] Zipes DP, Jackman WM, Heger JJ *et al.*
Clinical transvenous cardioversion of recurrent life-threatening ventricular tachyarrhythmias: Low energy synchronized cardioversion of ventricular tachycardia and termination of ventricular fibrillation in patients using a catheter electrode.
Am Heart J 1982; **103:** 789–94.

[42] Nathan AW, Bexton RS, Spurrell RAJ, Camm AJ.
Internal transvenous low energy cardioversion for the treatment of cardiac arrhythmias.
Br Heart J 1984; **52:** 377–84.

[43] Gomes JA.
Inducibility and reproducibility of ventricular arrhythmias: Therapeutic implications.
J Am Coll Cardiol 1986; **7:** 829–31.

[44] McPherson CA, Rosenfeld LE, Batsford WP.
Day-to-day reproducibility of responses to right
ventricular programmed electrical stimulation:
Implications for serial drug testing.
Am J Cardiol 1985; **55**: 689–95.

[45] Kudenchuk PJ, Kron J, Walance CG *et al.*
Reproducibility of arrhythmia induction with intracardiac electrophysiologic testing: Patients
with clinical sustained ventricular tachyarrhythmias.
J Am Coll Cardiol 1986; **7**: 819–28.

VALUE OF ELECTROPHYSIOLOGIC TESTING

[1] Long-term reproducibility of responses to programmed cardiac stimulation in spon-
taneous ventricular arrhythmias.
Schoenfeld MH, McGovern B, Garan H, Ruskin JN, Massachussetts Gen Hosp, Boston,
MA, USA.
Am J Cardiol 1984; **54**: 564–8.

[2] Daily reproducibility of electrophysiologic test results in malignant ventricular
arrhythmia.
Lombardi F, Stein J, Podrid PJ, Graboys TB, Lown B, Harvard Sch Public Hlth, Boston,
MA, USA.
Am J Cardiol 1986; **57**: 96–101.

[3] Reproducibility of arrhythmia induction with intracardiac electrophysiologic testing:
patients with clinical sustained ventricular tachyarrhythmias.
Kudenchuk PJ, Kron J, Walance CG, Murphy ES, Morris CD, Griffith KK, McAnulty JH, Por-
tland, OR, USA.
J Am Coll Cardiol 1986; : 819–28.

[4] A prospective comparison of triple extrastimuli and left ventricular stimulation in studies
of ventricular tachycardia induction.
Morady F, DiCarlo L, Winston S, Davis JC, Scheinman MM, Univ California, San Francisco,
CA, USA.
Circulation 1984; **70**: 52–7.

[5] Clinical significance of ventricular fibrillation-flutter induced by ventricular pro-
grammed stimulation.
DiCarlo LA Jr, Morady F, Schwartz AB *et al*, Univ Michigan Med Cent, Ann Arbor, MI,
USA.
Am Heart J 1985; **109**: 959–62.

[6] Prospective comparison of Holter monitoring and electrophysiologic study in patients
with coronary artery disease and sustained ventricular tachyarrhythmias.
Swerdlow CD, Peterson J, Deaconess Med Cent, Spokane, WA, USA.
Am J Cardiol 1985; **56**: 577–80.

[7] Survivors of cardiac arrest: prevention of recurrence by drug therapy as predicted by
electrophysiologic testing or electrocardiographic monitoring.
Skale BT, Miles WM, Heger JJ, Zipes DP, Prystowsky EN, Krannert Inst Cardiology,
Indianapolis, IN, USA.
Am J Cardiol 1986; **57**: 113–9.

[8] Is programmed stimulation of value in predicting the long-term success of anti-
arrhythmic therapy for ventricular tachycardias?
Kim SG, Seiden SW, Felder SD, Waspe LE, Fisher JD, Montefiore Med Cent, Bronx,
NY, USA.
N Engl J Med 1986; **315**: 356–62.

[9] Endocardial mapping in humans in sinus rhythm with normal left ventricles: activation patterns and characteristics of electrograms.
Cassidy DM, Vassallo JA, Marchlinski FE, Buxton AE, Untereker WJ, Josephson ME, Hosp Univ Pennsylvania, Philadelphia, PA, USA.
Circulation 1984; **70**: 37–42.

[10] The value of catheter mapping during sinus rhythm to localize site of origin of ventricular tachycardia.
Cassidy DM, Vassallo JA, Buxton AE, Doherty JU, Marchlinski FE, Josephson ME, Hosp Univ Pennsylvania, Philadelphia, PA, USA.
Circulation 1984; **69**: 1103–10.

[11] A prospective evaluation and follow-up of patients with syncope.
Kapoor WN, Karpf M, Wieand S, Peterson JR, Levey GS, Univ Pittsburgh, Pittsburgh, PA, USA.
N Engl J Med 1983; **309**: 197–204.

[12] Electrophysiologic testing in the upright position: improved evaluation of patients with rhythm disturbances using a tilt table.
Hammill SC, Holmes DR Jr, Wood DL *et al*, Mayo Clin and Mayo Found, Rochester, MN, USA.
J Am Coll Cardiol 1984; **4**: 65–71.

[13] Head-up tilt: a useful test for investigating unexplained syncope.
Kenny RA, Ingram A, Bayliss J, Sutton R, Westminster Hosp, London, UK.
Lancet 1986; i: 1352–5.

[14] Increased vagal tone as an isolated finding in patients undergoing electrophysiological testing for recurrent syncope: response to long term anticholinergic agents.
McLaran CJ, Gersh BJ, Osborn MJ *et al*, Mayo Clin and Mayo Found, Rochester, MN, USA.
Br Heart J 1986; **55**: 53–7.

Comment. Electrophysiologic study has become of increasing value in the management of ventricular arrhythmia. However, whereas the sensitivity and specificity of induced responses to programmed electrical stimulation has been defined, the important aspect of reproducibility has received little attention. Schoenfeld *et al* [1] examined the long-term reproducibility in 17 patients studied 2–24 months after a control electrophysiologic study. Of the 11 patients who had underlying coronary artery disease, all had ventricular tachycardia inducible at both studies.

These figures contrasted with the six remaining patients with cardiomyopathy, congenital heart disease or no underlying structural abnormality, and in whom only one patient had ventricular tachycardia inducible on both occasions. The daily reproducibility of electrophysiologic tests was examined in two studies [2,3]. Lombardi *et al* [2] examined the reproducibility on successive days in 42 patients presenting with a malignant ventricular arrhythmia, 17 with ventricular tachycardia and 25 with ventricular fibrillation. An arrhythmia was inducible in 32 patients (76%) at the first study, whereas a similar end-point was reached in only 22 patients (52%) at the second study. In this study, reproducibility seemed to be unrelated to the presence of coronary artery disease or presenting arrhythmia. Kudenchuk *et al* [3] repeated electrophysiologic testing within 6–24 hours in 114 patients with a variety of sustained ventricular arrhythmias. Inducibility of arrhytnmia increased (from 10% to 64%) as the number of extrastimuli required was increased from one to four. In parallel with these changes, non-reproducibility increased from 7% to 27%, although there was no significant difference between the levels of non-reproducibility using three or four extrastimuli when compared with those requiring two extrastimuli for induction.

These reports also highlight the problems of comparing studies that use different stimulation protocols as well as different subsets of patients. Morady *et al* [4] undertook a prospective comparison of two aggressive protocols for the induction of ventricular arrhythmia. By using two extra stimuli at multiple sites, and then three extra stimuli if no arrhythmia had been induced, a higher yield of clinical and a lower yield of non-clinical ventricular arrhythmias were produced when compared with protocols that started by using up to three extra stimuli at each site. Where non-clinical arrhythmias are inducible, the study of Dicarlo *et al* [5] indicated that they are non-specific responses to programmed stimulation and do not imply an underlying ventricular vulnerability. During 224 electrophysiologic studies undertaken in patients who had no prior documented serious ventricular arrhythmia, sustained ventricular flutter-fibrillation was induced in 18 patients. During follow-up for 25 ±14 months, nine patients received antiarrhythmic therapy, but there were no cardiac arrests or episodes of sudden death, either in those being treated or in those receiving no therapy.

Both electrophysiologic testing and ambulatory ECG monitoring have a role to play in the management of patients with serious ventricular arrhythmia. A prospective comparison of the two techniques was undertaken by Swerdlow *et al* [6] in 43 patients with sustained ventricular arrhythmia and coronary artery disease. As expected, ECG monitoring identified significantly fewer patients with arrhythmias that were suitable for drug assessment (50%) than did electrophysiologic study (82%). The value of drug testing was assessed in 62 survivors of cardiac arrest by Skale *et al* [7]. They found that 74% of patients had inducible arrhythmia at electrophysiologic study compared with only 31% who had spontaneous ventricular tachycardia on 48-hour (or more) continuous ECG monitoring. However, there was a subset of five patients who had arrhythmia on ambulatory monitoring, but no inducible ventricular tachycardia during electrophysiologic testing. Forty-one patients completed serial electrophysiologic drug testing, of whom 14 had successful suppression of ventricular tachycardia, and none of these had a recurrence of arrhythmia. Of the 27 failed drug studies, six patients subsequently died of cardiac arrest and four had recurrent ventricular tachycardia. In comparison, 20 patients had drug therapy guided by ECG monitoring, and in 4 of 9 in whom drug therapy suppressed ventricular tachycardia, sudden death subsequently occurred. This study suggests that the two techniques are probably appropriate for different subsets of patients. The possibility that the two methods could be complementary was raised by Kim *et al* [8] who demonstrated in a group of 52 patients with sustained ventricular tachycardia that persisting frequent ventricular extrasystoles predicted clinical outcome irrespective of whether ventricular tachycardia remained inducible.

In addition to induction of ventricular arrhythmias, the location of abnormal local electrograms may be important in identifying the origin of ventricular tachycardia prior to surgery. Two papers from Cassidy *et al* [9,10] described the characteristics of normal and abnormal local electrograms, and the value of catheter mapping during sinus rhythm in order to localize the site of origin of ventricular tachycardia.

Unexplained syncope remains an important clinical problem in which electrophysiologic testing may have an important diagnostic role. Kapoor *et al* [11] prospectively evaluated 204 patients with syncope. After standard clinical evaluation, patients underwent ambulatory ECG monitoring, electrophysiologic study, cardiac catheterization, cerebral angiography, electroencephalography and CT scanning only if the initial assessment pointed to a diagnosis for which such tests would be confirmatory.

In the 106 patients in whom a diagnosis could be established, it was made by history and physical examination in 52, routine ECG in 12, ECG monitoring in 29, electrophysiologic study in 3, cardiac catheterization in 7, cerebral angiography in 2 and electroencephalography in 1. After follow-up for 12 months, the overall mortality was 14%. It was significantly higher in those with cardiovascular disease (30%) than in those with a non-cardiovascular cause (12%) and those with syncope of unknown origin (6.4%). In 97 patients, the cause of syncope remained unknown. Sudden death occurred in 24% of those with a cardiovascular cause of syncope compared with 4% of those with a non-cardiovascular cause and 3% in those with syncope of unknown origin. Thus, these routine investigations did not enable a diagnosis to be made in nearly one-half of those presenting with syncope, although in this population the mortality is relatively low.

Recently introduced modifications to the tests for syncope, however, may improve the diagnostic yield. Hammill *et al* [12] undertook electrophysiologic testing with the patient on a tilt table, and obtained a better yield of sustained tachycardia and better reproduction of the clinical symptoms of the patient's spontaneous attacks in a group of patients with supraventricular arrhythmias, vasovagal syncope or carotid sinus hypersensitivity. Kenny *et al* [13] used a modification of this test, requiring head-up tilt at 40° for 60 minutes to act as a stimulus to vasovagal syncope, in patients with syncope that remained unexplained despite detailed clinical and electrophysiologic investigation. In patients in whom syncope developed during this test, pacemaker implantation resulted in freedom from recurrent symptoms. In these and other patients, increased vagal tone may be an important determinant of syncope. McLaran *et al* [14] identified 12 patients presenting with recurrent syncope who at electrophysiologic testing demonstrated abnormal atrioventricular nodal function which could be reversed by atropine. As a result, the patients were treated with the anticholinergic drug, propantheline bromide, and a marked reduction in the frequency of symptoms occurred, with six patients becoming asymptomatic. Recognition of this subgroup of patients may prevent the need for permanent cardiac pacing.

ELECTROPHYSIOLOGIC STUDIES IN PATIENTS AFTER MYOCARDIAL INFARCTION

Review: A.P. RAE, S.M. COBBE

In patients who survive the acute phase of myocardial infarction, the mortality rate in the first year is 10–20% [1–3] with 50% of these deaths being sudden [3–5]. Pathophysiologically, three mechanisms have been implicated in this mortality: left-ventricular dysfunction, myocardial ischemia and ventricular arrhythmia. Attempts at defining risk stratification have been directed towards the identification of these factors and have included exercise testing [6,7] and radionuclide angiography [8].

Ventricular Arrhythmias and Post-Infarction Mortality
The association of ventricular arrhythmias with subsequent mortality in patients after myocardial infarction is well recognized [9–11]; particularly the relationship between ventricular ectopy and sudden death [4,5,11,12]. Initial studies suggested that the presence of ventricular premature complexes (VPC) was not of independent prognostic value but was related more to the severity of left-ventricular dysfunction [9,13]. However, more recent studies have confirmed that ventricular arrhythmias are an independent risk factor and that their relationship with impaired ventricular function is of particular importance [5,12]. The complexity of ventricular ectopy has also been addressed. Although an increased risk of sudden death has been observed with a VPC frequency of more than 1 per hour [5], the presence of more complex forms, including repetitive VPCs and non-sustained ventricular tachycardia (>3 consecutive VPCs), has particular independent significance [5,12,14].

Despite the prognostic impact of ventricular ectopy, subsequent studies employing antiarrhythmic drug prophylaxis have generally been disappointing [15]. It is important to note that many of these studies have been too small to demonstrate a significant effect of antiarrhythmic therapy on mortality. Several factors may militate against the demonstration of the beneficial effect of suppression of ventricular arrhythmias. Although it is a sensitive index of subsequent sudden death, the demonstration of ventricular ectopy may not be sufficiently specific to identify the patient population at high risk, and any benefit is therefore diluted by the larger population of low-risk patients [16]. In addition, suppression of ventricular ectopy may not reflect protection from the development of ventricular tachycardia or fibrillation. A third factor that may offset the efficacy of antiarrhythmic drugs is the development in some patients of proarrhythmia or aggravation of arrhythmias due to the drug therapy itself [17].

Rationale for Electrophysiologic Testing
In patients with recurrent sustained ventricular tachycardia, programmed ventricular stimulation can reproducibly induce the clinical tachycardia [18,19]. The procedure involves the transvenous placement of electrode catheters with the introduction of timed extrastimuli during sinus rhythm and ventricular pacing. The rationale for this technique is that the introduction of extrastimuli can create the conditions of unidirectional block and slowed conduction necessary for the development of a re-entrant tachycardia in patients with an existing electrophysiological substrate [20]. Current

evidence suggests that subendocardial scarring caused by previous myocardial infarction provides this substrate [21–23]. Furthermore, since modification of arrhythmia induction by antiarrhythmic therapy has been shown to equate with the long term effect of that therapy, programmed stimulation is employed to define an effective drug regimen or alternative therapeutic modality.

In patients who have been resuscitated from sudden death, similar results have been obtained using programmed stimulation. In 70–80% of patients, ventricular tachycardia or ventricular fibrillation can be induced [24–26]. In cases of sudden death where the patient has been monitored, although the terminal arrhythmia was ventricular fibrillation, this was preceded by ventricular tachycardia [27,28].

On the basis of these observations, the use of electrophysiologic testing as a predictive technique for risk stratification has been investigated. Its potential for defining a subsequent treatment strategy has yet to be addressed.

Results of Electrophysiologic Testing in Post Myocardial Infarction Patients
The results from studies evaluating the prognostic significance of electrophysiologic testing in post-myocardial infarction patients have been very variable depending on patient selection, and specific aspects of individual protocols may influence results. These factors are discussed on page 276.

Programmed ventricular stimulation to assess ventricular electrical instability or ventricular vulnerability was first performed by Greene *et al* in 1978 [29]. In 48 patients studied <3 months after an acute myocardial infarction, single ventricular extrastimuli were introduced during atrial pacing at both the right ventricular apex and the right-ventricular outflow tract. Repetitive ventricular responses were observed in 39.6% of the patients. Within 1 year of follow-up, 15 of the 19 patients with repetitive ventricular responses had experienced either ventricular tachycardia or sudden death compared with only 4 of 29 patients without repetitive ventricular responses. However, the predictive value of the induction of repetitive ventricular responses could not be reproduced by other groups despite larger patient populations and the use of more sophisticated stimulation protocols [30–33].

Hamer *et al* [34] performed electrophysiological testing in 70 patients 7–20 days after acute myocardial infarction. In 37 patients, who underwent a stimulation protocol of up to two extrastimuli at two right-ventricular sites with stimulation amplitudes ranging from 2 to 10 V, >5 repetitive ventricular responses were induced in 12 patients, of whom 4 subsequently died suddenly during a 12-month follow-up period. In contrast, there was only 1 sudden death in 25 patients in whom 5 or fewer repetitive ventricular responses were induced ($P<0.05$). This group concluded that this type of response was potentially an important indicator of sudden death after myocardial infarction.

A similar result was reported by Richards *et al* [35]. In their study, ventricular instability was defined as the induction of ventricular fibrillation or ventricular tachycardia lasting at least 10 seconds. The stimulation protocol was somewhat unusual, in that two ventricular extrastimuli were introduced during a single paced cycle length at the right-ventricular apex and outflow tract at stimulation strengths of twice diastolic threshold and at 20 mA. The study population consisted of 165 patients evaluated 6–28 days after acute myocardial infarction. Ventricular electrical instability was observed in 38 (23%) of the patients. In the mean follow-up period of eight months, sudden death occurred in eight (21%) of these patients whereas no sudden deaths occurred in patients without electrical instability. The development of spontaneous ventricular tachycardia was also identified by this response, with two of the stable patients and four of the patients with electrical instability having sustained tachycardia over the follow-up period. The predictive accuracy for occurrence of sudden death or spontaneous ventricular tachycardia was 32% and the accuracy for the absence of electrical instability was 98%.

In contrast to these encouraging results, Marchlinski and colleagues [36] reported that, in a study of 46 patients investigated 8–60 days after infarction, the response to programmed stimulation was not of value. Using a limited stimulation protocol of up to two extrastimuli during sinus rhythm and ventricular pacing at only the right-ventricular apex at twice diastolic threshold, sustained or non-sustained ventricular tachycardia ($\geqslant$4 repetitive ventricular responses) was induced in 10 of the patients. During follow-up, six patients experienced sudden death but only one of these had been identified as having electrical instability. A similar conclusion was reached by Santarelli et al [37], although an association with non-sustained ventricular tachycardia on Holter monitoring was noted.

The study by Waspe et al [38] differed from the previous studies in two respects. The patient population consisted of 50 high-risk patients whose myocardial infarction had been complicated by the development of a new conduction disturbance, congestive heart failure or sustained ventricular tachyarrhythmias either alone or in combination. Secondly, the stimulation protocol was more aggressive using up to three extrastimuli at four times diastolic threshold at two right-ventricular sites. Two groups of patients were identified by their response to programmed stimulation. Group I patients had inducible sustained or non-sustained ventricular tachycardia (defined as >7 repetitive ventricular responses) and Group II patients had 7 or less repetitive ventricular responses following complete stimulation protocol. Group I patients had a higher incidence of anterior infarction and a lower ejection fraction (35% vs 48%) than Group II patients. During a mean follow-up of 23 months, none of the 33 patients in Group II experienced either sudden death or spontaneous ventricular tachycardia. Out of seven patients in Group I, six died suddenly and one developed sustained ventricular tachycardia ($P<0.001$). The sensitivity of the test was 100% with a specificity of 57%. Of particular note is the fact that triple extrastimuli were required to induce the tachyarrhythmia in five of the seven patients. Furthermore, although the patient population was small, the stongest clinical variable for the occurrence of sudden death was the response to programmed stimulation.

Using a similarly aggressive protocol, however, Bhandari et al [39] did not confirm these results. The major difference from the study by Waspe et al [38] is that this was a lower-risk population, as manifest by the low subsequent mortality and the higher mean ejection fraction of the two groups (45% and 50%).

Roy et al [40] evaluated a much larger patient population. Programmed stimulation was performed on 150 patients, at a mean of 12 days after infarction. This group employed a relatively non-aggressive stimulation protocol of up to 2 ventricular extrastimuli at two right-ventricular sites at a stimulus strength of twice diastolic threshold. Non-sustained ventricular tachycardia was induced in 17 patients and sustained tachycardia in 16 patients. During the 10-month follow-up, 4 of the 150 patients (3%)

experienced either sudden death or sustained ventricular tachycardia. Only two of these patients had evidence of electrical instability as determined by programmed stimulation.

Value of Electrophysiologic Testing in Association with Non-Invasive Testing
Denniss and colleagues [41] evaluated programmed stimulation and exercise testing in 228 patients 1–4 weeks after myocardial infarction. Programmed stimulation was performed in 175 of these patients. This was an update of the study reported by Richards *et al* [35] from the same group. With the same protocol and end-point, ventricular tachycardia or ventricular fibrillation was induced in 38 patients (22%), and these had a subsequent mortality rate of 26% over the follow-up period. In contrast, the mortality rate in patients without electrical instability was only 6% ($P<0.01$). In the 191 patients who underwent exercise testing, 61 (32%) had an ischemic response, as defined by ST-segment change of 2 mm or more. In the 138 patients who underwent both tests, there was no statistically significant relationship between the results of the two tests. The mortality rate if either or both tests were positive was 13% compared with 1% (1 of 85 patients) if both tests were negative. It was therefore concluded that programmed stimulation was a powerful predictor of sudden death but that the combination of tests allowed prediction of virtually all deaths during a one-year follow-up. It should be noted that this was a relatively low-risk group of patients since 111 patients had already been excluded from the study because of complications such as heart failure. The mortality of the excluded group was 22%, which was twice the rate of the study group.

Breithardt *et al* [42] investigated the combination of ventricular late potentials and electrophysiologic testing as a marker for sudden death or subsequent spontaneous ventricular tachycardia. The pathophysiologic mechanisms and the methodology for detection and registration of ventricular late potentials have recently been comprehensively reviewed [43,44]. Briefly, late potentials are low-amplitude fractionated activity occurring after the QRS complex of the surface electrocardiogram. Registration of these signals requires high-gain amplification and filtering in association with some form of computer-averaging procedure. Signal-averaging techniques help to reduce the degree of random noise by either summating the signals over many cardiac cycles (temporal averaging) or by registering simultaneous beat-to-beat signals from multiple electrodes in close proximity (spatial averaging). These signal-averaged recordings probably reflect areas of endocardial scarring which provide the anatomical substrate for ventricular arrhythmias. Breithardt *et al* [42] studied 379 patients with coronary artery disease of whom 132 patients were evaluated within six weeks of an acute myocardial infarction. During follow-up, 3% had sudden death and 6.8% developed sustained ventricular tachycardia. The induction of four or more repetitive ventricular responses or of ventricular tachycardia was not predictive of sudden death, but did predict the spontaneous development of ventricular tachycardia. A similar result was obtained for the presence of late potentials. The predictive value if both tests were positive was 20%. Furthermore, if the results of the positive tests were further defined by the combination of the presence of late potentials of 40 ms duration or more and induction of monomorphic sustained ventricular tachycardia at rates below 270 bpm, a predictive value of 50% was attained. These observations suggest that the combination of these two techniques may be useful in identifying a subgroup of post-infarction patients for whom prophylactic antiarrhythmic therapy might be beneficial.

The value of antiarrhythmic therapy was tested by Denniss *et al* [45] who randomized 96 patients with electrical instability either to an untreated control group or to receive quinidine, disopyramide or mexiletine with dosage titration to achieve therapeutic drug levels. During the mean follow-up of 18 months, there was no difference in either sudden death or development of spontaneous ventricular tachycardia between the two groups. This lack of benefit was attributed to the low efficacy of the selected antiarrhythmic agents in suppressing inducible arrhythmias.

Reasons for the Variable Results of Electrophysiologic Testing

The variability of results reported among electrophysiologic studies may be due to several different factors [46].

In order to test satisfactorily the hypothesis that ventricular electrical instability as determined by programmed ventricular stimulation can identify patients at high-risk of subsequent sudden death, a sufficiently large sample size is required to ensure that a meaningful number of end-point events occur over the follow-up period. In most of the studies reported, the incidence of sudden death has been too small. This has been compounded by the fact that, except for the study by Waspe *et al* [38], the study populations have been at low risk, thus reducing the pretest probability of sudden death. The majority of studies have excluded patients with sustained ventricular arrhythmias and poor left-ventricular function. Indeed, one study evaluating the response to programmed stimulation in patients undergoing thrombolytic therapy demonstrated that ventricular arrhythmias were less commonly induced in patients whose arteries were reperfused than in patients without reperfusion suggesting that the response to stimulation was related to the extent of myocardial damage [47].

Interstudy comparison of electrophysiologic testing is notoriously difficult because of the differing methods employed. The studies that have reported a positive predictive value for this technique have tended to employ the more aggressive stimulation protocols including the use of three extrastimuli or higher stimulus energies [34,35,37,41]. The argument for using less aggressive stimulation is based on observations from studies evaluating the specificity of arrhythmia induction in patients without ventricular arrhythmias. Non-specific or non-clinical ventricular tachyarrhythmias using aggressive protocols with three and four extrastimuli can be induced in up to 40% of patients [48,49]. The finding by Waspe *et al* [38] that the third extrastimulus was necessary to provide predictive significance appears to refute this argument, although further studies comparing stimulation protocols in the same patient population are required to select the optimum protocol.

A further aspect of the stimulation protocol which might influence the response to programmed stimulation is the development of myocardial ischemia produced by the protocol itself. Preliminary studies have suggested that, in some patients with coronary artery disease, concomitant myocardial ischemia during ventricular stimulation (as evidenced by coronary sinus lactate production) is required for the induction of arrhythmia [50,51]. Whether this factor is important in electrophysiological testing in postinfarction patients has not been reported.

The impact of the timing of testing in relation to the index infarction has recently been addressed by Roy *et al* [52]. Stimulation was performed in 21 patients who had an inducible tachyarrhythmia at a mean of 12 days after myocardial infarction and then repeated the same protocol at a mean of 8 months after infarction. Ventricular tachyarrhythmias could be reinitiated in 16 (76%) of these patients. Despite persistence of electrical instability, only one patient died suddenly over a mean follow-up period of 17 months. A similar lack of time-dependent change in response to stimulation was reported for the repetitive ventricular response by Pop and colleagues [53]. In contrast, Aonuma *et al* [54] found a decrease in the incidence of inducible non-sustained ventricular tachycardia in 19 patients from 53% during testing at 2–3 weeks after infarction to 21% at 12–14 weeks. This latter observation is supported indirectly by the study of Breithardt *et al* [42] who noted a markedly lower prevalence of inducible sustained ventricular tachycardia in patients studied more than three months after infarction compared with those studied within 4–8 weeks. A converse result was obtained by Kuck *et al* [55] in a small study of 18 patients in an earlier phase after infarction at 5 and 24 days. At 5 days, non-sustained ventricular tachycardia was induced in two patients and sustained tachycardia in two patients, compared with the responses at 24 days when non-sustained tachycardia was induced in two patients, sustained tachycardia in six patients and ventricular fibrillation in three patients. Over the follow-up of 24 months no arrhythmic event occurred in any patient. However, the induction of polymorphic tachycardia or monomorphic tachycardia with a short cycle length on the second study must raise the question of the specificity of these responses.

A further factor confounding the interpretation of the reported studies is the variability of subsequent antiarrhythmic and other cardioactive agents prescribed during follow-up which may influence the subsequent development of tachyarrhythmias.

Conclusions

The results from studies of the prognostic significance of the response to programmed stimulation are conflicting. A negative response is associated with a low risk of subsequent sudden death, but the specificity of a positive response has been too low in most studies to be of predictive value. However, this disappointing conclusion may reflect flawed study protocols and, before this technique can be dismissed, further studies are required incorporating much larger populations, comparisons of different stimulation protocols and longer and more rigorously controlled follow-up. It is much more likely, however, that the place of electrophysiologic testing is in those patients who have already been stratified by non-invasive testing as high risk. As an invasive technique with a small but inherent risk of complication, it cannot practically be applied to all survivors of myocardial infarction. Indeed, as programmed stimulation probably reveals only the potential anatomic-electrophysiologic substrate for ventricular tachyarrhythmias and does not identify the trigger factors, such as myocardial ischemia, that are necessary for subsequent spontaneous development of arrhythmia, it should be considered as an adjunct to other techniques, such as exercise testing, radionuclide ventriculography, ambulatory monitoring and the recording of late potentials. Since the etiology of sudden death is multifactorial, a multidisciplinary approach to risk stratification is therefore required.

References

[1] Kannel WB, Sorlie P, McNamara PM.
Prognosis after initial myocardial infarction: the Framingham Study.
Am J Cardiol 1979; **44**: 53–9.

[2] Moss AJ.
Prognosis after myocardial infarction.
Am J Cardiol 1983; **52**: 667–9.

[3] The Multicenter Postinfarction Research Group.
Risk stratification and survival after myocardial infarction.
N Engl J Med 1983; **309**: 331–6.

[4] Goldstein S, Friedman L, Hutchinson R *et al*, Aspirin Myocardial Infarction Study.
Timing, mechanism and clinical setting of witnessed deaths in postmyocardial infarction patients.
J Am Coll Cardiol 1984; **3**: 1111–7.

[5] Bigger JT Jr, Fleiss JL, Kleiger R, Miller VP, Rolnitzky LM. The Multicenter Postinfarction Research Group.
The relationships among ventricular arrhythmias, left ventricular dysfunction, and mortality in the 2 years after myocardial infarction.
Circulation 1984; **69**: 250–8.

[6] Theroux P, Waters DD, Halphen C, Debaisieux JC, Mizgala HF.
Prognostic value of exercise testing soon after myocardial infarction.
N Engl J Med 1979; **301**: 341–5.

[7] Weld FM, Chu KL, Bigger JT, Ronitzky LM.
Risk stratification with low-level exercise testing 2 weeks after acute myocardial infarction.
Circulation 1981; **64**: 306–14.

[8] Fioretti P, Brower RW, Simoons ML *et al*.
Prediction of mortality in hospital survivors of myocardial infarction. Comparison of predischarge exercise testing and radionuclide ventriculography at rest.
Br Heart J 1984; **52**: 292–8.

[9] Schultze RA Jr, Strauss HW, Pitt B.
Sudden death in the year following myocardial infarction: relation to ventricular premature contractions in the late hospital phase and left ventricular ejection fraction.
Am J Med 1977; **62**: 192–9.

[10] Moss AJ, Davis HT, DeCamilla J, Bayer LW.
Ventricular ectopic beats and their relation to sudden and non sudden cardiac death after myocardial infarction.
Circulation 1978; **60**: 998–1003.

[11] Ruberman W, Weinblatt E, Goldberg JD, Frank CW, Chaudhary BJ, Shapiro S.
Ventricular premature complexes and sudden death after myocardial infarction.
Circulation 1981; **64**: 297–305.

[12] Mukharji J, Rude RE, Poole WK *et al*.
Risk factors for sudden death following acute myocardial infarction (two year follow-up).
Am J Cardiol 1984; **54**: 31–6.

[13] Califf M, Burks SM, Behar VS, Margolis JR, Wagner GS.
Relationship among ventricular arrhythmias, coronary artery disease and angiographic and electrocardiographic indicators of myocardial fibrosis.
Circulation 1978; **57**: 725–32.

[14] Bigger JT Jr, Fleiss JL, Rolnitzky LM, Multicenter Post-Infarction Research Group.
Prevalence, characteristics and significance of ventricular tachycardia detected by 24-hour continuous electrocardiographic recordings in the late hospital phase of acute myocardial infarction.
Am J Cardiol 1986; **58**: 1151–60.

[15] May GS, Eberlein KA, Furberg CD, Passamani ER, DeMets DL.
Secondary prevention after myocardial infarction: a review of long-term trials.
Prog Cardiovasc Dis 1982; **24**: 331–52.

[16] Cowan C, Campbell RWF.
Antiarrhythmic therapy in post myocardial infarction patients.
Eur Heart J 1986; **7** (Suppl A): 145–7.

[17] Velebit V, Podrid P, Lown B, Cohen BH, Graboys TB.
Aggravation and provocation of ventricular arrhythmias by antiarrhythmic drugs.
Circulation 1986; **65**: 886–93.

[18] Vendepol CJ, Farshidi A, Spielman SR, Greenspan AM, Horowitz LN, Josephson ME.
Incidence and clinical significance of induced ventricular tachycardia.
Am J Cardiol 1980; **45**: 725–31.

[19] Livelli FD Jr, Bigger JT Jr, Reiffel JA *et al*.
Response to programmed ventricular stimulation: sensitivity, specificity and relation to heart disease.
Am J Cardiol 1982; **50**: 452–8.

[20] Josephson ME, Marchlinski FE, Buxton AE, Waxman HL, Doherty JU, Kienzle MG, Falcone R.
Electrophysiologic basis for sustained ventricular tachycardia - role of reentry.
In: *Tachycardias: Mechanism, diagnosis, treatment*. Philadelphia: Lea and Febiger 1984: 305-23.

[21] Mehra R, Zeiler RH, Gough WB, El-Sherif N.
Reentrant ventricular arrhythmias in the late myocardial infarction period. 9. Electrophysiologic-anatomic correlation of reentrant circuit.
Circulation 1983; **67**: 11-24.

[22] Josephson ME, Horowitz LN, Farshidi A.
Continuous local electrical activity. A mechanism of recurrent ventricular tachycardia.
Circulation 1986; **57**: 659-65.

[23] Horowitz LN, Josephson ME, Harben AH.
Epicardial and endocardial activation during sustained ventricular tachycardia in man.
Circulation 1980; **61**: 1227-38.

[24] Ruskin JN, DiMarco JP, Garan H.
Out-of-hospital cardiac arrest: electrophysiologic observations and selection of long-term antiarrhythmic therapy.
N Engl J Med 1980; **303**: 607-13.

[25] Morady F, Scheinman MM, Hess DS, Sung RJ, Shen E, Shapiro W.
Electrophysiologic testing in the management of survivors of out-of-hospital cardiac arrest.
Am J Cardiol 1983; **51**: 85-9.

[26] Benditt DG, Benson DW Jr, Klein GJ, Pritzker MR, Kriett JM, Anderson RW.
Prevention of recurrent sudden cardiac arrest: role of provocative electropharmacologic testing.
J Am Coll Cardiol 1983; **2**: 418-25.

[27] Pratt CM, Francis MJ, Luck JC, Wyndham CR, Miller RR, Quinones MA.
Analysis of ambulatory electocardiograms in 15 patients during spontaneous ventricular fibrillation with special reference to preceding arrhythmic events.
J Am Coll Cardiol 1983; **2**: 789-97.

[28] Panidis IP, Morganroth J.
Sudden death in hospitalized patients: cardiac rhythm disturbances detected by ambulatory electrocardiographic monitoring.
J Am Coll Cardiol 1983; **2**: 798-805.

[29] Greene HL, Reid PR, Schaeffer AH.
The repetitive ventricular response in man: a predictor of sudden death.
N Engl J Med 1978; **299**: 729-37.

[30] Troup PJ, Pederson DH, Zipes DP.
Effects of premature ventricular stimulation in patients with ventricular tachycardia.
Circulation 1978; **58**: 111-261.

[31] Mason JW.
Repetitive beating after single ventricular extrastimuli: incidence and prognostic significance in patients with recurrent ventricular tachycardia.
Am J Cardiol 1980; **45**: 1126-31.

[32] Breithardt G, Abendroth RR, Borggrefe M, Yeh HL, Haerten K, Seipel L.
Prevalence and clinical significance of the repetitive ventricular response during sinus rhythm in coronary disease patients.
Am Heart J 1984; **107**: 229-36.

[33] Treese N, Pop T, Meinertz T, Kasper W, Geibel A, Stienen U, Meyer J.
Prognostic significance of repetitive ventricular response in chronic coronary artery disease.
Eur Heart J 1985; **6**: 594-601.

[34] Hamer A, Vohra J, Hunt D, Sloman G.
Prediction of sudden death by electrophysiologic studies in high risk patients surviving acute myocardial infarction.
Am J Cardiol 1982; **50**: 223-9.

[35] Richards DA, Cody DV, Denniss AR, Russell PA, Young AA, Uther JB.
Ventricular electrical instability: a predictor of death after myocardial infarction.
Am J Cardiol 1983; **51**: 75-80.

[36] Marchlinski FE, Buxton AE, Waxman HL, Josephson ME.
Identifying patients at risk of sudden death after myocardial infarction: value of the response to programmed stimulation, degree of ventricular ectopic activity and severity of left ventricular dysfunction.
Am J Cardiol 1983; **52**: 1190-6.

[37] Santarelli P, Bellocci F, Loperfido F *et al*.
Ventricular arrhythmia induced by programmed ventricular stimulation after acute myocardial infarction.
Am J Cardiol 1985; **55**: 391-4.

[38] Waspe LE, Seinfeld D, Ferrick A, Kim SG, Matos JA, Fisher JD.
Prediction of sudden death and spontaneous ventricular tachycardia in survivors of complicated myocardial infarction: value of the response to programmed stimulations using a maximum of three ventricular extrastimuli.
J Am Coll Cardiol 1985; **5**: 1292-301.

[39] Bhandari AK, Rose JS, Kotlewski A, Rahimtoola SH, Wu D.
Frequency and significance of induced sustained ventricular tachycardia or fibrillation two weeks after acute myocardial infarction.
Am J Cardiol 1985; **56**: 737–42.

[40] Roy D, Marchand E, Theroux P, Waters DD, Pelletier GB, Bourassa MG.
Programmed ventricular stimulation in survivors of an acute myocardial infarction.
Circulation 1985; **72**: 487–94.

[41] Denniss AR, Baaijens H, Cody DV *et al*.
Value programmed stimulation and exercise testing in predicting one-year mortality after acute myocardial infarction.
Am J Cardiol 1985; **56**: 213–20.

[42] Breithardt G, Borggrefe M, Haerten K.
Ventricular late potentials and inducible ventricular tachyarrhythmias as a marker for ventricular tachycardia after myocardial infarction.
Eur Heart J 1986; **7** (Suppl A): 127–34.

[43] Breithardt G, Borggrefe M.
Pathophysiological mechanisms and clinical significance of ventricular late potentials.
Eur Heart J 1986; **7**: 364–85.

[44] El-Sherif N, Gomes JAC, Restivo M, Mehra R.
Late potentials and arrhythmogenesis.
PACE 1985; **8**: 440–62.

[45] Denniss AR, Ross DL, Cody DV, Richards DA, Russell PA, Young AA, Uther JB.
Randomised trial of antiarrhythmic drugs in patients with inducible ventricular tachyarrhythmias after recent myocardial infarction.
Circulation 1986; **74** (Suppl): II–213.

[46] Greenspan AM.
Can electrophysiologic testing predict mortality after myocardial infarction?
J Am Coll Cardiol 1986; **7**: 1243–4.

[47] Kersschot IE, Brugada P, Ramentol M *et al*.
Effects of early reperfusion in acute myocardial infarction on arrythmias induced by programmed stimulation: a prospective randomized study.
J Am Coll Cardiol 1986; **7**: 1234–42.

[48] Brugada P, Abdollah H, Heddle B, Wellens HJJ.
Results of a ventricular stimulation protocol using a maximum of 4 premature stimuli in patients without documented or suspected ventricular arrhythmias.
Am J Cardiol 1983; **52**: 1214–8.

[49] Mann DE, Luck JC, Griffin JC *et al*.
Induction of clinical ventricular tachycardia using programmed stimulation: value of third and fourth extrastimuli.
Am J Cardiol 1983; **52**: 501–6.

[50] Borggrefe M, Breithardt G.
Metabolic effects of programmed stimulation: relation to arrhythmia induction and response to revascularization.
Circulation 1986; **74** (Suppl): II–481.

[51] Morady F, Di Carlo L, Krol R, Annesley T, Baerman J, De Buitleir M, Kou W.
The role of myocardial ischemia during programmed stimulation in patients with aborted sudden death and coronary artery disease.
Circulation 1986; **74** (Suppl): II–481.

[52] Roy D, Marchand E, Theroux P, Waters DD, Pelletier GB, Cartier R, Bourassa MC.
Long-term reproducibility and significance of provokable ventricular arrhythmias after myocardial infarction.
J Am Coll Cardiol 1986; **8**: 32–9.

[53] Pop T, Treese N, Henkel B, Erbel R, von Olshausen K, Meyer J.
Stimulus-induced vulnerability in the early and late post-infarction phase.
Eur Heart J 1986; **7**: 866–70.

[54] Aonuma K, Iesaka Y, Ri K, Furukawa T, Nitta J, Taniguchi K, Lister JW.
Time dependent response to ventricular programmed stimulation in post acute myocardial infarction patients.
Circulation 1986; **74** (Suppl): II–189.

[55] Kuck K-H, Costard A, Schluter M, Kunze K-P.
Significance of Timing Programmed Electrical Stimulation after acute myocardial infarction.
J Am Coll Cardiol 1986; **8**: 1279–88.

INDICATIONS FOR THE TREATMENT OF VENTRICULAR ARRHYTHMIAS

Review: MICHAEL E. CAIN

For the purposes of this review, *sustained ventricular arrhythmias* are defined as episodes of ventricular tachycardia or ventricular fibrillation lasting longer than 30 seconds or associated with hemodynamic decompensation; *ventricular ectopy* refers to ventricular arrhythmias other than sustained ventricular tachycardia or ventricular fibrillation; *complex ventricular ectopy* includes frequent ventricular premature depolarizations (>30/hour), multiform ventricular premature depolarizations, couplets, and non-sustained ventricular tachycardia; and *simple ventricular ectopy* refers to uniform ventricular premature depolarizations that occur at a frequency of <30/hour.

Patients who develop sustained ventricular tachycardia or ventricular fibrillation require vigorous evaluation and aggressive therapy. Nevertheless, the management of patients who manifest ventricular ectopy alone remains controversial. Despite the recent advances in electrophysiologic techniques and monitoring capabilities that have helped to delineate the cellular and clinical electrophysiologic derangements accompanying ventricular arrhythmias, decisions concerning the treatment of patients with ventricular ectopy are based, unfortunately, on empiricism. This review focuses on the indications for treating patients with ventricular ectopy detected during ambulatory ECG monitoring.

Indications for Therapy

Theoretic objectives for treating patients who manifest ventricular ectopy include the prevention of sustained ventricular tachycardia or ventricular fibrillation and the reduction of symptoms that may accompany an irregular heart rhythm, such as anxiety secondary to awareness of an irregular heart rhythm or reduction in forward cardiac output. The latter may result in: (i) angina; (ii) precipitation or exacerbation of symptoms of congestive heart failure; (iii) derangements of central nervous system function, including altered mental status, lightheadedness and presyncope; or (iv) fatigue.

The severity of symptoms varies widely. Definitive documentation of a cause-and-effect relationship is best achieved by correlating the symptoms experienced clinically with spontaneous rhythm. Prolonged and repeated ambulatory ECG monitoring is often necessary. Patient-activated transtelephonic ECG monitors are particularly useful in patients in whom symptoms occur capriciously. Patients with symptoms documented as being due to ventricular ectopy shoud be treated with antiarrhythmic agents and the alleviation of symptoms used as a therapeutic end-point. Antiarrhythmic agents should be continued as long as they remain effective, and as long as adverse reactions do not become evident which result in symptoms more severe than those attributed to ventricular ectopy.

Prevention of Sustained Ventricular Arrhythmias

The decision to treat patients with asymptomatic ventricular ectopy should be made only after careful consideration of the benefit/risk ratio of administering potentially toxic antiarrhythmic agents to asymptomatic individuals. The benefit/risk ratio can best be considered in terms of the following questions.

1. Which patients are at highest risk for developing sustained ventricular tachycardia or ventricular fibrillation?
2. Is ventricular ectopy a specific progenitor of sudden arrhythmic death?
3. Does treatment of ventricular ectopy prevent the occurrence of sustained ventricular arrhythmias?
4. Can antiarrhythmic agents be deleterious?

Cardiovascular Status of Patients Developing Sustained Ventricular Tachycardia/ Ventricular Fibrillation

Each year, more than 400 000 Americans die suddenly from sustained ventricular arrhythmias. The electrophysiologic derangements underlying sustained ventricular tachycardia or ventricular fibrillation may be present transiently during episodes of acute myocardial ischemia with or without infarction, metabolic or electrolyte imbalance, neurologic abnormalities, or treatment with antiarrhythmic agents. Conversely, the arrhythmogenic substrate may be present persistently as a consequence of prior infarction or myocardial injury. The relative incidences of the two disparate circumstances are unclear.

The clinical characteristics of 116 consecutive patients referred to the arrhythmia service at Barnes Hospital, St Louis, for sustained ventricular tachycardia or ventricular fibrillation not associated with acute myocardial infarction, electrolyte abnormalities, or toxicity to antiarrhythmic drugs, are shown in Table I. Most patients (80%) had coronary artery disease, prior myocardial infarction, and severe left-ventricular dysfunction; 20 (17%) had cardiomyopathies. These findings are comparable to those reported by others [1–6]. Although sustained ventricular tachycardia or ventricular fibrillation ocurs in patients with structural heart disease other than coronary artery disease and with myopathic derangements (including mitral valve prolapse [7,8]), and

Table I: Barnes Hospital Arrhythmia Service: Characteristics of 116 consecutive patients with sustained ventricular arrhythmias.

Cardiac diagnosis	Patients	Age (yrs)	Left-ventricular ejection fraction (%)
Coronary artery disease/ myocardial infarction	93 (80%)	63 ± 11	31 ± 4
Cardiomyopathy	20 (17%)	57 ± 12	25 ± 8
Other			
S/P repair TOF	1 (1%)	28	60
Normal	2 (2%)	52 ± 3	63 ± 3
TOF = Tetralogy of Fallot			

even in apparently normal individuals [9–11], such occurrences are exceedingly uncommon. Overall, sustained ventricular arrhythmias occur only rarely in patients without organic heart disease or in patients with organic heart disease but with well-preserved ventricular function.

Because of the prevalence of coronary artery disease, the largest group of patients at risk for developing sustained ventricular arrhythmias comprises those who have survived myocardial infarction, in whom there is a 3%–8% incidence of sudden cardiac death during the first year following infarction and an incidence of 2%–4% per year thereafter. The patients at highest risk for sudden cardiac death, however, are those with hypertrophic or congestive cardiomyopathies: results of studies in patients with hypertrophic cardiomyopathy have demonstrated the incidence of sudden death to be 2%–8% per year [12–14]. Sudden cardiac death constitutes 30%–50% of all deaths in patients with congestive cardiomyopathies [15–22].

Relationship between Ventricular Ectopy and Sudden Cardiac Death
At present, one of the most challenging problems in clinical cardiology to address is which patient recovering from myocardial infarction is at highest risk for developing a sustained ventricular arrhythmia: (i) the patient without ventricular ectopy; (ii) the patient with infrequent or simple ventricular ectopy; (iii) the patient with complex ventricular ectopy, including multiform ventricular premature depolarizations or couplets; or (iv) the patient with non-sustained ventricular tachycardia. Conventional teaching has favored the view that ventricular ectopy, especially in its complex forms, portends sustained ventricular arrhythmias. As new data emerge, however, this concept is being challenged.

The relationship between the presence of ventricular ectopy and mortality has been the subject of many studies [23–38], most of which have demonstrated that, in addition to left-ventricular dysfunction, patients recovering from myocardial infarction who manifest ventricular ectopy – especially when frequent or with complex forms – have a higher mortality than patients with absent, or simple, ventricular ectopy. These findings do not, however, necessarily imply a cause-and-effect relationship between the presence of ventricular ectopy and the occurrence of sustained ventricular arrhythmias or sudden death – both may reflect other factors such as left-ventricular dysfunction or on-going ischemia. Because left-ventricular dysfunction is both a major predictor of mortality and an important determinant of ventricular ectopy [39,40], some have argued that ventricular ectopy does not contribute independently to the risk of mortality, but is an epiphenomenon of severe myocardial damage [29]. Results of larger studies have demonstrated that the presence of ventricular ectopy in patients surviving an acute myocardial infarction *does* provide prognostic information independent of left-ventricular function [31,33,35–38]. These results indicate, however, that residual left-ventricular function is the major prognostic index of survival. Manifest ischemia and complex ventricular ectopy are less powerful descriptors.

Although certain patterns of ventricular ectopy may predict higher cardiac mortality in large groups, none specifically predicts sudden arrhythmic death when applied to individuals. The results of several studies pertinent to this issue have recently been reviewed [41,42]. Ruberman *et al* compared the cumulative incidence of sudden cardiac death and death due to other cardiac causes in a large number of patients with prior

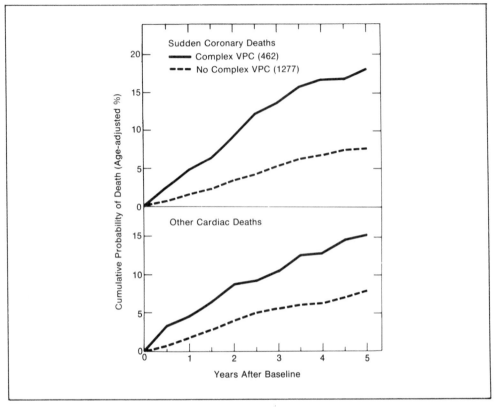

FIGURE 1: Sudden and non-sudden cardiac death over five years in male survivors of myocardial infarction, in relation to the presence of complex ventricular premature complexes (VPC) during one hour of baseline monitoring. (Reprinted, with permission, from Ruberman et al [34].)

myocardial infarction with and without complex ventricular ectopy (Fig. 1) [33]. Among the 1739 patients studied, 462 had complex ventricular ectopy and were identified as a high-risk group; the 1277 patients without complex ectopy were defined as a low-risk group. Sixty-eight patients (15%) in the high-risk and 71 patients (6%) in the low-risk group died suddenly. However, the percentage that was sudden of the total deaths (49% vs 40%) did not differ significantly between the groups. Thus, although patients who manifest complex ventricular ectopy following myocardial infarction are at higher risk of death, the presence of complex ventricular ectopy did not differentiate the risk of sudden cardiac death from that of death due to other cardiac causes. More importantly, over half of all the patients dying suddenly were from the group without complex ventricular ectopy. In the context of these results, if antiarrhythmic agents were prescribed for patients with complex ventricular ectopy for the purpose of preventing sudden cardiac death, 85% of those alleged to be at risk would be treated inappropriately with costly and potentially toxic antiarrhythmic agents, and more than half of those who were to die suddenly would not be treated.

There are several factors making the interpretation of epidemiologic studies difficult. The occurrence of ventricular ectopy demonstrates marked day-to-day and hour-to-hour variability [43,44]. Consequently, the incidence of ventricular ectopy varies directly with the duration of the monitoring period [45]. In the Ruberman study, a single one-hour ECG recording was used to distinguish patients with from those without complex ventricular ectopy, and complex ventricular ectopy was identified in 27% of the study population [33]. However, with the increasing availability of telemetry units, patients recovering from myocardial infarction are currently being monitored more extensively. Results from the telemetry unit at Barnes Hospital (shown in Table II) indicate that 58% of hospitalized patients manifest complex ventricular ectopy during the convalescent phase after myocardial infarction [42]. Paradoxically, as a greater number of arrhythmias are being detected, assessment of the role ventricular ectopy plays in identifying patients at increased risk for developing sustained ventricular tachycardia or ventricular fibrillation has become more difficult.

Results of epidemiologic studies have demonstrated that the incidence of sudden cardiac death is highest during the first 3–6 months after infarction [23–38]. In the study by Ruberman, for example, patients were recruited a mean interval of three months after infarction [33]. The incidence of ventricular ectopy in patients with and without structural heart disease increases as a function of age [46], and antiarrhythmic agents influence the incidence and complexity of ventricular arrhythmias at any age.

Studies purported to establish a relationship between ventricular ectopy and sudden cardiac death have utilized ECG-monitoring durations ranging from *seconds* to *48 hours*, recruited patients days to months after the reference infarction, failed to control for the administration of antiarrhythmic agents, and variably included and excluded patients with marked left-ventricular dysfunction. Thus, uniform interpretation is impossible.

Another factor clouding the interpretation of results of studies examining the relationship between ventricular ectopy and sudden death is the definition of sudden cardiac death. In my opinion, the term 'sudden cardiac death' should be restricted to *instantaneous* death. Investigators have variously defined sudden cardiac death as instantaneous, or as death occurring within 1 hour, 2 hours, 12 hours or 24 hours of the onset of symptoms. It is inappropriate to compare one patient with ventricular ectopy who dies suddenly three months after a myocardial infarction because of the spon-

Table II. Barnes Hospital Telemetry Unit: 1983 data*

Category	Patients
Post-myocardial infarction	277
Complex VEA	161 (58%)
Non-sustained VT	92 (33%)
VEA = ventricular ectopic activity; VT = ventricular tachycardia.	
* Modified from Cain [42].	

taneous occurrence of sustained ventricular tachycardia or ventricular fibrillation, with another patient with ventricular ectopy who succumbs 24 hours after a second acute myocardial infarction due to profound heart failure or myocardial rupture.

Although the limitations already noted can confound interpretation of studies of patients with hypertrophic and congestive cardiomyopathies as well, patients with hypertrophic cardiomyopathy and asymptomatic non-sustained ventricular tachycardia detected during ambulatory ECG monitoring have a yearly incidence of sudden death of 9% – markedly greater than that of patients without non-sustained ventricular tachycardia [12–14]. Mortality in patients with congestive cardiomyopathy has been correlated with hemodynamic measurements, echocardiographic left-ventricular mass and relative wall thickness, and the extent of ventricular arrhythmias [15–22]. Results with ambulatory ECG monitoring indicated that 60%–90% of these patients had ventricular ectopy, and that 40%–60% exhibited non-sustained ventricular tachycardia. Similar to results in patients with myocardial infarction, results of studies in patients with congestive cardiomyopathy have demonstrated that prognosis is related primarily to the degree of left-ventricular dysfunction, and that, although the presence of complex ventricular ectopy can indicate a poor prognosis, its presence does not distinguish between total mortality and mortality from sudden cardiac death [20,22].

Mitral valve prolapse is a common clinical entity, often occurring in otherwise healthy individuals. Ventricular ectopy may be seen in over 60% of these patients [47,48]. However, because sudden death occurs only rarely [49], the prognostic significance of ventricular ectopy in this population is quite low.

Ventricular ectopy, including complex forms of it, has been detected in 40%–70% of normal subjects, as assessed during 24–48-hour ambulatory ECG monitoring [50–53]. The incidence and frequency of ventricular ectopy increases with age. Results of several studies have shown that the long-term prognosis of asymptomatic healthy subjects with frequent and complex ventricular ectopy is similar to that of healthy subjects without detectable ventricular ectopy [54,55].

Absence of Beneficial Effects despite Treatment with Antiarrhythmic Drugs
Even if ventricular ectopy is related to sustained ventricular arrhythmias and sudden cardiac death, no data indicate that prophylaxis with antiarrhythmic agents is protective. Possible explanations for the failure to demonstrate a favorable effect include: (i) inadequate study designs with inclusion of patients at low risk, inadequate doses of antiarrhythmic drugs, or small sample sizes; (ii) patient non-compliance with prescribed antiarrhythmic regimens, due to the high incidence of side-effects and the need for multiple-dosing intervals; (iii) the low efficacy of available antiarrhythmic agents; (iv) the proarrhythmic effects of antiarrhythmic agents, which may facilitate the spontaneous occurrence of sustained ventricular arrhythmias; and (v) the fact that suppression of ventricular ectopy *per se* may not prevent sustained ventricular tachycardia or ventricular fibrillation unless the suppressing agent is antifibrillatory.

Suppression of Ventricular Ectopy and Prevention of Sustained Ventricular Tachycardia/Ventricular Fibrillation. The conventional wisdom that the suppression of ventricular ectopy in patients who have already experienced a sustained ventricular arrhythmia represents an objective end-point against which the efficacy of antiarrhythmic agents can be judged has been challenged: (i) many patients with recurrent sustained ventricular tachycardia or ventricular fibrillation do not manifest complex ventricular ectopy between episodes; (ii) some patients in whom sustained ventricular arrhythmias have been prevented by medical or surgical therapy continue to manifest complex ventricular ectopy [56]; (iii) sustained ventricular tachycardia or ventricular fibrillation may occur despite suppression of spontaneous ventricular ectopy [57,58]; and (iv) there may be a disparity between the plasma concentration of an antiarrhythmic agent required to suppress ventricular ectopy and that required to prevent sustained ventricular tachycardia or ventricular fibrillation [59,60].

Figure 2 depicts the clinical course of a patient with sustained ventricular tachycardia during treatment with procainamide who was evaluated at Barnes Hospital. As demonstrated here, suppression of ventricular ectopy during treatment with antiarrhythmic agents may not correlate with prevention of sustained ventricular tachycardia. Therefore, the presence or absence of ventricular ectopy does not necessarily predict whether patients will exhibit sustained ventricular tachycardia: ventricular tachycardia may occur when ectopy is absent or scanty or, conversely, ventricular tachycardia may not occur despite marked ventricular ectopy.

In contrast, Lown and co-workers have continued to champion the concept that ventricular ectopy foreshadows the occurrence of sustained ventricular arrhythmias, and that the suppression of ventricular ectopy provides a reliable and objective endpoint for defining the efficacy of antiarrhythmic agents [61]. Criticisms of this approach have been focused on biased selection of patients in the studies reported, the fact that the approach is not applicable to patients who manifest only simple forms of ventricular

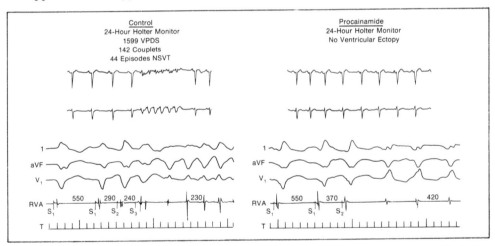

FIGURE 2: Clinical course of a patient with recurrent sustained ventricular tachycardia. In the absence of antiarrhythmic agents (left panels), complex ventricular ectopy, including frequency ventricular premature depolarizations (VPDs), ventricular couplets, and episodes of nonsustained VT (NSVT) occurred spontaneously. Sustained ventricular tachycardia with a cycle length of 230 ms was induced, using double ventricular extrastimuli. During treatment with procainamide (right panels), no ventricular ectopy was detected by 24-hour ECG monitoring. However, sustained ventricular tachycardia could still be induced, and initiation required only a single ventricular extrastimulus.

ectopy or none at all, and the failure by other investigators to corroborate such favorable results [57,58].

The debate regarding suppression of complex forms of ventricular ectopy and protection against the recurrence of sustained ventricular arrhythmias in patients with known sustained ventricular tachycardia or ventricular fibrillation has recently been fueled by comparisons of the predictive power of the response to programmed ventricular stimulation and ambulatory ECG monitoring [57,58,62,63]. Although preclusion of initiation of sustained ventricular tachycardia or ventricular fibrillation by treatment is the most powerful predictor of the efficacy of an antiarrhythmic agent, results of some studies demonstrate that selected patients with sustained ventricular arrhythmias in whom an antiarrhythmic agent suppresses complex forms of ventricular ectopy but who remain inducible to sustained ventricular tachycardia or ventricular fibrillation have a relatively favorable prognosis when compared with patients who remain inducible and continue to minifest complex ventricular ectopy. Figure 3, from a retrospective study by Kim *et al* [63], illustrates a favorable prognosis in this group of patients, although results of other studies have differed [57,58]. No prospective study has yet been performed in which assessment of drug efficacy has been randomized to programmed ventricular stimulation or ambulatory ECG monitoring.

Thus, in patients with documented sustained arrhythmias, relationships between suppression of ventricular ectopy and the prevention of sustained ventricular tachycardia or ventricular fibrillation are not yet clear. Moreover, the correlation between the two may differ for different antiarrhythmic drugs, and results in patients with documented sustained ventricular arrhythmias may not be applicable to patients with

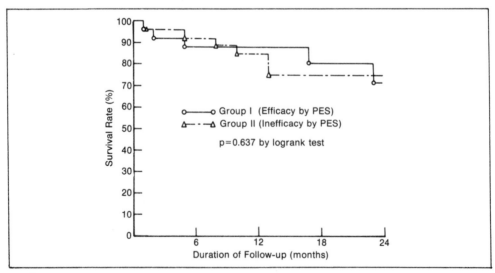

FIGURE 3: Rates of arrhythmia-free survival, in patients (Group I) with a history of sustained ventricular tachycardia or ventricular fibrillation discharged on an antiarrhythmic regimen defined to be effective by programmed electrical stimulation (PES), and in patients (Group II) with sustained ventricular tachycardia or ventricular fibrillation discharged on an antiarrhythmic regimen which was not effective by PES criteria but was effective by criteria using Holter monitoring. (Reproduced, with permission, from Kim *et al* [63].)

ventricular ectopy who have not manifested sustained ventricular tachycardia or ventricular fibrillation.

Surprisingly, there is a paucity of well-controlled, prospective clinical studies on the administration of antiarrhythmic agents to patients recovering from myocardial infarction who manifest ventricular ectopy but have not suffered episodes of sustained ventricular tachycardia or ventricular fibrillation [64–71], and none has demonstrated a favorable effect on the incidence of sustained ventricular arrhythmias or mortality. Figure 4 compares the mortality rates from one study in which patients were randomized to mexiletine or placebo [70]. There were no significant differences in the incidence of sudden or non-sudden cardiac death between the two groups of patients during a 14-month follow-up. Similar results with aprindine as the active agent have recently been presented [71]. To date, the only agents shown to exert a favorable effect on the incidence of sudden cardiac death are beta-blocking agents [72], administered to decrease myocardial oxygen requirements rather than to suppress arrhythmias.

Efficacy of Antiarrhythmic Drugs. Figure 2 shows that the available antiarrhythmic agents are often not effectve in preventing sustained ventricular arrhythmias. A comparison of the efficacy of conventional antiarrhythmic drugs in preventing the initiation of sustained ventricular tachycardia is shown in Figure 5. The data are from a study of 50 patients evaluated at the University of Pennsylvania, Philadelphia [73]. Procainamide appears to be the single most effective drug among the conventional antiarrhythmic agents, preventing the initiation of sustained ventricular tachycardia in 30%–35% of cases. Newer drugs, including flecainide, tocainide, encainide, lorcainide and mexiletine, do not appear to be better. Amiodarone is the single most effective antiarrhythmic agent for the prevention of recurrent sustained ventricular tachycardia. Judging from an intention-to-treat analysis, amiodarone has been effective in 62% of our patients

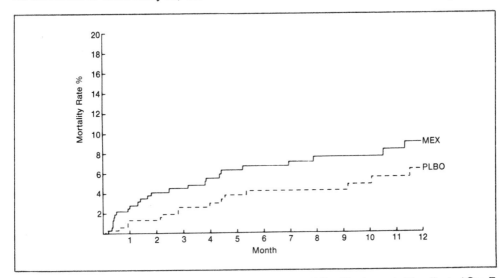

FIGURE 4: Life-table analysis for total mortality. Unadjusted Cox Z value = 1.47; adjusted Cox Z value = 1.47; Mex = mexiletine; PLBO = placebo. (Reprinted, with permission, from Impact Research Group [70].)

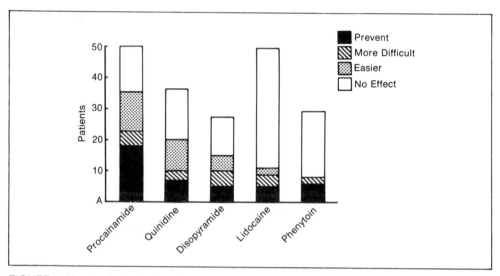

FIGURE 5: Effects of standard and antiarrhythmic agents on the initiation of sustained ventricular tachycardia. Antiarrhythmic drugs are indicated on the abscissa and number of patients on the ordinate. Results are shown of programmed stimulation following the administration of each of the agents. (Reprinted, with permission, from Horowitz *et al* [73].)

with documented sustained ventricular tachycardia or ventricular fibrillation who were refractory or intolerant to other antiarrhythmic agents. The relative efficacy of newer investigational agents, including primenol, propafenone, ethmozin and sotalol, has not yet been definitively determined.

Dosage. The successful prevention of sustained ventricular arrhythmias in patients recovering from myocardial infarction requires accurate identification of the patient at risk, selection of an effective antiarrhythmic agent, and the administration of the drug at appropriate doses.

Figure 6 illustrates the results of increasing doses (1000 mg, 1500 mg, 1750 mg) of procainamide in a patient with sustained ventricular tachycardia. During the control study (Fig. 6A), performed in the absence of procainamide, sustained ventricular tachycardia was induced following the introduction of double ventricular extrastimuli. During treatment with procainamide, which resulted in a plasma level of 8.3 µg/ml (Fig. 6B), the initiation of sustained ventricular tachycardia was facilitated, requiring only a single extrastimulus, although the rate of the tachycardia was slowed markedly. At a plasma level of 12.9 µg/ml (Fig. 6C), sustained ventricular tachycardia was still induced with a single extrastimulus, although the rate of the tachycardia slowed modestly. Finally, at a plasma procainamide level of 14.6 µg/ml (Fig. 6D), sustained ventricular tachycardia was no longer induced. This pharmacodynamic property decreases the chance that any given antiarrhythmic regimen selected empirically will reduce the incidence of sustained ventricular tachycardia or ventricular fibrillation.

Deleterious Effects of Antiarrhythmic Drugs. All antiarrhythmic agents have a high incidence of adverse effects, some of which are life-threatening. Treatment often

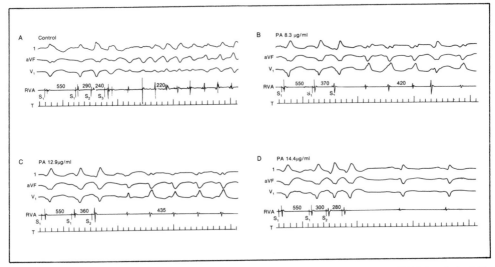

FIGURE 6: Dose-response relationship for procainamide. Each panel shows ECG leads I, aVF, V_1, a right-ventricular electrogram (RVA), and time lines (T). A: In the control study, sustained ventricular tachycardia with a cycle length of 220 ms was initiated by two ventricular extrastimuli (S_2 and S_3). B: During treatment with procainamide that resulted in a plasma level of 8.3 µg/ml, sustained ventricular tachycardia was induced more easily and required only a single extrastimulus (S_2); the rate of tachycardia slowed markedly (420 ms). C: At a procainamide level of 12.9 µg/ml, initiation of sustained ventricular tachycardia again required only a single extrastimulus. The rate of tachycardia slowed modestly (435 ms). D: At a procainamide level of 14.4 µg/ml, tachycardia could no longer be initiated.

results in symptoms in previously asymptomatic subjects. All antiarrhythmic agents can be proarrhythmic, and may therefore precipitate arrhythmias more complex than those being treated [74]. Figure 7 shows the response of a patient with asymptomatic non-sustained ventricular tachycardia to procainamide. During the control study performed in the absence of antiarrhythmic drugs, only non-sustained ventricular tachycardia was induced in response to programmed ventricular stimulation. During treatment with procainamide, however, sustained ventricular tachycardia was easily induced. Overall, proarrhythmic effects occur in approximately 13% of patients in drug trials. Results of studies with the new Class Ic drugs, including flecainide [75] and encainide [76], indicate that they are particularly likely to aggravate ventricular arrhythmias.

Treating Patients with Asymptomatic Ventricular Ectopy
The decision to treat a patient with asymptomatic ventricular ectopy for the purpose of preventing a sustained ventricular arrhythmia should be based on consideration of the benefit/risk ratio. Even though certain patterns of ventricular ectopy predict higher cardiac mortality in large groups, none specifically predicts sudden arrhythmic death when applied to individual patients. A decision to treat patients with antiarrhythmic agents based solely on the presence or absence of ventricular ectopy would subject many patients needlessly to potentially toxic drugs, and more than 50% of patients destined to develop sustained ventricular tachycardia or ventricular fibrillation would

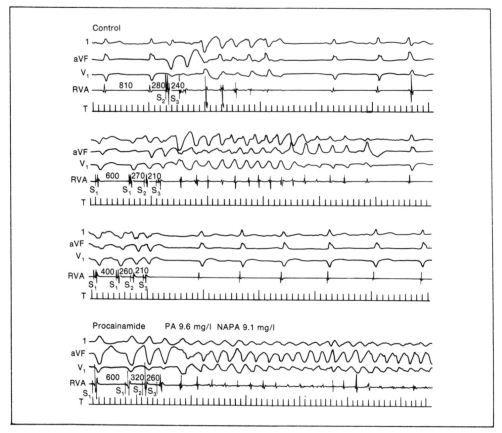

FIGURE 7: Results of programmed ventricular stimulation in a patient with clinically non-sustained ventricular tachycardia. Each panel is organized from top to bottom with ECG leads I, aVF, V₁, and an intracardiac recording from the right-ventricular apex (RVA) and time lines (T). During the control study, only non-sustained ventricular tachycardia was induced. During treatment with procainamide, sustained ventricular tachycardia was readily induced.

not be identified or treated. Left-ventricular function is the single most powerful descriptor of survival. Patients at highest risk for sudden and non-sudden cardiac death are those with marked left-ventricular dysfunction (ejection fraction <30%) and complex ventricular ectopy. Patients with ventricular ectopy but with normal or well-preserved left-ventricular function belong to a group that is statistically at low risk for developing sustained ventricular tachycardia or ventricular fibrillation.

It has been proposed and hoped that treatment of complex ventricular ectopy in high-risk groups will reduce mortality. At present, however, there are no data to demonstrate that such treament favorably alters the incidence of sudden or non-sudden cardiac death. Because of the potential physiologic importance of residual left-ventricular function, first-line therapy should consist of optimizing left-ventricular performance and eliminating factors known to precipitate ventricular arrhythmias, including recurrent ischemia and electrolyte abnormalities (particularly hypokalemia).

If there were antiarrhythmic drugs available that were effective, not proarrhythmic, and free from significant side-effects, the threshold for treating patients with asymptomatic ventricular ectopy could be lowered. No such agent is available – nor is one likely to become available in the foreseeable future. The benefit/risk ratio of treating complex ventricular ectopy in asymptomatic patients in the high-risk group with poor left-ventricular function appears equivocal, provided that complex centricular ectopy is suppressed without deleterious effects. In this circumstance, the physician can conclude that at least he has done no harm. If antiarrhythmic agents are not effective in suppressing complex forms of ventricular ectopy, are proarrhythmic, or are associated with significant side-effects, then the benefit/risk ratio does not justify treatment, even in this high-risk group of patients. At present, the benefit/risk ratio does not favor the administration of antiarrhythmic agents to patients with asymptomatic ventricular ectopy who are not in a high-risk group.

Elucidation of the indications for treating patients with asymptomatic ventricular ectopy requires delineation of the relationship between ventricular ectopy and the propensity for developing sustained ventricular arrhythmias. The Cardiac Arrhythmia Pilot Study (CAPS) has beeen designed to address this issue [77]. Results of this prospective multicenter trial are eagerly awaited.

Recent Advances in Identifying Patients at Risk for Developing Sustained Ventricular Tachycardia or Ventricular Fibrillation
Recently, investigators have developed and evaluated new methods for characterizing the risk for development of sustained ventricular arrhythmias, including invasive electrophysiologic studies and advanced non-invasive interrogation of signal-averaged ECGs.

Programmed Ventricular Stimulation
Sustained ventricular tachycardia identical to that occurring clinically can be reproducibly initiated in up to 95% of patients who experience this arrhythmia spontaneously [78]. This approach has also been found useful in patients surviving a cardiac arrest [4,5], which has led to the implementation of ventricular stimulation protocols in patients recovering from myocardial infarction, to test the hypothesis that the initiation of sustained ventricular tachycardia or ventricular fibrillation in patients not yet experiencing these arrhythmias clinically presages sudden cardiac death. This hypothesis is being tested in two groups of patients – those recovering from acute myocardial infarction, and those with organic heart disease and complex ventricular ectopy.

Although results from initial studies demonstrated that the response to programmed ventricular stimulation distinguished patients recovering from infarction who subsequently developed sustained ventricular tachycardia or ventricular fibrillation from those who did not [79,80], more recent results using more conventional stimulation protocols have not been corroborative [81,82]. Results of studies performed in patients with organic heart disease and complex ventricular ectopy have shown that sustained ventricular tachycardia or ventricular fibrillation are induced only occasionally [83]. Gomes *et al* found that the initiation of sustained ventricular tachycardia or ventricular fibrillation in such patients had prognostic implications [84]. Obviously, a much larger number of patients (particularly those with depressed left-ventricular function) must be studied, with a uniform stimulation protocol, before the role of electrophysiologic testing in identifying those patients recovering from myocardial infarction or with complex ventricular ectopy who are at high risk of developing sustained ventricular arrhythmias can be ascertained definitively.

Analysis of Signal-Averaged ECGs
Results of studies using advanced signal-processing systems in the time and frequency domains have demonstrated distinguishing features in signal-averaged ECGs obtained during sinus rhythm that differentiate between patients with and without documented sustained ventricular tachycardia [85–90]. These distinguishing features appear to reflect occult derangements of ventricular activation not readily apparent in ECGs obtained and analyzed conventionally [91,92]. Figure 8 illustrates the results of frequency analysis of the terminal QRS and ST segments from signal-averaged X, Y and Z ECG leads from a patient with a history of infarction with sustained ventricular tachycardia (left) and from a patient with a history of infarction without ventricular

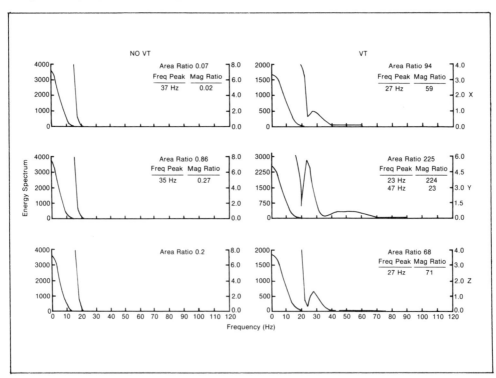

FIGURE 8: Energy spectra of the terminal QRS and ST segments, from a patient with prior myocardial infarction and sustained ventricular tachycardia (VT) (right), and from a patient with prior myocardial infarction without sustained ventricular tachycardia (left). Shown in each panel are the initial (left scale) and magnified (right scale) evergy *vs* frequency plots of the terminal QRS and ST segment of signal-averaged X, Y and Z ECG leads; values for the area ratio; peak frequencies; and values for the magnitude ratios. In each lead, the combined terminal QRS and ST segment from the patient with sustained ventricular tachycardia contains a 10- to 100-fold greater proportion of components in the 20–50-Hz range, compared with the patient without ventricular tachycardia. (Reprinted, with permission, from Cain *et al* [89].)

tachycardia (right) [89]. In each lead, the terminal QRS and ST segments from the patient with ventricular tachycardia contains a 10- to 100-fold greater proportion of frequencies in the 20–50-Hz range, compared with corresponding values in the patient without ventricular tachycardia. These differences are independent of left-ventricular ejection fraction, complexity of spontaneous ventricular ectopy, and QRS duration.

The clinical value of this and other advanced signal-processing techniques depends ultimately on the extent to which prospective detection of vulnerability to the development of life-threatening ventricular arrhythmias is possible. The hypothesis that the results of frequency analysis of signal-averaged ECGs would improve selection of patients for programmed ventricular stimulation was recently tested [90]. The relationship between the results of frequency analysis and the response to programmed ventricular stimulation was defined in patients with non-sustained ventricular tachycar-

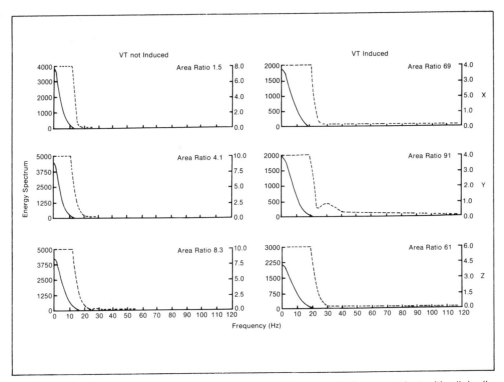

FIGURE 9: Energy spectra of the terminal QRS and ST segments from a patient with clinically non-sustained ventricular tachycardia (VT) in whom sustained ventricular tachycardia was induced during programmed ventricular stimulation (right), and from a patient with clinically non-sustained ventricular tachycardia in whom sustained ventricular tachycardia was not induced (left). Shown in each panel are the initial (left scale, solid curve) and magnified (right scale, broken curve) energy vs frequency plots of the terminal 40 ms of the QRS complex and ST segment of signal-averaged X, Y and Z leads, and values for the area ratio. In each lead, the terminal QRS complex and ST segment from the patient in whom sustained ventricular tachycardia was induced contain a substantially larger fraction of components in the 20–50-Hz range, compared with corresponding ECG segments from the patient in whom sustained ventricular tachycardia was not induced. (Reprinted, with permission, from Lindsay et al [90].)

dia or syncope but without documented sustained ventricular arrhythmias. Results of frequency analysis correctly predicted the results of programmed ventricular stimulation in 82% of the patients. In none of the 26 patients with a normal frequency content was ventricular tachycardia inducible. Sustained ventricular tachycardia was induced in 5 of 12 patients demonstrating an abnormal frequency content.

Figure 9 shows representative spectral plots of the terminal QRS and ST segments from a patient with clinically non-sustained ventricular tachycardia in whom sustained ventricular tachycardia was induced (right) and from a patient with clinically non-sustained ventricular tachycardia in whom sustained ventricular tachycardia was not induced (left). Denniss et al have recently completed a study to determine whether the results of analysis of signal-averaged ECGs performed in patients convalescing from myocardial infarction distinguish between patients who subsequently develop ventricular tachycardia or ventricular fibrillation and those who do not [93]. Results demonstrate that this approach may provide improved non-invasive definition of risk for development of sustained ventricular arrhythmias. Studies to determine the applicability of these techniques for assessing the efficacy of antiarrhythmic drugs, defining risk for developing sustained ventricular arrhythmias in patients having bundle branch block during sinus rhythm, and defining risk in patients with non-ischemic heart disease are in progress.

Acknowledgment

Supported in part by NIH Grant HL 17646, SCOR in Ischemic Heart Disease.

References

[1] Perper JA, Kuller LH, Cooper M.
Arteriosclerosis of coronary arteries in sudden, unexpected deaths.
Circulation 1975; 51 (Suppl 3): III27–33.

[2] Weaver WD, Lorch GS, Alvarez HA et al.
Angiographic findings and prognostic indicators in patients resuscitated from sudden cardiac death.
Circulation 1976; 54: 895–900.

[3] Myerburg RJ, Conde CA, Sung RJ et al.
Clinical, electrophysiologic and hemodynamic profile of patients resuscitated from prehospital cardiac arrest.
Am J Med 1980; 68: 568–76.

[4] Ruskin JN, DiMarco JP, Garan H.
Out-of-hospital cardiac arrest. Electrophysiologic observations and selection of long-term antiarrhythmic therapy.
N Engl J Med 1980; 303: 607–13.

[5] Josephson ME, Horowitz LN, Spielman SR et al.
Electrophysiologic and hemodynamic studies in patients resuscitated from cardiac arrest.
Am J Cardiol 1980; 46: 948–55.

[6] Goldstein S, Landis R, Leighton R et al.
Characteristics of the resuscitated out-of-hospital cardiac arrest victim with coronary heart disease.
Circulation 1981; 64: 977–84.

[7] Winkle RA, Lopes MG, Popp RL et al.
Life-threatening arrhythmias in the mitral valve prolapse syndrome.
Am J Med 1976; 60: 961–7.

[8] Wei JY, Bulkley BH, Schaeffer AH et al.
Mitral-valve prolapse syndrome and recurrent ventricular tachyarrhythmias. A malignant variant refractory to conventional drug therapy.
Ann Intern Med 1978; 89: 6–9.

[9] Wu D, Kou HC, Hung JS.
Exercise-triggered paroxysmal ventricular tachycardia. A repetitive rhythmic activity possibly related to afterdepolarizations.
Ann Intern Med 1981; 95: 410–4.

[10] Rahilly GT, Prystowsky EN, Zipes DP et al.
Clinical and electrophysiologic findings in patients with repetitive monomorphic ventricular tachycardia and otherwise normal electrocardiogram.
Am J Cardiol 1982; 50: 459–68.

[11] Lin FC, Finley CD, Rahimtoola SH et al.
Idiopathic paroxysmal ventricular tachycardia
with a QRS pattern of right bundle branch block
and left axis deviation: A unique clinical entity
with specific properties.
Am J Cardiol 1983; **52**: 95–100.

[12] Maron BJ, Savage DD, Wolfson JK et al.
Prognostic significance of 24-hour ambulatory
electrocardiographic monitoring in patients
with hypertrophic cardiomyopathy: A prospective study.
Am J Cardiol 1981; **48**: 252–7.

[13] McKenna W, Deanfield J, Faruqui A et al.
Prognosis in hypertrophic cardiomyopathy:
Role of age and clinical, electrocardiographic
and hemodynamic features.
Am J Cardiol 1981; **47**: 532–8.

[14] Maron BJ, Roberts WC, Epstein SE.
Sudden death in hypertrophic car-
diomyopathy: A profile of 78 patients.
Circulation 1982; **65**: 1388–94.

[15] Hamby RI.
Primary myocardial disease: A prospective clinical and hemodynamic evaluation of 100 patients.
Medicine 1970; **49**: 55–78.

[16] Shugoll GI, Bowen PJ, Moore JP et al.
Follow-up observations and prognosis in prim-
ary myocardial disease.
Arch Intern Med 1972; **129**: 67–72.

[17] Fuster V, Gersh BJ, Giuliani ER et al.
The natural history of idiopathic dilated car-
diomyopathy.
Am J Cardiol 1981; **47**: 525–31.

[18] Massie B, Ports T Chatterjee K et al.
Long-term vasodilator therapy for heart failure:
Clinical response and its relationship to
hemodynamic measurements.
Circulation 1981; **63**: 269–78.

[19] Meinertz T, Hofmann H, Kasper W et al.
Significance of ventricular arrhythmias in
idiopathic dilated cardiomyopathy.
Am J Cardiol 1981; **53**: 902–7.

[20] Wilson JR, Schwartz JS, Sutton MSJ et al.
Prognosis in severe heart failure: Relation to
hemodynamic measurements and ventricular
ectopic activity.
J Am Coll Cardiol 1983; **2**: 403–10.

[21] Franciosa JA, Wilen M, Ziesche S et al.
Survival in men with severe chronic left ventricular failure due to either coronary heart disease or idiopathic dilated cardiomyopathy.
Am J Cardiol 1983; **51**: 831–6.

[22] Holmes J, Kubo SH, Cody R et al.
Arrhythmias in ischemic and nonischemic dilated cardiomyopathy: Prediction of mortality
by ambulatory electrocardiography.
Am J Cardiol 1985; **55**: 146–51.

[23] Tominaga S, Blackburn H.
The coronary drug project research group:
Prognostic importance of premature beats fol-
lowing myocardial infarction.
JAMA 1973; **223**: 116–24.

[24] Schulze RA Jr, Rouleau J, Rigo P et al.
Ventricular arrhythmias in the late hospital
phase of acute myocardial infarction: Relation
of left ventricular function detected by gated
cardiac blood pool scanning.
Circulation 1975; **52**: 1006–11.

[25] Schulze RA Jr, Strauss HW, Pitt B.
Sudden death in the year following myocardial
infarction. Relation to ventricular premature
contractions in the late hospital phase and left
ventricular ejection fraction.
Am J Med 1977; **62**: 192–8.

[26] Vismara LA, Vera Z, Foerster JM et al.
Identification of sudden death risk factors in
acute and chronic coronary artery disease.
Am J Cardiol 1977; **39**: 821–8.

[27] Anderson KP, DeCamilla J, Moss AJ.
Clinical significance of ventricular tachycardia
(3 beats or longer) detected during ambulatory
monitoring after myocardial infarction.
Circulation 1978; **57**: 890–7.

[28] deSoyza N, Bennett FA, Murphy ML et al.
The relationship of paroxysmal ventricular
tachycardia complicating the acute phase and
ventricular arrhythmia during the late hospital
phase of myocardial infarction to long-term survival.
Am J Med 1978; **64**: 377–81.

[29] Califf RM, Burks JM, Behar VS et al.
Relationships among ventricular arrhythmias,
coronary artery disease, and angiographic and
electrocardiographic indicators of myocardial
fibrosis.
Circulation 1978; **57**: 725–32.

[30] Davis HT, DeCamilla J, Bayer LW et al.
Survivorship patterns in the posthospital phase
of myocardial infarction.
Circulation 1979; **60**: 1252–8.

[31] Moss AJ, Davis HT, DeCamilla J et al.
Ventricular ectopic beats and their relation to
sudden and nonsudden cardiac death after
myocardial infarction.
Circulation 1979; **60**: 998–1003.

[32] DeBusk RF, Davidson DM, Houston N et al.
Serial ambulatory electrocardiography and treadmill exercise testing following uncomplicated myocardial infarction.
Am J Cardiol 1980; 45: 547–54.

[33] Ruberman W, Weinblatt E, Goldberg JD et al.
Ventricular premature complexes and sudden death after myocardial infarction.
Circulation 1981; 64: 297–305.

[34] Ruberman W, Weinblatt E, Frank CW et al.
Repeated 1 hour electrocardiographic monitoring of survivors of myocardial infarction at 6 month intervals: Arrhythmia detection and relation to prognosis.
Am J Cardiol 1981; 47: 1197–204.

[35] Bigger JT Jr, Weld FM, Rolnitzky LM.
Prevalence, characteristics and significance of ventricular tachycardia (three or more complexes) detected with ambulatory electrocardiographic recording in the late hospital phase of acute myocardial infarction.
Am J Cardiol 1981; 48: 815–23.

[36] Moss AJ and the Multicenter Postinfarction Research Group.
Risk stratification and survival after myocardial infarction.
N Engl J Med 1983; 309: 331–6.

[37] Bigger JT Jr, Fleiss JL, Kleiger R et al.
The relationships among ventricular arrhythmias, left ventricular dysfunction, and mortality in the 2 years after myocardial infarction.
Circulation 1984; 69: 250–8.

[38] Mukharji J, Rude RE, Poole WK et al.
Risk factors for sudden death after acute myocardial infarction: Two year follow-up.
Am J Cardiol 1984; 54: 31–6.

[39] Geltman EM, Ehsani AA, Campbell MK et al.
The influence of location and extent of myocardial infarction on long-term ventricular dysrhythmia and mortality.
Circulation 1979; 60: 805–14.

[40] Kleiger RE, Miller JP, Thanavaro S et al.
Relationship between clinical features of acute myocardial infarction and ventricular runs 2 weeks to 1 year after infarction.
Circulation 1981; 63: 64–70.

[41] Josephson ME.
Treatment of ventricular arrhythmias post myocardial infarction.
Circulation 1986; 74: 653–8.

[42] Cain ME.
Management of ventricular arrhythmias occurring in patients after myocardial infarction.
Angiology 1986/7 (in press).

[43] Winkle RA.
Antiarrhythmic drug effect mimicked by spontaneous variability of ventricular ectopy.
Circulation 1978; 57: 1116–21.

[44] Michelson EL, Morganroth J.
Spontaneous variability of complex ventricular arrhythmias detected by long-term electrocardiographic recording.
Circulation 1980; 61: 690–5.

[45] Kennedy HL, Chandra V, Sayther KL et al.
Effectiveness of increasing hours of continuous ambulatory electrocardiography in detecting maximal ventricular ectopy. Continuous 48 hour study of patients with coronary heart disease and normal subjects.
Am J Cardiol 1978; 42: 925–30.

[46] Moss AJ.
Clinical significance of ventricular arrhythmias in patients with and without coronary artery disease.
Prog Cardiovasc Dis 1980; 223: 33–52.

[47] Winkle RA, Lopes MG, Fitgerland JW et al.
Arrhythmias in patients with mitral valve prolapse.
Circulation 1975; 52: 73–81.

[48] DeMaria AN, Amsterdam EA, Vismara LA et al.
Arrhythmias in the mitral valve prolapse syndrome.
Ann Intern Med 1976; 84: 656–60.

[49] Mills P, Rose J, Hollingsworth J et al.
Long-term prognosis of mitral-valve prolapse.
N Engl J Med 1977; 297: 13–8.

[50] Clarke J, Shelton J, Hamer J et al.
The rhythm of the normal human heart.
Lancet 1976; i: 508–12.

[51] Brodsky M, Wu D, Denes P et al.
Arrhythmias documented by 24 hour continuous electrocardiographic monitoring in 50 male medical students without apparent heart disease.
Am J Cardiol 1977; 39: 390–5.

[52] Glasser S, Clark P, Applebaum H.
Occurrence of frequent complex arrhythmias detected by ambulatory monitoring.
Chest 1979; 75: 565–8.

[53] Kennedy H, Underhill S.
Frequent or complex ventricular ectopy in apparently healthy subjects: A clinical study of 25 cases.
Am J Cardiol 1976; 38: 141–8.

[54] Hinkle L, Carver S, Arovrus D.
The prognostic significance of ventricular premature contractions in healthy people and in people with coronary heart disease.
Acta Cardiol 1974; 43 (Suppl): 5–32.

[55] Kennedy HL, Whitlock JA, Sprague MK *et al.*
Long-term follow-up of asymptomatic healthy subjects with frequent and complex ventricular ectopy.
N Engl J Med 1985; **312**: 193–7.

[56] Herling IM, Horowitz LN, Josephson ME.
Ventricular ectopic activity after medical and surgical treatment for recurrent sustained ventricular tachycardia.
Am J Cardiol 1980; **45**: 633–9.

[57] Platia EV, Reid PR.
Comparison of programmed electrical stimulation and ambulatory electrocardiographic (Holter) monitoring in the management of ventricular tachycardia and ventricular fibrillation.
J Am Coll Cardiol 1984; **4**: 493–500.

[58] Skale BT, Miles WM, Heger JJ *et al.*
Survivors of cardiac arrest: Prevention of recurrence by drug therapy as predicted by electrophysiologic testing or electrocardiographic monitoring.
Am J Cardiol 1986; **57**: 113–9.

[59] Myerburg RJ, Conde C, Sheps DS *et al.*
Antiarrhythmic drug therapy in survivors of prehospital cardiac arrest: Comparison of effects on chronic ventricular arrhythmias and recurrent cardiac arrest.
Circulation 1979; **49**: 855–63.

[60] Myerburg RJ, Zaman L, Kessler KM, Castellanos A.
Evolving concepts of management of stable and potentially lethal arrhythmias.
Am Heart J 1982; **103**: 615–25.

[61] Grayboys TB, Lown B, Podrid PJ, DeSilva R.
Long-term survival of patients with malignant ventricular arrhythmia treated with antiarrhythmic drugs.
Am J Cardiol 1982; **50**: 437–43.

[62] Kim SG, Seiden SW, Matos JA *et al.*
Discordance between ambulatory monitoring and programmed stimulation in assessing efficacy of class IA antiarrhythmic agents in patients with ventricular tachycardia.
J Am Coll Cardiol 1985; **6**: 539–44.

[63] Kim SG, Seiden SW, Felder SD *et al.*
Is programmed stimulation of value in predicting the long-term success of antiarrhythmic therapy for ventricular tachycardias?
N Engl J Med 1986; **315**: 356–62.

[64] Collaborative Group.
Phenytoin after recovery from myocardial infarction: Controlled trial in 568 patients.
Lancet 1971; **ii**: 1055–7.

[65] Peter T, Ross D, Duffield A *et al.*
Effect on survival after myocardial infarction of long-term treatment with phenytoin.
Br Heart J 1978; **40**: 1356–60.

[66] Hugenholtz PG, Hagemeijer F, Lubsen J *et al.*
One year follow-up in patients with persistent ventricular dysrhythmias after myocardial infarction treated with aprindine or placebo. In: Sandoe E, Julian DG, Pell JE, eds. *Management of Ventricular Tachycardia: Role of Mexiletine.* Amsterdam: Excerpta Medica, 1978; pp. 572–8.

[67] Bastian BC, MacFarlane PW, McLaughlan JH *et al.*
A prospective randomized trial of tocainide in patients following myocardial infarction.
Am Heart J 1980; **100**: 1017–22.

[68] Chamberlain DA, Julian DG, Boyle D *et al.*
Oral mexiletine in high-risk patients after myocardial infarction.
Lancet 1980; **ii**: 1324–7.

[69] Ryden L, Arnman K, Conradson TB *et al.*
Prophylaxis of ventricular tachyarrhythmias with intravenous and oral tocainide in patients with and recovering from acute myocardial infarction.
Am Heart J 1980; **100**: 1006–12.

[70] Impact Research Group.
International mexiletine and placebo antiarrhythmic coronary trial: I. Report on arrhythmias and other findings.
J Am Coll Cardiol 1984; **4**: 1148–63.

[71] Gottlieb SH, Achuff SC, Baughman KL *et al.*
Prophylactic antiarrhythmic therapy of high risk post infarction patients: Mortality is delayed but not reduced [Abstract].
Circulation 1985; **72** (Suppl): III–358.

[72] The Norwegian Multicenter Study Group.
Timolol-induced reduction in mortality and reinfarction in patients surviving acute myocardial infarction.
N Engl J Med 1981; **304**: 801–7.

[73] Horowitz LN, Josephson ME, Kastor JA.
Intracardiac electrophysiologic studies as a method for the optimization of drug therapy in chronic ventricular arrhythmia.
Prog Cardiovasc Dis 1980; **23**: 81–97.

[74] Velebit V, Podrid P, Lown B *et al.*
Aggravation and provocation of ventricular arrhythmias by antiarrhythmic drugs.
Circulation 1982; **65**: 886–94.

[75] Morganroth J, Horowitz LN.
Flecainide: Its proarrhythmic effect and expected changes on the surface electrocardiogram.
Am J Cardiol 1984; **53**: 89B–94B.

[76] Horowitz LN.
Encainide in lethal ventricular arrhythmias evaluated by electrophysiologic testing and decrease in symptoms.
Am J Cardiol 1986; **58**: 83C–86C.

[77] The CAPS Investigators.
The Cardiac Arrhythmia Pilot Study.
Am J Cardiol 1986; **57**: 91–5.

[78] Josephson ME, Horowitz LN.
Electrophysiologic approach to therapy of recurrent sustained ventricular tachycardia.
Am J Cardiol 1979; **43**: 631–42.

[79] Hamer A, Vohra J, Hunt D.
Prediction of sudden death by electrophysiologic studies in high risk patients surviving acute myocardial infarction.
Am J Cardiol 1982; **50**: 223–9.

[80] Richards DA, Cody DV, Denniss AR et al.
Ventricular electrical instability: A predictor of death after myocardial infarction.
Am J Cardiol 1983; **51**: 75–80.

[81] Marchlinski FE, Buxton AE, Waxman HL et al.
Identifying patients at risk of sudden death after myocardial infarction: Value of the response to programmed stimulation, degree of ventricular ectopic activity and severity of left ventricular dysfunction.
Am J Cardiol 1983; **52**: 1190–6.

[82] Roy D, Marchand E, Théroux P et al.
Programmed ventricular stimulation in survivors of an acute myocardial infarction.
Circulation 1985; **72**: 487–94.

[83] Buxton AE, Waxman HL, Marchlinski FE et al.
Electrophysiologic studies in nonsustained ventricular tachycardia: Relation to underlying heart disease.
Am J Cardiol 1983; **52**: 985–91.

[84] Gomes JAX, Hariman RI, Kang PS et al.
Programmed electrical stimulation in patients with high-grade ventricular ectopy: Electrophysiologic findings and prognosis for survival.
Circulation 1984; **70**: 43–51.

[85] Simson MB.
Use of signals in the terminal QRS complex to identify patients with ventricular tachycardia after myocardial infarction.
Circulation 1981; **64**: 235–42.

[86] Breithardt G, Becker R, Seipel L et al.
Noninvasive detection of late potentials in man. A new marker for ventricular tachycardia.
Eur Heart J 1981; **2**: 1–6.

[87] Denes P, Santarelli P, Hauser RG, Uretz EF.
Quantitative analysis of the high frequency components of the terminal portion of the body surface QRS in normal subjects and in patients with ventricular tachycardia.
Circulation 1983; **67**: 1129–38.

[88] Cain ME, Ambos HD, Witkowski FX, Sobel BE.
Fast-Fourier transform analysis of signal-averaged electrocardiograms for identification of patients prone to sustained ventricular tachycardia.
Circulation 1984; **69**: 711–20.

[89] Cain ME, Ambos HD, Markham J, Fisher AE, Sobel BE.
Quantification of differences in frequency content of signal-averaged electrocardiograms between patients with and without sustained ventricular tachycardia.
Am J Cardiol 1985; **55**: 1500–5.

[90] Lindsay BD, Ambos HD, Schechtman KB, Cain ME.
Improved selection of patients for programmed ventricular stimulation by frequency analysis of signal-averaged electrocardiograms.
Circulation 1986; **73**: 675–83.

[91] Simson MB, Untereker WJ, Spielman SR et al.
The relationship between late potentials on the body surface and directly recorded fragmented electrograms in patients with ventricular tachycardia.
Am J Cardiol 1983; **51**: 105–12.

[92] Josephson ME, Simson MB, Harken AH, Horowitz LN, Falcone RA.
The incidence and clinical significance of epicardial late potentials in patients with recurrent sustained ventricular tachycardia and coronary artery disease.
Circulation 1982; **66**: 1199–204.

[93] Denniss AR, Richards DA, Cody DV et al.
Prognostic significance of ventricular tachycardia and fibrillation induced at programmed stimulation and delayed potentials detected on signal-averaged electrocardiograms of survivors of acute myocardial infarction.
Circulation 1986; **74**: 731–45.

THE SURGICAL APPROACH TO THE TREATMENT OF ARRHYTHMIAS

Review: JAMES L. COX

The surgical treatment of cardiac arrhythmias has continued to expand and diversify during the past two years. Although most of the clinical reports have described refinements in established surgical techniques, perhaps the most important have focused on the development of entirely new surgical approaches to treat refractory arrhythmias for which there were previously no satisfactory surgical options. The results of most types of arrhythmia surgery are dependent upon rapid and accurate intraoperative electrophysiologic studies. Thus, recent developments in data acquisition and display are of particular importance. Technologic advances involving implantable antiarrhythmia devices have changed the indications for their use. Both pharmacologic therapy and surgical intervention are based on the concept of ablating arrhythmogenic tissue, or at least suppressing the likelihood that subsequent arrhythmias will develop. Certain exceptions include the use of digitalis preparations in patients with persistent atrial fibrillation and surgical isolation procedures. In both, the primary arrhythmia is not ablated although its effects on cardiac hemodynamics are minimized. Antitachycardia pacemakers, internal cardiovertors, and automatic defibrillators are designed to terminate arrhythmias only after they have continued sufficiently long to allow 'diagnosis' by the device (the so-called 'rescue' approach). Thus, the concept of true arrhythmia prevention (or cure) is not intrinsic to the use of implantable antiarrhythmia devices. Certain of these devices, although they have had a major impact on the treatment of some types of arrhythmias during the past two years, will not be discussed further here, as their implantation does not represent a surgical procedure designed to stop arrhythmias permanently.

Recent Advances in the Techniques of Intraoperative Mapping
The specific method of intraoperative mapping employed depends on the type of arrhythmia being characterized. For example, the mapping technique used to locate the accessory atrioventricular connection in patients with the Wolff-Parkinson-White syndrome is useless in a patient with ventricular tachycardia, although the hardware employed may be the same. In the early years of arrhythmia surgery, virtually the only arrhythmia curable by surgery was the Wolff-Parkinson-White syndrome: a single hand-held exploring electrode was used to map multiple sites on the heart sequentially until the accessory pathway was located. This invariably necessitated cardiopulmonary bypass support, because of excessive manipulation of the heart for exposure during the mapping procedure. The technique usually worked quite well, except in Wolff-Parkinson-White patients with atrial fibrillation or in patients with only intermittent pre-excitation. Another problem was iatrogenic conduction block in the accessory pathway caused by cardiac manipulation, which resulted in an inability to map intraoperatively.

When surgery for ventricular tachycardia became feasible, it was immediately apparent that the old system for mapping was inadequate – these arrhythmias often last for only a few cycles intraoperatively, and they may be multifocal in origin. The desirability of a mapping system capable of recording electrograms simultaneously from multiple sites was obvious. Since such a system lent itself to automation, several groups designed various electrode arrays and computer-systems for data acquisition and display. The major problem, however, was user interaction with the system in an on-line, real-time fashion.

In 1984, three separate mapping systems that were 'user-interactive' intraoperatively were described [1–3]. The Amsterdam group was at the leading edge of this technology. They placed inflatable balloons uniformly covered with electrode terminals directly into the left-ventricular cavity to record 16 simultaneous endocardial electrograms during ventricular tachycardia. After gross localization of the apparent site of origin of the arrhythmia, a rectangular grid with up to 64 electrode terminals was placed over the region of arrhythmogenesis for refined resolution. Witkowski and Corr from Washington University in St Louis described an automated transmural cardiac mapping system that could record a virtually unlimited number of electrograms simultaneously and analyze and display the data within 120 seconds [2]. In animal experiments the system recorded 240 channels simultaneously from 60 plunge-needle electrodes, with four bipolar terminals located along the shaft of each needle from endocardium to epicardium. Clinically, 16 channels of a 48-channel system were first used for mapping patients with the Wolff-Parkinson-White syndrome [3]. This clinical system has now been expanded to 160 channels, and is employed for constructing endocardial, intramural and epicardial maps in patients with ventricular tachycardia.

Parson and Downar took a different approach to the need for an on-line intraoperative mapping system capable of recording data from multiple sites simultaneously: their battery-operated multiplexed system analyzed analog data and incorporated a marker-matrix visual display of the epicardial activation sequence recorded from an epicardial sock-electrode array [4]. A digital computer was not employed. The same system has subsequently been used to display endocardial activation data recorded from inflatable cavitary balloons similar to those employed by the Amsterdam group.

The development of these intraoperative mapping systems has greatly enhanced our ability to localize the specific sites of arrhythmogeneses in both supraventricular and ventricular tachycardia, and has dramatically decreased the time required for intraoperative mapping.

Surgery for Supraventricular Tachycardia
Wolff-Parkinson-White Syndrome
After 18 years of slowly accumulating experience in the surgical treatment of the Wolff-Parkinson-White syndrome, we have witnessed a sharp increase in the variety of surgical approaches to this electrophysiologic abnormality. Originally, accessory pathways were accessed from outside the heart with an epicardial approach. With accumulating experience, it was learned that, although this technique was satisfactory for most patients, 20% required reoperation because of early or late postoperative recurrence of conduction across the pathway. In the early 1970s, both Dr Sealy at Duke University, Durham, North Carolina, and Dr Iwa in Kanazawa, Japan began to employ an endocardial approach to the accessory pathways, reasoning that the plane of dissection between the atrioventricular groove fat pad and either the atrium or ventricle could thereby be dissected more precisely. More importantly, this technique was believed to be safer

because of the protection afforded by the fat pad to the coronary vessels during dissection. Because the anatomy of the accessory pathways was not completely understood, however, recurrence after initial operation continued to be a problem. As a result, we began to utilize not only the endocardial approach but combined this with the epicardial approach and adjuvant cryosurgery, in hopes of interrupting conduction by whatever means possible at the time of initial operation.

In 1981 we decided to address the persistent problem of postoperative recurrence of the Wolff-Parkinson-White syndrome by converting from a physiologic to an anatomic operation. The standard operation at the time was first to localize the accessory pathway by intraoperative mapping techniques and then to dissect the local regions in the atrioventricular groove by one of the methods mentioned above. This usually involved dissecting an area in the atrioventricular groove, which included the precise location of the accessory pathway plus approximately 1-2 cm on either side of the pathway. (Although the anatomic boundaries of the atrioventricular groove were known, they were actually seen infrequently at the time of surgery because of limited dissection.) The latter technique was based on a firm faith in the electrophysiologic maps to localize precisely the position of any and all anatomic accessory pathways. However, we had observed that, when we were forced to reoperate for recurrence, it was always necessary to extend the margins of dissection rather widely from the actual site of the functional pathway - in addition, to dissect the entire plane between the fat pad and the ventricle and/or atrium, in order to be certain that the pathway had been interrupted. Moreover, unless the intraoperative mapping had been grossly erroneous (an extremely unusual occurrence), it was not necessary to dissect more than the one anatomic space to which the accessory pathway had been traced. In other words, if the pathway had mapped to the left free-wall space during the initial surgery, it would be found in the same space at reoperation, and would be permanently ablated only if the entire left free-wall space were adequately dissected; however, it would not be necessary to dissect other anatomic spaces.

These observations suggested that an individual accessory pathway might actually be accompanied by broad bands of tissue connecting the atrium to the ventricle in that area, and that the electrophysiologic maps were detecting only the portion of tissue which was functional or dominant because of its specific conduction characteristics. Surgical interruption of this functional portion of accessory tissue might then result merely in a temporary 'cure' of the problem until another adjacent portion of the accessory tissue began to conduct postoperatively. Believing this to be the case, we decided to perform a meticulous dissection of the entire anatomic space identified as harbouring the specific pathway in every patient – regardless of the precise location of the pathway within that given space. The dissection included unequivocal identification of all anatomic boundaries of each dissected space. This approach improved the results of surgery for the Wolff-Parkinson-White syndrome immediately and dramatically. By 1985, we were able to report that 137 of 137 accessory pathways had been divided successfully with a single operation in 110 consecutive patients, with no recurrences during a four-year follow-up period [5].

Iwa reported the Kanazawa experience with surgery for the Wolff-Parkinson-White syndrome in 160 patients, with 140 cures, 14 recurrences, and 6 operative deaths [6]. Guiraudon *et al* prefer to employ the epicardial approach exclusively, and add cryosurgery in order to ablate any accessory pathways that might have been missed during the course of surgical dissection [7]. The authors have termed this approach a 'new closed-heart technique', although cardiopulmonary bypass is employed in all but a few cases to support the circulation while the heart is retracted for surgical dissection. In 53 patients, 52 were cured at the time of initial operation; the remaining patient had persistent conduction across the accessory pathway despite two separate operations [8]. The role of cryosurgery in this approach is unclear, since, in the 47 patients with left free-wall pathways, the delta wave disappeared during the course of dissecting the fat pad away from the left atrium. This would indicate that cryosurgical ablation of the mitral valve annulus following dissection of the fat pad is unnecessary. However, when an imprecise anatomic dissection is employed for this recalcitrant problem, it is perhaps wise to add cryosurgery as an adjunctive measure, despite the precautions necessary to avoid thermal injury to the coronary arteries.

Although the necessity for cryosurgery adjunctive to the epicardial approach is suspect, a true cryosurgical ablative technique was described in 1985 by Bredikis and co-workers [9,10]. Specialized cryoprobes were designed for each anatomic space in which accessory pathways could be located; the cryoprobes were then inserted either into the coronary sinus (for left free-wall pathways) or into the right atrium (for all other pathways). Cryosurgical ablation can be performed without any need for cardiopulmonary bypass. Accordingly, this technique is a true closed-heart technique. Bredikis cured all 24 patients with right free-wall or septal pathways and 19 of 21 patients with left free-wall pathways.

Several short reports have appeared in the past two years describing attempts at ablating accessory pathways by an electric shock delivered via a catheter positioned in the vicinity of the pathway. Morady *et al* summarized the results of catheter ablation in 1985, and reported their results in eight additional patients [11]. They correctly emphasized the dismal results with left free-wall, right free-wall, and anterior septal pathways. The results are slightly more promising with posterior septal pathways, although the pathway clearly cannot be located in the vicinity of the His bundle, which also resides in the posterior septal space. If the accessory pathway is well posterior to and close to the os of the coronary sinus, the chances of a successful catheter ablation are markedly enhanced. Long-term success was calculated at 75%.

Atrioventricular Node Re-Entry Tachycardia
Prior to 1981, the only surgical option available for the treatment of medically refractory atrioventricular node re-entry tachycardia was ablation of the His bundle. This was accomplished by an open-heart operation in which the right atrium was opened, the His bundle identified with a hand-held electrode, and the bundle ablated by either cryosurgery or surgical dissection. In 1981, Scheinman first reported a non-surgical method of ablating the atrioventricular node-His bundle complex by delivering an electric shock through the tip of a catheter positioned over the His bundle. This technique immediately replaced surgical ablation of the His bundle, for the obvious reason that it avoided the necessity for an open-heart operation. However, the major long-term disadvantage of both surgical and catheter ablation of atrioventricular conduction was the necessity for a permanent pacemaker system. Because of this undesirable side-effect of His bundle ablation, we had started to develop a more direct

approach to the treatment of the arrhythmia even before the advent of catheter ablative techniques. We applied discrete 3-mm cryolesions to the atrial tissue immediately surrounding the atrioventricular node, in an attempt either to modify the input pathways to the node or to interrupt one of the limbs of the re-entrant circuit responsible for the tachycardia. After extensive laboratory investigation, we first applied this technique to a 35-year-old female patient in August 1982. We have since applied the procedure to six other patients, all of whom have been cured of their tachycardia and have maintained normal atrioventricular conduction postoperatively.

In 1984, Johnson and associates initiated a slightly different approach, but one with the same goal – i.e. surgical cure of the tachycardia without interruption of normal atrioventricular conduction [12]. The Sydney group performs a surgical dissection of the region of the atrioventricular node similar to the endocardial approach to posterior septal pathways for the Wolff-Parkinson-White syndrome. By December 1985, they reported 10 consecutive patients who had undergone this procedure, with cure of the tachycardia in all patients and no recurrences during a follow-up period of 2–14 months [12].

Automatic Atrial Tachycardias
Automatic tachycardias originating in the atria pose a unique challenge for the surgeon. These arrhythmias are frequently suppressed by general anesthesia and, thus, may be impossible to map in the operating room. Because of this problem, surgeons were frequently forced in the past to resort to His bundle ablation to confine the tachycardia to the atria. In 1980, we described an alternative to His bundle ablation when automatic left-atrial tachycardia could not be induced and mapped intraoperatively. By surgically isolating the left atrium, the sinoatrial node would no longer be suppressed by the tachycardia, and could then drive the remainder of the heart in the normal manner. We emphasized that, if the left-atrial tachycardia could be mapped intraoperatively, local excision or cryoablation should be the procedure of choice over left-atrial isolation. Because of improved anesthetic practices and more sophisticated mapping systems, it is now usually possible to map automatic atrial tachycardias intraoperatively and, therefore, their sites of origin are simply ablated. Thus, Gillette *et al* reported their surgical results in 16 patients with automatic atrial tachycardia, all of whom underwent some type of ablative procedure (cryoablation, catheter ablation, or excision): 11 patients had right-atrial foci and 5 had left-atrial foci [13].

The Gillette study is an important one, because it suggests that the long-term results (mean, 2.2 years) of ablative therapy are excellent. Our experience with both left-atrial and right-atrial tachycardia is similar, but we found the right-atrial tachycardias to be much more difficult to ablate intraoperatively, as they are frequently multifocal in origin. Our concern is that, with time, new sites in the body of the right atrium that were not apparently arrhythmogenic at the time of surgery might give rise to new automatic foci, resulting in late recurrence of the right-atrial tachycardia. We have therefore recently developed a technique to isolate the body of the right atrium from the remainder of the heart, while maintaining continuity of the sinoatrial node and atrial pacemaker complex with the heart to preserve normal sinus rhythm [14]. Because of their multifocal characteristics, all right-atrial tachycardias can be treated satisfactorily without concern about long-term recurrences.

Surgery for Ventricular Tachycardia

Non-Ischemic Ventricular Tachycardia

Few important developments have occurred in the surgical treatment of non-ischemic ventricular tachycardia over the past few years. As the evolution of new therapeutic modalities depends to a large extent upon the accumulation of experience, it is understandable that progress in the treatment of these rare arrhythmias has been slow. It has now become apparent, however, that the best approaches to refractory non-ischemic ventricular tachycardia are surgical isolation procedures rather than ablative techniques. Of course, isolation procedures can be applied only in the right ventricle but, fortunately, most ventricular arrhythmias that are not attributable to ischemia do not involve the left ventricle. In 1985, we described the surgical technique for both localized isolation procedures and for total isolation of the entire right ventricle in patients with right-ventricular tachycardia due either to cardiomyopathy or to arrhythmogenic right-ventricular dysplasis [15]. The follow-up period for patients with localized isolation of a portion of the right ventricle is now nearly eight years, and no adverse sequelae have developed. However, a four-year follow-up on two teenagers who required total isolation of the right ventricle for multifocal ventricular tachycardia has revealed a progressive dilatation of the right ventricle that may eventually become detrimental to overall cardiac performance. As a result, we no longer recommend isolation of the entire right ventricle for these life-threatening arrhythmias, unless there is absolutely no other way to correct the problem. In such a situation, serious consideration should be given to cardiac transplanation. Fortunately, with the automated intraoperative mapping systems now available, even multifocal non-ischemic ventricular tachycardias can generally be mapped and treated with more localized isolation techniques.

Ventricular Tachycardia Secondary to Ischemia

A clearer understanding of the best surgical approach for treating refractory ischemic ventricular tachycardia has emerged during the past two years. In the previous edition of this publication, I described the three basic surgical approaches to these arrhythmias that had been developed: (i) the encircling endocardial ventriculotomy; (ii) the endocardial resection procedure (frequently called 'subendocardial resection'); and (iii) endocardial cryoablation [16]. Modifications of these three techniques included removal of all visible endocardial scar associated with the infarct or aneurysm (the 'extended' endocardial resection procedure) and the so-called 'partial' encircling endocardial ventriculotomy. To this list must now be added laser photoablation.

The standard encircling endocardial ventriculotomy as originally described by Guiraudon in 1978 has been abandoned because of a high incidence of postoperative low-output syndrome and the associated perioperative mortality. However, Oster-meyer *et al* continue to report excellent long-term results using the modified, or 'partial' encircling endocardial ventriculotomy [17]. Likewise, the standard (localized) endocardial resection procedure, as originally described by Harken *et al* in 1979, is now usually modified to include much larger areas of scar resection because of the high rate of postoperative tachycardia inducibility. The addition of cryosurgery as an adjunct to the extended endocardial resection may further improve the results of surgery.

Although little information is available at present on the results of laser ablation for the treatment of ventricular tachycardia associated with ischemia, two groups have recently reported their preliminary experiences with this new therapeutic modality. Selle *et al* presented their results in five patients in whom the Nd-YAG laser was used to photoablate ventricular tachycardia, with no operative mortality or complications and with a 100% success rate [18]. Gallagher, from the same group, updated their series at a recent international symposium, stating that 17 patients had now undergone this procedure, with three operative deaths (17%) but with relief of the tachycardia in the survivors (unpublished data). The technique of laser photoablation described by these authors differs from that previously described by Mesnildrey, who performs an 'encircling thermo-exclusion' that is quite comparable in principle to the encircling endocardial ventriculotomy [19]. Other authors have proposed the use of both carbon dioxide and argon lasers for the treatment of ventricular tachycardia because of the precision of tissue destruction [20], yet, paradoxically, this characteristic of lasers probably represents a disadvantage rather than an advantage: even the most sophisticated mapping system is incapable of localizing the site of origin of tachycardia to a minute area [21].

In summary, current procedures of choice for the treatment of refractory tachycardia secondary to ischemia comprise either the partial encircling endocardial ventriculotomy or an extended subendocardial resection, with or without the addition of cryosurgery for the latter.

References

[1] de Bakker JMT, Janse MJ, van Capelle FJL, Durrer D.
An interactive computer system for guiding the surgical treatment of life-threatening ventricular tachycardias.
IEEE Trans Biomed Eng 1984; **BME-31**: 362–8.

[2] Witkowski FX, Corr PB.
An automated transmural cardiac mapping system.
Am J Physiol 1984; **247**: H661–8.

[3] Kramer JB, Corr PB, Cox JL, Witkowski FX, Cain ME.
Arrhythmia and conduction disturbances: Simultaneous computer mapping to facilitate intraoperative localization of accessory pathways in patients with Wolff-Parkinson-White syndrome.
Am J Cardiol 1985; **56**: 571–6.

[4] Parson I, Downar E.
Clinical instrumentation for the intraoperative mapping of ventricular arrhythmias.
Pace 1984; **7**: 683–92.

[5] Cox JL, Gallagher JJ, Cain ME.
Experience with 118 consecutive patients undergoing operation for the Wolff-Parkinson-White syndrome.
J Thorac Cardiovasc Surg 1985; **90**: 490–501.

[6] Iwa T, Mitsui T, Misaki T, Mukai K, Magara T, Kamata E.
Radical surgical cure of Wolff-Parkinson-White syndrome: The Kanazawa experience.
J Thorac Cardiovasc Surg 1986; **91**: 225–33.

[7] Guiraudon GM, Klein GJ, Gulamhusein S *et al*.
Surgical repair of Wolff-Parkinson-White syndrome: A new closed-heart technique.
Ann Thorac Surg 1984; **37**: 67–71.

[8] Guiraudon GM, Klein GJ, Sharma AD, Jones DL, McLellan DG.
Surgery for Wolff-Parkinson-White syndrome: Further experience with an epicardial approach.
Circulation 1986; **74**: 525.

[9] Bredikis J, Bredikis A.
Cryosurgical ablation of left parietal wall accessory atrioventricular connections through the coronary sinus without the use of extracorporeal circulation.
J Thorac Cardiovasc Surg 1985; **90**: 199–205.

[10] Bredikis J, Bukauskas F, Zebrauskas R *et al*.
Cryosurgical ablation of right parietal and septal accessory atrioventricular connections without the use of extracorporeal circulation.
J Thorac Cardiovasc Surg 1985; **90**: 206–11.

[11] Morady F, Scheinman MM, Winston SA et al.
Efficacy and safety of transcatheter ablation of posteroseptal accessory pathways.
Circulation 1985; **72**: 170–7.

[12] Ross DL, Johnson DC, Denniss AR, Cooper MJ, Richards DA, Uther JB.
Curative surgery for atrioventricular junctional (AV nodal) reentrant tachycardia.
J Am Coll Cardiol 1985; **6**: 1383–92.

[13] Gillette PC, Wampler DG, Garson A Jr, Zinner A, Ott D, Cooley D.
Treatment of atrial automatic tachycardia by ablation procedures.
J Am Coll Cardiol 1985; **6**: 405–9.

[14] Harada A, D'Agostino HJ Jr, Scafuri A, Boineau JP, Cox JL.
Isolation of the right atrium with preservation of the sinoatrial node: A new technique for the treatment of supraventricular tachycardia.
Surg Forum 1986; **37**: 300–1.

[15] Cox JL, Bardy GH, Damiano RJ Jr et al.
Right ventricular isolation procedures for nonischemic ventricular tachycardia.
J Thorac Cardiovasc Surg 1985; **90**: 212–24.

[16] Cox JL.
Treatment of ventricular arrhythmias. In: Sobel BE, Julian DG, Hugenholtz PG. *Perspectives in Cardiology 1984*. London: Current Medical Literature, 1984; pp. 234–9.

[17] Ostermeyer J, Breithardt G, Borggrefe M, Godehardt E, Seipel L, Bircks W.
Surgical Treatment of Ventricular tachycardias: Complete versus partial encircling endocardial ventriculotomy.
J Thorac Cardiovasc Surg 1984; **87**: 517–25.

[18] Selle JG, Svenson RH, Sealy WC et al.
Successful clinical laser ablation of ventricular tachycardia: A promising new therapeutic modality. Presented at *22nd Annual Meeting of the Society of Thoracic Surgeons*, Washington, DC, January 1986.

[19] Mesnildrey P, Laborde F, Piwnica A, Lareboisiere H.
Encircling thermo-exclusion by the Nd-YAG laser without mapping: A new surgical technique for ischemic ventricular tachycardia.
Circulation 1985; **72** (Suppl 3): 389.

[20] Isner JM, Michlewitz H, Clarke RH et al.
Laser photoablation of pathological endocardium: In-vitro findings suggesting a new approach to the surgical treatment of refractory arrhythmias and restrictive cardiomyopathy.
Ann Thorac Surg 1985; **39**: 201.

[21] Cox JL.
Laser photoablation for the treatment of refractory ventricular tachycardia and endocardial fibroelastosis [Editorial].
Ann Thorac Surg 1985; **39**: 100.

ANTIARRHYTHMIC DRUG THERAPY

[1] Usefulness of electrophysiologic testing in evaluation of amiodarone therapy for sustained ventricular tachyarrhythmias associated with coronary heart disease.
Horowitz LN, Greenspan AM, Speilman SR *et al*, Hahnemann Univ Hosp and Sch Med, Philadelphia, PA, USA.
Am J Cardiol 1985; **55**: 367–71.

[2] Long-term clinical outcome of ventricular tachycardia or fibrillation treated with amiodarone.
McGovern B, Garan H, Malacoff RF *et al*, Massachusetts Gen Hosp, Boston, MA, USA.
Am J Cardiol 1984; **53**: 1558–63.

[3] Results of late programmed electrical stimulation and long-term electrophysiological effects of amiodarone therapy in patients with refractory ventricular tachycardia.
Veltri EP, Reid PR, Platia EV, Griffith LSC, Johns Hopkins Med Insts, Baltimore, MD, USA.
Am J Cardiol 1985; **55**: 375–9.

[4] Amiodarone in the treatment of life-threatening tachycardia: role of Holter monitoring in predicting longterm clinical efficacy.
Veltri EP, Reid PR, Platia EV, Griffith LSC, Johns Hopkins Med Insts, Baltimore, MD, USA.
J Am Coll Cardiol 1985; **6**: 806–13.

[5] Amiodarone: risk factors for recurrence of symptomatic ventricular tachycardia identified at electrophysiologic study.
Naccarelli GV, Fineberg NS, Zipes DP, Heger JJ, Duncan G, Prystowsky EN, Krannert Inst Cardiol, Indianapolis, IN, USA.
J Am Coll Cardiol 1985; **6**: 814–21.

[6] Steady-state serum amiodarone concentrations: relationships with antiarrhythmic efficacy and toxicity.
Rotmensch HH, Belhassen B, Swanson BN *et al*, Jefferson Med Coll, Philadelphia, PA, USA.
Ann Intern Med 1984; **101**: 462–9.

[7] Amiodarone: correlation of serum concentration with suppression of complex ventricular ectopic activity.
Mostow ND, Rakita L, Vrobel TR, Noon DL, Blumer J, Cleveland Metropolitan Gen Hosp, Cleveland, OH, USA.
Am J Cardiol 1984; **54**: 569–74.

[8] Adverse reactions during treatment with amiodarone hydrochloride.
McGovern B, Garan H, Kelly E, Ruskin JN, Massachusetts Gen Hosp, Boston, MA, USA.
Br Med J 1983; **287**: 175–80.

[9] Amiodarone: clinical efficacy and toxicity in 96 patients with recurrent, drug-refractory arrhythmias.
Fogoros RN, Anderson JP, Winkle RA, Swerdlow CD, Mason JW, Stanford Univ Med Cent, Stanford, CA, USA.
Circulation 1983; **68**: 88–94.

[10] Long-term efficacy and toxicity of high-dose amiodarone therapy for ventricular tachycardia or ventricular fibrillation.
Morady F, Sauve MJ, Malone P *et al*, Univ California, San Francisco, CA, USA.
Am J Cardiol 1983; **52**: 975–9.

[11] Amiodarone: the experience of the past decade.
McKenna WJ, Rowland E, Krikler DM, Royal Postgrad Med Sch, London, UK.
Br Med J 1983; **287**: 1654–6.

[12] The QT interval: a predictor of the plasma and myocardial concentrations of amiodarone.
Debbas NMG, du Cailar C, Bexton RS, Demaille JG, Camm AJ, Puech P, St Bartholomew's Hosp, London, UK.
Br Heart J 1984; **51**: 316–20.

[13] QT Prolongation and the antiarrhythmic efficacy of amiodarone.
Torres V, Tepper D, Flowers D *et al*, Einstein Coll Med, Bronx, NY, USA.
J Am Coll Cardiol 1986; **7**: 142–7.

[14] Evaluation by serial electrophysiologic studies of an abbreviated oral loading regimen of amiodarone.
Kennedy EE, Rosenfeld LE, McPherson CA, Batsford WP, Yale Univ Sch Med, New Haven, CT, USA.
Am J Cardiol 1985; **56**: 867–71.

[15] Clinical efficacy and electropharmacology of continuous intravenous amiodarone infusion and chronic oral amiodarone in refractory ventricular tachycardia.
Saksena S, Rothbart ST, Shah Y, Cappello G, Newark Beth Israel Med Cent, Newark, NJ, USA.
Am J Cardiol 1984; **54**: 347–52.

[16] Hemodynamic effects of intravenous amiodarone.
Kosinski EJ, Albin JB, Young E, Lewis SM, LeLand OS Jr, New England Deaconess Hosp, Boston, MA, USA.
J Am Coll Cardiol 1984; **4**: 565–70.

[17] Cardiac function in patients on chronic amiodarone therapy.
Ellenbogen KA, O'Callaghan WG, Colavita PG, Smith MS, German LD, Duke Univ Med Cent, Durham NC, USA.
Am Heart J 1985; **110**: 376–81.

[18] Amiodarone for refractory atrial fibrillation.
Gold RL, Haffajee CI, Charos G, Sloan K, Baker S, Alpert JS, Univ Massachusetts Med Cent, Worcester, MA, USA.
Am J Cardiol 1986; **57**: 124–7.

[19] Long-term tolerance of amiodarone treatment for cardiac arrhythmias.
Smith WM, Lubbe WF, Whitlock RM, Mercer J, Rutherford JD, Roche AH, Green Lane Hosp, Auckland, New Zealand.
Am J Cardiol 1986; **57**: 1288–93.

[20] Amiodarone treatment of critical arrhythmias in children and young adults.
Garson A Jr, Gillette PC, McVey P *et al*, Texas Children's Hosp, Houston, TX, USA.
J Am Coll Cardiol 1984; **4**: 749–55.

[21] Cardiac electrophysiologic effects of flecainide acetate for paroxysmal reentrant junctional tachycardias.
Hellestrand KJ, Nathan AW, Bexton RS, Spurrell RAJ, Camm AJ, St Bartholomew's Hosp, London, UK.
Am J Cardiol 1983; **51**: 770–6.

[22] Flecainide: electrophysiologic and antiarrhythmic properties in refractory ventricular tachycardia.
Platia EV, Estes NAM, Heine DL *et al*, Johns Hopkins Med Insts, Baltimore, MD, USA.
Am J Cardiol 1985; **55**: 956–2.

[23] Comparative study of encainide and quinidine in the treatment of ventricular arrhythmias.
Morganroth J, Somberg JC, Poole PE, Hsu P-H, Lee IK, Durkee J, for the Encainide-Quinidine Research Group, Hahneman Univ Hosp, Philadelphia, PA, USA.
J Am Coll Cardiol 1986; **7**: 9–16.

[24] The role of beta blocking agents as adjunct therapy to membrane stabilizing drugs in malignant ventricular arrhythmia.
Hirsowitz G, Podrid PJ, Lampert S, Stein J, Lown B, Harvard Sch Public Hlth, Boston, MA, USA.
Am Heart J 1986; **111**: 852–9.

[25] Incidence and clinical features of quinidine-associated long QT syndrome: implications for patient care.
Roden DM, Woosley RL, Primm RK, Vanderbilt Univ Sch Med, Nashville, TN, USA.
Am Heart J 1986; **111**: 1088–94.

[26] Intramuscular lidocaine for prevention of lethal arrhythmias in the prehospitalization phase of acute myocardial infarction.
Koster RW, Dunning AJ, Academic Med Cent, Amsterdam, Netherlands.
N Engl J Med 1985; **313**: 1105–10.

[27] Lidocaine to prevent ventricular fibrillation: easy does it (Editorial).
Lown B, Harvard Sch Public Hlth, Boston, MA, USA.
N Engl J Med 1985; **313**: 1154–6.

Comment. Amiodarone is an effective drug for the treatment of both ventricular and supraventricular arrhythmias. The value of electrophysiologic study for determining long-term efficacy may be less useful with amiodarone than with other anti-arrhythmic drugs. Horowitz *et al* [1] found electrophysiologic testing to be of value, but noted that the hemodynamic response to induced tachycardia on amiodarone was as important as its continuing inducibility. Other groups have also found serial electrophysiologic testing to be of value [2], but other workers [3] did not find that restudy predicted efficacy whereas ambulatory ECG monitoring was specific, and reasonably sensitive for assessing clinical response in patients with life-threatening ventricular tachycardia [4]. Naccarelli [5] used a discriminant analysis approach to predict clinical outcome in patients with ventricular tachycardia, and found that estimates based on prolongation of ventricular effective refractory period, change in corrected QT interval, induction of repetitive ventricular responses and ease of ventricular tachycardia reinduction identified overall clinical efficacy in 90% of patients.

High maintenance doses of amiodarone may be necessary for patients with malignant ventricular arrhythmia but are undoubtedly associated with an increased incidence of adverse reactions. A variety of studies has evaluated the relationship between plasma concentration of amiodarone and both efficacy and toxicity, drawing attention to the incidence of serious toxicity and demonstrating the benefits of dose reduction to a minimum essential maintenance dose [6–11]. Two studies [12,13] have examined the close relationship between the QT interval with plasma and myocardial concentrations of amiodarone and show that, where the QT can be measured, it is a useful marker for electrophysiologic effect and possibly antiarrhythmic efficacy.

A more prompt onset of action of amiodarone may be achieved by intravenous loading, but this can also be achieved by a higher dose oral loading regimen [13]. Using 1200 mg/day, significant changes in refractory periods were seen, although prevention of inducibility of ventricular tachycardia was less impressive. The correlation between intravenous infusion and chronic oral use of amiodarone was shown by Saksena *et al* [15] who failed to show any change in ventricular effective refractory period with the intravenous infusion. Any influence that may have occurred may have been antagonized by the hemodynamic effects of intravenous amiodarone [16] which can produce clinically important myocardial depression in the severely compromised left ventricle. In contrast, a study of 41 patients evaluated by radionuclide angiography before and after at least three months' oral therapy with amiodarone showed that blood pressure and ejection fraction were unchanged in the majority — there was a fall in ejection fraction of >10% in three patients [17].

Amiodarone remains one of the most effective drugs for the treatment of refractory atrial fibrillation, being effective in 79% of a study of 68 patients by Gold *et al* [18]. Interestingly, the results of a long-term study [19] suggested that, when patients with supraventricular arrhythmias were grouped together, the probability of surviving and continuing with amiodarone therapy at 50 months was only 19%. Adverse effects attributable to the drug were recorded in 59% and resulted in withdrawal of therapy in 26%.

Amiodarone may also be of value in pediatric practice. In a wide-ranging group of 39 patients with both supraventricular and ventricular arrhythmia, its efficacy ranged

311

from 55%–94% [20]. Adverse effects were mild and uncommon, although the authors cautioned that the long-term effects of the drug are not known.

There remains the need for alternative effective antiarrhythmic drugs. Flecainide and encainide have been shown to be effective in supraventricular and ventricular arrhythmias [21–23]. It has also been shown that both may cause important pro-arrhythmic effects.

Whether combination therapy may increase efficacy while reducing adverse effects is still open to question. Hirsowitz [24] demonstrated improved efficacy when beta-blocking drugs were added to class I antiarrhythmic agents and, as none of the underlying ventricular arrhythmias were significantly altered by beta-blocking drugs alone, the author suggests that synergistic benefit accrued from the combination rather than a summation of individual effects.

Although quinidine is a common cause of the acquired long QT syndrome, there is a paucity of clinical data on such cases. In a paper by Roden *et al* [25], 24 patients with long QT syndrome following quinidine therapy are described — 20 of them had tor-sade de pointes. The authors estimate the risk of quinidine-associated long QT syndrome as being at least 1.5% per year; it was found to be most common in patients with *non-sustained* ventricular arrhythmia or atrial fibrillation or flutter. A feature of QT prolongation in those treated for atrial fibrillation was the appearance of torsade de pointes only after conversion to sinus rhythm. In 20 of the 24 patients, at least one other major risk factor for QT prolongation was also present, which included hypokalemia, serum potassium between 3.5 and 3.9 mmol/litre, high-grade atrioventricular block and underlying pre-existent QT prolongation. Plasma quinidine concentrations were either at or below the lower limit of the therapeutic range in 50% of patients. QRS widening was usually absent. Clearly, close attention to factors that may aggravate QT prolongation in association with quinidine treatment is important, but whether the risk is greater than with other classs I antiarrhythmic drugs remains to be established.

There is still a lack of convincing evidence that lidocaine administered in hospital to patients with myocardial infarction prevents ventricular fibrillation. Use of paramedical community services to treat patients with suspected myocardial infarction offers the prospect of reducing the mortality of those high-risk patients whose death from arrhythmia occurs before they would otherwise reach hospital. It is therefore disappointing that of 6024 patients with chest pain randomized to treatment by paramedics with intramuscular lidocaine in the prehospitalization phase of suspected acute myocardial infarction or control (32% were subsequently proven to have had acute myocardial infarction), no statistically significant overall difference in the incidence of ventricular fibrillation during the 60-minute observation phase was noted (8 episodes in the treatment group, 17 in the control patients; $P=0.08$) [26]. However, analysis of the data from 15 minutes after randomization (the time taken for plasma lidocaine levels to reach therapeutic range) showed that lidocaine conferred statistical benefit (2 *vs* 12 patients; $P<0.01$). The majority of patients had plasma lidocaine levels within the therapeutic range; only 3% had toxic levels of the drug. In the accompanying editorial [27], Lown outlines the current role of lidocaine in preventing primary ventricular fibrillation and highlights some of the potential benefits and risks, particularly the suggestion made by Koster and Dunning [26] that "lidocaine self-injection by patients with prolonged chest pain ... may be of value."

THE PHYSICAL ASPECTS OF CATHETER ABLATION

Review: A. DAVID CUNNINGHAM

Catheter ablation to control or manage cardiac arrhythmias is a recent, fast-moving therapeutic approach. It represents to the electrophysiologist — much as angioplasty does to the angiographer — an opportunity to extend investigative techniques towards definitive cure in conditions previously amenable only to the cardiac surgeon, and with the obvious attractions of avoiding chronic drug therapy.

Catheter ablation may be used to produce complete heart block, thus allowing control of ventricular rate in drug-refractory supraventricular arrhythmias, or it may be targeted directly at the myocardial site responsible for an arrhythmia, such as a ventricular tachycardia focus, or at an accessory pathway.

The first report of atrioventricular block induced by electric shock in man came from Vedel in Paris [1]. During electrophysiologic study, a patient required six external shocks of 360 J for conversion of a malignant ventricular arrhythmia; subsequently, the patient was found to be in persistent complete heart block. The presence of a His bundle recording catheter was implicated in the production of the heart block, and, since mechanical damage seemed unlikely, it appeared that some phenomenon of electrical induction was responsible. The presence of a conducting surface (such as catheter electrodes) in an electric field causes a threefold local amplification of the field intensity [2]. This still represents a very small current density, and it must be presumed that critical positioning of the electrode allowed six-minute 'local shocks' to create permanent heart block.

Intentional ablation of atrioventricular conduction was developed in dogs by Gonzales [3] using a standard defibrillator connected to an electrode catheter, which was modified by partially insulating the electrodes to encourage directional current flow. Complete block was produced in 9 out of 10 dogs, and Gonzales *et al* were encouraged to attempt the technique in man for control of drug-refractory supraventricular arrhythmias. The first reports in man showed that persistent complete block could be achieved, using synchronized discharges of up to 500 J stored energy [4,5]. The delivered shocks were unipolar, using a back paddle as an indifferent electrode. The patients required permanent pacing after ablation.

Current Usage and Usefulness

Many groups have taken up this novel form of treatment, perceiving that it could obviate open-heart surgery in certain patients. A worldwide registry was set up in 1984 [6]; its most recent report, on 209 patients, demonstrated that persistent complete block was achieved in 70% of cases [7]. In an additional 8%, although atrioventricular conduction returned, it was modified in such a way that the arrhythmia was controlled without the need for drug therapy; in 13%, previously ineffective drug regimens

313

now provided effective control; and in the remaining 9%, ablation was ineffective. A single shock (150–400 J) proved effective in 45 of 127 patients in the initial report of the World Registry [6]. In contrast, one in seven patients received a cumulative energy of over 1000 J during attempted ablation.

The acute complications associated with ablation, as reported by various groups, include elevation of serum creatine kinase, and its MB fraction, in over 90% of cases [6,8]: mean CK-MB levels in the World Registry were 31 IU/l [7]. Other complications included induction of ventricular tachycardia or fibrillation in 2% [7], perforation and tamponade [7,9,10], transient hypotension, pericarditis, and asystole [7]. None of these complications has had chronic sequelae, but there is a late mortality of 7% (mean follow-up, 8 months) [7]. Death has been sudden in 2%, but other cardiac death has also been reported, albeit in patients with pre-existing cardiac failure. Diffuse myocardial damage caused by ablation, and a subsequent reduction in cardiac function, may be implicated: a study in 24 patients after atrioventricular junctional ablation showed a reduction in exercise tolerance to 45% of the predicted value for a permanently paced patient, when corrected for age and sex [11]. Even in patients with rate-responsive pacemakers, exercise tolerance only reached 67% of the predicted norm. Concern has been expressed about the use of ablative techniques which result in complete heart block [12,13] because of the patients' pacemaker dependency and associated risks.

After initial reports of His bundle ablation, the technique was applied by other groups to accessory pathways [14], ventricular tachycardia [15] and focal atrial tachycardia [16]. Safety concerns become even more crucial in these groups of patients. Although Morady and Scheinman have had considerable success with the ablation of posteroseptal pathways [7,17], the worldwide success rate for all accessory pathway ablations is probably well below 50%, and serious complications are more frequent in these patients: 43 cases have been reported to the World Registry [7], and in four of these the coronary sinus was ruptured by the ablative shock, resulting in tamponade, and death in one patient. Clearly, the delivery of high energies in this small vessel is dangerous and potentially lethal, and ablation in the coronary sinus is currently contraindicated.

In ventricular tachycardia, success rates have varied from group to group [10,15,18–22]. Of 91 patients reported by these groups, 33 (35%) had no recurrence of tachycardia during follow-up without drug therapy. In 26 patients (20%), tachycardia was controlled successfully using previously ineffective drugs, and in 32 (45%) ablation was unsuccessful. The mean number of shocks delivered (3.6), and their mean energy (350 J), was higher than during atrioventricular junctional ablation, and this may help to explain the higher complication rate: ventricular tachycardia or fibrillation occurred in 40%, perforation of apex or outflow tract in two patients, one of whom died acutely, and acute or early death in seven other cases. Again, serum cardiac enzyme levels were usually raised. Total mortality for these groups is difficult to assess, but it may be as high as 25% in the first year. Ablation of ventricular tachycardia appears, in its present form, to be associated with an unacceptably high complication rate.

The relationship between the degree of ablative myocardial damage and resultant myocardial dysfunction or mortality has yet to be explored adequately for any of the forms of ablation.

Physical Effects in Vitro

When a high-energy pulse is delivered by a defibrillator through a standard electrode catheter to the endocardial surface of the heart, there are a number of dramatic effects. Phenomena include the formation of an electrical arc, a high-pressure shock wave, and significant volumes of gas. The radiographic appearance of a 'black hole' surrounding the electrode during ablation [8] suggests that high-energy photons are being emitted. Examination of electrodes reveals a characteristic pitting [23,24] of the surface, which is usually platinum. This damage is generally considered to be caused by the high-temperature electrical arc, and suggests that local temperatures exceed 1700°C, the melting point of platinum. It is therefore likely that the majority of gas formation is due to boiling; however, collection and mass spectroscopy [25,26] of the non-condensable gases shows a difference between the gas formed by cathodal and anodal shocks, suggesting that some electrolysis may be taking place. Formation of a plasma (a hot, ionized vapor) may occur [25], which would be associated with extremely high ($\sim 5000°C$) temperatures and consequent rapid gas production.

Gas bubble nucleation and growth, due primarily to local liquid superheating near the electrode surface, is theoretically not associated with large pressure changes in the medium [27]: after a short initial rapid phase, bubble growth is essentially isobaric. However, the eventual accelerating collapse of the gas bubble is associated with a rapid-onset, high-pressure transient — in excess of 10 atm (7600 mmHg) [25]. The phenomenon of shock-wave formation due to collapsing bubbles is a well-known cause of damage to structures such as propeller blades [28]. Damage is caused by a combination of asymmetric bubble collapse — which results in emission of a high-velocity liquid 'microjet' — and direct shock-wave damage. The shock wave will be minimally attenuated in body fluids, which are incompressible, but there may be some absorption (in addition to transmission and reflection) by solid structures, such as myocardium. The shock wave may be followed by a trailing negative-pressure (rarefaction) wave. If the negative pressure falls below the vapor pressure of the blood, secondary microbubble formation may occur (cavitation [28]). Widespread microbubbles have been seen in the right ventricle during His bundle ablation [29], and their additional presence in the left ventricle suggests that the shock wave and subsequent negative-pressure undershoot are partially transmitted through the interventricular septum. It is possible that diffuse tissue damage may be caused by this pressure transient during ablation, or by cavitation erosion due to microbubble collapse. It is also possible that the shock wave of the primary bubble collapse contributes to the observed electrode pitting.

Holt and Boyd showed that high-energy anodal shocks produced significantly more hemolysis and gas production than did cathodal shocks [26]. The explanation for this lies in the basic principle that arcing can only occur at a cathode [30]. When a unipolar anodal shock is delivered, the surface of the gas bubble which develops around the electrode will act as a 'virtual cathode', creating a more diffuse 'fireball'. The mean incident power during arcing is greater at an anode than at a cathode (due to electron bombardment), and hence an anode will reach a higher mean temperature, with greater associated boiling and hemolysis. Rapid local oxidation of biological tissue has also been suggested as an explanation for the increased violence of high-energy anodal shocks [26]. The electrical arc, which burns over a very small sur-

315

face area (a 'cathode spot' [31]), would be expected to produce microscopically discrete erosion craters; anodal 'hot spots' have a much larger surface area. This has been shown using electron microscopy [26], although the authors have interpreted the results somewhat differently. The virtual cathode will also have a greater surface area than the anode, and at a given current there will be a lower current density. Thus, at lower energies, an arc will preferentially form at a cathode (rather than an anode). This has been shown experimentally in saline and blood [25] and in high-speed cinematographic studies [32]. At low energies, anodal ablation will reduce electrical arcing and bubble formation, but at energies above 100 J anodal arcing is associated with violent shock waves, and cathodal ablation undoubtedly becomes safer.

Analysis of evolved gas has produced conflicting results. Although similar gas volumes were collected for various energy settings [25,26], Bardy *et al* found that the collected gas was predominantly (>85%) composed of nitrogen and oxygen [25]. Holt and Boyd found significant quantities of hydrogen in the collected gas, ranging from 50% to 68% depending on energy and polarity [26]. During our own studies at the National Heart Hospital, London, UK, significant volumes of hydrogen were collected (unpublished data). These important discrepancies may be related to the method of gas collection, and in particular to the diffusivity of the collection apparatus to hydrogen.

Catheter Effects

In addition to electrode pitting, multipolar catheters are prone to breakdown of the dielectric insulation, resulting in electrical continuity between different poles (internal breakdown) or a hole in the insulation (external breakdown). The ability of catheters to withstand high-energy shocks varies according to catheter size and construction [24], and is not consistent. Damage may affect both the electrodes and the adjacent insulation. The most commonly used electrode for these procedures, the USCI temporary pacing catheter, has recently undergone a change in construction; the 'modular' construction is much less likely to withstand an ablative discharge. Fisher *et al* concluded that most catheters can safely be used up to 100 J [24], but above this level there is great variability in electrical strength.

Fontaine reported that, of 32 USCI catheters tested, only five were able to withstand repeated shocks with a peak voltage of 2000 V and only three could be used repeatedly at 3500 V [33]. He also showed that the current measured during a catheter shock showed a characteristic 'dip' after approximately 2–5 ms, and that it could fall virtually to zero for a brief period and then recover to continue its previous course (that of a damped sinusoidal waveform). This may be related to gas production around the electrode, which effectively insulates it from the conductive medium, thus reducing current flow. The voltage developed across this gas bubble may exceed the breakdown voltage and initiate an electrical arc, with associated high temperature and pressure wave. Bardy *et al* extended these studies to measure the dielectric breakdown voltage of 24 catheters [23]. In eight new catheters, breakdown occurred between 2200 and 3500 V; thus, some of these catheters would not withstand a 400-J discharge, which has a peak voltage >3000 V. A further 16 catheters were used to deliver a single shock in dogs. The proximal electrode was rendered electrically open circuit in six catheters, and the dielectric strength was considerably reduced (to as low as 70 V) in one. Pitting occurred on all electrodes, but in seven cases pitting was seen on an electrode not connected to the defibrillator, showing that energy had been shunted through the insulation and had resulted in inappropriate energy delivery, which could be potentially hazardous with ablation near the coronary sinus os [7,17]. This phenomenon will also reduce energy delivery at the appropriate electrode, diminishing the efficacy of the procedure. Reduced dielectric strength after the first shock clearly makes further shocks even more hazardous from this point of view. Existing catheters obviously have insufficient dielectric strength for conventional ablative procedures; either the energy requirements for ablation must be reduced, or catheters of higher dielectric strength must be developed.

The use of non-standard catheters to deliver ablative discharges has been limited. Holt *et al* used a unipolar Helifix permanent pacing electrode, and reported that permanent His bundle ablation was achieved with four shocks of 50 J, in 7 out of 10 patients [34]. The active fixation properties of this lead and its different geometry were suggested to make it superior to the USCI electrode. The delivered energy in these patients was less than one-third of the mean delivered energy in the World Registry [7]; however, the high line-resistance of this lead means that energy is dissipated in the lead material (in fact, the energy delivered to the patient may have been considerably less than 50 J), and secondly the increased total impedance prolongs energy delivery time. Leaving the guidewire in place during ablation might lower the resistance of the lead, but its stiffness engenders the risk of mechanically perforating the septum, as has been seen with conventional catheters at both apex and outflow tract of the right ventricle [9]. The considerable time required for accurate placement of the electrode is a further disadvantage.

Scheinman *et al* achieved a low rate of complete block using a barbed active fixation electrode in dogs [35]. Polgar *et al* also reported limited success in man, using a suction electrode catheter to deliver the shock [36]. The small surface area of these electrodes might mean that little energy is delivered before arcing occurs, and it will thus be difficult to avoid barotrauma. An improved design of suction electrode has recently been described which uses a high melting-point tungsten/rhenium electrode; complete heart block was obtained in dogs using 20 J [37].

Clearly, further catheter development is required to combine the ideal geometry (which is yet to be determined), low line-resistance and suitable maneuverability in one catheter.

Electrical Characteristics in Vivo
There are few studies which have measured the electrical characteristics of ablative discharges *in vivo*, due to technical difficulties associated with the measurement of voltage and current. Trantham *et al* reported on His bundle ablation in 23 patients [38]: 200-J shocks had a peak voltage of 2160 V and peak current of 42 A; these values increased to 2400 V and 58 A at 300 J. Electrode pitting was seen in 22 cases. They noted that the current peaks later than the voltage, suggesting the presence of a non-linear impedance. The impedance reached a minimum value of around 50Ω during the shock. Results in dogs showed higher voltages, and lower currents, at both 200 and 360 J [39], consistent with a mean impedance of $>100\Omega$.

It is important to note that a 'dip' in the delivered current waveform is always seen when arcing occurs [25,33]; we can thus identify even minimal in-vivo arcing by measuring delivered current, when direct visualization is obviously impossible.

Catheter Ablation: In-Vivo Histology
A number of studies have looked at acute and chronic effects of high-energy shocks on tissue — both in dogs, and in man at post-mortem. Ablation of the atrioventricular junction is associated with acute deformation of cell shape, pyknotic nuclei, interstitial edema and hemorrhage, and sarcomere disruption [7]. An inflammatory reaction develops within days [7,39,40], with diffuse hematoma and congested vasculature. Necrosis with local fatty infiltration has been described [3], and fibrotic changes can be seen as early as 5–7 days after ablation. There appears to be little chronic damage to the atrioventricular nodal artery [39,41]. Ward and Davies described an absence of apparent atrioventricular nodal fibers, rather than preservation of a damaged nodal structure, and suggested that this appearance may be consistent with damage due to the pressure wave (barotrauma) [41]. The size of chronic lesion has been reported at between 2 and 20 mm in diameter [40,42].

Coronary sinus lesions follow a similar course [43,44]. There is transmural atrial injury at the site of the shock, with no evidence of damage to the annulus or circumflex coronary artery; the lesions are between 7 and 23 mm long. Coltorti *et al* described thrombotic stenosis of the coronary sinus in 6 of 12 dogs and complete occlusion in 3; all 12 dogs had evidence of damage or rupture of the internal elastica of the sinus, without gross rupture [44]. They suggest that the mechanism of therapeutic success may be disconnection of the atrial end of the accessory pathway, rather than damage to the pathway itself. In support of this, Fisher *et al* described two cases where attempted ablation failed [45]; at surgery the accessory pathway was intact, but was inserted into the left atrium at a point where fibrosis due to catheter shock was clearly seen. An interesting insight into the inflammatory reaction was provided by identification of platinum deposits in the atrial wall via spectroscopy [44], presumably due to the melting of the platinum electrode during the shock. This might explain the occasional finding in several studies of giant cell formation in the region of injury.

Animal studies of ventricular ablation [46–49] consistently showed sub-endocardial damage with shocks under 100 J, and transmural necrosis for energies of 200 J and above; no perforation was seen in any of these studies. As with other sites, hematoma and interstitial edema is a common finding: Lee *et al* [48] and Lerman *et al* [49] described the appearance of contraction band necrosis — a reaction typical of irreversibly damaged cells which continue to be perfused. The volume of tissue damaged is in the region of 0.5–5 ml, demonstrating that gross anatomic lesions are focal; however, evidence of focal necrosis cannot be considered proof that global myocardial damage is not occurring, as this may be histologically undetectable. The degree of enzyme elevation [6,8] supports the view that diffuse damage is occurring.

Non-Conventional Power Sources
There is, of course, no reason *a priori* why an external defibrillator should be the ideal source of power for use in catheter ablation; indeed it is quite unlikely to be so, since

its waveform (a damped sinusoid) was designed to produce global myocardial depolarization while minimizing trauma due to intense current flow at the paddles [50] — quite the reverse of the ideal ablation power source, where discrete local damage is desirable. The widespread use of conventional defibrillators can probably be attributed more to availability than suitability. Investigation into new power sources for ablation has developed along several different avenues.

The use of lasers in arrhythmia therapy has aroused recent interest. Lasers are, by definition, highly focal in application, and do not involve subjecting the entire heart to a high electrical field. Both argon and Nd-YAG lasers have been used to produce lesions in specimens of ventricular tissue, and in live dogs and man [48,51–53]. Lee *et al* showed that Nd-YAG produced larger lesions *in vivo* than on tissue specimens [48]. They produced a similar lesion size for less energy than electrical ablation, and suggested that laser photoablation was associated with fewer ventricular arrhythmias and wall-motion abnormalities. Saksena *et al* concluded that pulsed argon lasers may be useful during intraoperative ablation procedures [51]. They suggest that the bulky energy delivery system and the fragility of the optical fiber are potential disadvantages. Gallagher *et al* used Nd-YAG laser energy during surgery for ventricular tachycardia in six patients [52]. They ablated 18–42 cm^2 of tissue, and were unable to induce tachycardia in these patients at up to two months follow-up. Isner *et al* produced controlled lesions *in vitro*, using both carbon dioxide and argon lasers [53]; 5 cm^2 of tissue could be ablated in 40 seconds, and they conclude that the technique may have application, not only for surgery but also for transcatheter arrhythmia ablation.

Transcatheter use of laser energy has been studied by Narula *et al* [54], who caused tamponade with 8-W continuous-wave argon laser energy in two dogs but were able to produce progressive degrees of heart block with 10–60-s application of 2.5-W laser energy. In all dogs the fiber was positioned against the right-ventricular septum. Histology did, however, show edema at the aortic annulus and surrounding tissue. The channel of laser-damaged tissue was extremely narrow (<0.5 mm wide). In a further series of six dogs [55], total delivered energies of 30–40 J caused variable degrees of heart block, related to the cumulative dose. Narula suggests that modification of atrioventricular nodal conduction may be achieved with laser energy, and might thus be useful in treating arrhythmias without producing complete heart block. It is perhaps surprising that such a focal technique can produce graded effects. Ablation of a very small section of the atrioventricular node or His bundle possibly allows a smaller remaining tissue area for conduction (effectively, an 'impedance mismatch' may be produced). Echocardiography has demonstrated intracavitary microbubble formation during laser energy delivery [48], presumably due to the boiling of surrounding body fluids and release of gas from photoablated tissue [56].

Recently there have been preliminary reports of the use of radio-frequency energy for atrioventricular junctional ablation, by 'desiccation' of the tissue [57]. The energy is delivered at a frequency of 750 kHz, which is well above frequencies liable to cause any cardiac stimulation. Power levels are much lower than with conventional electrical ablation, and consequently energy is delivered over longer periods (typically 5 s at 35-W power). No ventricular arrhythmias were induced in dogs using this method [57]. This technique is of great interest, because the low power levels employed raise the possibility of ablation procedures being performed without general anesthesia. However, the long energy delivery time may also considerably increase the area of damage, by allowing thermal equilibrium to be established, and it remains to be seen if the extent of damage caused by this technique will be appropriate for the ablation of different arrhythmias.

A direct attempt to address the problem of electrical arcing, and consequent pressure-wave formation, has been made by two groups. Bardy *et al* have used high-intensity (15-A), short-duration discharges at a repetition rate of up to 5 kHz, and have shown that pressure-wave formation is absent or much less than for conventional, damped sinusoid waveforms at the same energy [58]. Our own work has been based on modification of a conventional defibrillator, by removing series inductance and reducing energy delivery time, giving greatly increased peak current for the same energy [59]. We have successfully produced complete heart block with as little as 3.1 J delivered energy. Delivered current waveforms showed that no arcing took place, and thus barotrauma played no part in these low-energy ablations. The mechanism of damage is likely to be thermal [60].

Future Directions

Catheter ablation of the atrioventricular junction is now the preferred method of producing complete heart block in patients in whom such a procedure is indicated. The method is safer than surgical techniques and has a similar success rate [7,61]. The long-term fate of ablated patients is still of concern, and reduction in energy requirement to provide a greater safety margin between therapeutic and dangerous levels of myocardial damage must be considered an important goal. Improved power source and electrode design may considerably extend these safety margins, and lead to improved success rates for other ablation targets. Research into the basis of the beneficial 'damage' caused by ablation must also provide direction for future technical developments.

References

[1] Vedel J, Frank R, Fontaine G, Gournial JF, Grosgogeat Y.
Bloc auriculo-ventriculaire intra-hisien definitif induit au cours d'une exploration endoventriculaire droite.
Arch Mal Coeur 1979; **72**: 107–12.

[2] Lorrain P, Corson D.
Electromagnetic Fields and Waves. San Francisco: W.H. Freeman, 1970; p. 169.

[3] Gonzales R, Scheinman MM, Margaretten W, Rubinstein M.
Closed chest electrode-catheter technique for His bundle ablation in dogs.
Am J Physiol 1981; **241**: H283–H7.

[4] Scheinman MM, Morady F, Hess S, Gonzalez R.
Catheter-induced ablation of the atrioventricular junction to control refractory supraventricular arrhythmias.
JAMA 1982; **248**: 851–5.

[5] Gallagher JJ, Svenson RH, Kasell JH et al.
Catheter technique for closed-chest ablation of the atrioventricular conduction system: A therapeutic alternative for the treatment of refractory SVT.
N Engl J Med 1982; **306**: 194–200.

[6] Scheinman MM, Evans-Bell T and the Executive Committee of the Percutaneous Cardiac Mapping and Ablation Registry.
Catheter ablation of the atrioventricular junction.
Circulation 1984; **70**: 1024–9.

[7] Scheinman MM.
Catheter ablation for patients with cardiac arrhythmias.
PACE 1986; **9**: 551–64.

[8] Nathan AW, Bennett DH, Ward DE, Camm AJ.
Catheter ablation of atrioventricular conduction.
Lancet 1984; **i**: 1280–4.

[9] Fisher JD, Kim SG, Matos JA *et al.*
Complications of catheter ablation of tachyarrhythmias: Occurrence, protection and prevention.
Clin Prog Electrophysiol Pacing 1985; **3**: 292–8.

[10] Leclercq JF, Cauchemez B, Chouty F, Attuel P, Coumel P.
Importance of electrical shunt-effect during closed chest ablation procedure using multipolar catheters.
New Trends Arrhyt 1986; **2**: 277–82.

[11] Schofield PM, Bowes RJ, Bennett DH.
Exercise capacity and heart rhythm following transvenous fulguration of atrio-ventricular conduction [Abstract].
Br Heart J 1985; **54**: 614.

[12] Rosen K, Dhingra RC, Wyndham CRC.
Trading arrhythmia for atrioventricular block.
Circulation 1980; **61**: 16–7.

[13] Surawicz B.
A tactic of last resort.
N Engl J Med 1982; **306**: 234–6.

[14] Fisher JD, Brodman R, Kim SG, Matos JA.
Nonsurgical Kent bundle ablation via the coronary sinus in patients with the Wolff-Parkinson-White syndrome [Abstract].
Circulation 1982; **66**: II–375.

[15] Hartzler GO.
Electrode catheter ablation of refractory focal ventricular tachycardia.
J Am Coll Cardiol 1983; **2**: 1107–13.

[16] Silka MJ, Gillette PC, Garson A, Zinner A.
Transvenous catheter ablation of a right atrial automatic ectopic tachycardia.
J Am Coll Cardiol 1985; **5**: 999–1002.

[17] Morady F, Scheinman MM, Winston SA *et al.*
Efficacy and safety of transcatheter ablation of posteroseptal accessory pathways.
Circulation 1985; **72**: 170–7.

[18] Toet JL, Fontaine G, Frank R, Grosgogeat Y.
Treatment of refractory ventricular tachycardias by endocardial fulguration [Abstract].
Circulation 1985; **2**: III–388.

[19] Breithardt G, Borggrefe M, Karbenn U, Schwarzmejer J.
Catheter ablation of ventricular tachycardia.
New Trends Arrhyt 1986; **2**: 253–6.

[20] Klein H, Trappe HJ, Hartwig CA, Kuhn E, Lichtlen PR.
Problems and pitfalls with catheter ablation of ventricular tachycardia.
New Trends Arrhyt 1986; **2**: 257–64.

[21] Davies DW, Nathan AW, Camm AJ.
Three deaths after attempted high energy ablation of ventricular tachycardia [Abstract].
Br Heart J 1986; **55**: 506.

[22] Belhassen B, Miller HI, Geller E, Laniado S.
Transcatheter electrical ablation of ventricular tachycardia.
J Am Coll Cardiol 1986; **7**: 1347–55.

[23] Bardy GH, Coltorti F, Ivey TD, Yerkovich D, Greene HL.
Effect of damped sine-wave shocks on catheter dielectric strength.
Am J Cardiol 1985; **56**: 769–72.

[24] Fisher JD, Brodman R, Johnston DR *et al.*
Nonsurgical ablation of tachycardias: Importance of prior in vitro testing of catheter leads.
PACE 1984; **7**: 74–81.

[25] Bardy GH, Coltorti F, Ivey TD *et al.*
Some factors affecting bubble formation with catheter mediated defibrillator pulses.
Circulation 1986; **73**: 525–38.

[26] Holt PM, Boyd EGCA.
Hematological effects of the high-energy endocardial ablation technique.
Circulation 1986; **73**: 1029–36.

[27] Tong LS.
Boiling Heat Transfer and Two-Phase Flow.
New York: Wiley, 1965; Ch. 2.

[28] Hammitt FG.
Cavitation and Multiphase Flow Phenomena.
New York: McGraw-Hill, 1980; Ch. 2.

[29] Rowland E, Foale R, Nihoyannopoulos P, Perelman M, Krikler DM.
Intracardiac contrast echoes during transvenous His bundle ablation.
Br Heart J 1985; **53**: 240–2.

[30] Duffin WJ.
Electricity and Magnetism. London: McGraw-Hill, 1973; p. 288.

[31] Cobine JD.
Introduction to vacuum arcs. In: Laffert JM, ed.
Vacuum Arcs: Theory and Application. New York: Wiley, 1980.

[32] Downar E, Harris L, Parson ID, Easty A.
Characterisation of catheter ablation with high speed cinematography [Abstract].
J Am Coll Cardiol 1986; **7**: 131A.

[33] Fontaine G, Cansell A, Lechat Ph *et al.*
Les chocs electriques endocavitaires: Problemes lies au materiel.
Arch Mal Coeur 1984; **77**: 1307–14.

[34] Holt PM, Boyd EGCA, Crick J, Sowton E.
Low energies and Helifix electrodes in the successful ablation of atrioventricular conduction.
PACE 1985; **8**: 639–45.

[35] Scheinman MM, Bharati S, Wang YS, Shapiro WA, Lev M.
Electrophysiologic and anatomic changes in the atrioventricular junction of dogs after direct-current shocks through tissue fixation catheters.
Am J Cardiol 1985; **55**: 194–8.

[36] Polgar P, Worum F, Kovacs P, Lorincz I, Bekassy Sz, Peterffy A.
A new technique for closed-chest human His bundle ablation using suction electrode catheter and DC shock. In: Perez-Gomez F, ed. *Cardiac Pacing, Electrophysiology, Tachyarrhythmias*. New York: Futura, 1985; pp. 1582–7.

[37] Cohen D, Taran PP, Boveja BK, Joubert TF, Kovacs T.
A novel catheter design for low energy ablation [Abstract].
PACE 1986; **9**: 287.

[38] Trantham JL, Gallagher JJ, German LD *et al*.
Effects of energy delivery via a His bundle catheter during closed-chest ablation of the atrioventricular conduction system.
J Clin Invest 1983; **72**: 1563–74.

[39] Bardy GH, Ideker RE, Kasell J *et al*.
Transvenous ablation of atrio-ventricular conduction system in dogs: Electrophysiologic and histologic observations.
Am J Cardiol 1983; **51**: 1775–82.

[40] Martinez Fabra J, Camanas A, Cosin J *et al*.
Experimental study of His bundle ablation: Evolution of junctional automaticity and anatomical lesions. In: Perez-Gomez F, ed. *Cardiac Pacing, Electrophysiology, Tachyarrhythmias*. New York: Futura, 1985; pp. 1560–7.

[41] Ward DE, Davies M.
Transvenous high energy shocks for ablating atrioventricular conduction in man: Observations on the histological effects.
Br Heart J 1984; **51**: 175–8.

[42] Critelli G, Gallagher JJ, Thiene G *et al*.
Histologic observations after closed chest ablation of the atrioventricular conduction system.
JAMA 1984; **252**: 2604–6.

[43] Brodman R, Fisher JD.
Evaluation of a catheter technique for ablation of accessory pathways near the coronary sinus using a canine model.
Circulation 1983; **67**: 923–9.

[44] Coltorti F, Bardy GH, Reichenbach D *et al*.
Catheter-mediated electrical ablation of the posterior septum via the coronary sinus: Electrophysiologic and histologic observations in dogs.
Circulation 1985; **72**: 612–22.

[45] Fisher JD, Brodman R, Kim SG *et al*.
Attempted nonsurgical ablation of accessory pathways via the coronary sinus in the Wolff-Parkinson-White syndrome.
J Am Coll Cardiol 1984; **4**: 685–94.

[46] Chapman PD, Klopfenstein S, Troup PJ, Brooks HL.
Evaluation of a percutaneous catheter technique for ablation of ventricular tachycardia in a canine model.
Am Heart J 1985; **110**: 1–8.

[47] Kempf FC, Falcone RA, Iozzo RV, Josephson ME.
Anatomic and hemodynamic effects of catheter-delivered ablation energies in the ventricle.
Am J Cardiol 1985; **56**: 373–7.

[48] Lee BI, Gottdiener JS, Fletcher RD, Rodriguez ER, Ferrans VJ.
Transcatheter ablation: Comparison between laser photoablation and electrode shock ablation in the dog.
Circulation 1985; **71**: 579–86.

[49] Lerman BB, Weiss JL, Bulkley BH, Becker LC, Weisfeldt ML.
Myocardial injury and induction of arrhythmia by direct current shock delivered via endocardial catheters in dogs.
Circulation 1984; **69**: 1006–12.

[50] Lown B, Crampton RS, DeSilva R.
The energy for ventricular fibrillation defibrillation – Too little or too much?
N Engl J Med 1978; **298**: 1252.

[51] Saksena S, Gadhoke A, Hussan M.
Feasibility of intraoperative laser ablation of ventricular tachycardia: Studies in intact animal ventricle and in diseased human ventricle resected from patients with ventricular tachycardia.
New Trends Arrhyt 1986; **2**: 285–92.

[52] Gallagher JJ, Svenson RH, Selle S *et al*.
Use of the Nd-YAG laser in the surgical treatment of ventricular tachycardia.
New Trends Arrhyt 1986; **2**: 293–8.

[53] Isner JM, Michelwitz H, Clarke RH *et al*.
Laser photoablation of pathological endocardium: In vitro findings suggesting a new approach to the surgical treatment of refractory arrhythmias and resistant cardiomyopathies.
Ann Thorac Surg 1985; **39**: 201–6.

[54] Narula OS, Bharati S, Chan MC, Embi AA, Lev M.
Microtransection of the His bundle with laser radiation through a pervenous catheter: Correction of histologic and electrophysiologic data.
Am J Cardiol 1984; **54**: 186–93.

[55] Narula OS, Boveja BK, Cohen DM, Narula JT, Tarjan PP.
Laser catheter-induced atrioventricular nodal delays and atrio-ventricular block in dogs: Acute and chronic observations.
J Am Coll Cardiol 1985; **5**: 259–67.

[56] Saksena S, Gadhoke A.
Laser therapy for tachyarrhythmias: A new frontier.
PACE 1986; **9**: 531–50.

[57] Huang SK, Jordan N, Graham A *et al*.
Closed-chest catheter desiccation of atrioventricular junction using radiofrequency energy - A new method of catheter ablation [Abstract].
Circulation 1985; **72**: III–389.

[58] Bardy GH, Coltorti F, Stewart R *et al*.
The role of duty factor in preventing voltage breakdown during delivery of modulated electric pulses to a catheter [Abstract].
PACE 1986; **9**: 298.

[59] Cunningham D, Rowland E, Rickards AF.
Low energy ablation and dump time factor – An effective new design and a power source index [Abstract].
PACE 1986; **9**: 287.

[60] Levine JH, Spear JF, Weisman HF, Kadish AH, Siu CO, Moore EN.
Myocardial damage due to electrical ablation is related to the current density delivered [Abstract].
PACE 1986; **9**: 287.

[61] German LD, Pressley J, Smith MS *et al*.
Comparison of cryoablation of the atrioventricular node versus catheter ablation of the His bundle.
Circulation 1984; **70**: II–412.

CURRENT STATUS OF LATE POTENTIALS

Review: MICHAEL B. SIMSON

Late potentials are microvolt-level, electrocardiographic waveforms, continuous with the QRS complex, which can be recorded frequently during sinus rhythm from patients prone to ventricular tachyarrhythmias. They were first recorded in 1978, and have been the subject of active investigation by many groups. This article briefly reviews the techniques needed to record late potentials, and discusses their incidence and clinical significance.

Methodology

Advanced signal processing of the electrocardiogram is necessary to detect late potentials. Signal averaging is used to reduce the noise level that contaminates the electrocardiogram [1,2]. The primary sources of noise are skeletal muscle activity, electrodes, power-line interference and amplifiers. Noise amplitude is typically 5–20 μV under optimal conditions before averaging.

Ensemble averaging is the most frequently used form of signal averaging. A small computer averages multiple beats of the electrocardiogram; random noise, not synchronized with the QRS complex, tends to be cancelled out [2]. The noise level in most studies is 1 μV or less after averaging 100–500 cycles – the equivalent of 1/100 mm on a standard ECG display scale. Ensemble averaging requires that the late potential must repeat precisely, and that it be linked in time with the higher-amplitude portions of the

QRS complex that are used to align the beats before averaging. If the late potential lacks a fixed temporal relationship with the large-amplitude portions of the QRS complex, then ensemble averaging will not reliably extract the late potential, and high-frequency details will be lost [2]. Most signal-averaging systems use template matching or cross-correlation before averaging in order to exclude ectopic or grossly noisy beats.

A second type of signal averaging is spatial averaging [3,4]. Potentials from 4 to 16 independent electrodes are summed together, yielding a theoretical 2- to 4-fold noise reduction. Spatial averaging has the advantage that transient, beat-by-beat events can be recorded. There is a practical limit, however, to the number of electrodes if all are to record the same ECG vector; moreover, the multiple, closely spaced electrodes may record a common noise source such as muscle activity. If noise is coherent between channels, then noise reduction is impaired [5]. Recently, Flowers *et al* have developed a variation on spatial averaging which improves noise reduction by rejecting those leads in which the signal is not in phase with the signals in the majority of leads [3].

Once averaged, the ECG is usually high-pass filtered to extract the relative high frequencies generated by the depolarization of cells and to minimize the lower frequencies which correspond to the slowly changing plateau or repolarization phases of the action potential. High-pass filtering aids the detection of microvolt late potentials arising from depolarization of very small areas of the myocardium. Most investigators use filter corner frequencies of 25–100 Hz, although some use no high-pass filtering [6]. The fast-Fourier transform has been applied to signal-averaged ECGs to extract diagnostic high-frequency (20–50 Hz) content [7,8]. High-pass filtering and the fast-Fourier transform have restrictions in accuracy and are prone to errors, such as smearing of the frequency spectrum or filter overshoot. A special digital filter, the bidirectional filter, has been developed to control filter artefacts [9].

To date there is little standardization in the methods used to record and analyze late potentials: wide variation obtains in the number and location of leads, the type of signal averaging, and the means to extract high-frequency information. The measurements used to classify the recordings differ among investigators. A recent study comparing four signal-averaging systems and interpretation techniques showed corresponding results among all four systems in only 73% of patients [10]. Two studies of reproducibility have shown, however, that there is no significant day-to-day variability in recordings from normal subjects when the same system and interpretation technique are used [6,11]. Clearly, further work is needed to refine the methodology used in recording late potentials.

Late Potentials
Ventricular late potentials are microvolt-level, high-frequency (>25 Hz) waveforms which are continuous with the QRS complex and persist for tens of milliseconds into the ST segment [7–15]. Late potentials correspond to delayed and disorganized ventricular activation, which has been observed with direct electrogram recordings in patients with ventricular tachycardia. The amplitude of the delayed electrograms, which occur in only a few areas of the heart, is typically under 1 mV when recorded directly [16]; conventional ECG techniques cannot detect those signals reliably from the body surface because they are masked by noise.

324

Figure 1 shows examples of signal-averaged electrocardiograms in two patients, one with and one without ventricular tachycardia. Both patients had a prior transmural (Q wave) myocardial infarction. The patient with ventricular tachycardia had repeated, sustained episodes of the arrhythmia; here, ventricular tachycardia could be induced reliably. The patient without ventricular tachycardia had no complex ventricular ectopy on prolonged ECG monitoring. The filtered QRS complex (bottom) in the patient without ventricular tachycardia shows an abrupt onset, a peak of high-frequency voltage 40–50 ms after QRS onset, and an abrupt decline to noise level at the end of the QRS complex. There is no high-frequency signal above noise level (<1 µV) in the ST segment. In the patient with ventricular tachycardia, the initial portion of the filtered QRS complex is generally similar to that of the control patient. At the end of the filtered QRS complex, however, there is a low-amplitude late potential (arrow), which corresponds to fine ripples and notches in the unfiltered leads (top). The amplitude of the late

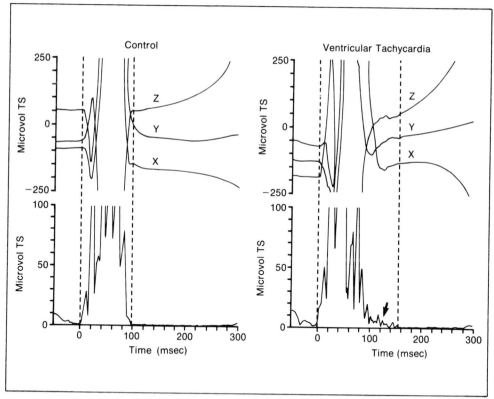

FIGURE 1: Signal-averaged ECGs from two patients with anterior myocardial infarctions during sinus rhythm. Unfiltered bipolar leads are shown at high gain (top). The filtered QRS complex (bottom) is the vector magnitude of the three leads after high-pass filtering (>25 Hz). The control patient had no complex ventricular ectopy on prolonged ECG monitoring. The patient with ventricular tachycardia had sustained, inducible ventricular tachycardia, and the recording demonstrates a late potential (arrow) at the end of the filtered QRS complex. The voltage in the last 40 ms was 50 µV for the control patient and 5 µV for the patient with ventricular tachycardia.

potential varies from 1 to 25 μV with 25-Hz filtering. Investigators use various criteria to classify signal-averaged ECGs as abnormal and to define late potentials. The most commonly used measurements include the duration of the filtered QRS complex, which is approximately 45 ms longer in patients with ventricular tachycardia, the duration of low-amplitude terminal waveforms, and voltage in terminal portions of the filtered QRS complex [9,11].

Since 1978, many groups have recorded late potentials with signal averaging from patients with ventricular tachycardia [4,7–19]. The results are fairly consistent. Patients with sustained and inducible ventricular tachycardia after myocardial infarction have abnormal signal-averaged ECGs in 73%–92% of cases. In contrast, 7%–15% of patients without ventricular tachycardia after myocardial infarction and Lown class 0–1 ventricular ectopy have abnormal signal-averaged ECGs. Only 0%–6% of normal volunteers have abnormal signal-averaged ECGs; most studies report no late potentials in healthy subjects [6,7,9,11,17,18,20,21]. Late potentials have been recorded from patients with other diseased states associated with ventricular tachycardia, such as arrhythmogenic right-ventricular dysplasia [12,22,24], non-ischemic cardiomyopathies [20,23] or postoperative tetralogy of Fallot [25]. Spatial signal averaging has revealed examples of late potentials with Wenckebach conduction patterns, and late potentials that span diastole between normal and ventricular premature beats [4,26].

Late potentials appear to originate from small areas of delayed and in-homogeneous ventricular activation. Prolonged, fragmented electrograms that often last beyond the apparent end of the QRS complex have been recorded in patients with ventricular tachycardia after myocardial infarction [27,28]. Studies in animals and man have shown that delayed ventricular activation can outlast diastole, and that it relates to the onset and maintenance of ventricular tachycardia [29–32]. Several groups have reported examples of delayed epicardial activation during sinus rhythm in patients with late potentials [12,14,15,17]. Electrogram mapping in patients with ventricular tachy-cardia after myocardial infarction established that late potentials correspond in time to fragmented and delayed electrograms recorded predominantly from the endocardium [16,33]. Studies in animals with experimental infarcts have shown a similar relationship between delayed, inhomogeneous ventricular activation and late potentials [34,35]. Recently, Gardner et al recorded fragmented electrograms in infarcted canine hearts in regions where infarct healing caused wide separation of individual myocardial fibres with distorted orientation; the multicomponent fragmented electrograms represented slow and inhomogeneous activation of the muscle fibres [36]. Fenoglio et al found a similar histology in human endocardium resected at the site of origin of ventricular tachycardia [37].

Abnormalities on a signal-averaged ECG often disappear after successful surgical control of ventricular tachycardia [13–15,17,20,38,39]. In our experience with 24 patients in whom ventricular tachycardia could not be induced after endocardial excision, the filtered QRS duration shortened from a mean of 137 ms to 121 ms, and the incidence of late potentials decreased (from 71% to 33%) [39]. The incidence of late potentials and the filtered QRS complex were not changed in 13 patients in whom ventricular tachycardia could be induced after operation. Surgical control of ventricular tachycardia may eliminate late potentials and the loss of the late potential associates with successful outcome. Persistence of the late potential in some cases, despite successful control of ventricular tachycardia, however, argues that the operation need not remove all areas of delayed activation in order to control the arrhythmia. This concept is supported by the finding that up to half of the endocardial sites with delayed activation occur in areas distant from the site of origin of ventricular tachycardia [40].

Antiarrhythmic drug therapy, in general, lengthens filtered QRS duration and decreases high-frequency content throughout the QRS complex; late potentials are not, however, abolished with drug therapy [1,14,15,18,41]. Cain et al have reported that effective drug therapy was associated with a relative decrease in the 20–50 Hz content of the terminal QRS and early ST segment [42]. In 8 of 10 successful trials, the 20–50-Hz components decreased – a change that was seen in only 1 of 10 unsuccessful trials. Other investigators have not detected changes in signal-averaged ECGs which would indicate a successful response to antiarrhythmic agents [1,15,18,41]. Additional studies are needed to resolve the differences.

Most, but not all, studies show a correlation between the presence of late potentials and ventricular dysfunction [1,19,20,21,43–45].

Recent studies have addressed the question of whether the signal-averaged ECG offers diagnostic information which is independent of other clinical findings, including low ejection fraction or wall-motion abnormalities. Denes et al studied the determinants of an abnormal signal-averaged ECG (late potentials or filter QRS complex >120 ms) in 166 patients with coronary artery disease [43]. An abnormal signal-averaged ECG had a univariate correlation with age, prior myocardial infarction, previous ventricular tachycardia or ventricular fibrillation, left-ventricular wall-motion abnormalities and ejection fraction. Multivariate analysis revealed, however, that a history of sustained ventricular tachycardia or ventricular fibrillation and prior myocardial infarction, were the only independent determinants of an abnormal signal-averaged ECG.

The question of whether the signal-averaged ECG provided independent information useful in identifying patients with ventricular tachycardia was addressed in a retrospective study which compared findings on signal-averaged ECG, Holter monitoring, and cardiac catheterization [46]. Logistic regression analysis showed that only three variables provided significant independent information in identification of patients with ventricular tachycardia: an abnormal signal-averaged ECG; a peak premature ventricular contraction rate >100/hour; and the presence of a left-ventricular aneurysm. This study suggested that the signal-averaged ECG should be combined with other clinical information to provide a more accurate identification of patients with ventricular tachycardia after myocardial infarction. Recently, Lindsay et al demonstrated that the signal-averaged ECG, as analyzed by the fast-Fourier transform, could prospectively identify those patients in whom sustained ventricular tachycardia could be induced at electrophysiologic study [47]. Multivariate analysis showed that an abnormal signal-averaged ECG was independent of other determinants of inducibility, including left-ventricular ejection fraction and prior myocardial infarction. In summary, these studies demonstrate that the non-invasive signal-averaged ECG provides unique and independent information useful in the identification of patients with ventricular tachycardia.

The predictive value of late potentials in patients after acute myocardial infarction has been evaluated in a few prospective studies. Breithardt et al studied 160 patients a median of 25 days after acute myocardial infarction: 48 patients (30%) had late potentials 20 ms or longer in duration [48]. The incidence of sustained ventricular tachycardia during a mean follow-up of 7.5 months was 8.3% (4 of 48) in patients with late potentials and 0% in 112 patients without late potentials ($P<0.01$). The incidence of ventricular tachycardia increased to 16.6% (3 of 18) if only those patients with late potentials longer than 40 ms were considered. A more recent study by Breithardt *et al* of 132 patients after acute myocardial infarction with a mean follow-up of 13 months showed similar results [49]. The presence of late potentials was not predictive of subsequent sudden death in either study, although the incidence of sudden death (3.0% and 4.4%) was low. Gomes *et al* prospectively studied 50 patients after acute myocardial infarction for one month; signal-averaged ECG was recorded a mean of three days after the myocardial infarction [50]. All five patients with sustained ventricular tachycardia/ventricular fibrillation or sudden death had late potentials; the specificity of late potentials was 62% for ventricular tachycardia/ventricular fibrillation or sudden death. Denniss *et al* followed 306 patients after myocardial infarction and found that those with an abnormal signal-averaged ECG had a 2-year probability of remaining free of cardiac death or ventricular tachycardia/ventricular fibrillation of 0.73, in contrast to 0.95 for patients with a normal signal-averaged ECG [51]. Kuchar *et al* prospectively studied 210 patients after myocardial infarction and determined that a low ejection fraction and an abnormal signal-averaged ECG had a sensitivity of 80% and a specificity of 89% to detect those patients who later had sudden death or sustained ventricular tachycardia [52]. Additional prospective studies are necessary to evaluate whether abnormalities on signal-averaged ECGs are an independent risk factor for sudden death or ventricular tachycardia after myocardial infarction, and to establish the role of the signal-averaged ECG, along with other non-invasive tests, in the accurate identification of patients at high risk for lethal arrhythmias.

Acknowledgment
Supported in part by Grant HL27925 from the National Heart, Lung and Blood Institute.

References

[1] Hombach V, Braun V, Hopp H-W *et al*.
The applicability of the signal averaging technique in clinical cardiology.
Clin Cardiol 1982; **5**: 107–24.

[2] Ros HH, Koeleman ASM, van den Akker TJ.
The technique of signal averaging and its practical application in the separation of atrial and His Purkinje activity. In: Hombach V, Hilger HH, eds. *Signal Averaging Technique in Clinical Cardiology*. Stuttgart: F.K. Stuttgart Verlag, 1981; p. 3.

[3] Flowers NC, Shvartsman V, Kennelly BM, Sohi GS, Horan LG.
Surface recording of His-Purkinje acitivity on an every-beat basis without digital averaging.
Circulation 1981; **63**: 948–52.

[4] El-Sherif N, Mehra R, Gomes JAC, Kelen G.
Appraisal of a low noise electrocardiogram.
J Am Coll Cardiol 1983; **1**: 456–67.

[5] Mehra R, Restivo M, El-Sherif N.
Electromyographic noise reduction for high resolution electrocardiography. In: Gerhard GC, Miller WT, eds. *Frontiers of Engineering and Computing in Health Care – 1983*. New York, NY: IEEE, 1983; p. 248.

[6] Denniss AR, Ross DL, Uther JB.
Reproducibility of measurements of ventricular activation time using the signal-averaged frank vectorcardiogram.
Am J Cardiol 1986; **57**: 156–60.

[7] Cain ME, Ambos D, Witkowski FX, Sobel BE.
Fast-Fourier transform analysis of signal-averaged electrocardiograms for the identification of patients prone to sustained ventricular tachycardia.
Circulation 1984; **69**: 711–20.

[8] Cain ME, Ambos HD, Markham J, Fischer AE, Sobel BE.
Quantification of differences in frequency content of signal- averaged electrocardiograms in patients with compared to those without sustained ventricular tachycardia.
Am J Cardiol 1985; **55**: 1500–5.

[9] Simson MB.
Use of signals in the terminal QRS complex to identify patients with ventricular tachycardia after myocardial infarction.
Circulation 1981; **64**: 235–42.

[10] Oeff M, von Leitner ER, Sthapit R *et al*.
Methods for non-invasive detection of ventricular late potentials – A comparative multicenter study.
Eur Heart J 1986; **7**: 25–33.

[11] Denes P, Santarelli P, Hauser RG, Uretz EF.
Quantitative analysis of the terminal portion of the body surface QRS in normal subjects and in patients with ventricular tachycardia.
Circulation 1983; **67**: 1129–38.

[12] Fontaine G, Guiraudon G, Frank R *et al*.
Stimulation studies and epicardial mapping in ventricular tachycardia. Study of mechanisms and selection for surgery. In: Kulbertus H, ed. *Reentrant Arrhythmias*. Lancaster: MTP Press, 1977; p. 334.

[13] Uther JB, Dennett CJ, Tan A.
The detection of delayed activation signals of low amplitude in the vectorcardiogram of patients with recurrent ventricular tachycardia by signal averaging. In: Sandoe E, Julian DJ, Bell JW, eds. *Management of Ventricular Tachycardia – Role of Mexiletine*. Amsterdam: Excerpta Medica, 1978; p. 80.

[14] Rozanski JJ, Mortara D, Myerburg RJ *et al*.
Body surface detection of delayed depolarization in patients with recurrent ventricular tachycardia and left ventricular aneurysm.
Circulation 1981; **63**: 1172–8.

[15] Breithardt G, Becker R, Seipel L *et al*.
Noninvasive detection of late potentials in man – A new marker for ventricular tachycardia.
Eur Heart J 1981; **2**: 1–11.

[16] Simson MB, Untereker WJ, Spielman SR *et al*.
The relationship between late potentials on the body surface and directly recorded fragmented electrograms in patients with ventricular tachycardia.
Am J Cardiol 1983; **51**: 105–12.

[17] Kertes PJ, Glabus M, Murray A, Julian DG, Campbell RWF.
Delayed ventricular depolarization — Correlation with ventricular activation and relevance to ventricular fibrillation in acute myocardial infarction.
Eur Heart J 1984; **5**: 974–83.

[18] Zimmerman M, Adamec R, Simonin P, Richez J.
Prognostic significance of ventricular late potentials in coronary artery disease.
Am Heart J 1985; **109**: 725–32.

[19] Freedman RA, Gillis AM, Keren A, Soderholm-Difatte V, Mason JW.
Signal-averaged electrocardiographic late potentials in patients with ventricular fibrillation or ventricular tachycardia: Correlation with clinical arrhythmia and electrophysiologic study.
Am J Cardiol 1985; **55**: 1350–3.

[20] Breithardt G, Borggrefe M, Karbenn U *et al*.
Prevalence of late potentials in patients with and without tachycardia: Correlation and angiographic findings.
Am J Cardiol 1982; **49**: 1932–7.

[21] Coto H, Maldonado C, Palakurthy P, Flower NC.
Late potentials in normal subjects and in patients with ventricular tachycardia unrelated to myocardial infarction.
Am J Cardiol 1985; **55**: 384–90.

[22] Abboud S, Belhassen B, Laniado S, Sadeh D.
Non-invasive recording of late ventricular activity using an advanced method in patients with a damaged mass of ventricular tissue.
J Electrocardiol 1983; **16**: 245–52.

[23] Poll DS, Marchlinski FE, Falcone RA, Simson MB.
Abnormal signal averaged ECG in nonischemic congestive cardiomyopathy: Relationship to sustained ventricular tachyarrhythmias.
Circulation 1985; **72**: 1308–13.

[24] Edvardsson N, Hirsch I, Lindblad A, Olsson SB.
Properties of late potentials in arrhythmogenic right ventricular dysplasia [Abstract].
Circulation 1984; **70**: II–373.

[25] Danford DA, Garson A Jr.
Abnormal conduction related to ventricular dysrrhythmias by signal averaged electrocardiography in postoperative tetralogy of Fallot [Abstract].
Circulation 1984; **70**: II–207.

329

[26] Hombach V, Kebbel U, Hopp H-W, Winter U, Hirche H.
Non-invasive beat-by-beat registration of ventricular late potentials using high resolution electrocardiography.
Int J Cardiol 1984; **6**: 167–83.

[27] Wiener I, Mindich B, Pitchon R.
Determinants of ventricular tachycardia in patients with ventricular aneurysms: Results of intraoperative epicardial and endocardial mapping.
Circulation 1982; **65**: 856–61.

[28] Klein H, Karp RB, Kouchoukos NT, Zorn GL, James TN, Waldo AL.
Intraoperative electrophysiologic mapping of the ventricles during sinus rhythm in patients with previous myocardial infarction. Identification of the electrophysiologic substrate of ventricular arrhythmias.
Circulation 1982; **66**: 847–53.

[29] Boineau JP, Cox JL.
Slow ventricular activation in acute myocardial infarction: A source of reentrant premature ventricular contraction.
Circulation 1973; **48**: 702–13.

[30] Waldo AL, Kaiser G.
A study of ventricular arrhythmias associated with acute myocardial infarction in the canine heart.
Circulation 1973; **3**: 1222–8.

[31] El-Sherif N, Scherlag BJ, Lazzara R *et al*.
Reentrant ventricular arrhythmias in the late myocardial infarction period: II. Patterns of initiation and termination of reentry.
Circulation 1977; **55**: 702.

[32] Josephson ME, Horowitz LN, Farshidi A.
Continuous local electrical activity. A mechanism of recurrent ventricular tachycardia.
Circulation 1978; **57**: 659.

[33] Josephson ME, Simson MB, Harken AH, Horowitz LN, Falcone RA.
The incidence and clinical significance of epicardial late potentials in patients with recurrent sustained ventricular tachycardia and coronary artery disease.
Circulation 1982; **66**: 1199–204.

[34] Berbari EJ, Scherlag BJ, Hope RR *et al*.
Recording from the body surface of arrhythmogenic ventricular activity during the ST segment.
Am J Cardiol 1978; **41**: 697.

[35] Simson MB, Euler D, Michelson EL *et al*.
Detection of delayed ventricular activation on the body surface in dogs.
Am J Physiol 1981; **241**: H363–9.

[36] Gardner PI, Ursell PC, Fenoglio JJ Jr, Wit AL.
Electrophysiologic and anatomic basis for fractionated electrograms recorded from healed myocardial infarcts.
Circulation 1985; **72**: 596–611.

[37] Fenoglio JJ Jr, Pham TD, Harken AH, Horowitz LN, Josephson ME, Wit AL.
Recurrent sustained ventricular tachycardia: Structure and ultrastructure of subendocardial regions in which tachycardia originates.
Circulation 1983; **68**: 518–33.

[38] Breithardt G, Seipel L, Ostermeyer J *et al*.
Effects of antiarrhythmic surgery on late ventricular potentials recorded by precordial signal averaging in patients with ventricular tachycardia.
Am Heart J 1982; **104**: 996–1003.

[39] Marcus NH, Falcone RA, Harken AH, Josephson ME, Simson MB.
Body surface late potentials: Effects of endocardial resection in patients with ventricular tachycardia.
Circulation 1984; **70**: 632–7.

[40] Vassallo JA, Cassidy D, Simson MB, Buxton AE, Marchlinski FE, Josephson ME.
Relation of late potentials to site of origin of ventricular tachycardia associated with coronary heart disease.
Am J Cardiol 1985; **55**: 985–9.

[41] Simson MB, Waxman HL, Falcone R, Marcus NH, Josephson ME.
Effects of anti-arrhythmic drugs on noninvasively recorded late potentials. In: Breithardt G, Loogen F, eds. *New Aspects in the Medical Treatment of Tachyarrhythmias*. Munich: Urban & Schwarzenberg, 1983; pp. 80–6.

[42] Cain ME, Ambos HD, Fischer AE, Markham J, Schechtman KB.
Noninvasive prediction of antiarrhythmic drug efficacy in patients with sustained ventricular tachycardia from frequency analysis of signal averaged ECGs [Abstract].
Circulation 1984; **70**: II-252.

[43] Denes P, Uretz E, Santarelli P.
Determinants of arrhythmogenic ventricular activity detected on the body surface QRS in patients with coronary artery disease.
Am J Cardiol 1984; **53**: 1519–23.

[44] Breithardt G, Borggrefe M, Quantius B, Karbenn U, Seipel L.
Ventricular vulnerability assessed by programmed ventricular stimulation in patients with and without late potentials.
Circulation 1983; **68**: 275–81.

[45] Pollak SJ, Kertes PJ, Bredlau CE, Walter PF.
Influence of left ventricular function on signal averaged late potentials in patients with coronary artery disease with and without ventricular tachycardia.
Am Heart J 1985; **110**: 747.

[46] Kanovsky MS, Falcone RA, Dresden CA, Josephson ME, Simson MB.
Identification of patients with ventricular tachycardia after myocardial infarction: Signal-averaged electrocardiogram, Holter monitoring, and cardiac catheterization.
Circulation 1984; **70**: 264–70.

[47] Lindsay BD, Ambos HK, Schechtman B, Cain ME.
Improved selection of patients for programmed ventricular stimulation by frequency analysis of signal-averaged electrocardiograms.
Circulation 1986; **73**: 675–83.

[48] Breithardt G, Schwarzmaier J, Borggrefe M, Haerten K, Seipel L.
Prognostic significance of late ventricular potentials after acute myocardial infarction.
Eur Heart J 1983; **4**: 487–95.

[49] Breithardt G, Borggrefe M, Haerten K.
Ventricular late potentials and inducible ventricular tachyarrhythmias as a marker for ventricular tachycardia after myocardial infarction.
Eur Heart J 1986; **7** (Suppl A): 127–34.

[50] Gomes JA, Mehra R, Barreca P, El-Sherif N, Hariman R, Holtzman R.
Quantitative analysis of the high-frequency components of the signal-averaged QRS complex in patients with acute myocardial infarction: A prospective study.
Circulation 1985; **72**: 105–11.

[51] Denniss AR, Richards DA, Cody DV *et al.*
Prognostic significance of ventricular tachycardia and fibrillation induced at programmed stimulation and delayed potentials detected on the signal-averaged electrocardiograms of survivors of acute myocardial infarction.
Circulation 1986; **74**: 731–45.

[52] Kuchar DL, Thorburn CW, Sammel NL.
Prediction of serious arrhythmic events after myocardial infarction: signal-averaged electrocardiogram, Holter monitoring and radionuclide ventriculography.
J Am Coll Cardiol 1987; **9**: 531–8.

PHYSIOLOGIC RATE-RESPONSIVE PACING

Review: E. JOHN PERRINS

Physiologic pacing includes two radically different philosophies. The first is dual-chamber rate-response, with the atrium as a physiologic indicator (the DDD pacemaker). The second is a single-chamber pacing device, usually in the ventricle, the rate of which is increased according to a sensor indicating some physiologic need other than the atrial rate. The last two years have seen a number of papers confirming the clinical advantages of DDD pacing over the fixed-rate VVI device, together with initial clinical experience with single-chamber rate-responsive devices. In addition, considerable progress has been made in sensor design and the refinement of clinical algorithms based upon individual sensor technologies.

Dual-Chamber Rate-Responsive Pacing
Little is known about the ability of physiologic pacing modes to prolong survival compared with VVI pacemakers. Alpert *et al* examined the five-year cumulative survival of 132 patients with VVI pacemakers and 48 with DVI or DDD units implanted [1]. All patients had atrioventricular block. There were no significant differences in overall survival, but if only those patients with pre-existing congestive cardiac failure were analyzed, the five-year survival was 47% for VVI and 69% for DVI/DDD ($P = 0.02$). Although this is a small study, it is the first to present data suggesting a prognostic

331

advantage for dual-chamber pacemakers. Sutton and Kenny have undertaken an extensive review of the literature relating to atrial pacing and sick sinus syndrome, and have concluded that there is good pooled evidence that atrial-demand pacing reduces the incidence of atrial fibrillation and systemic thromboembolism in sinus node disorders [2]. Rosenqvist has also confirmed the clinical advantages of atrial stimulation in sick sinus syndrome [3].

Initial reports, primarily from the USA, reported a high incidence of pacemaker-induced tachycardias with DDD pacemakers. Fontaine *et al* have shown that this incidence can greatly be reduced by non-invasive evaluation of retrograde conduction using pacemaker telemetry of the atrial electrogram [4]. This allows precise programming of the atrial refractory period, allowing the most effective use to be made of the upper tracking rate facility. The authors have also confirmed the effectiveness of automatic pacemaker-induced tachycardia algorithms within the implanted pacemaker. Pacemaker-induced tachycardia is caused by detection by the pacemaker of a retrograde P wave. Furman's group showed that anterograde and retrograde P waves could be discriminated on the basis of amplitude and slew rate [5]. In some patients in whom the retrograde P wave was much smaller in amplitude than the anterograde one, simply programming the atrial sensitivity was sufficient to abolish pacemaker-induced tachycardia [6].

The clinical benefits in terms of exercise performance in patients with DDD pacemakers is now established, but the importance of the atrioventricular delay (a programmable option in most DDD units) is not known. Three studies have shown that there is an optimal atrioventricular delay in individual patients, and that this can be determined non-invasively [7–9]. However, the authors do not provide any evidence that this is of clinical relevance.

Jones *et al*, using invasive ambulatory arterial pressure monitoring, have shown that in patients with dominant sinus rhythm and VVI pacemakers very frequent swings in blood pressure occur [10]. They have also demonstrated that dual-chamber pacemakers drastically reduce these swings, and that this is associated with clinical improvement in patients with the pacemaker syndrome.

Dual-chamber pacemakers are undoubtedly more costly at implant than VVI devices. In a careful cost analysis Harthorne's group has shown that this cost disadvantage increases with length of follow-up due to (in their experience) shorter device lifetimes in the DDD group [11]. This analysis may not be directly applicable to health-care systems outside the USA.

Single-Chamber Rate-Responsive Pacemakers
Many physiologic sensors are currently under development. The topic is the subject of frequent review articles, and two recent contributions are worthy of note [12,13].

Clinical experience has been obtained with the QT-sensing pacemaker [14,15], confirming earlier reports of increased effort capacity with this device. Similar excellent results in terms of effort capacity have been demonstrated with the activity-sensing pacemaker [16,17] and the respiratory-dependent unit [18]. The work from Rossi's group dealing with the respiratory-dependent device is an important contribution to the hemodynamics and cardiorespiratory responses of patients with heart block. Rossi was able to show that during exercise, when the pacemaker rate algorithm was correctly set, there were no important differences in terms of oxygen uptake between atrial synchronous and non-synchronous rate-responsive pacing modes. He also suggests that in individual patients there is an optimal change of rate with exercise which is closely allied to maximal oxygen uptake and anerobic threshold.

The long-term reliability of implanted sensor systems is important. Clinical studies have suggested that activity and respiration are reliable [14–18]. Some doubts have arisen concerning the QT-sensing pacemaker and particularly its algorithm, and marked variations in heart rate response to identical exercise protocols have been observed during repeated stress testing in the same patients [19]. The long-term reliability of T-wave sensing (as opposed to the algorithm) would appear to be satisfactory, this being 94.1% in a series of 1500 patients [20].

Preliminary papers have appeared describing the potential use of central venous blood temperature sensed with a thermistor-tipped pacing lead [21–23] and also central venous oxygen saturation [24]. Sensing of the latter presents considerable technical problems regarding long-term reliability. The present design of respiratory-dependent pacemakers requires the use of an additional chest-wall electrode to measure intrathoracic impedance changes during respiration. Maloney has suggested that it may be possible to implement a single-lead design [25].

Although rate-responsive pacemakers have been shown to increase exercise capacity, a recent study failed to show any real differences in patients' self-perceived symptoms compared with fixed-rate ventricular pacing [16]. This may reflect loss of atrioventricular synchrony at lower heart rates with hemodynamic consequences. A logical step will be incorporation of sensor technology in a dual-chamber device, and Kappenberger has reported his initial encouraging experience with a prototype in three patients [26].

References

[1] Alpert MA, Curtis JJ, Sanfelippo JF et al.
Comparative survival after permanent ventricular and dual chamber pacing for patients with chronic high degree atrioventricular block with and without preexistent congestive heart failure.
J Am Coll Cardiol 1986; 7: 925–32.

[2] Sutton R, Kenny R-A.
The natural history of sick sinus syndrome.
PACE 1986; 9: 1110–4.

[3] Rosenqvist M, Brandt J, Schuller H.
Atrial versus ventricular pacing in sinus node disease: A treatment comparison study.
Am Heart J 1986; 3: 292–6.

[4] Fontaine JM, Maloney JD, Castle LW, Morant VA.
Noninvasive assessment of ventriculo-atrial conduction and early experience with the tachycardia termination algorithm in pacemaker-mediated tachycardia.
PACE 1986; 9: 212–22.

[5] Pannizzo F, Amikam S, Bagwell P, Furman S.
Discrimination of antegrade and retrograde atrial depolarization by electrogram analysis.
Am Heart J 1986; 112: 780–6.

[6] Klementowicz PT, Furman S.
Selective atrial sensing in dual chamber pacemakers eliminates endless loop tachycardia.
J Am Coll Cardiol 1986; 7: 590–4.

[7] Forfang K, Otterstad JE, Ihlen H.
Optimal atrioventricular delay in physiological pacing determined by Doppler echocardiography.
PACE 1986; 9: 17–20.

[8] Haskell RJ, France WJ.
Optimum AV interval in dual chamber pacemakers.
PACE 1986; 9: 670–5.

[9] Toeda T.
Atrial contribution to ventricular filling in patients with coronary artery disease as assessed by cardiac pacing.
Jpn Circ J 1986; 50: 385–95.

[10] Jones RI, Cashman PMM, Hornung RS, Prince H, Bassein L, Raftery EB.
Ambulatory blood pressure and assessment of pacemaker function.
Br Heart J 1986; **55**: 462–8.

[11] Eagle KA, Mulley AG, Singer DE, Schoenfeld D, Harthorne JW, Thibault GE.
Single-chamber and dual-chamber cardiac pacemakers.
Ann Intern Med 1986; **105**: 264–71.

[12] Fearnot NE, Smith HJ.
Trends in pacemakers which physiologically increase rate: DDD and rate responsive.
PACE 1986; **9**: 939–47.

[13] Anderson KM, Moore AA.
Sensors in pacing.
PACE 1986; **9**: 954–9.

[14] Maisch B, Langenfeld H.
Rate adaptive pacing – clinical experience with three different pacing systems.
PACE 1986; **9**: 997–1004.

[15] Zegelman M, Beyersdorf F, Kreuzer J, Cieslinski G.
Rate responsive pacemakers: Assessment after two years.
PACE 1986; **9**: 1005–9.

[16] Lindemans FW, Rankin IR, Murtaugh R, Chevalier PA.
Clinical experience with an activity sensing pacemaker.
PACE 1986; **9**: 978–86.

[17] Humen DP, Kostuk WJ, Klein GJ.
Activity-sensing, rate-responsive pacing: Improvement in myocardial performance with exercise.
PACE 1985; **8**: 52–9.

[18] Rossi P, Rognoni G, Occhetta E *et al*.
Respiration-dependent ventricular pacing compared with fixed ventricular and atrial-ventricular synchronous pacing: Aerobic and hemodynamic variables.
J Am Coll Cardiol 1985; **6**: 646–52.

[19] Fananapazir L, Rademaker M, Bennett DH.
Reliability of the evoked response in determining the paced ventricular rate and performance of the QT or rate responsive (TX) pacemaker.
PACE 1985; **8**: 701.

[20] Boute W, Derrien Y, Wittkampf FHM.
Reliability of evoked endocardial T-wave sensing in 1,500 pacemaker patients.
PACE 1986; **9**: 948–53.

[21] Alt E, Hirgstetter C, Heinz M, Theres H.
Measurement of right ventricular blood temperature during exercise as a means of rate control in physiological pacemakers.
PACE 1986; **9**: 970–7.

[22] Baker RG Jr, Phillips RE, Frey ML, Calfee RV.
A central venous temperature sensing lead.
PACE 1986; **9**: 965–9.

[23] Alt E, Hirgstetter C, Heinz M, Blomer H.
Rate control of physiologic pacemakers by central venous blood temperature.
Circulation 1986; **6**: 1206–12.

[24] Stangl K, Wirtzfeld A, Gobl G *et al*.
Rate control with an external SO$_2$ closed loop system.
PACE 1986; **9**: 992–6.

[25] Nappholtz T, Valenta H, Maloney J, Simmons T.
Electrode configurations for a respiratory impedance measurement suitable for rate responsive pacing.
PACE 1986; **9**: 960–4.

[26] Kappenberger LJ, Herpers L.
Rate responsive dual chamber pacing.
PACE 1986; **9**: 987–91.

PACING

[1] Indications for pacing in the treatment of bradyarrhythmias. Report of an independent study group.
Phibbs B, Friedman HS, Graboys TB *et al*, Kino Community Hosp, Tucson, AZ, USA.
J Am Med Assoc 1984; **252**: 1307–11.

[2] Guidelines for permanent cardiac pacemaker implantation. May 1984. A report of the Joint American College of Cardiology/American Heart Association Task Force on Assessment of Cardiovascular Procedures (Sub-committee on Pacemaker Implantation).
Field DJ (Director), Am Coll Cardiol, Bethesda, MD, USA.
J Am Coll Cardiol 1984; **4**: 432–42.

[3] Survival time and course after pacemaker implantation: a comparison of patients with sick-sinus syndrome, AV block or brady-arrhythmia (In German).
Alt E, Dechand E, Wirtzfeld A, Ulm K, Univ, Munich, FRG.
Dtsch Med Wochenschr 1983; **108**: 331-5.

[4] Survival in second degree atrioventricular block.
Shaw DB, Kekwick CA, Veale D, Gowers J, Whistance T, Royal Devon and Exeter Hosp (Wonford), Exeter, UK.
Br Heart J 1985; **53**: 587-93.

[5] Atrial versus ventricular pacing in sinus node disease: a treatment comparison study.
Rosenqvist M, Brandt J, Schuller H, Huddinge Univ Hosp, Huddinge, Sweden.
Am Heart J 1986; **111**: 292-6.

[6] Permanent exclusive atrial pacing: clinical experience in 65 cases with a follow up of 1 to 5 years.
Barnay C, Coste A, Quittet F, Medveldowsky JL.
Stimulation Auriculaire Exclusive 1986; **79**: 1703.

[7] Atrial pacing in the management of sick sinus syndrome; long-term observation for conduction disturbances and supraventricular tachyarrhythmias.
Bellinder G, Nordlander R, Pehrsson SK, Astrom H, Karolinska Hosp, Stockholm, Sweden.
Eur Heart J 1986; **7**: 105-9.

[8] Stability of AV conduction in sick sinus node syndrome patients with implanted atrial pacemakers.
Hayes DL, Furman S, Montefiore Med Cent, Bronx, NY, USA.
Am Heart J 1984; **107**: 644-7.

[9] Randomised controlled trial of physiological and ventricular pacing.
Perrins EJ, Morley CA, Chan SL, Sutton R, Westminster Hosp, London UK.
Br Heart J 1983; **50**: 112-7.

[10] Carotid sinus hypersensitivity: beneficial effects of dual-chamber pacing.
Madigan NP, Flaker GC, Curtis JJ, Reid KJ, Murphy TJ, Missouri-Columbia Hosp and Clins, Columbia, MO, USA.
Am J Cardiol 1984; **53**: 1034-40.

[11] Single lead atrial synchronised pacing in patients with cardiogenic shock after acute myocardial infarction.
Fowler MB, Crick JCP, Tayler DI *et al*, Royal Sussex County Hosp, Brighton, UK.
Br Heart J 1984; **51**: 622-5.

[12] Atrial synchronous ventricular pacing in ischaemic heart disease.
Kristensson BE, Arnman K, Ryden L, Central Hosp, Skovde, Sweden.
Eur Heart J 1983; **4**: 668-73.

[13] Optimum pacing mode for patients with angina pectoris.
Kenny RA, Ingram A, Mitsuoka T, Walsh K, Sutton R, Westminster Hosp, London, UK.
Br Heart J 1986; **56**: 463-8.

[14] Rate responsive pacing using the evoked QT principle. A physiological alternative to atrial synchronous pacemakers.
Donaldson RM, Richards AF, Nat Heart Hosp, London, UK.
PACE 1983; **6**: 1344-9.

[15] Respiration as a reliable physiological sensor for controlling cardiac pacing rate.
Rossi P, Plicchi G, Canducci G, Rognoni G, Aina F, Osp Maggiore della Carita, Novara, Italy.
Br Heart J 1984; **51**: 7-14.

[16] Clinical experience with an activity sensing pacemaker.
Lindemans FW, Rankin IR, Murtaugh R, Chevalier PA, Medtronic Inc, Minneapolis, MN, USA.
PACE 1986; **9**: 978.

[17] Single-chamber cardiac pacing with activity-initiated chronotropic response: evaluation by cardiopulmonary exercise testing.
Benditt DG, Mianulli M, Fetter J *et al,* Univ Minnesota Med Sch, Minneapolis, MN, USA.
Circulation 1987; **75**: 184–91.

[18] Measurement of right ventricular blood temperature during exercise as a means of rate control in physiological pacemakers.
Alt E, Hirgstetter C, Heinz M, Theres H, Univ Munich, Munich, Germany.
PACE 1986; **9**: 970.

[19] Mortality in patients with implanted automatic defibrillators.
Morowski M, Reid PR, Wrinkle RA *et al,* Johns Hopkins Med Insts, Baltimore, MD, USA.
Ann Intern Med 1983; **98**: 585–8.

[20] The automatic implantable cardioverter-defibrillator: efficacy, complications and device failures.
Marchlinski FE, Flores BT, Buxton AE *et al,* Hosp Univ Pennsylvania, Philadelphia, PA, USA.
Ann Intern Med 1986; **104**: 481–8.

Comment. Two important studies have set out guidelines for permanent pacemaker implantation. An independent study group [1], composed mainly of conservative physicians, reviewed the arrhythmias for which pacing might be indicated. The Joint Report of the Sub-committee on Pacemaker Implantation formed by the Joint American College of Cardiology and American Heart Association Task Force on Cardiovascular Procedures [2], in addition to discussing the various arrhythmias for which pacing might be considered, lists the conditions for which various pacing models might be selected. There is considerable similarity in the recommendations of these two reports, both stressing the need to rule out transient disturbances and drug effects before permanent pacing is undertaken, and both emphasizing the need to confirm the relationship between an arrhythmia and symptoms. The benign course of sick-sinus syndrome was confirmed by Alt *et al* [3] who showed that the survival of patients with the sick-sinus syndrome was comparable with that in the general population, irrespective of whether they were paced. This finding was first shown by Shaw *et al* who continued their pacing survey and published important data on survival in second degree atrioventricular block [4]. In this prospective study, the fate of 77 patients with chronic second degree type 1 atrioventricular block was compared with the outcome of patients with type 2 block. The overall survival figures for the groups were not statistically different, and the prognosis was not influenced by concomitant bundle branch block. Paced and unpaced subgroups were compared, and in each group the survival of the paced patients was significantly improved (78% *versus* 41% at five years). Small age differences between paced and unpaced patient groups were counteracted by comparison with matched controls, and improved survival of the paced groups was maintained. This study suggests that, contrary to previous and questionable evidence, type 1 second degree atrioventricular block does not have a more benign prognosis than type 2, and similar criteria for deciding the necessity of permanent pacing in the form of atrioventricular block should be used.

Improvements in pacemaker technology have increased the reliability of atrial pacing. There has been interest in using atrial pacing alone for the management of sick-sinus syndrome because it is thought that atrial support may stabilize atrial irritability. However, the results so far have been conflicting. Rosenqvist *et al* [5], who compared AAI against VVI pacing, showed significantly less chronic atrial fibrillation and fewer cases of congestive heart failure with AAI.

Barnay *et al* [6] also reported the benefit of atrial pacing; 10 of their 15 patients had no further supraventricular arrhythmias, although in the majority of cases concomitant (previously ineffective) antiarrhythmic therapy was required. Bellinder *et al* [7] failed to show any decline in the incidence of supraventricular arrhythmias with atrial-demand pacing. Both these studies, as well as the study of Hayes *et al* [8], also addressed the question of whether atrial pacing alone is a satisfactory mode in patients with sick-sinus syndrome, because it was thought that sinoatrial disease and atrioventricular disease often coexist. In all these studies the rate of progression to atrioventricular block was low and suggested that simple assessment of atrioventricular conduction by incremental atrial pacing at the time of pacemaker implant is adequate for the detection of those patients who require dual-chamber units.

Dual-chamber (AV sequential) pacemakers are the most physiologic available when sinoatrial function is intact. Their hemodynamic superiority over conventional VVI pacing was demonstrated by Perrins *et al* [9]. This form of pacing has been shown to be of particular value in carotid-sinus hypersensitivity as shown by Madigan *et al* [10], who also drew attention to the exacerbation of the vasodepressor component by VVI pacing. Maintenance of atrioventricular synchrony may also be of value in patients with cardiogenic shock after myocardial infarction, in whom Fowler *et al* [11] showed that it was possible to achieve a 27% higher cardiac output, when compared with conventional ventricular pacing at a rate of 100 beats/minute, and a blood pressure persistently higher than the peak achieved with ventricular pacing. Kristensson [12] also showed that atrial synchronous ventricular pacing, contrary to popular belief, may be of value in patients with ischemic heart disease because they were able to demonstrate an improvement of exercise capacity. In comparison with VVI pacing, exacerbation of angina was found and patients preferred the atrial synchronous ventricular pacing mode. The problem of pacing in patients with coronary artery disease was also addressed by Kenny *et al* [13], who conducted a double-blind trial in 10 patients with angina who had dual chamber pacemakers implanted. They were studied in VVI mode, in DDD mode with the rate limited to 100 beats/minute and in DDD with the rate limited to 150 beats/minute. The order of pacing mode was randomized. The preferred mode was found to be DDD with an upper rate limit of 100 beats/minute in seven of the 10 patients. The difference in measured exercise capacity did not reach statistical signficance, and was lowest with the DDD-150 beats/minute mode.

Where sinoatrial function is inadequate for providing the physiologic stimulus to ventricular pacing, alternative sensors have been developed, which include the evoked QT interval [14], respiration [15], muscle activity [16,17], and temperature [18]. Which sensor is the most physiologic remains debatable.

Considerably more experience has been gained with the automatic implantable cardiovertor-defibrillator [19] which has shown a significant reduction in anticipated death rate, based upon a calculated mortality. However, complications may occur and those seen in a series of 33 patients have been reported by Marchlinski *et al* [20].

ATRIAL FIBRILLATION

[1] Characteristics and prognosis of lone atrial fibrillation. 30 year follow-up in the Framingham Study.
Brand FN, Abbott RD, Kannel WB, Wolf PA, Univ Hosp, Boston Univ Sch Med, Boston, MA, USA.
J Am Med Assoc 1985; **254**: 3449–53.

[2] Duration of atrial fibrillation and imminence of stroke: the Framingham Study.
Wolf PA, Kannel WB, McGee DL, Meeks SL, Bharucha NE, McNamara PM, Boston Univ Sch Med, Boston, MA, USA.
Stroke 1983; **14**: 664–7.

[3] Alcohol-related acute atrial fibrillation. A case-control study and review of 40 patients.
Rich EC, Siebold C, Campion B, St Paul-Ramsey Med Cent, St Paul, MN, USA.
Arch Intern Med 1985; **45**: 830–3.

[4] Exercise heart rates at different serum digoxin concentrations in patients with atrial fibrillation.
Beasley R, Smith DA, McHaffie DJ, Wellington Clin Sch, Wellington, New Zealand.
Br Med J 1985; **290**: 9–11.

[5] Superiority of oral verapamil therapy to digoxin in treatment of chronic atrial fibrillation.
Lang R, Klein HO, Weiss E *et al*, Meir Hosp, Kfar Saba, Israel.
Chest 1983; **83**: 491–9.

[6] Efficacy and safety of high-dose diltiazem alone and in combination with digoxin for control of heart rate at rest and during exercise in patients with chronic atrial fibrillation.
Roth A, Harrison E, Mitani G, Cohen J, Rahimtoola SH, Elkayam U.
Circulation 1986; **73**: 316–24.

[7] Verapamil improves exercise capacity in chronic atrial fibrillation: double-blind crossover study.
Lang R, Klein HO, Di Segni E *et al*, Meir Gen Hosp, Kfar Saba, Israel.
Am Heart J 1983; **105**: 820–5.

[8] Noninvasive support for and characterization of multiple intranodal pathways in patients with mitral valve disease and atrial fibrillation.
Olsson SM, Cai N, Dohnal M, Talwar KK, Sahlgrenska Hosp, Goteborg, Sweden.
Eur Heart J 1986; **7**: 320–33.

[9] Absence of cardioversion-induced ventricular arrhythmias in patients with therapeutic digoxin levels.
Mann DL, Maisel AS, Atwood JE, Engler RL, LeWinter MM, San Diego VA Med Cent, San Diego, CA, USA.
J Am Coll Cardiol 1985; **5**: 882–8.

[10] Advance prediction of transthoracic impedance in human defibrillation and cardioversion: importance of impedence in determining the success of low-energy shocks.
Kerber RE, Kouba C, Martins J *et al*, Univ Iowa Hosp, Iowa City, IA, USA.
Circulation 1984; **70**: 303–8.

Comment. The Framingham Study has given rise to two important reports on the clinical characteristics of atrial fibrillation. In the first [1], 32 men and 11 women were identified with "lone" atrial fibrillation among a population of 5209 followed over 30 years. The mean age at diagnosis was 70.6 years for men and 68.1 years for women; predisposing characteristics were identified by comparison with age- and sex-matched controls. No differences were found with respect to caffeine intake, smoking habits or alcohol consumption. Significantly more non-specific T-wave and ST-segment abnormalities were present in patients than in controls. The majority of patients were followed (mean follow-up 10.9 years) and, when compared with controls, the rate of stroke development was four times higher in the "lone" atrial fibrillation group, whereas there was no difference in the rates of development of coronary artery disease or cardiac failure, either in men or women. Thus, "lone" atrial fibrillation cannot be considered to be a benign condition, although whether these findings also apply to younger groups of patients without any pre-existing ECG abnormalities remains open to question.

The second Framingham report examined the role of atrial fibrillation as a precursor of stroke [2]. During the period of follow-up, 501 strokes occurred, 59 of which were associated with atrial fibrillation. The risk of stroke was increased fivefold by atrial fibrillation, and the excess risk was found to be independent of the frequently associated cardiac failure and coronary heart disease. The contribution of atrial fibrillation to stroke risk was also at least as powerful as that of the other cardiovascular precursors. Importantly, there was a distinct clustering of stroke events at the time of onset of atrial fibrillation, but recurrence of stroke in those who had atrial fibrillation was slightly, but not significantly, more frequent. Stroke recurrence in the first six months following initial stroke was more than twice as common in the atrial fibrillation group.

Lack of association of alcohol with "lone" atrial fibrillation was not shown by a case-control study [3] in which 64 cases of acute "lone" atrial fibrillation were compared with 64 randomly selected, but matched, general medical patients. Sixty-two per cent of cases and 33% of controls were found to have heavy alcohol intake, although no differences were found when congestive heart failure, ECG abnormalities, heart size, electrolyte disturbance or response to therapy were examined.

Treatment with digoxin has proved the mainstay for the control of heart rate in established atrial fibrillation. However, recent studies have demonstrated that, although digoxin controls the heart rate at rest, it is much less effective in modifying exercise heart rate [4]. The calcium antagonists verapamil [5] and diltiazem [6] have been shown to provide adequate control of heart rate at rest, and superior control of heart rate on exercise. In the case of verapamil, a double-blind crossover study showed that the calcium antagonist was better able than digoxin to improve exercise capacity as judged by multistage ergometry [7].

There have been few studies that have examined the ventricular rate in atrial fibrillation in any detail. Olsson *et al* [8] used computer modelling of RR intervals to show that bimodal or trimodal RR-interval distributions were common — they were seen in 16 of the 22 patients examined. This adds further weight to the suggestion that dual atrioventricular nodal pathways occur frequently and may reflect the dual atrial input into the atrioventricular node.

The practice of discontinuing digoxin for 24 hours prior to cardioversion is widespread. Mann *et al* [9] determined the incidence of cardioversion-induced ventricular arrhythmias and, having excluded patients with electrolyte disturbances, myocardial ischemia or those receiving class I antiarrhythmic drugs, found that no patient developed malignant ventricular arrhythmia after cardioversion and that there was no relationship between serum digoxin level and the change in frequency of ventricular extrasystoles. Provided that the serum digoxin level is within the therapeutic range, there seems no need to discontinue digoxin prior to cardioversion.

The amount of energy required for cardioversion, as well as defibrillation, is in part dependent on transthoracic impedance. Kerber *et al* [10] have shown that the success rate with low-energy shocks was significantly lower when there was a high thoracic impedence than when impedence was low or average. They have shown that transthoracic impedence can be a useful measurement for predicting the patients in whom low-energy shocks will have a high chance of success and, equally, for detecting those with high transthoracic impedence in whom it would be inappropriate to start at low energy levels.

ARRHYTHMOGENIC RIGHT-VENTRICULAR DYSPLASIA

[1] Chronic recurrent right ventricular tachycardia in patients without ischemic heart disease: clinical, hemodynamic and angiographic findings.
Pietras RJ, Lam W, Bauernfeind R *et al*, Univ Illinois Hosp, Chicago, IL, USA.
Am Heart J 1983; **105**: 357–65.

[2] Ventricular tachycardia of left bundle branch block configuration in patients with isolated right ventricular dilatation. Clinical and electrophysiological features.
Rowland E, McKenna WJ, Sugrue D, Barclay R, Foale RA, Krikler DM, Royal Postgrad Med Sch, London, UK.
Br Heart J 1984; **51**: 15–24.

[3] Usefulness of noninvasive studies for diagnosis of right ventricular dysplasia.
Manyari DE, Duff HJ, Kostuk WJ *et al*, Foothills Hosp, Calgary, Alb, Canada.
Am J Cardiol 1986; **57**: 1147–53.

[4] Right ventricular abnormalities in ventricular tachycardia of right ventricular origin: relation to electrophysiological abnormalities.
Foale RA, Nihoyannopoulos P, Ribeiro P *et al*, St Mary's Hosp, London, UK.
Br Heart J 1986; **56**: 45–54.

[5] Arrhythmogenic right ventricular dysplasia in a family.
Ruder MA, Winston SA, Cavis JC, Abbott JA, Eldar M, Scheinman MM, Univ California, San Francisco, CA, USA.
Am J Cardiol 1985; **56**: 799–801.

[6] Familial arrhythmogenic right ventricular disease.
Rakovec P, Rossi L, Fontaine G, Sasel B, Markez J, Voncina D.
Am J Cardiol 1985; **56**: 377–79.

[7] Left ventricular abnormalities in arrhythogenic right ventricular dysplasia.
Webb J, Kerr C, Huckell V, Mizgala H, Ricci D.
Am J Cardiol 1986; **58**: 568–70.

Comment. This unusual but frequently under-diagnosed condition has received increasing attention. It is commonly complicated by ventricular tachycardia and has important prognostic implications. The diagnosis should always be suspected in patients who have ventricular tachycardia of left bundle branch block configuration. The frequency with which right-ventricular disease underlies right-ventricular tachycardia was assessed by Pietras *et al* [1] who evaluated 38 consecutive patients with this abnormality. Just under one-half had selective right-ventricular abnormalities, such as localized or generalized angiographic right-ventricular wall-motion abnormalities. The clinical electrophysiologic characteristics of those with right-ventricular tachycardia in the presence of isolated right-ventricular dilatation was addressed by Rowland *et al* [2]. Both groups of workers [1,2] stressed the requirement for specific investigations of right-ventricular structure and function, issues that were addressed in greater detail by two further studies [3,4]. Manyari *et al* [3] compared the value and limitations of echocardiography and cardiac scintigraphy, respectively, for establishing the diagnosis of right-ventricular dysplasia and arrived at diagnostic criteria based on right-ventricular volumes, ejection fractions and wall-motion scores. Foale *et al* [4] evaluated the role of echocardiography as a screening test for right-ventricular tachycardia and compared the results between a group of eight patients who had isolated abnormalities of right-ventricular structure and function and the remainder who had normal right ventricles; the patients had been previously categorized by electrophysiologic features, contrast angiography and radionuclide angiography. The results of these two studies [3,4] suggest that, if particular attention is paid to the right ventricle, echocardiography is an important screening test for identifying patients with right-ventricular dysplasia.

The etiology of right-ventricular dysplasia remains obscure, but a familial propensity has been noted [5–7], as well as further evidence that left-ventricular abnormalities may occur [7].

ARRHYTHMIAS IN CONGENITAL HEART DISEASE

[1] Ventricular arrhythmias and biventricular dysfunction after repair of tetralogy of Fallot.
Webb Kavey R-E, Deaver Thomas F, Byrum CJ, Blackman MS, Sondheimer HM, Bove EL, State Univ New York, Syracuse, NY, USA.
J Am Coll Cardiol 1984; 4: 126–34.
[2] Analysis of adults with and without complex ventricular arrhythmias after repair of tetralogy of Fallot.
Burns RJ, Liu PP, Druck MN, Seawright SJ, Williams WG, McLaughlin PR, Toronto Gen Hosp, Toronto, Ont, Canada.
J Am Coll Cardiol 1984; 4: 226–33.
[3] Ventricular arrhythmia in unrepaired and repaired tetralogy of Fallot. Relation to age, timing of repair, and haemodynamic status.
Deanfield JE, McKenna WJ, Presbitero P, England D, Graham GR, Hallidie-Smith K, Hammersmith Hosp, London, UK.
Br Heart J 1984; 52: 77–81.

[4] Local abnormalities of right ventricular depolarization after repair of tetralogy of Fallot: a basis for ventricular arrhythmia.
Deanfield J, McKenna W, Rowland E, Hammersmith Hosp, London, UK.
Am J Cardiol 1985; **55**: 522–5.

[5] Cardiac arrhythmias in patients with surgical repair of Ebstein's anomaly.
Oh JK, Holmes DR Jr, Hayes DL, Porter C-BJ, Danielson GK, Mayo Clin and Mayo Found, Rochester, MN, USA.
J Am Coll Cardiol 1985; **6**: 1351–7.

[6] Electrophysiologic abnormalities of children with ostium secundum atrial septal defect.
Ruschhaupt DG, Khoury L, Thilenius OG, Replogle RL, Arcilla RA, Univ Chicago, Chicago, IL, USA.
Am J Cardiol 1984; **53**: 1643–7.

[7] Long-term follow-up of dysrhythmias following the Mustard procedure.
Duster MC, Bink-Boelkens ThE, Wampler D, Gillette PC, McNamara DG, Cooley DA, Texas Children's Hosp, Houston, TX, USA.
Am Heart J 1985; **109**: 1323–6.

Comment. Among the congenital heart defects that may be associated with arrhythmia, tetralogy of Fallot has received the most attention. Two studies [1,2] examined the characteristics of patients with and without ventricular arrhythmia after repair of tetralogy of Fallot. Webb Kavey *et al* [1] demonstrated a significantly lower left-ventricular ejection fraction in the arrhythmia group, but no difference in right-ventricular function, and suggested that evaluation of ventricular function allows those at risk of developing potentially lethal arrhythmias to be selected. Conversely, Burns *et al* [2] found a higher right-ventricular systolic blood pressure, a higher incidence of residual left-to-right intracardiac shunts, and more frequently abnormal left-ventricular ejection fraction in the arrhythmia group. They suggested that patients with ventricular arrhythmia have subclinical left-ventricular dysfunction consequent either to a fibrotic process or right-ventricular overload.

Deanfield *et al* [3] examined the problem by comparing a preoperative group with a group who had undergone repair at various ages. Twenty per cent of the unoperated group had ventricular arrhythmia, the prevalence increasing with age. The higher incidence of ventricular arrhythmia in the corrected group was associated with age at repair, but not with hemodynamic status, era of surgery or duration of follow-up. Further evidence for the widespread nature of the myocardial disturbance, consequent to the underlying defect, rather than surgery, was supplied by a further study from this group on local abnormalities of right-ventricular depolarization [4].

Cardiac arrhythmia has been an important problem in patients with Ebstein's anomaly. Oh *et al* [5] provided data on the influence of operative procedures on these arrhythmias in 52 patients. Although paroxysmal supraventricular tachycardia was the most frequent arrhythmia, ventricular arrhythmia occurred in 13, and high-grade atrioventricular block in 3. During follow-up of this group, there were seven deaths between 1 day and 27 months after the operation, of which five were sudden, four patients having had perioperative ventricular tachycardia or ventricular fibrillation. Of those with preoperative paroxysmal supraventricular tachycardia, 22% continued to have symptomatic episodes over a mean follow-up period of 40 months; a similar percentage (30%) of those with paroxysmal atrial fibrillation or atrial flutter continued to be symptomatic. In contrast, none of the 11 patients without preoperative arrhythmia died suddenly or developed symptomatic arrhythmia postoperatively.

Ruschhaupt *et al* [6] studied 49 patients with secundum atrial septal defect and found preoperative abnormalities in 40% of the patients, although none were seen in those <2.5 years old. Although there was a non-significant increase in the number having induction abnormalities postoperatively, these findings may favor early surgical intervention in those with hemodynamically significant defects.

The high incidence of sinus node dysfunction after the Mustard procedure led to modification of the operation, aimed at protecting the integrity of the sinus node. The initial result was that a higher proportion of patients remained in sinus rhythm. Duster *et al* [7] report the long-term results of these operative modifications in terms of both sino-atrial and atrioventricular arrhythmias. Three eras of operation were examined, and at 2-year follow-up the incidence of maintenance of sinus rhythm was higher in those patients who had operations that protected sinus node integrity. After 8 years, <50% of patients were in sinus rhythm and both bradycardia and symptomatic tachycardia were common in all groups. A high proportion of patients undergoing Mustard correction have arrhythmias that appear to be unaffected by operations to preserve sinus node function.

7. Examination and Diagnostic Procedures

MAGNETIC RESONANCE IMAGING OF THE CARDIOVASCULAR SYSTEM

Review: S. RICHARD UNDERWOOD

Magnetic resonance imaging now has an established place in diagnostic imaging of the brain and spinal cord [1]. Its value lies in high soft-tissue contrast and high resolution, and in the fact that that contrast is determined partly by the biochemical environment of the protons forming the image. The process of imaging moving organs in the thorax and abdomen requires additional techniques such as electrocardiographic or respiratory gating, but images of the heart with excellent anatomic definition can be produced using electrocardiographic gating alone [2–4]. This has been widely applied only in the last three years, but many advances have been made in this time.

The physical principles underlying magnetic resonance are complex; a brief description of some of the concepts follows. (More complete descriptions are available elsewhere [5].)

Physical Principles of Magnetic Resonance Imaging

Nuclear Magnetism

The hydrogen nucleus, in common with some other nuclei, possesses both charge and spin, and in an external magnetic field it behaves like a bar magnet, aligning with the field. Quantum physics describes only two allowed orientations – parallel or anti-parallel to the field, a small majority being in the lower, parallel energy state. The individual axes of spin are not in fact parallel to the field, but at an angle of 55°, and, in the same way that a spinning top precesses about a gravitational field, the nuclear spin axes precess about the magnetic field, at a rate proportional to the field strength (the resonant or Larmor frequency).

Magnetic resonance is most easily understood by considering only the net effect of many millions of nuclei. The sum of the individual magnetic moments is called the 'net magnetization vector', M, and at equilibrium it is parallel to the external field (Fig. 1a). If this vector is disturbed from equilibrium by a radio pulse at the resonant frequency, it too precesses about the field, and its subsequent behavior can be described in terms of two components – one in the direction of the field, M_z, and the other in the plane perpendicular to this, M_{xy} (Fig. 1b).

The rotation of M_{xy} leads to the emission of a radio signal, and a map of the amplitude of this signal at each point in a selected plane produces an image. (The techniques used for mapping are beyond the scope of this article, but they rely upon magnetic field gradients in each of the three dimensions.)

344

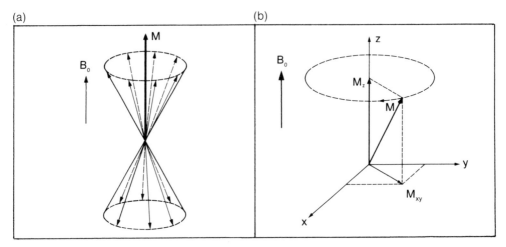

FIGURE 1: (a) In an external magnetic field, certain nuclei align at an angle with the field and precess around it. The sum of the individual nuclear magnetization vectors is the net magnetization vector, M, which at equilibrium is in the direction of the external field (B_o). (b) The net magnetization vector can be displaced from equilibrium, and it then also precesses about the external field. It is best considered as two components – one in the direction of the field, M_z, and one perpendicular to it, M_{xy}.

Relaxation

After disturbance, M_z and M_{xy} return to equilibrium because of spin–lattice and spin–spin relaxation, respectively, and the observed signal decays along with M_{xy}. These processes are so named because they are the result of interaction of the nuclear spins with their surrounding lattice and with each other. They are both exponential decays with time constants T_1 and T_2. Depending upon the sequence of radio pulses used to disturb the net magnetization vector, and the time at which the magnetic resonance signal is recorded, the magnitude of signal and hence the contrast in the image can be made to reflect proton density, T_1, T_2, or mixtures of each (the images are 'T_2-weighted', etc.). The ability to vary contrast, and the fact that T_1 and T_2 depend upon the biochemical environment of the hydrogen nuclei forming the image, introduces the functional information which sets magnetic resonance apart from X-ray computed tomography.

Spectroscopy

The frequency of the emitted signal is determined by the magnetic field experienced by the nucleus. As nuclei in different chemical environments are screened from an external field by surrounding electrons to varying extents, the same nucleus in different chemical environments will emit signal at different frequencies. The spectrum of frequencies gives important information, because the position of the peaks identifies chemical species and the size of each is proportional to the number of emitting nuclei.

Magnetic resonance imaging is almost entirely restricted to the hydrogen nucleus because of its abundance and the need for a strong signal. Although hydrogen spectroscopy is possible, the number of different chemical environments in which it is found makes interpretation difficult. Phosphorus-31 spectroscopy is more common, and its value lies in the importance of phosphorus-containing compounds in cellular metabolism. The ratio of high-energy phosphates (phosphocreatine and adenosine triphosphate) to inorganic phosphate is a measure of tissue energetics, and the position of the inorganic phosphate peak reflects intracellular pH [6].

Cardiac Anatomy and Pathology

Because conventional sequences usually give no signal from moving blood, the images have high contrast between blood and other structures, without injection of contrast media. A wide variety of cardiovascular disease can be investigated using magnetic

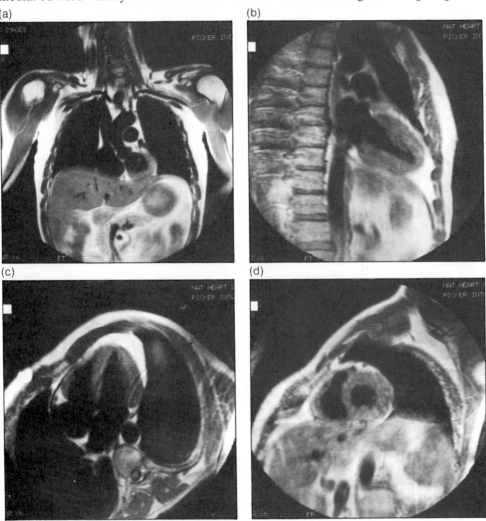

FIGURE 2: Systolic magnetic resonance images: (a) coronal plane through the aortic valve; (b) vertical long-axis plane, which is equivalent to the right anterior oblique projection; (c) horizontal long axis, which is identical to the apical four-chamber view of echocardiography; and (d) short axis, perpendicular to (b) and (c).

resonance imaging, including congenital heart disease, ischemic heart disease, cardiomyopathy, neoplastic disease and diseases of the pericardium and great vessels. Several centers have published reviews of their experience [7–11].

The ability to image in any plane makes the technique particularly versatile (Fig. 2). Oblique planes are important in cardiac imaging [12], and although they can be acquired by tilting the patient within the machine [13–15] it is simpler and more reproducible to tilt the imaging gradients to alter acquisition planes [16–18].

Congenital Disease

Simple congenital anomalies, such as atrial and ventricular septal defects, are readily seen with magnetic resonance imaging (Fig. 3) [19–21] although, as in echocardiography, care is necessary in the diagnosis of atrial defects because the septum is very thin in the region of the foramen secundum. Specificity is improved by oblique images or a ciné sequence.

(a)

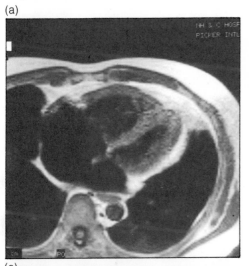

(b)

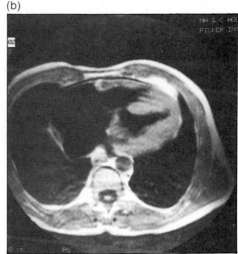

(c)

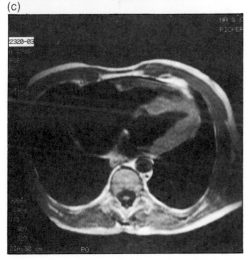

FIGURE 3: Transverse images, showing (a) ostium secondum atrial septal defect; (b) ventricular septal defect; and (c) Gerbode defect in the same patient as (b).

Even complex congenital disease can be assessed [22–25] and magnetic resonance imaging is particularly valuable for the pulmonary vessels (Fig. 4); these are often not accessible to echocardiography and, in tricuspid or pulmonary atresia, for instance, may also present difficulties for invasive angiography. Because slowly moving blood does give magnetic resonance signal [26], a semi-quantitative measurement of pulmonary vascular resistance is possible, since velocity and resistance appear to be related [27]. More promising, however, are direct flow measurements by velocity mapping (described below).

(a)   (b)

(c)   (d)

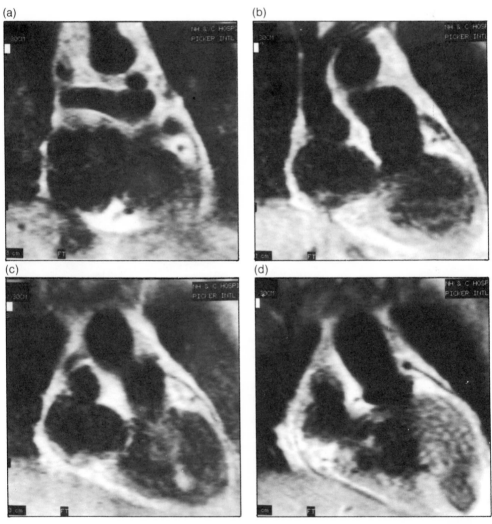

FIGURE 4: Contiguous 1-cm coronal sections from posterior (a) to anterior (b) in a patient with transposition of the great arteries and a previous Mustard operation. The aorta arises anteriorly from the right ventricle (c) and (d), and the pulmonary artery posteriorly from the left ventricle (b).

Tumors and Thrombi

Tumors and thrombi within the heart [28–31] and mediastinum [32,33] may be visualized with magnetic resonance imaging and, although echocardiography will remain the first investigation in such cases, magnetic resonance imaging will play an important role in cases of doubt or in difficult echocardiographic subjects. One problem with image interpretation is the signal from static blood, which can be confused with thrombus or tumour, but ciné imaging and the use of different sequences help simplify interpretation (Fig. 5).

Pericardium

The pericardium usually shows as a dark line between high signal from pericardial and epicardial fat; thickening or effusion are well demonstrated by magnetic resonance imaging [34–37]. One drawback is that calcification is not seen, because calcium gives no magnetic resonance signal; supplementary investigation may be needed.

(a)

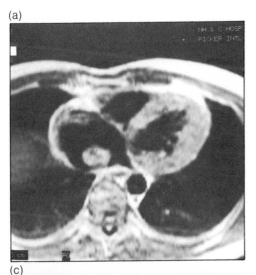

(b)

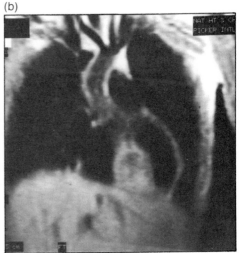

(c)

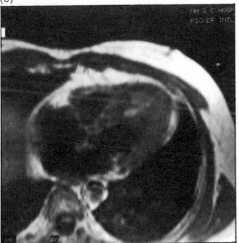

FIGURE 5: Magnetic resonance images showing (a) right atrial myxoma; (b) benign septal fibroma; and (c) apical thrombus following acute myocardial infarction.

Great Vessels

X-Ray computed tomography is valuable in the assessment of aortic aneurysms and dissection, and it appears that magnetic resonance imaging will be equally useful for visualizing aneurysms of the abdominal aorta [38,39] and the thoracic aorta (Fig. 6) [40–45]. It is particularly helpful in sick patients to avoid contrast agents; however, if the patient is very ill, imaging may be impractical because of the relatively long acquisition time and difficulty in accommodating metallic resuscitation equipment close to the scanner.

Emboli in the central pulmonary arteries have been described [46–48], but it does not appear likely that magnetic resonance will be sensitive in the detection of embolic disease: without respiratory gating the peripheral lung is not well seen.

Valves

Heart valves can be visualized with magnetic resonance imaging and, although the thickening of abnormal valves is usually apparent, resolution is not adequate to define pathology well. Prosthetic valves are not seen, because no signal is obtained from metallic nuclei; although it was initially feared that magnetic fields might affect valve function, this is not a problem because nearly all modern valves are non-ferromagnetic [49]. However, currents induced in the valves by the changing magnetic field gradients may distort the image for a small area around the valve.

Ventricular Function

Global Function

Dimensions can be measured very accurately from the images, and several studies have compared magnetic resonance imaging results with measurements obtained using other techniques [50,51]. To determine wall thickness, it is important to use oblique images, because true thickness will not be measured if the ventricle does not pass perpendicularly through the image [52]. Volumes are calculated by summing the areas of the chambers in multiple contiguous sections, or, more rapidly, the volume of the left ventricle is calculated from the area and length of the chamber in an oblique image

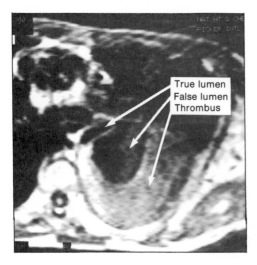

True lumen
False lumen
Thrombus

FIGURE 6: Transverse image through the descending aorta in a patient with aortic dissection. The true lumen is compressed to a slit by a large, false lumen which is lined with thrombus.

containing the long axis. The multiple-slice method is accurate to within approximately 2% [53], but the single-slice method is suitable for the routine measurement of left-ventricular ejection fraction, provided the ventricle is not too irregular [54].

Subtraction of end-diastolic from end-systolic volumes leads to stroke volumes, ejection fractions, and determination of cardiac output for both ventricles. The accuracy of these measurements has provided a standard by which to judge other techniques – particularly for the right ventricle, which is difficult to assess by other methods. Equilibrium radionuclide ventriculography, for instance, has been shown to underestimate right-ventricular stroke volume and ejection fraction, and to overestimate the ratio of left- and right-ventricular stroke volumes which is used to quantify valvular regurgitation [55]. The degree of shunting through atrial septal defects can also be calculated from this ratio, and, while first-pass radionuclide ventriculography is accurate, oximetry performed at cardiac catheterization is not, because of the difficulty of estimating mixed venous saturation [56].

Regional Function
By comparing endocardial contours at end-diastole and end-systole, wall motion can be assessed with magnetic resonance imaging, although it is important to use oblique planes with the wall passing perpendicularly through the image. Wall motion agrees well with the conventional techniques of X-ray contrast and radionuclide ventriculography, and the combination of wall-motion and thickness measurements makes magnetic resonance imaging highly specific in the detection of previous infarction (Fig. 7) [57].

Tissue Characterization
The spin–lattice and spin–spin relaxation times, T_1 and T_2, depend upon local biochemistry, and may be measured and displayed as maps showing relaxation times throughout the myocardium. There are several sources of inaccuracy in these measurements,

(a)   (b)

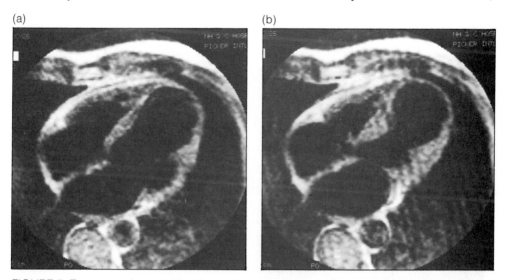

FIGURE 7: Transverse images showing an apical aneurysm. The infarcted region is thin, and superimposition of diastolic (a) and systolic contours (b) shows it to be dyskinetic.

with the results depending upon the method used; however, because the amplitude of signal in spin-echo images depends partly upon T_2, the brightness of the image is a simple way of assessing changes.

These changes could help in the assessment of acute [58–60] and chronic infarction [61], in interventions aimed at limiting the extent of infarction [62,63] and in the detection of cardiac-transplant rejection [64]. Both T_1 and T_2 increase early after coronary occlusion, due in part to an increase in myocardial water content, and changes are apparent in images between 30 minutes and 3 hours after infarction [65,66]. T_2 may remain elevated for at least 5 hours – even with reperfusion and without eventual infarctions – presumably because of edema [67]. In established infarction, relaxation times are prolonged for several weeks, slowly returning to normal or below [68].

Paramagnetic contrast agents may be helpful in studies of myocardial ischemia. Gadolinium is a rare earth which shortens relaxation times; when complexed to diethylene triamine penta-acetic acid (DTPA), it is distributed in the vascular compartment in the same way as are the iodine-containing media used to provide contrast in X-rays [69]. This provides additional contrast in the detection of myocardial ischemia [70-72], and suggests the prospect of myocardial perfusion maps through the comparison of images with and without contrast enhancement.

Angiography and Blood Flow
Magnetic Resonance Angiography
Many different factors determine the amplitude of the magnetic resonance signal, but flow usually abolishes signal from blood, providing high contrast in the heart and blood vessels [73]. Peripheral and central arteries show well, with sufficient resolution to detect disease in vessels down to about the size of the popliteal artery (Fig. 8) [74,75]. Coronary artery bypass grafts may be assumed to be patent if they are seen without intraluminal signal [76]. Conventional imaging has its limitations in the detection of vascular disease [77], but a number of techniques have been developed to improve reliability.

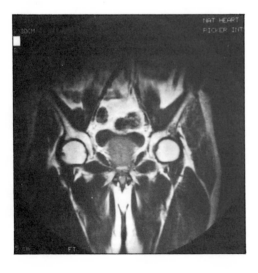

FIGURE 8: Coronal spin echo image, showing disease of the right external iliac artery.

Because of a phenomenon called even-echo rephasing, flowing blood gives a higher signal in the second image of a multiple-echo sequence, and a computed T_2 map using the two images gives spuriously long values of T_2 from flowing blood. Computer reconstruction from these maps provides a pseudo three-dimensional display of the vessel from which disease can be demonstrated [78,79].

A second method involves the use of pulsatile arterial flow by subtracting a systolic from a diastolic image. In the latter, blood will give a signal because it is relatively static, and the result will be an arteriogram with signal only from arterial blood. Summation of contiguous tomographic images obtained in this way gives the equivalent of a projection arteriogram [80], and the technique has been used successfully in patients with vascular disease [81].

A short-field echo sequence gives high signal even from rapidly moving blood, and provides more versatile magnetic resonance angiography. A modification of the sequence abolishes signal from the blood, and subtraction of the two images provides an angiogram which overcomes the problems of vessel motion between diastole and systole (Fig. 9) [82]. Coronary arteriograms can be produced, although resolution is not yet sufficient to see stenoses of any but the major coronary arteries (Fig. 10). The particular strength of this technique is that the same sequence can be used to map velocity at any point within the vessel, thus providing an assessment of function as well as anatomy (see below).

Blood Flow

A number of different methods have been developed for the measurement of blood flow [83–87], but the most versatile uses a short-field echo sequence with phase-encoding to display a map of velocity either in the plane of the image or perpendicular to it [82,88]. The technique is accurate over a wide range of velocities [89] and is compatible with ciné imaging [90]. Colour-coding of the velocities with superimposition upon a conventional image demonstrates anatomy and blood flow in a single display [91].

Velocity measurements have proved useful in a number of situations, such as the assessment of coronary artery bypass grafts (Fig. 11), stenoses in peripheral and central

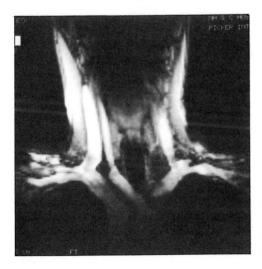

FIGURE 9: Magnetic resonance angiogram using a short-field echo sequence. The right common carotid and innominate arteries are seen, also the jugular veins on both sides.

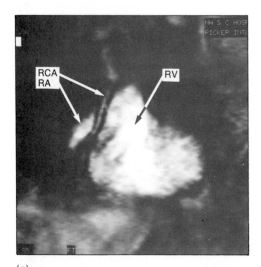

(a)

FIGURE 10: Arteriogram of the right coronary artery, acquired using the short-field echo sequence. RCA = right coronary artery; RV = right ventricle; RA = right atrium.

(b)

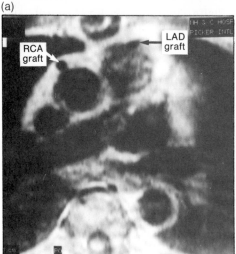

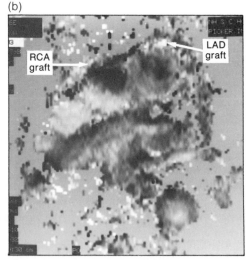

FIGURE 11: (a) Transverse image, showing vein grafts to the right coronary artery (RCA graft) and the left anterior descending artery (LAD graft). (b) Map of velocity perpendicular to the plane in (a). Midgrey = zero velocity; white = cranial velocities; black = caudal velocities. High velocity (326 mm/s) is seen in the LAD graft, very low velocities (74 mm/s) in the RCA graft.

vessels, intracardiac shunting, valvular regurgitation and flow in the great vessels in congenital heart disease [92]. The most exciting prospect is that of non-invasive coronary arteriography with flow measurements.

The Future

As magnetic resonance becomes more widely available, its use in the management of all forms of cardiovascular disease will increase. It is unlikely to displace echocardiography as the initial investigation in congenital heart disease, but a combination of echocardiography and magnetic resonance imaging could almost eliminate the need for inva-

354

sive investigation. As rapid imaging techniques [93] and real-time imaging [94] become available even echocardiography may be threatened, although magnetic resonance will always be more expensive because of the technology involved, and its cost-effectiveness is yet to be determined.

In the detection and management of vascular disease, magnetic resonance imaging will gain further importance. The non-invasive assessment of anatomy and flow in peripheral and coronary artery disease appears possible, although we must remember the lesson of digital subtraction radiography, which held out the promise of coronary arteriograms from a venous injection of contrast but has failed to fulfil this promise.

The machines of the future need not be large and expensive. Magnets will become smaller and less restricted for patient access. Already the cost of a scanner is the same as that of a modern catheter laboratory, and the cheapest machines are approaching the cost of an X-ray tomography scanner. The future of magnetic resonance, as an imaging technique, is assured.

References

[1] Bydder GM, Steiner RE, Young IR et al.
Clinical MR imaging of the brain: 140 cases.
Am J Roentgenol 1982; **139**: 215–36.

[2] Crooks LE, Barker B, Chang H et al.
Magnetic resonance imaging strategies for heart studies.
Radiology 1984; **153**: 459–65.

[3] Lanzer P, Barta C, Botvinick EH, Wiesendanger HUD, Modin G, Higgins CB.
ECG-synchronised cardiac MR imaging: Method and evaluation.
Radiology 1985; **155**: 681–6.

[4] Lanzer P, Botvinick E, Schiller NB et al.
Cardiac imaging using gated magnetic resonance.
Radiology 1984; **150**: 121–7.

[5] Pykett IL, Newhouse JH, Buonanno FS et al.
Principles of nuclear magnetic resonance imaging.
Radiology 1982; **143**: 157–68.

[6] Radda GK, Bore PJ, Rajagopalan B.
Clinical aspects of ^{31}P NMR spectroscopy.
Br Med Bull 1983; **40**(No. 2).

[7] Higgins CB, Byrd BF, McNamara MT et al.
Magnetic resonance imaging of the heart: A review of the experience in 172 subjects.
Radiology 1985; **155**: 671–9.

[8] Higgins CB, Kaufman L, Crooks LE.
Magnetic resonance of the cardiovascular system.
Am Heart J 1985; **109**: 136–52.

[9] Steiner RE, Bydder GM, Selwyn A et al.
Nuclear magnetic resonance imaging of the heart. Current status and future prospects.
Br Heart J 1983; **50**: 202–8.

[10] Lieberman JM, Alfidi RJ, Nelson AD et al.
Gated magnetic resonance imaging of the normal and diseased heart.
Radiology 1984; **152**: 465–70.

[11] Rees RSO, Underwood SR, Firmin DN et al.
Clinical studies of the heart by magnetic resonance.
Br Heart J 1987 (submitted for publication).

[12] Akins EW, Hill JA, Fitzsimmons JR, Pepine CJ, Williams CM.
Importance of imaging plane for magnetic resonance imaging of the normal left ventricle.
Am J Cardiol 1985; **56**: 366–72.

[13] Dinsmore RE, Wismer GL, Levine RA, Okada RD, Brady TJ.
Magnetic resonance imaging of the heart: Positioning and gradient angle selection for optimal imaging planes.
Am J Roentgenol 1984; **143**: 1135–42.

[14] Dinsmore RE, Wismer GL, Miller SW et al.
Magnetic resonance imaging of the heart using image planes oriented to cardiac axes: Experience with 100 cases.
Am J Roentgenol 1985; **145**: 1177–83.

[15] Huber DJ, Mueller E, Heubes P.
Oblique magnetic resonance imaging of normal structures.
Am J Roentgenol 1985; **145**: 843–6.

[16] Edelman RR, Stark DD, Saini S et al.
Oblique planes of section in MR imaging.
Radiology 1986; **159**: 807–10.

[17] Feiglin DH, George CR, MacIntyre WJ et al.
Gated cardiac magnetic resonance structural imaging: Optimization by electronic axial rotation.
Radiology 1985; **154**: 129–32.

[18] Murphy WA, Gutierrez FR, Levitt RG, Glazer HS, Lee JKT.
Oblique views of the heart by magnetic resonance imaging.
Radiology 1985; **154**: 225–6.

[19] Jacobstein MD, Fletcher BD, Goldstein S, Riemenschneider TA.
Evaluation of atrioventricular septal defect by magnetic resonance imaging.
Am J Cardiol 1985; **55**: 1158–61.

[20] Dinsmore RE, Wismer GL, Guyer D *et al*.
Magnetic resonance imaging of the interatrial septum and atrial septal defects.
Am J Roentgenol 1985; **145**: 697–703.

[21] Lowell DG, Turner DA, Smith SM *et al*.
The detection of atrial and ventricular septal defects with electrocardiographically synchronized magnetic resonance imaging.
Circulation 1986; **73**: 89–94.

[22] Didier D, Higgins CB, Fisher MR, Osaki L, Silverman NH, Cheitlin MD.
Congenital heart disease: Gated MR imaging in 72 patients.
Radiology 1986; **158**: 227–35.

[23] Fletcher BD, Jacobstein MD.
MRI of congenital abnormalities of the great arteries.
Am J Roentgenol 1986; **146**: 941–8.

[24] Fletcher BD, Jacobstein MD, Nelson AD, Riemenschneider TA, Alfidi RJ.
Gated magnetic resonance imaging of congenital cardiac malformations.
Radiology 1984; **150**: 137–40.

[25] Fisher MR, Hricak H, Higgins CB.
Magnetic resonance imaging of developmental venous anomalies.
Am J Roentgenol 1985; **145**: 705–9.

[26] Edelstein WA, Hutchinson JMS, Johnson G *et al*.
Gated MR imaging of the heart: Intracardiac signals in patients and healthy subjects.
Radiology 1985; **156**: 125–32.

[27] Didier D, Higgins CB.
Estimation of pulmonary vascular resistance by MRI in patients with congenital cardiovascular shunt lesions.
Am J Roentgenol 1986; **146**: 919–24.

[28] Dooms GC, Higgins CB.
MR imaging of cardiac thrombi.
J Comput Assist Tomogr 1986; **10**: 415–20.

[29] Pizzarello RA, Goldberg SM, Goldman MA *et al*.
Tumour of the heart diagnosed by magnetic resonance imaging.
J Am Coll Cardiol 1985; **5**: 989–91.

[30] Go RT, O'Donnell JK, Underwood DA *et al*.
Comparison of gated cardiac MRI and 2D echocardiography of intracardiac neoplasms.
Am J Roentgenol 1985; **145**: 21–5.

[31] Conces DJ, Vox VA, Klatte EC.
Gated MR imaging of left atrial myxomas.
Am J Roentgenol 1985; **156**: 445–7.

[32] Amparo EG, Higgins CB, Farmer D, Gamsu G, McNamara M.
Gated MRI of cardiac and paracardiac masses: Initial experience.
Am J Roentgenol 1984; **143**: 1151–6.

[33] von Schulthess GK, McMurdo K, Tscholakoff D, DeGeer G, Gamsu G, Higgins CB.
Magnetic resonance imaging of mediastinal masses.
Radiology 1986; **158**: 289–97.

[34] Soulen RL, Stark DD, Higgins CB.
Magnetic resonance imaging of constrictive pericardial disease.
Am J Cardiol 1985; **55**: 480–4.

[35] Schiavone WA, O'Donnell JK.
Congenital absence of the left portion of parietal pericardium demonstrated by magnetic resonance imaging.
Am J Cardiol 1985; **55**: 1439–40.

[36] Stark DD, Higgins CB, Lanzer P *et al*.
Magnetic resonance imaging of the pericardium: Normal and pathologic findings.
Radiology 1984; **150**: 469–74.

[37] McMurdo KK, Webb WR, von Schulthess GK, Gamsu G.
Magnetic resonance imaging of the superior pericardial recesses.
Am J Roentgenol 1985; **145**: 985–8.

[38] Amparo EG, Hoddick WK, Hricak H *et al*.
Comparison of magnetic resonance imaging and ultrasonography in the evaluation of abdominal aortic aneurysms.
Radiology 1985; **154**: 451–6.

[39] Flak B, Li DKB, Ho BYD *et al*.
Magnetic resonance imaging of aneurysms of the abdominal aorta.
Am J Roentgenol 1985; **144**: 991–6.

[40] Moore EH, Webb WR, Verrier ED *et al*.
MRI of chronic posttraumatic false aneurysms of the thoracic aorta.
Am J Roentgenol 1984; **143**: 1195–6.

[41] Dinsmore RE, Liberthson RR, Wismer GL *et al*.
Magnetic resonance imaging of thoracic aortic aneurysms: Comparison with other imaging methods.
Am J Roentgenol 1986; **146**: 309–14.

[42] Amparo EG, Higgins CB, Shafton EP.
Demonstration of coarctation of the aorta by magnetic resonance imaging.
Am J Roentgenol 1984; **143**: 1192–4.

[43] Amparo EG, Higgins CB, Hoddick W *et al.*
Magnetic resonance imaging of aortic disease: Preliminary results.
Am J Roentgenol 1984; **143**: 1203–9.

[44] Amparo EG, Higgins CB, Hricak H, Sollitto R.
Aortic dissection: Magnetic resonance imaging.
Radiology 1985; **155**: 399–406.

[45] Boxer RA, LaCorte MA, Singh S *et al.*
Nuclear magnetic resonance imaging in evaluation and follow-up of children treated for coarctation of the aorta.
J Am Coll Cardiol 1986; **7**: 1095–8.

[46] Fisher MR, Higgins CB.
Central thrombi in pulmonary arterial hypertension detected by MR imaging.
Radiology 1986; **158**: 223–6.

[47] Gamsu G, Hirji M, Moore EH, Webb WR, Brito A.
Experimental pulmonary emboli detected using magnetic resonance.
Radiology 1984; **53**: 467–70.

[48] Moore EH, Gamsu G, Webb WR, Stulbarg MS.
Pulmonary embolus: Detection and followup using magnetic resonance.
Radiology 1984; **153**: 471–2.

[49] Soulen R, Higgins CB, Budinger RF.
Magnetic resonance imaging of prosthetic heart valves.
Radiology 1985; **154**: 705–7.

[50] Fisher MR, von Schulthess GK, Higgins CB.
Multiphasic cardiac magnetic resonance imaging: Normal regional left ventricular wall thickening.
Am J Roentgenol 1985; **145**: 27–30.

[51] Byrd BF III, Schiller NB, Botvinick EG, Higgins CB.
Normal cardiac dimensions by magnetic resonance imaging.
Am J Cardiol 1985; **55**: 1440–2.

[52] Kaul S, Wismer GL, Brady TJ *et al.*
Measurement of normal left heart dimensions using optimally oriented MR images.
Am J Roentgenol 1986; **146**: 75–9.

[53] Longmore DB, Klipstein RH, Underwood SR *et al.*
Dimensional accuracy of magnetic resonance in studies of the heart.
Lancet 1985; i: 1360–2.

[54] Underwood SR, Firmin DN, Klipstein RH *et al.*
Rapid measurement of left ventricular volume from single oblique magnetic resonance images.
Radiology 1985; **157**(P): 309.

[55] Underwood SR, Klipstein RH, Firmin DN *et al.*
Magnetic resonance assessment of aortic and mitral regurgitation.
Br Heart J 1986; **56**: 455–62.

[56] Underwood SR, Klipstein RH, Firmin DN *et al.*
Magnetic resonance assessment of the accuracy of radionuclide methods for the quantification of valvular regurgitation and atrial shunting. In: Hoefer R, Bergman H, eds. *Radioactive Isotopes in Medicine and Research, Vol. 17.* Vienna: H. Egerman, 1986; pp. 299–305.

[57] Underwood SR, Rees RSO, Savage PE, Firmin DN, Klipstein RH, Longmore DB.
The assessment of regional left ventricular function by magnetic resonance.
Br Heart J 1986; **56**: 334–40.

[58] McNamara MT, Higgins CB, Schechtmann N *et al.*
Detection and characterization of acute myocardial infarction in man with use of gated magnetic resonance.
Circulation 1985; **71**: 717–24.

[59] Brown JJ, Strich G, Higgins CB, Gerber KH, Slutsky RA.
Nuclear magnetic resonance analysis of acute myocardial infarction in dogs: The effects of transient coronary ischemia of varying duration and reperfusion on spin lattice relaxation times.
Am Heart J 1985; **109**: 486–90.

[60] Pflugfelder PW, Wisenberg G, Prato FS, Carroll E, Turner KL.
Early detection of canine myocardial infarction by magnetic resonance imaging in vivo.
Circulation 1985; **71**: 587–94.

[61] Higgins CB, Lanzer P, Stark O *et al.*
Imaging by nuclear magnetic resonance in patients with chronic ischemic heart disease.
Circulation 1984; **69**: 523–31.

[62] Johnston DL, Brady TJ, Ratner AV *et al.*
Assessment of myocardial ischemia with proton magnetic resonance: Effects of a three hour coronary occlusion with and without reperfusion.
Circulation 1985; **71**: 595–601.

[63] Ratner AV, Okada RD, Newell JB, Pohost GM.
The relationship between proton nuclear magnetic resonance relaxation parameters and myocardial perfusion with acute coronary arterial occlusion and reperfusion.
Circulation 1985; **71**: 823–8.

[64] Ratner AV, Barrett LV, Okada RD, Gang JL.
Alterations of the proton nuclear magnetic resonance spin-lattice relaxation time (T1) in rejecting cardiac allografts [Abstract].
J Am Coll Cardiol 1984; **3**: 538.

[65] Been M, Smith MA, Ridgeway JP et al.
Characterisation of acute myocardial infarction by gated magnetic resonance imaging.
Lancet 1985; ii: 348–50.

[66] Tscholakoff D, Higgins CB, McNamara MT, Derugin N.
Early-phase myocardial infarction: Evaluation by MR imaging.
Radiology 1986; **159**: 667–72.

[67] Tscholakoff D, Higgins CB, Sechtem U, Caputo G, Derugin N.
MRI of reperfused myocardial infarct in dogs.
Am J Roentgenol 1986; **146**: 925–30.

[68] Pflugfelder PW, Wisenberg G, Prato FS, Turner KL, Carroll E.
Serial imaging of canine myocardial infarction by in vivo nuclear magnetic resonance.
J Am Coll Cardiol 1986; **7**: 843–9.

[69] Weinman HJ, Brasch RC, Press WR, Wesbey GE.
Characteristics of gadolinium–DTPA complex: A potential NMR contrast agent.
Am J Roentgenol 1984; **142**: 619–29.

[70] Rehr RB, Peshock RM, Malloy CR et al.
Improved in vivo magnetic resonance imaging of acute infarction after intravenous paramagnetic contrast agent administration.
Am J Cardiol 1986; **57**: 864–8.

[71] Wesbey GE, Higgins CB, McNamara MT et al.
Effects of gadolinium–DTPA on the magnetic relaxation times of normal and infarcted myocardium.
Radiology 1984; **153**: 165–9.

[72] McNamara MT, Higgins CB, Ehman RL et al.
Acute myocardial ischaemia: Magnetic resonance contrast enhancement with gadolinium–DTPA.
Radiology 1984; **153**: 157–63.

[73] Axel L.
Blood flow effects in MRI.
Am J Roentgenol 1984; **143**: 1167–74.

[74] Herfkens RJ, Higgins CB, Hricak H et al.
Nuclear magnetic resonance imaging of atherosclerotic disease.
Radiology 1983; **148**: 161–6.

[75] Wesbey GE, Higgins CB, Amparo EG, Hale JD, Kaufman L, Pogany AC.
Peripheral vascular disease: Correlation of MR imaging and angiography.
Radiology 1985; **156**: 733–9.

[76] Jenkins JPR, Love HG, Foster CJ, Isherwood I, Rowlands DJ. Magnetic resonance imaging in the assessment of coronary artery bypass graft patency [Abstract]. In: *Proc 44th Annual Congress British Institute of Radiology*. London: British Institute of Radiology, 1986; p. 158.

[77] Miller DL, Reinig JW, Volkman DJ.
Vascular imaging with MRI: Inadequacy in Takayasu's arteritis compared with angiography.
Am J Roentgenol 1986; **146**: 949–54.

[78] Valk PE, Hale JD, Kaufman L, Crooks LE, Higgins CB.
MR imaging of the aorta with three dimensional image reconstruction: Validation by angiography.
Radiology 1985; **157**: 721–5.

[79] Valk PE, Hale JD, Crooks LE, Kaufman L, Higgins CB.
MR imaging of aortoiliac atherosclerosis with 3D image reconstruction.
J Comput Assist Tomogr 1986; **10**: 439–44.

[80] Wedeen VJ, Meuli RA, Edelman RR et al.
Projective imaging of pulsatile flow with magnetic resonance.
Science 1985; **230**: 946–8.

[81] Meuli RA, Wedeen VJ, Geller SC et al.
MR gated subtraction angiography: Evaluation of lower extremities.
Radiology 1986; **159**: 411–8.

[82] Nayler GL, Firmin DN, Longmore DB.
Cine MR blood flow imaging.
J Comput Assist Tomogr 1986; **10**: 715–22.

[83] van Dijk P.
Direct cardiac NMR imaging of heart wall and blood flow velocity.
J Comput Assist Tomogr 1984; **8**: 429–36.

[84] Wedeen VJ, Rosen BR, Chesler D, Brady TJ.
MR velocity imaging by phase display.
J Comput Assist Tomogr 1985; **9**: 530–6.

[85] Bradley WG Jr, Waluch V.
Blood flow: Magnetic resonance imaging.
Radiology 1985; **154**: 443–50.

[86] O'Donnell M.
NMR blood flow imaging using multiecho phase contrast sequences.
Med Phys 1985; **12**: 59–64.

[87] Moran PR, Moran RA, Karstaedt N et al.
Verification and evaluation of internal flow and motion. True magnetic resonance imaging by the phase gradient modulation method.
Radiology 1985; **154**: 433–41.

[88] Bryant DJ, Payne JA, Firmin DN, Longmore DB.
Measurement of flow with NMR imaging using a gradient pulse and phase difference technique.
J Comput Assist Tomogr 1984; **8**: 588–93.

[89] Longmore DB, Firmin DN, Nayler GL, Underwood SR, Klipstein RH.
Cine magnetic resonance blood flow imaging in clinical use.
Mag Res Imag 1986; **4**: 157.

[90] Waterton JC, Jenkins JPR, Zhu XP, Love HG, Isherwood I, Rowlands DJ.
Magnetic resonance (MR) cine imaging of the human heart.
Br J Radiol 1985; **58**: 711–6.

[91] Klipstein RH, Firmin DN, Underwood SR, Nayler GL, Rees RSO, Longmore DB.
Colour display of quantitative blood flow and cardiac anatomy in a single magnetic resonance cine loop.
Br J Radiol 1987 (in press).

[92] Underwood SR, Firmin DN, Klipstein RH, Rees RSO, Longmore DB.
Magnetic resonance velocity mapping: Clinical application of a new technique.
Br Heart J 1987 (submitted for publication).

[93] Frahm J, Haase A, Matthaei D.
Rapid three-dimensional MR imaging using the FLASH technique.
J Comput Assist Tomogr 1986; **10**: 363–8.

[94] Rzedzian R, Mansfield P, Doyle M *et al*.
Real-time nuclear magnetic resonance imaging in paediatrics.
Lancet 1983; **ii**: 1281–2.

DOPPLER ULTRASOUND

[1] Comparison of Doppler-derived pressure gradient to that determined at cardiac catheterization in adults with aortic valve stenosis: implications for management.
Yeager M, Yock P, Popp RL, Stanford Univ Sch Med, Stanford, CA, USA.
Am J Cardiol 1986; **57**: 644–8.

[2] Doppler hemodynamic evaluation of prosthetic (Starr-Edwards and Bjork-Shiley) and bioprosthetic (Hancock and Carpentier-Edwards) cardiac valves.
Williams GA, Labovitz AJ, St Louis Univ Hosp, St Louis, MO, USA.
Am J Cardiol 1985; **56**: 325–32.

[3] Valvar prosthetic dysfunction. Localisation and evaluation of the dysfunction using the Doppler technique.
Veyrat C, Witchitz S, Lessana A, Ameur A, Abitbol G, Kalmanson D, Fond A de Rothschild, Paris, France.
Br Heart J 1985; **54**: 273–84.

[4] Non-invasive assessment by Doppler ultrasound of 155 patients with bioprosthetic valves: a comparison of the Wessex porcine, low profile Ionescu-Shiley, and Hancock pericardial bioprostheses.
Simpson IA, Reece IJ, Houston AB, Hutton I, Wheatley DJ, Cobbe SM, Royal Infirm, Glasgow, UK.
Br Heart J 1986; **56**: 83–8.

Comment. Doppler ultrasound can be used as a non-invasive method of assessing the severity of aortic stenosis. Although there are considerable data available showing the accuracy of Doppler ultrasound in measuring aortic stenosis in children, there is less information available with respect to the assessment of this condition in adults. In a study by Yeager *et al* [1], cardiac catheterization was perfomed in 58 patients (mean age 66 years) within a mean of eight days of having been found to have elevated aortic blood flow velocity (>1.7 m/second) on continuous Doppler-wave echocardiography. The aortic-valve mean pressure gradients at catheterization ranged from 0 to 93 mmHg. The linear correlation coefficient (r value) between the mean pressure gradient determined by Doppler echocardiography and catheterization was 0.87. This correlation was maintained in 15 patients with aortic regurgitation ($r=0.91$) and in 16 patients with significant coronary artery disease ($r=0.93$). In the 16 patients with reduced cardiac output (mean 3.2 litres/minute, range 2.2–3.9), the correlation was 0.81. The authors derived a strategy for using the Doppler echo-calculated pressure gradient to manage patients with valvular aortic stenosis by investigating the relation of the Doppler echo gradient to the aortic-valve area in 35 patients with no aortic regurgitation detected at catheterization. All 12 patients with a Doppler echo mean gradient of <30 mmHg had an aortic-valve area of >0.75 cm^2; all patients with a Doppler echo mean gradient of >50 mmHg had an aortic-valve area of <0.75 cm^2. Nine patients with an aortic-valve area of <0.75 cm^2 and 3 patients with an aortic-valve area of >0.75 cm^2 had a Doppler echo mean gradient of between 30 and 50 mmHg. These data suggest that Doppler echocardiography is useful for distinguishing subgroups of patients with critical (mean gradient >50 mmHg) and non-critical (mean gradient <30 mmHg) aortic stenosis. However, when the mean gradient is intermediate (30–50 mmHg), additional data are necessary for the accurate non-invasive assessment of aortic stenosis.

Following cardiac valve replacement in patients with heart failure, catheterization is often required to exclude the possibility of dysfunction of the prosthesis. It is in this field that Doppler techniques may have their greatest potential for reducing the need for invasive investigation. The authors of these two papers report the results of Doppler examinations in a large number of patients with a variety of normal and malfunctioning prosthetic valves. Williams and Labovitz [2] established the range of Doppler-derived aortic gradients (from maximal velocity) and mitral areas (by the pressure half-time method) for Björk-Shiley, porcine and Starr-Edwards valves. They found evidence of mild regurgitation in 11–42% of cases, depending on the type of valve and its site of implantation. Abnormal function was detected in 11 valves, and confirmed by subsequent investigation or surgery in all cases. Veyrat *et al* [3] correctly diagnosed prosthetic valvular dysfunction in 35 of 37 patients. They were able to quantify, with a high degree of precision, the severity of regurgitation and determine its origin (para-prosthetic or leaflet tear) by jet mapping. In contrast to the study of Williams and Labovitz [2], however, evidence of regurgitation was found in only three of 88 apparently normal prostheses, and all appeared to be 'false-positive' findings [3].

In another study [4], Doppler ultrasound was used to assess the prosthetic function of 167 bioprosthetic valves (68 Wessex porcine, 54 Hancock pericardial and 45 low-profile Ionescu-Shiley pericardial valves) in 155 patients. The modified Bernoulli equation was used to calculate valve gradients from the mitral and aortic flow velocities. The mean mitral gradients were found to be significantly smaller across the Ionescu-Shiley valves than across either the Wessex or Hancock valves. However, mitral pressure half-time was found to be significantly longer in the Hancock pericardial valve than in the Wessex porcine or Ionescu-Shiley pericardial valves. There were

360

no significant differences among the aortic bioprostheses, although the comparable size of Wessex porcine valves showed significantly higher gradients. Doppler ultrasound detected bioprosthetic regurgitation in 13 of 103 mitral valves and in 11 of 59 aortic valves; regurgitation had been suspected clinically in 12 mitral and six aortic bioprostheses. The use of Doppler ultrasound to assess prosthetic function *in vivo* has much to recommend it; however, the use of the Bernoulli equation could be regarded as a limiting factor of this technique.

POSITRON EMISSION TOMOGRAPHY

[1] Reversibility of cardiac wall-motion abnormalities predicted by positron tomo-graphy.
Tillisch J, Brunken R, Marshall R *et al*, UCLA Med Cent, Los Angeles, CA, USA.
N Engl J Med 1986; **314**: 884–8.
[2] Identification of impaired metabolic reserve by atrial pacing in patients with significant coronary artery stenosis.
Grover-McKay M, Schelbert HR, Schwaiger M *et al,* Univ California Sch Med, Los Angeles, CA, USA.
Circulation 1986; **74**: 281–92.

Comment. Previous studies have shown that regional myocardial dysfunction at rest improves after adequate blood flow had been restored. The results of experimental studies have demonstrated that severe reductions in coronary flow may result in the loss of regional contractility with no evidence of myocardial infarction. Other studies have suggested that transient reductions in flow may lead to impaired contractility that persists beyond the duration of ischemia in the absence of frank myocardial necrosis. Thus, clinically, abnormalities of regional cardiac wall motion at rest may be due to persistently depressed blood flow, prolonged myocardial cellular dysfunction following transient ischemia or myocardial infarction. To estimate regional myocardial blood flow, positron emission tomography can be used with nitrogen-13-ammonia; to measure exogenous glucose uptake by the myocardium, it can be used with fluorine-18-deoxyglucose. In a study of 17 patients who underwent coronary artery bypass surgery [1], positron emission tomography was used to predict whether preoperative abnormalities of left ventricular wall motion are reversible. Radionuclide or contrast angiography or both were used to measure abnormalities before and after grafting. Images using positron emission tomography were obtained preoperatively. Abnormal wall motion in regions in which positron emission tomography had shown preserved glucose uptake was predicted to be reversible; abnormal motion in regions with depressed glucose uptake was predicted to be irreversible. Using these criteria, abnormal contraction in 35 of 41 segments was correctly predicted to be reversible (85% predictive accuracy); abnormal contraction was correctly predicted to be irreversible in 24 of 26 regions (92% predictive accuracy). By contrast, ECGs with pathological Q waves in the region of asynergy predicted reversibility in only 43% of regions. From these results, positron emission tomography is a useful technique for assessing blood flow and the metabolic viability of myocardium and it can predict the reversibility of wall-motion abnormalities after myocardial re-vascularization.

Positron emission tomography has also been used to investigate myocardial ^{11}C-palmitate clearance kinetics at resting heart rate and during pacing in 10 patients with significant coronary artery narrowing (>70%) and evidence of exercise-induced ischemia [2]. Serial ^{11}C-palmitate images were acquired at rest and during pacing for myocardiuim at risk, i.e. that supplied by a stenosed coronary artery, and normal myocardium, i.e. that supplied by a normal coronary artery. At rest, the average rate of myocardial ^{11}C-palmitate clearance was found to be similar for the normal myocardium and the myocardium at risk, which suggests that there was a similar rate and amount of myocardial fatty acid oxidation in the normal and the at-risk myocardium. However, on pacing, although clearance half-times were shorter and the residual fractions were decreased for both normal and at-risk myocardium, the clearance half-times were found to be 17% longer and the residual fractions were 14% higher in the myocardium at risk when compared with the normal myocardium (P<0.005 and P<0.01, respectively). This suggests there was impaired fatty acid metabolism in the myocardium at risk during pacing. As metabolic reserve can be measured by the increase in substrate utilization in response to an increase in workload, these data indicate that the metabolic reserve for free fatty acid oxidation is impaired in myocardium that is supplied by a significantly stenosed coronary artery (as demonstrated by analysis of myocardial ^{11}C-palmitate clearance kinetics). This study provides an elegant demonstration of processes of myocardial metabolism in ischemic heart disease.

8. Surgery

HEMODYNAMICS

PHARMACOLOGIC AGENTS

[1] Beneficial hemodynamic effects of oral levodopa in heart failure. Relation to the generation of dopamine.
Rajfer SI, Anton AH, Rossen JD, Goldberg LI, Univ Chicago, Chicago, IL, USA.
N Engl J Med 1984; **310**: 1357–62.

[2] Combined hemodynamic effects of dopamine and dobutamine in cardiogenic shock.
Richard C, Ricome JL, Rimailho A, Bottineau G, Auzepy P, Hop Bicetre, Le Kremlin Bicetre, France.
Circulation 1983; **67**: 620–5.

Comment. There is no inotropic agent available for oral use. Patients in need of inotropic support necessarily require the support of intravenous infusion. Thus, the paper of Rajfer *et al* [1] is of interest. They report on a useful pilot study with important potential and implications for both surgeons and physicians in cardiovascular medicine in which oral levodopa (1.5–2.0 g), which is decarboxylated to form dopamine, was given to 10 patients with severe congestive heart failure. Peak hemodynamic responses occurred one hour after the ingestion of levodopa, and the mean ($\pm$SEM) cardiac index increased from 1.8 $\pm$0.1 to 2.4 $\pm$0.2 l/min/m^2 of body-surface area ($P<0.01$), with systemic vascular resistance declining from 1905 $\pm$112 to 1513 $\pm$121 dyn/s/cm^{-5} ($P<0.01$). These effects persisted for 4–6 hours. Left-ventricular filling pressure, heart rate and mean arterial pressure were unchanged. Plasma concentrations of dopamine rose to a peak level of 34 $\pm$5 ng/ml one hour after drug ingestion, and decreased toward baseline over the following five hours. A significant correlation was observed between plasma dopamine levels and changes in cardiac index ($r = 0.8$; $P<0.02$). Five patients who were enrolled in a trial to evaluate the effectiveness of long-term therapy with levodopa had similar hemodynamic responses to the drug after 6.8 $\pm$1.7 months of treatment. Thus, oral administration of levodopa to patients with severe heart failure was found to produce a sustained improvement in cardiac function. The hemodynamic responses that were observed can be attributed to the activation of beta$_1$-adrenergic, dopamine$_1$ and dopamine$_2$ receptors by dopamine derived from levodopa.

Richard *et al* [2] explored the combined hemodynamic effects of dopamine and dobutamine in cardiogenic shock. In a small series of mechanically ventilated patients in cardiogenic shock, the hemodynamic effects of an infusion of dopamine and dobutamine in combination were compared with the effects of administering each alone. Stroke-volume index increased similarly with all infusions. However, the dopamine-dobutamine combination increased mean arterial pressure more than dobutamine alone, the maintenance of pulmonary capillary wedge pressure within normal limits was better than with dopamine alone, and the worsening of hypoxemia induced by dopamine was prevented. This study has important clinical applications of interest to the cardiac surgeon as well as to all cardiologists.

CARDIAC PHYSIOLOGY

[1] Influence of atrial systole on the Frank-Starling relation and the end-diastolic pressure-diameter relation of the left ventricle.
Linderer T, Chatterjee K, Parmley WW, Sievers RE, Glantz SA, Tyberg JV, Univ California, San Francisco, CA, USA.
Circulation 1983; **67**: 1045-53.
[2] Atrial transport function in coronary artery disease: relation to left ventricular function.
Hamby RI, Noble WJ, Murphy DH, Hoffman I, St Francis Hosp, Roslyn, NY, USA.
J Am Coll Cardiol 1983; **1**: 1011-7.

Comment. The contribution of atrial systole to hemodynamic performance has been assessed of late. In a study on dogs [1], Linderer *et al* attempted to explain previously reported observations that withdrawal of the atrial contribution to left-ventricular filling reduces left-ventricular stroke volume without simultaneously reducing filling pressure (i.e. it causes a downward shift in the conventional ventricular function curve). Data were obtained from open-chest anesthetized dogs during different volume loads with the pericardium open and closed. The mechanical contribution of atrial systole was varied by controlling atrioventricular synchrony. Left-ventricular end-diastolic pressure-diameter relations were measured in addition to the usual stroke volume-filling pressure curve.

Hamby *et al* [2] provide a good hemodynamic study in which atrial contribution to ventricular stroke volume was evaluated in normal subjects and in 50 patients with diseased myocardium. All patients underwent complete hemodynamic and angiographic studies to determine the atrial contribution to stroke volume, end-systolic volume and ejection fraction. In normal subjects and patients with coronary disease, the atrial contribution to stroke volume was 20% ±7% and 33% ±11%, respectively ($P<0.05$). The combination of congestive heart failure and cardiomegaly was the only clinical aspect associated with a significantly higher ($P<0.05$) atrial contribution to stroke volume than that in the remaining patients with coronary disease (46% *vs* 31%). No patient with an ejection fraction (>0.50) had an atrial contribution greater than 40% of stroke volume. The ratio of peak left-ventricular systolic pressure/end-systolic volume (mmHg/ml) was 2.7 ±1.5 in patients ($n=14$) with an atrial contribution $>40\%$ of stroke volume, compared with 5.3 ±3.4 in patients with an atrial contribution of $<40\%$ of stroke volume ($P<0.01$). These findings indicate that atrial contribution to stroke volume is inversely related to left-ventricular function. This study is of particular importance to cardiac surgery, where the necessity of maintaining sinus rhythm in the postoperative phase in those patients with poor ventricular function has been underestimated.

TECHNIQUES OF PRESERVATION

MYOCARDIAL PRESERVATION

CLINICAL

[1] Accelerated myocardial metabolic recovery with terminal warm blood cardioplegia.
Teoh KH, Christakis GT, Weisel RD *et al*, Toronto Gen Hosp, Toronto, Ontario, Canada.
J Thorac Cardiovasc Surg 1986; **91**: 888–95.

[2] A randomized comparison of crystalloid and blood-containing cardioplegic solutions in 60 patients.
Buttner EE, Karp RB, Reves JG *et al*, Univ Alabama Sch Med, Birmingham, AL, USA.
Circulation 1984; **69**: 973–82.

[3] Myocardial protection: a comparison of cold blood and cold crystalloid cardioplegia.
Iverson LIG, Young JN, Ennix CL Jr *et al*, Oakland, CA, USA.
J Thorac Cardiovasc Surg 1984; **87**: 509–16.

[4] Preservation of human cardiac contractility during anoxic arrest with glucose-containing cardioplegia.
Lolley DM, Regional Medical Cent, Madisonville, KY, USA.
Am Surg 1985; **51**: 256–61.

[5] First report of intramyocardial pH in man. II. Assessment of adequacy of myocardial preservation.
Khuri SF, Josa M, Marston W *et al*, Veterans Administration Med Cent, West Roxbury, MA, USA.
J Thorac Cardiovasc Surg 1983; **86**: 667–78.

[6] Cardioplegic protection of the child's heart.
Bull C, Cooper J, Stark J, Hosp Sick Children, London, UK.
J Thorac Cardiovasc Surg 1984; **88**: 287–93.

Comment. The methods of myocardial preservation using various cardioplegic techniques are now extremely complicated such that their importance may rival the cardiac operation itself (they take almost as long to perform as the operation). Blood cardioplegia has been shown to provide excellent myocardial protection. However, it is known to delay myocardial metabolic recovery, a factor that has limited its use. Teoh *et al*[1] conducted a prospective randomized trial of 20 patients undergoing elective coronary artery bypass grafting to assess the use of a terminal warm cardioplegic infusion after cold blood cardioplegia. Eleven patients received cold blood cardioplegia and nine received cold blood cardioplegia and warm blood cardioplegia before the removal of the aortic cross-clamp. The warm blood was found to provide oxygen and remove excess lactate from the arrested heart. After the warm blood cardioplegia, lactate was extracted by the heart, and tissue levels of adenosine triphosphate and glycogen were preserved. Atrial pacing and volume loading three and four hours postoperatively were found to decrease myocardial lactate extraction after cold blood cardioplegia but they increased lactate extraction after the warm blood. Left atrial pressures were higher at similar end-diastolic volumes (as measured by nuclear ventriculography), which suggests there was a decrease in diastolic compliance after cold blood cardioplegia. Thus, terminal warm blood cardioplegia accelerated myocardial metabolic recovery, preserved the high-energy phosphates, improved the myocardial metabolic response to postoperative hemodynamic stress and reduced the left atrial pressure.

The use of blood-containing cardioplegic solutions is, however, controversial. Buttner et al [2] carried out a randomized prospective trial of 60 patients undergoing coronary revascularization, and compared the effects of a crystalloid potassium cardioplegic solution with those of a similar solution to which blood had been added according to a modified Buckerg technique. Indices of myocardial metabolism (lactate, inorganic phosphate, base deficit release, glucose and lactate uptake, and oxygen extraction) and damage (creatine kinase-MB levels) were measured. The cardioplegic solution with added blood had a significantly greater oxygen content ($P<0.05$), a lower pH and higher concentrations of potassium, calcium, sodium and glucose. Although the authors found a greater uptake of oxygen in the patients with blood-containing cardioplegic solution ($P<0.06$) during the initial stages of cardioplegic infusion, this was not maintained at effective temperatures for myocardial protection. Furthermore, during myocardial reperfusion, no differences were found in any of the indices of myocardial metabolism or damage between the two groups of patients. The authors stress that within the limits of the system they found no additional protective effect when using a blood-containing cardioplegic solution. It should be borne in mind that such overall comparisons are difficult to make because of the variability among surgeons in their cardioplegic techniques. Nonetheless, this was a good attempt at rationalizing the relative merits of two cardioplegic solutions.

Iverson et al [3] carried out a well-designed study of 207 consecutive patients who were randomized into four groups on the basis of left-ventricular end-diastolic pressure, and subsequently into groups receiving either crystalloid cardioplegia or blood cardioplegia. They found that blood cardioplegia offered a slight but statistical advantage over crystalloid cardioplegia with respect to left-ventricular stroke work index, and also that levels of creatine kinase and serum glutamic oxaloacetic transaminase were slightly but significantly better with blood cardioplegia.

From these two studies [2,3] it would appear that the discrepancies observed probably result from the differences between individual surgeons and not from any differences in the solutions under evaluation.

In a study of 102 patients undergoing coronary artery surgery [4], patients were randomized to a control group or to myocardial protection in which the aortic root was infused with a hypothermic solution containing glucose, insulin and potassium (GIK) during aortic cross-clamping and anoxic arrest. This form of myocardial protection resulted in a significant preservation of human myocardial contractility indices. Control coronary artery surgery patients had acute post-cardiopulmonary bypass dp/dt_{max} depressed to 79.8% of pre-bypass levels and maintained only 73.0% of pre-bypass Vpm. Patients with aortic root GIK maintained 148.1% of pre-bypass dp/dt_{max} and 157.2% of pre-bypass Vpm, which were significantly better than control values ($P<0.001$). These patients also required significantly less vasopressor ($P<0.05$). Patients who maintained at least 85% of pre-bypass dp/dt_{max} or Vpm had less need of vasopressor in the recovery period ($P<0.05$). Peak quantified subsequent vasopressor need was found to be negatively correlated with the percentage of pre-bypass Vpm that was maintained ($P<0.05$). GIK root infusion enhanced anaerobic metabolism. The coronary wash-out of acidotic byproducts and direct cardiac buffer combined with an improved glycolytic flux and better global hypothermia would appear to be the mechanisms of contractility preservation. Contractility indices seem to be useful in determining subsequent vasopressor needs. This new technique has been well documented, and the results of its implementation are impressive; as such it merits inclusion in surgical practice.

Khuri et al [5] report an important experimental study of patients undergoing aortic cross-clamping during cardiac surgery. The adequacy of myocardial protection produced by systemic hypothermia and multidose potassium cardioplegia at $4°C$ was monitored using intramyocardial pH. The magnitude of the rise of intramyocardial pH produced by cardioplegia related directly to the adequacy of the myocardial protection produced. This was assessed by subsequent creatine phosphokinase-MB levels, ECG changes and radionuclide ventriculography. There was no relationship between myocardial temperature and either intramyocardial pH or recovery score. The authors conclude that, with aortic cross-clamping times >40 minutes during cardioplegic arrest, myocardial temperature is a poor indicator of the adequacy of myocardial preservation, because progressive tissue acidosis may occur despite low temperatures.

Bull et al [6] evaluated cardioplegia as a method of myocardial preservation in pediatric cardiac surgery in a consecutive series of 200 patients. Cytochemical and biophysical assessment of 129 pairs of right-ventricular biopsy specimens taken on bypass, before cardioplegic arrest and from the beating heart just prior to the cessation of bypass, usually demonstrated deterioration of the myocardium despite cardioplegia, and poor scores were found to be predictive of hospital death. The authors then compared early mortality related to ischemic time in the cardioplegia series with a previous consecutive series of 200 patients who had undergone intermittent ischemia as a method of myocardial preservation. (This comparison seems to be of doubtful value.) Finally, they performed a logistic analysis of the data, which they say suggest that "about half of the hospital deaths were attributable to inadequate myocardial preservation despite cardioplegia". This statement seems unequivocal and incautious, when one considers that the data presented in this paper are from a heterogeneous series.

EXPERIMENTAL

[1] Optimal intraoperative protection of myocardium distal to coronary stenoses.
Silverman NA, Schmitt G, Levitsky S, Feinberg H, Univ Illinois, Coll Med, Chicago, IL, USA.
J Thorac Cardiovasc Surg 1984; 88: 424–31.
[2] Comparison of distribution beyond coronary stenoses of blood and asanguineous cardioplegic solutions.
Robertson JM, Buckberg GD, Vinten-Johanden J, Leaf JD, UCLA Med Cent, Los Angeles, CA, USA.
J Thorac Cardiovasc Surg 1983; 86: 80–6.

[3] Myocardial preservation: effect of venous drainage.
Bennett EV Jr, Fewel JG, Grover FL, Trinkle JK, Univ Texas Health Sci Cent, San Antonio, TX, USA.
Ann Thorac Surg 1983; **36**: 132–42.

[4] Comparison of flow differences among venous cannulas.
Bennett EV Jr, Fewel JG, Ybarra J, Grover FL, Trinkle JK, Univ Texas Health Sci Cent, San Antonio, TX, USA.
Ann Thorac Surg 1983; **36**: 59–65.

[5] Cardiac performance during reperfusion improved by pretreatment with oxygen free-radical scavengers.
Otani H, Engelman Rm, Rousou JA, Breyer RH, Lemeshow S, Das DK, Univ Connecticut Hlth Cent, Framington, CT, USA.
J Thorac Cardiovasc Surg 1986; **91**: 290–5.

[6] Protective metabolic effects of propranolol during total myocardial ischemia.
Veronee CD, Lewis WR, Takla MW, Hull-Ryde EA, Lowe JE, Duke Univ Med Cent, Durham, NC, USA.
J Thorac Cardiovasc Surg 1986; **92**: 425–33.

[7] Effect of oxygenated crystalloid cardioplegia on the functional and metabolic recovery of the isolated perfused rat heart.
Coetzee A, Kotze J, Louw J, Lochner A, Univ Stellenbosch Med Sch, Tygerberg, South Africa.
J Thorac Cardiovasc Surg 1986; **91**: 259–69.

Comment. Silverman *et al* [1] studied 40 dogs to obtain metabolic evidence of improved delivery of cardioplegic solutions by the adjuvant use of nitroglycerin during cold cardioplegic arrest. Adenosine triphosphate was found to be preserved in the myocardium distal to a patent coronary artery, whether nitroglycerin was added to the cardioplegic solution or not. Moreover, nitroglycerin did not prevent the 26%–34% ($P<0.05$) decline observed in adenosine triphosphate levels when the left anterior descending coronary artery remained obstructed throughout ischemia. The metabolic reperfusion injury, manifested by a 37% ($P<0.01$) decline in adenosine triphosphate levels after aortic unclamping, was prevented when nitroglycerin was added to the cardioplegic solution. Surprisingly, the depletion of cardioplegic solution stores during ischemia was more severe in dogs which received nitroglycerin than in controls ($P<0.05$), and these metabolic changes did not correlate with regional myocardial temperature gradients. The data indicate that myocardium jeopardized by coronary stenoses can be preserved as well as that supplied by a patent coronary artery, if nitroglycerin is used as an adjuvant and if the mode of delivery of the cardioplegic solution is varied.

Robertson *et al* [2] reported on a canine study in which they compared the different efficiencies of asanguineous and blood cardioplegic solutions in the myocardium distal to critical stenoses. Blood cardioplegia resulted in more rapid arrest and lower myocardial temperatures distal to the stenosis than did asanguineous cardioplegia. This is primarily a function of the higher aortic pressures produced during cardioplegic delivery. It is a pity that these workers did not normalize aortic pressures to obtain a truer comparison.

Bennett and co-workers [3] assessed myocardial performance and damage after cardiopulmonary bypass in dogs in which the venous drainage was established using either a single atriocaval cannula or separate caval cannulae, either snared or unsnared. With single-dose cardioplegia, the single cannula produced the lowest myocardial temperatures ($P<0.001$). Myocardial rewarming to $20°C$ was not significantly different with either cannulation. Coronary blood flow was determined with microspheres; myocardial metabolites and left-ventricular function were measured before and after bypass. The authors found better postischemic blood flow, glycogen levels and ventricular compliance differences in the dogs with a single atriocaval cannula.

In another canine study, Bennett et al [4] showed that venous drainage was better and caval pressure lower using double-snared caval cannulae but that this method was poorest at right-heart decompression. The latter improved proportionately using unsnared cavae and a USCI size 40F atrial cannula. The Sarns 51F atriocaval cannula had the most efficient right-heart decompression.

It has recently been suggested that oxygen-derived free radicals play a significant role in reperfusion injury of the myocardium following ischemia. In an experimental study [5], two groups of isolated pig hearts were subjected to 60 minutes of regional ischemia at normothermia by occlusion of the left anterior descending coronary artery, followed by 60 minutes of hypothermic cardioplegic arrest and 60 minutes of normothermic reperfusion; one group acted as controls, the other received the oxygen free-radical scavengers, superoxide dismutase and catalase, before occlusion of the left anterior descending coronary artery. During reperfusion, there was a significant generation of free radicals in the untreated group (measured by the level of malondialdehyde in the perfusate), which was associated with an increase in creatine kinase. However, in the treated group, superoxide dismutase and catalase were found to slow significantly the appearance of malondialdehyde and the release of creatine kinase during reperfusion. Although the oxygen free-radical scavengers did not alter coronary blood flow and myocardial oxygen extraction or consumption during occlusion, coronary flow and oxygen consumption during reperfusion were significantly higher in the hearts treated with anti-oxidants. Moreover, the decline in left ventricular developed pressure and its maximum first derivative observed in the untreated group were significantly inhibited in the group treated with superoxide dismutase and catalase; left ventricular end diastolic pressure was not altered significantly. These results further implicate oxygen-derived free radicals in the reperfusion injury of ischemic myocardium, and they indicate that free-radical scavengers are an effective protection against such injury. It is interesting to note that the use of mannitol during cardiopulmonary bypass for its effect on the renal system must have had a dual role for years without the significance of its effect on the production of oxygen-derived free radicals being recognized.

It is thought that beta-blockers exert their protective effect in patients with coronary heart disease primarily by decreasing heart rate and subsequent myocardial work, and it is standard clinical practice to continue beta-blockade until a patient undergoes coronary artery bypass surgery. In a study of 24 anesthetized dogs subjected to total myocardial ischemia at $37°C$, the primary protective effects of beta-blockade on the globally ischemic myocardium were determined [6]. The levels of high-energy nucleotide and lactate were determined at control, 15-minute intervals and the onset of ischemic contracture. Seventeen of the dogs had been treated with propranolol before ischemia. Propranolol was found to reduce the time to ischemic contracture: it was 63.3 ± 1.4 minutes in control dogs and 75.9 ± 2.2 minutes in the dogs treated with propranolol ($P<0.01$). Propranolol was also found to decrease the rate of anaerobic glycolysis during ischemia: the control dogs had an average adenosine triphosphate level of 1.25 ± 10.08 mol/g wet weight ($P<0.0025$). These results suggest that the protective effects of beta-blockade may be related to a beneficial effect on the metabolism of the ischemic myocardium enabling the myocardium to survive at lower levels of adenosine triphosphate.

The oxygenation of crystalloid cardioplegic solution has never been regarded as a viable surgical practice for the preservation of the myocardium. However, the results of a study of the efficacy of oxygenated crystalloid cardioplegia, using isolated per-fused rat heart as a model, should stimulate a re-evaluation of this proposition [7]. The experiments were conducted at 4°C and 20°C. The average oxygen tension of the non-oxygenated cardioplegic solution was 117 mmHg; it was 440 mmHg for the oxygenated solution. The adenosine triphosphate content of hearts subjected to 120 minutes of oxygenated cardioplegia at 4°C was significantly higher than that of hearts subjected to non-oxygenated cardioplegia; however, the functional recovery during reperfusion was found to be the same for both groups. At 20°C, myocardial adenosine triphosphate concentration decreased at a significantly faster rate during ischemia in the group receiving non-oxygenated cardioplegia than it did in the group receiving oxygenated cardioplegia. Hearts subjected to 180 minutes of ischemia with oxygenated cardioplegia were found to have a normal ultrastructural appearance, whereas those hearts subjected to only 120 minutes of non-oxygenated cardioplegia were found to have undergone severe ischemic damage. Functional recovery of the myocardium was greater in the group receiving an oxygenated cardioplegic solution. Myocardial adenosine triphosphate concentration at the end of ischemia was found to be a predictor of subsequent cardiac output, peak systolic blood pressure and total myocardial work.

SPINAL CORD PRESERVATION

[1] Relationship of spinal cord blood flow to vascular anatomy during thoracic aortic cross-clamping and shunting.
    Svensson LG, Rickards E, Coull A, Rogers G, Fimmel CJ, Hinder RA, Univ Witwatersrand, Johannesburg, South Africa.
    J Thorac Cardiovasc Surg 1986; 91: 71-8.
[2] The arteria radicularis magna anterior as a decisive factor influencing spinal cord damage during aortic occlusion.
    Wadouh F, Lindemann E-V, Arndt CF, Hetzer R, Borst HG, Hanover Med Sch, Hanover, GFR.
    J Thorac Cardiovasc Surg 1984; 88: 1-10.
[3] Acute spinal cord ischemia: prevention of paraplegia with verapamil.
    Gelbfish JS, Phillips T, Rose DM, Wait R, Cunningham JN, Maimonides Med Cent, Brooklyn, NY, USA.
    Circulation 1986; **74** (Suppl I): 1-5.

Comment. There is no satisfactory explanation for the occurrence of paraplegia following thoracic aortic interruption despite the practice of distal aortic perfusion. Svensson *et al* [1] used radioactive microspheres to study the hemodynamics, paraplegia rate and spinal cord blood flow of 17 baboons divided into three groups: control animals, animals subjected to cross-clamping for 60 minutes and those subjected to aortic-aortic shunts for 60 minutes. Shunting was found to increase significantly lumbar spinal cord blood flow, which correlated with distal aortic mean pressure. However, lower thoracic spinal cord blood flow was not found to increase during shunting nor did it correlate with distal aortic pressure. These results can be explained in terms of the vascular anatomy of the anterior spinal artery (and those of the baboon and man are the same), which is smaller above than below the entry of the arteria radicularis magna. Using Poiseuille's equation, it was calculated that the resistance to flow was 51.7 times greater up the anterior spinal artery than down it. Thus, it can be seen that distal aortic perfusion protects the spinal cord below but not above the arteria radicularis magna.

Wadouh *et al* [2] assessed damage to the spinal cord in 47 pigs which underwent occlusion of the descending aorta for 45 minutes and one of the following five protocols: no reduction in arterial blood pressure proximal to the site of occlusion; no reduction in arterial blood pressure proximal to the site of occlusion plus drainage of the cerebrospinal fluid; reduction in arterial blood pressure; reduction in arterial blood pressure plus drainage of the cerebrospinal fluid; or permanent ligation of the artery of Adamkiewicz. The authors did not find any significant difference in the degree of permanent spinal cord damage observed among the various protocols, which varied from 71.4% to 85.7%. The frequency of spinal cord damage was found to be independent of arterial blood pressure, intracranial pressure and intraspinal pressure, and the intracranial pressure and intraspinal pressure were significantly dependent upon the central venous pressure but independent of the arterial blood pressure. This interesting study is more relevant to conditions during surgery for thoracic aneurysm than to those during surgery for coarctation of the aorta, in which the collateral vessels are likely to play a more protective role.

The occurrence of injury to the spinal cord as a result of cardiac surgery is unpredictable. Recently, the suggestion that calcium-mediated metabolic events are responsible for the damage to neuronal cells during reperfusion has been put forward. In an experimental study using a canine model [3], the effect of verapamil on the neurologic sequelae of spinal cord ischemia was investigated by monitoring somatosensory evoked potentials. Five dogs were pretreated with 0.4 mg/kg verapamil and five dogs acted as the control group. The thoracic aorta was occluded; 17 minutes after the complete loss of somatosensory evoked potentials, flow was restored. Additional doses of verapamil were given to the experimental group on reperfusion and at 1, 2, 3, 4, 5, 6 and 10 hours after reperfusion. Four of the 5 verapamil-treated dogs were able to walk postoperatively whereas all the control animals developed paraplegia. Obviously, this investigation is only preliminary; however, it does provide a strong case for assessing this relatively safe therapy clinically.

CORONARY ARTERY BYPASS SURGERY

CORONARY ARTERY BYPASS SURGERY IN MILD ANGINA

Myocardial infarction and mortality in the Coronary Artery Surgery Study (CASS) randomized trial.
CASS Principal Investigators and their Associates, Univ Washington, Seattle, WA, USA.
N Engl J Med 1984; **310**: 750-8.

Comment. The long-term benefit of coronary bypass surgery in terms of longevity and prevention of major ischemic events in patients who have mild angina is not well defined. The randomized Coronary Artery Surgery Study (CASS) was designed to evaluate this issue; it consists of 780 patients who were considered operable and who had mild stable angina pectoris or who were free of angina after infarction. Patients were randomly assigned to medical or surgical treatment groups. The likelihood of death in the five-year period after randomization was 8% in the medical cohort, as compared with 5% in the surgical cohort (not significant). The likelihood of non-fatal Q-wave myocardial infarction was 11% and 14%, respectively (not significant). The five-year probability of remaining alive and free of infarction was 82% in the patients assigned to medical therapy and 83% in the patients assigned to surgery (not significant). There were no statistically significant differences in the survival rate or in the myocardial infarction rate between subgroups of patients randomly assigned to medical and to surgical therapy when they were analyzed according to initial group assignment, number of diseased vessels or ejection fraction. Therefore, as compared with medical therapy, coronary bypass surgery appears neither to prolong life nor to prevent myocardial infarction in patients who have mild angina or who are asymptomatic after infarction in the five-year period after coronary angiography. However, it is important to note that patients with left main stenosis were excluded from the trial and that approximately 25% of the so-called 'medical group' underwent coronary bypass surgery during the study. The message of CASS is that it is safe to delay the decision for surgery if left main stenosis is excluded and the angina is mild.

INTERNAL THORACIC (MAMMARY) ARTERY GRAFTS IN CORONARY ARTERY SURGERY

Review: FLOYD D. LOOP

Approximately 15 years of coronary artery surgery were to elapse from initial developments before reports about the internal thoracic (mammary) artery conduit demonstrated the unequivocal superiority of that (arterial) graft over the aortocoronary saphenous vein graft. Until recently, few surgeons have used the internal thoracic artery graft; the procedure is tedious and, in inexperienced hands, fraught with technical complications. In 1984, only 11% of nearly 200 000 coronary artery operations involved an internal thoracic artery graft. Because saphenous vein degeneration frequently occurs after the seventh postoperative year, it takes follow-up at least that long to document significant patency differences, and probably up to 10 years to show improvement in survival and freedom from certain cardiac events.

The vein graft is intrinsically prone to intimal degeneration. Vein-graft attrition after the first postoperative year averages 2% per year until the fifth to seventh postoperative year, when it accelerates to 5% per year [1]. At 10–12 years, approximately half of the aortocoronary saphenous vein grafts will be open and, of those still patent, half will show wall alterations consistent with vein-graft atherosclerosis. Elevated serum cholesterol and triglyceride concentrations, low levels of high-density lipoproteins, and diabetes appear to predispose to vein-graft atherosclerosis [1,2]. Degeneration of the vein graft has become the leading cause of coronary artery reoperation [3].

Patency and Physiologic Response
Many reports attest to the high early patency of internal thoracic artery grafts. Recently, a large number of single internal thoracic artery grafts, sequential internal thoracic artery grafts to the circumflex system, and isolated free and free sequential grafts were studied shortly after surgery up to 32 weeks [4,5]. The early patency rates approached 100%, the only exception occurring in grafts placed through the transverse sinus. It is likely that compression from the size of the pedicle, and tension or twisting of the anastomosis, accounted for the reduced patency rates under these circumstances. The left internal thoracic artery appears to yield a higher patency rate than the right internal thoracic artery [6–9]. We at The Cleveland Clinic Foundation believe that use of the right internal thoracic artery frequently involves grafting at the most distal point on the pedicle to reach the right coronary branches, the anterior descending artery, or the circumflex system through the transverse sinus. The distance required may lead to tension in reaching the point of anastomosis, which could account for the lower patency. There is clearly a learning curve related to extension of the use of internal thoracic artery grafts.

In contrast to the vein graft, the internal thoracic artery graft has shown consistently high patency rates up to 12 years postoperatively which far exceed late patency for vein grafts, even when conduits are matched with the recent bypassed anterior descending artery. The patency of anterior descending vein grafts is significantly higher than that of grafts to other major coronary arteries. When we compared 841 internal thoracic artery grafts to the anterior descending artery with 1445 vein grafts to that vessel, overall patency was 96% and 81%, respectively ($P<0.0001$) [10]. Internal thoracic artery patency was consistently above 90% (Fig. 1), compared with the downward trend in time for vein grafts performed to the anterior descending artery.

The sequential internal thoracic artery graft is often used to gain additional revascularization from a single conduit. The best combinations are diagonal/anterior descending or vice versa, and circumflex/circumflex. Initial reports indicate satisfactory patency correlated with negative postoperative exercise stress tests [11].

The free internal thoracic artery graft is useful for avoiding the crossing of the midline and for gaining length. In 156 consecutive patients who received the free

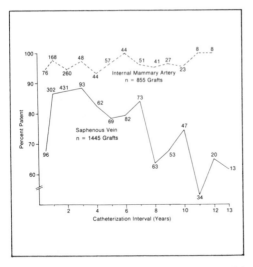

FIGURE 1: The patency of internal thoracic (mammary) artery and saphenous vein grafts to the anterior descending coronary artery at one-year intervals. The number of patients restudied at each interval is noted. (Reprinted by permission of *The New England Journal of Medicine* 1986; **314**: 1–6.)

arterial conduit in the aortocoronary position, 84% of 75 free thoracic arteries restudied a mean of four years postoperatively were patent [12]. Whereas only 77% of free grafts studied within 18 months were open, 92% of those studied more than five years postoperatively were patent, with no sign of late graft atherosclerosis. The lower early patency rate is attributable to technical problems in the construction of the aortic anastomosis, which have largely been solved.

Patency is not necessarily synonymous with nutritive perfusion. However, judging from the results of numerous non-invasive studies, it is apparent that the internal thoracic artery provides sufficient blood flow to meet oxygen demands of the myocardium. We found that patients with one-vessel disease who received either a single internal thoracic artery graft or a single vein graft had comparably improved physiologic performance, as judged by graded exercise testing [13]. The use of the internal thoracic artery graft in patients with multi-vessel disease who received one or more arterial grafts alone or in combination with vein grafts was associated with improved exercise tolerance also, which was attributed to the additional arterial perfusion [14]. Radioactive xenon washout studies of regional myocardial perfusion with patients at rest and after infusion of isoproterenol have shown comparable perfusion in the distribution of arterial and vein grafts [15]. Recently, Johnson *et al* have reviewed studies testing the sufficiency of internal thoracic artery blood flow [16]. After adding their results with exercise thallium-201 scintigraphy, the internal thoracic artery compared favorably with the vein graft during periods of peak myocardial oxygen demand. These authors conclude that prior concerns about inadequate peak flow from the internal thoracic artery are unfounded. This information, coupled with sequential arteriography showing that the internal thoracic artery may increase in size *in situ* [17], indicates that the internal thoracic artery may adapt to provide blood flow adequate to meet oxygen demands, even at peak exercise capacity.

The low incidence of atherosclerosis in the internal thoracic artery graft is puzzling, and possibly related to the vasoactive properties of the arterial wall that are protective against atherosclerosis. The persistent consequent patency appears to be the major reason for the discrepancy in late results between patients who have had an internal thoracic artery graft to the anterior descending artery and those who have received vein grafts only.

Influence on Survival and Cardiac Events

Clinical results in terms of relief of angina indicate consistently satisfactory performance with the internal thoracic artery graft [6,18]. These results, coupled with the better prolonged patency and relief of ischemia, prompted us to compare clinical results in two coronary artery surgical groups operated on between 1971 and 1978: (i) patients who had received an internal thoracic artery graft to the anterior descending artery alone or combined with vein grafts to other coronary arteries; and (ii) patients who had undergone vein graft surgery only. Patients in both groups were followed for a mean of nine years. Since the internal thoracic artery graft is performed mainly to the anterior descending coronary artery, we included patients with severe narrowing or occlusion of that vessel. In the years of observation, we recognized that early patency was higher among the internal thoracic artery grafts, but did not know whether these grafts improved survival or reduced cardiac events postoperatively. Toward the end of the 1970s, it was clear that a substantial difference in late patency existed, and that the internal thoracic artery was therefore preferable as a bypass graft. This led to the preferential use of the conduit subsequently. Accordingly, we did not include patients operated on after 1979 in the comparative study. We excluded left main stenosis >70%, emergency cases, reoperations, and bilateral, sequential, and free internal thoracic artery grafts throughout.

The analysis included 2306 patients with an internal thoracic artery graft to the anterior descending artery with or without vein grafts to other coronary arteries, and 3625 with vein grafts only. After adjustment for demographic and clinical differences among the two groups, the presence of an internal thoracic artery graft to the anterior descending artery was found to improve 10-year survival significantly (Fig. 2a-c). In the one-vessel disease subset (anterior descending), those who received an arterial graft had a 93.4% 10-year survival, compared with 88% in patients with a vein graft to the anterior descending artery. For two-vessel disease, the 10-year survival was 90% and

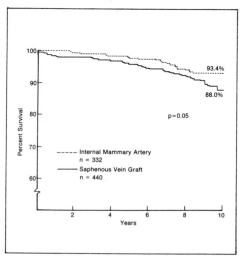

FIGURE 2a: Ten-year survival of patients with one-vessel (anterior descending artery) disease who had either an isolated internal thoracic artery graft or a vein graft. The survival difference was statistically significant by univariate analysis; however, when preoperative multivariate characteristics were entered, significance was lost. (Reprinted by permission of *The New England Journal of Medicine* 1986; **314:** 1–6.)

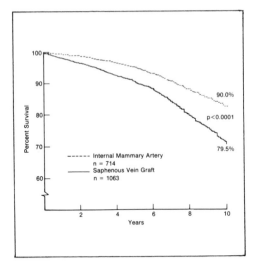

FIGURE 2b: Ten-year survival of patients with two-vessel disease, including those with lesions of the proximal anterior descending artery. The difference in survival between the patients who received internal thoracic artery grafts and those who received saphenous vein grafts was significant according to univariate and multivariate analysis. (Reprinted by permission of *The New England Journal of Medicine* 1986; **314**: 1–6.)

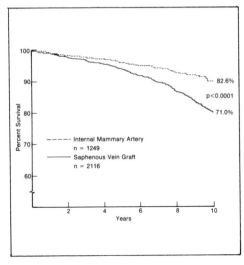

FIGURE 2c: Ten-year survival of patients with three-vessel disease. The internal thoracic artery group contained those who had one internal thoracic artery graft and one or more saphenous vein grafts. The saphenous vein graft group had vein grafts only. The differences between the two groups were significant according to univariate and multivariate analysis. (Reprinted by permission of *The New England Journal of Medicine* 1986; **314**: 1–6.)

79%, respectively, and for three-vessel disease, survival was 82.6% and 71.0%, respectively. All of these figures were highly significant, regardless of left-ventricular function.

The incidence of late myocardial infarction, reoperation, and death was reduced significantly by use of the internal thoracic artery graft. Patients in the internal thoracic artery graft group did not experience a significant influence on recurrence of severe angina or hospitalization for cardiac arrhythmia. This analysis and that of Okies *et al* [19] indicate that fewer cardiac events occur after an internal thoracic artery graft to the anterior descending artery than after vein grafts only.

Subsequently, Cameron *et al* reviewed 748 patients operated on by Green, who were divided into 532 with one or two internal thoracic artery grafts and 216 with vein grafts only [20]. The 14-year survival rate for the internal thoracic artery graft group was 72%, as against 57% for the vein-graft group. These patients, who were followed for up to 15 years, had significantly better cumulative survival, less early recurrence of angina, fewer myocardial infarctions, fewer reoperations, and better cumulative event-free survival, when the internal thoracic artery graft was used. Furthermore, these investigators found that patients with postoperative angina had a better cumulative survival after internal thoracic artery grafts than after vein grafts alone. Patients with double internal thoracic artery grafts had the best survival rates and the highest event-free survival of all. Bilateral internal thoracic artery grafting yielded an 86% 14-year survival, which confirms the 83% survival at 10 years reported by Galbut *et al* [8].

Contraindications are relative, but one should give consideration to *not* using the internal thoracic artery graft in the following situations: (i) advanced age (>75 years); (ii) emergency surgery in unstable patients; (iii) unusually large coronary arteries associated with left-ventricular hypertrophy; (iv) extensive brachiocephalic atherosclerosis; (v) poor left-ventricular function with left-ventricular ejection fraction <30%; (vi) endarterectomy because of lengthened arteriotomy site; (vii) higher-risk combined operations (e.g. simultaneous carotid endarterectomy, ventricular aneurysmectomy, or valve repair and replacement); (viii) left main trunk cases in which only an anterior descending graft is feasible; and (ix) previous chest-wall irradiation.

The above studies have shown that internal thoracic artery grafts for focal proximal atherosclerotic narrowing of the anterior descending artery are the preferable conduits, and should be used whenever clinically indicated and technically feasible. The most likely reason for the increased survival and significantly improved freedom from important cardiac events postoperatively is that the anterior descending is strategically the most important artery. Narrowing of the anterior descending artery is a greater determinant of survival than that of any other artery, with the exception of the left main artery [21]. High-grade proximal stenosis is a risk factor for premature death [22], and is more likely to cause fatal myocardial infarction than are acute obstructions of any other coronary artery - again with the exception of the left main artery [23].

Finally, these favorable late results are not achieved at increased perioperative risk. In internal thoracic artery grafts to the anterior descending artery, there have been no additional wound or pulmonary complications reported from our earlier experience [24]. Lytle *et al*, in dealing with the risk of bilateral internal thoracic artery grafting, found only eight major wound complications among 500 consecutive patients; however, a greater percentage of wound complications occurred among diabetics [25].

Conclusions

The excellent results achieved with one internal thoracic artery graft to the anterior descending artery suggest that expanded use to sequential, bilateral, and free grafts is warranted as long as morbidity and mortality are not increased. Late results with these techniques, particularly bilateral internal thoracic artery grafting, justify their continued application. Thus far, our experience with the single arterial graft indicates that: (i) it can be performed without significant increase in morbidity; (ii) it provides adequate flow to relieve ischemia; (iii) the long-term patency rate of grafts to the anterior descending artery exceeds 90%; (iv) this arterial graft will increase in size depending upon the peripheral coronary resistance; (v) the performance of grafting to the anterior descending artery significantly improves 10-year survival in categories of one-, two- and three-vessel disease, regardless of preoperative left-ventricular function; and (vi) performance of left internal thoracic artery grafting to the anterior descending artery decreases late incidence of myocardial infarction, cardiac hospitalization, and cardiac reoperation.

The therapeutic implications are that these arterial conduits should be performed to revascularize the most critical areas of arterial underperfusion. The internal thoracic artery graft deserves the widest application in younger patients. Surgeons using this arterial graft should document their results, especially with expanded usage.

References

[1] Campeau L, Enjalbert M, Lespérance J et al. The relation of risk factors to the development of atherosclerosis in saphenous-vein bypass grafts and the progression of disease in the native circulation: A study 10 years after aorto-coronary bypass surgery. *N Engl J Med* 1984; **311**: 1329–32.

[2] Lytle BW, Loop FD, Cosgrove DM, Ratliff NB, Easley K, Taylor PC. Long-term (5 to 12 years) serial studies of internal mammary artery and saphenous vein coronary bypass grafts. *J Thorac Cardiovasc Surg* 1985; **89**: 248–58.

[3] Loop FD, Lytle BW, Gill CC, Golding LAR, Cosgrove DM, Taylor PC. Trends in selection and results of coronary artery reoperations. *Ann Thorac Surg* 1983; **36**: 380–8.

[4] Rankin JS, Newman GE, Bashore TM et al. Clinical and angiographic assessment of complex mammary artery bypass grafting. *J Thorac Cardiovasc Surg* 1986; **92**: 832–46.

[5] Russo P, Orszulak TA, Schaff HV, Holmes DR Jr. Use of internal mammary artery grafts for multiple coronary artery bypasses. *Circulation* 1986; **74** (Suppl 3): 48–52.

[6] Barner HB, Swartz MT, Mudd JG, Tyras DH. Late patency of the internal mammary artery as a coronary bypass conduit. *Ann Thorac Surg* 1982; **34**: 408–12.

[7] Lytle BW, Cosgrove DM, Saltus GL, Taylor PC, Loop FD. Multivessel coronary revascularization without saphenous vein: Long-term results of bilateral internal mammary artery grafting. *Ann Thorac Surg* 1983; **36**: 540–7.

[8] Galbut DL, Traad EA, Dorman MJ et al. Twelve year experience with bilateral internal mammary artery grafts. *Ann Thorac Surg* 1985; **40**: 264–70.

[9] Huddleston CB, Stoney WS, Alford WC Jr et al. Internal mammary artery grafts: Technical factors influencing patency. *Ann Thorac Surg* 1986; **42**: 543–9.

[10] Loop FD, Lytle BW, Cosgrove DM et al. Influence of the internal-mammary-artery graft on 10-year survival and other cardiac events. *N Engl J Med* 1986; **314**: 1–6.

[11] Tector AJ, Schmahl TM, Canino VR, Kallies JR, Sanfilippo D. The role of the sequential internal mammary artery graft in coronary surgery. *Circulation* 1984; **70** (Suppl 1): 222–5.

[12] Loop FD, Lytle BW, Cosgrove DM, Golding LAR, Taylor PC, Stewart RW. Free (aorto-coronary) internal mammary artery graft: Late results. *J Thorac Cardiovasc Surg* 1986; **92**: 827–31.

[13] Siegel W, Loop FD. Comparison of internal mammary artery and saphenous vein bypass grafts for myocardial revascularization: Exercise test and angiographic correlations. *Circulation* 1976; **54** (Suppl 3): 1–3.

[14] Vogel JHK, McFadden RB, Spence R, Jahnke EJ Jr, Love JW. Quantitative assessment of myocardial performance and graft patency following coronary bypass with the internal mammary artery. *J Thorac Cardiovasc Surg* 1978; **75**: 487–98.

[15] Schmidt DH, Blau F, Hellman C, Grzelak L, Johnson WD. Isoproterenol-induced flow responses in mammary and vein bypass grafts. *J Thorac Cardiovasc Surg* 1980; **80**: 319–26.

[16] Johnson AM, Kron IL, Watson DD, Gibson RS, Nolan SP. Evaluation of postoperative flow reserve in internal mammary artery bypass grafts. *J Thorac Cardiovasc Surg* 1986; **92**: 822–6.

[17] Singh RN, Beg RA, Kay EB.
Physiological adaptability: The secret of suc-
cess of the internal mammary artery grafts.
Ann Thorac Surg 1986; **41**: 247–50.

[18] Tector AJ, Schmahl TM, Janson B, Kallies JR,
Johnson G.
The internal mammary artery graft: Its longevity
after coronary bypass.
J Am Med Assoc 1981; **246**: 2181–3.

[19] Okies JE, Page US, Bigelow JC, Krause AH,
Salomon NW.
The left internal mammary artery: The graft of
choice.
Circulation 1984; **70** (Suppl 1): 213–21.

[20] Cameron A, Kemp HG Jr, Green GE.
Bypass surgery with the internal mammary
artery graft: 15 year follow-up.
Circulation 1986; **74** (Suppl 3): 30–6.

[21] Klein LW, Weintraub WS, Agarwal JB *et al.*
Prognostic significance of severe narrowing of
the proximal portion of the left anterior descending coronary artery.
Am J Cardiol 1986; **58**: 42–6.

[22] European Coronary Surgery Study Group.
Long-term results of prospective randomised
study of coronary artery bypass surgery in
stable angina pectoris.
Lancet 1982; ii: 1173–80.

[23] Schuster EH, Griffith LS, Bulkley BH.
Preponderance of acute proximal left anterior
descending coronary arterial lesions in fatal
myocardial infarction: A clinicopathologic
study.
Am J Cardiol 1981; **47**: 1189–96.

[24] Cosgrove DM, Loop FD, Lytle BW *et al.*
Does mammary artery grafting increase sur-
gical risk?
Circulation 1985; **72** (Suppl 2): 170–4.

[25] Lytle BW, Cosgrove DM, Loop FD, Borsh J,
Goormastic M, Taylor PC.
Perioperative risk of bilateral internal mammary
artery grafting: Analysis of 500 cases from
1971 to 1984.
Circulation 1986; **74** (Suppl 3): 37–41.

ASPIRIN AND VEIN GRAFTS

Review: PHILIP C. ADAMS, JAMES H. CHESEBRO, VALENTIN FUSTER

Aortocoronary venous bypass grafting provides effective relief from symptoms of
angina due to obstructive atherosclerotic coronary artery disease, and in important
subgroups of patients improves life-expectancy. However, the success of coronary
artery grafting is limited by vein-graft closure. At one month, 15%–30% of patients not
receiving antithrombotic therapy will have at least one occluded vein graft, while about
10% of distal anastomoses are associated with an occluded graft [1–3].

Mechanisms of Graft Closure

Three mechanisms contribute to graft closure – thrombosis, intimal hyperplasia and
true atherosclerosis.

Early Thrombotic Occlusion

Early occlusion is generally thrombotic [4,5], the thrombosis being stimulated by
damage to the vein-graft wall. Platelet deposition onto the vein graft begins during
surgery [6], the venous endothelium being unavoidably damaged during harvesting,
preparation and insertion. Damage may be produced by sudden exposure to the
high-pressure arterial system, and a reduction in the nutrition of the wall of the vein may
also contribute to thrombosis. Thrombus is most commonly found around the distal
anastomosis, where the arteriotomy and venotomy have, of necessity, produced deep
damage to the vessel wall, thus stimulating thrombus formation [7]. Recently, inaccu-

rate suturing has been shown by angioscopy to be a cause of local problems, while other technical factors – for example, kinking of the graft and inappropriate graft length – are well-known contributors to early graft closure.

The importance of platelet deposition in the production of thrombosis is demonstrated by studies in which labeled platelets have been detected on the canine coronary vein graft [6]. However, fibrin is also commonly detected on the surface of vein grafts at autopsy early after grafting, emphasizing that the coagulation system (as well as platelets) is stimulated at this time [7]. Further support for this comes from the ability of fibrinolytic agents to lyse thrombi responsible for early vein-graft closure [8].

Intimal Hyperplasia

Up to one year after surgery, intimal hyperplasia develops in vein grafts. This produces a diffuse reduction in graft caliber of 25%–30% when compared with an early postoperative evaluation. The reduction in diameter is due to the proliferation of intimal smooth muscle cells, which begins within 30 days of surgery [5,9], and progresses so that the intima may be several-fold thicker than the media and may obstruct the graft [10].

It is likely that hyperplasia is stimulated by platelet deposition, with release of mitogens, including platelet-derived growth factor. Other cells – for example, newly grown endothelial cells – may also release growth factors. Continuing platelet deposition may well be responsible for continuing stimulation of intimal hyperplasia. Studies of vein grafts to the carotid in rabbits [11], and of coronary bypass grafts in dogs [12], up to one month after operation show continuing platelet deposition. Normally, when the subendothelium or neointima alone is exposed, an injured vessel loses its thrombogenicity within about eight hours [13]. Why, then, does continuing platelet deposition occur? One possibility is that damage continues, due perhaps to arterial pressure in the venous graft. Other factors related to the effect of vessel size or geometry on the pattern of blood flow may be important.

An appearance similar to that of intimal hyperplasia may be produced by the organization of mural thrombi, intially formed perioperatively. Although some studies suggest that organized mural thrombus bears 'no resemblance' to intimal hyperplasia [10], other workers suggest that the two are difficult to distinguish [14].

Late Stage of Atherosclerosis

By the end of the first year after surgery, there is considerable connective-tissue synthesis by intimal smooth muscle cells. Later, lipid accumulates in intra- and extracellular sites, leading to changes which closely resemble atherosclerosis [10]. At this stage, the disease progresses slowly, like atherosclerosis, with unpredictable occlusive events. However, by 10 years after surgery, the majority of grafts will be diseased or occluded [15].

Antithrombotic Treatment

Results of studies to examine the issue of vein-graft closure must be considered in the light of the above three stages in the pathology of vein-graft closure. The method of assessment used has been almost exclusively graft angiography. Studies in which angiography has been performed early after surgery usually examine only the role of thrombus formation, while those performed at six months to one year are concerned with the role of intimal hyperplasia as well. The small number of studies in which angiography has been carried out after this time, up to 10 years later, are more revealing regarding the problem of true graft atherosclerosis (*cf.* p. 387).

Anticoagulant Treatment
Although recent studies have emphasized the role of platelets in the production of the changes outlined above [16], fibrin is an important component of thrombosis in vein grafts, and oral anticoagulants have become routine therapy in the postoperative management of coronary artery bypass graft patients, particularly in Europe [17–19]. Oral anticoagulant treatment would be expected to have its greatest effect on the earlier phase of graft closure, that due to thrombosis, but it may also reduce thrombus formation related to the subsequent processes, intimal hyperplasia and atherosclerosis. However, anticoagulants alone might not be adequate [20]: they do not prevent platelet deposition onto exposed subendothelium, or onto deeper tissues exposed by the trauma associated with vein handling, although they may reduce thrombus mass.

Heparin, for example, has no effect on the deposition of the platelet monolayer onto exposed subendothelium. However, the platelet monolayer is soon replaced by a neointima, the new luminal lining which develops from smooth muscle cells following loss of endothelium. Heparin has been found, in some hands, to reduce platelet deposition onto damaged neointima [21], although the properties of oral anticoagulants in this regard are not known. As a neointima would be expected to form over the damaged vein graft during the first 4–7 days after removal of the endothelium, the properties of neointima may be important in determining the response to the continuing trauma that probably occurs following grafting.

Three randomized controlled trials have assessed the ability of oral anticoagulants to reduce the rate of closure of vein grafts after coronary artery grafting [22–24]. In the first, dipyridamole and subcutaneous heparin were given for one week after surgery, oral anticoagulants being introduced on the seventh day [22]. At two months' follow-up, all grafts were patent in 81% of patients receiving oral anticoagulants, while this finding was made in only 67% of controls. In the treatment group, 90% of 251 grafts were patent, while in controls 84% of 238 grafts were patent ($P<0.015$). The benefit produced by anticoagulation was limited to grafts with low flow, a condition favoring fibrin deposition. In two other studies, oral anticoagulants were started on the third postoperative day. No advantage was gained from therapy in either study, with follow-up at 6 months [23] or 24 months [24]. In a non-randomized study from the Netherlands, oral anticoagulants appeared effective in reducing graft closure, whereas aspirin and dipyridamole started after surgery had little effect [25]. In the trial of Brooks *et al*, anticoagulation for 3–12 months was associated with a low risk of graft occlusion in all patients, including those with endarterectomy [17]. There is therefore evidence that anticoagulants might be effective in reducing the frequency of graft closure, if given early after surgery.

It should be noted that all patients routinely receive heparin or another agent (for example, PGI_2) at the time of cardiopulmonary bypass. In two studies, anticoagulants were given together with antiplatelet agents [17,18]. The pre- and perioperative use of such powerful antithrombotic agents as the oral anticoagulants may be undesirable because of the risk of surgical bleeding [26], and anticoagulants, with their need for monitoring, are more expensive and troublesome to use than are antiplatelet agents. Thus, although oral anticoagulants may be effective, their use is unlikely to be popular for the majority of patients receiving coronary artery grafts. However, the use of more powerful antithrombotic regimens, perhaps using both anticoagulants and platelet inhibitors, may be valuable in high-risk patients, particularly in the setting of anastomoses to small arteries (<1.5 mm diameter), if the risk of bleeding can be minimized, for example by careful surgical hemostasis.

Antiplatelet Agents
The importance of platelets in the pathogenesis of thrombosis indicates that antiplatelet agents should reduce thrombus formation, might reduce intimal hyperplasia and perhaps retard the development of late clinical events due to complicated graft atherosclerosis. Animal experiments have shown a clearcut reduction in platelet deposition and formation of mural thrombus early after operation [6,27], although there was no benefit in treated animals at 90 days, when platelet deposition in all animals was very low [27]. These results were achieved with dipyridamole given perioperatively, and thereafter aspirin and dipyridamole. The degree of intimal hyperplasia at six months was reduced in the same model by a combination of aspirin and dipyridamole [27].

Several trials have been performed to test the efficacy of platelet-inhibiting therapy in the prevention of coronary vein-graft closure, with follow-up time ranging between one week and one year. Overall, the results demonstrate that antiplatelet agents can reduce graft occlusion (see Table I) when used optimally, particularly in the early phase after surgery. However, several issues regarding their use must still be resolved.

Aspirin versus *dipyridamole plus aspirin*. Both dipyridamole and aspirin are antithrombotic in experimental situations. On the basis of results of platelet survival studies in which the antithrombotic effect of aspirin was potentiated by dipyridamole, the combination has been widely used in clinical medicine with no unequivocal evidence of its efficacy. When added to warfarin, dipyridamole reduces the rate of emboli in patients with prosthetic heart valves [34], but no clinical study shows a clearcut benefit of dipyridamole where the thrombogenic surface is biologic. For example, in the AICLA study [35], the benefit of aspirin/dipyridamole was the same as that of aspirin alone, and in the Persantine–aspirin trial in cerebral ischemia [36] dipyridamole did not add significantly to the effect of aspirin, but this may not apply to arteries to other organs.

Recent clinical trials provide further data to support the suggestion that aspirin provides most of the protection gained in the studies in which the combination of dipyridamole and aspirin is antithrombotic. Aspirin alone was found to be effective in reducing vein-graft closure at the low dose of 100 mg/day in the study reported by Lorenz *et al* [29]. This study was unfortunately characterized by a high rate of graft occlusion in the placebo group – 32% at four months, compared with the 10%–20% in most centers. The reasons for this are not clear: no anticoagulants were given except for the heparin administered during cardiopulmonary bypass. In the VA/Wadsworth study reported by Brown *et al*, both aspirin and aspirin/dipyridamole had a similar efficacy [33]. The only suggestion of an advantage of the addition of dipyridamole was that the rate of perianastomotic stenosis was slightly lower in the group receiving both drugs

Table I: Antiplatelet treatment in patients receiving coronary artery bypass grafts*

Reference	% Patients with angiogram	Daily dose of antiplatelet agent	Day started	Follow-up	Patency rate of grafts Control[†]	Treated[†]	
Baur et al 1982 [2]	71	800 mg sulfinpyrazone	1	7–14 d	90% (219)	96% (212)	Sig
Chevigné et al 1984 [28]	25§	500 mg ticlopidine	1	3 m	78% (55)	93% (70)	Sig
Lorenz et al 1984 [29]	77	100 mg aspirin	1	4 m	68% (53)	90% (40)	Sig
Mayer et al 1981 [30]	64	1300 mg aspirin	1	3–6 m	78% (92)	92% (75)	Sig
Chesebro et al 1982 [1]	88	400 mg dipyridamole	−2	8 d median	85% (520)	96% (488)	Sig
1984 [31]	84	After surgery: 225 mg dipyridamole 975 mg aspirin	1	11–18 m	75% (486)	89% (478)	Sig
Rajah et al 1985 [18]	82	990 mg aspirin 225 mg dipyridamole	−1	4–7.5 m	75% (118)	92% (95)	Sig
Pantley et al 1979 [23]	77	975 mg aspirin 225 mg dipyridamole	3	6 m	82% (61)	82% (33)	NS
McEnany et al 1982 [24]	51	600 mg aspirin	3–4	1–47 m	73% (74)	80% (81)	NS
Sharma et al 1983 [32]	80	975 mg aspirin 225 mg dipyridamole	3–5	12 m	80% (95)	83% (89)	NS
Brooks et al 1985 [17]	83	990 mg aspirin 225 mg dipyridamole	2–3	11–14 m	87% (352)	89% (385)	NS
Brown et al 1985 [33]	86	975 mg aspirin or 975 mg aspirin plus 225 mg dipyridamole	2–3	12 m	79% (147) 79% (147)	88% (114) 86% (138)	Sig Sig

* Adapted, with permission, from Verstraete et al [20] with additional data.
† Total numbers of grafts in parentheses.
§ Assessment also based on treadmill testing.

than in the aspirin group. Many patients would have to be studied to prove the advantages of this combination. It is unlikely that the small potential advantage outweighs the side-effects and extra cost of the additional therapy.

Reservations regarding the role of dipyridamole are specifically addressed to its use in chronic therapy. However, its value in preventing platelet deposition onto artificial surfaces, and the results of the animal experiments mentioned above, suggest that perioperative use of dipyridamole may inhibit the platelet activation occasioned by components of cardiopulmonary bypass, and that it may have a role in perioperative therapy (see below).

Timing of therapy. Several factors act to reduce platelet counts [37] and platelet adhesiveness [38] during the perioperative period. Similarly, the activity of the coagulation system is depressed – by the heparin given for bypass, for instance. The patient is therefore at a potentially higher risk of bleeding at this time. The time of treatment with platelet inhibitors needs to be examined with this risk in mind.

Preoperative treatment with aspirin increases bleeding in dogs [6,27], and in some studies in man [26] but not in others [39]. The study of Torosian *et al* was not randomized [26], and it is possible that other factors, associated with aspirin therapy, were partly responsible for the increased bleeding. A recent randomized study, however, does suggest increased blood loss in patients treated with 100 mg aspirin preoperatively, compared with anticoagulants following surgery (M. Weber, personal communication). One randomized comparative study has used preoperative aspirin and dipyridamole (330 mg and 75 mg, respectively, for one dose), with a non-significant increase in perioperative blood loss and no increase in either reoperation for bleeding or late tamponade [18]. Overall, the data suggest that on occasion, particularly under difficult surgical conditions, preoperative aspirin is likely to increase the risk of excessive blood loss.

The same reservations do not hold for the preoperative use of dipyridamole. In dogs, dipyridamole does not prolong bleeding time or increase blood loss in cardiopulmonary bypass [6,27]. In man, there were no adverse effects when it was given preoperatively [1,31]. As grafts occasionally thrombose a few hours after coronary artery grafting, it seems appropriate to try to prevent this with pre- or intraoperative therapy.

Dipyridamole was given preoperatively in the Mayo Clinic study for two days, at 400 mg/day [1,31]. In the study of Rajah *et al*, aspirin and dipyridamole were given preoperatively, and this treatment produced a similar marked benefit [18]. In the Wadsworth/VA study, when aspirin alone was started on the second, third or fifth postoperative day, graft occlusion rates at one year were 8%, 12% and 17%, respectively; with aspirin and dipyridamole, 12%, 12% and 18%; and with placebo, about 21% in each case [33]. Grafts at high risk of occlusion (low flow, coronary lumen <1.5 mm) were not protected by therapy in this study, whereas they were protected in The Mayo Clinic study, in which therapy was given preoperatively [1]. These findings indicate that early therapy was of greater benefit than therapy started later after surgery. In earlier studies in which no benefit was observed, therapy was generally started later than the third day (Table I).

Although the perioperative use of heparin and the iatrogenic platelet dysfunction that occurs at the time of coronary surgery produce a hemostatic defect, early anti-thrombotic therapy is clearly important. As dipyridamole is safe when administered preoperatively and the results obtained at The Mayo Clinic suggest so clearly that the regimen used there was efficacious in grafts at both high and low risk of occlusion [1,31], the protocol used in that study can be recommended. Dipyridamole (400 mg/day) is started two days preoperatively (one day may be sufficient), and is then given at 06.00 on the day of surgery. One hour after surgery it can be given by nasogastric tube, and six hours later aspirin (325 mg) and dipyridamole (75 mg) three times daily can be started. It is strongly suspected that there is no benefit from the long-term use of dipyridamole and, indeed, that it can be discontinued in hospital.

Dosage of aspirin. An important factor in promoting platelet activation and irreversible platelet aggregation is the generation of thromboxane A_2 from platelet arachidonate by a mechanism involving platelet fatty acid cyclo-oxygenase. Aspirin acts by acetylating this enzyme, thereby rendering it inactive [39]; thromboxane A_2 generation is blocked and aggregation is inhibited. Acetylation is irreversible and, as the platelet cannot synthesize protein, thromboxane A_2 generation by platelets is only restored by the production of new platelets. It is important to recall that aspirin does not block other pathways by which platelets are activated (ADP or platelet-activating factor), nor does it block the formation of a monolayer via the adhesion of platelets to a damaged surface. Thus, it does not completely inhibit platelet deposition at the site of vascular damage.

Acetylation of platelet cyclo-oxygenase is dose dependent [39,40]. In most normal subjects, after a single oral dose of aspirin (100 mg) 100% inhibition of the production of platelet thromboxane B_2 (the more stable product of thromboxane A_2 metabolism) occurs, with maximal platelet-inhibiting effects. On the other hand, during chronic therapy, lower doses of aspirin also completely suppress thromboxane B_2 production. With 0.45 mg/kg aspirin (about 30 mg/day for the average man), a greater than 95% reduction in thromboxane B_2 generation occurs, the full effect being reached after 4–6 days of therapy [40].

The effect of aspirin on other cyclo-oxygenase systems is also dose dependent, but the concentrations of aspirin required for full inhibition of the enzyme in these other sites are higher [39]. Unlike synthesis in the platelet, the synthesis of cyclo-oxygenase in other tissues recovers rapidly, and the effects are more short-lived. Cyclo-oxygenase in the vessel wall is necessary for the production of PGI_2, the antiaggregatory prostaglandin, which may help maintain the non-thrombogenic properties particularly of the abnormal vessel wall [41]. Low doses of aspirin may spare this vessel-wall enzyme and thus maintain the capacity of the vessel wall to prevent thrombus formation. A further mechanism for selective inhibition of platelet cyclo-oxygenase may be presystemic exposure of circulating platelets as they pass through the portal system, where they can be exposed to higher concentrations of aspirin than are reached in the systemic circulation [42].

Low-dose aspirin also has the advantage of an absence of adverse effects. Aspirin-induced inhibition of PGI_2 production in gastric mucosa and glomeruli has been proposed to account for at least some of the adverse effects, and gastric adverse effects are a particular problem with normal doses of aspirin [43]. These effects are dose dependent, a fact clearly illustrated by two large studies of aspirin in unstable angina. In the McMaster study, in which the dose was 1300 mg/day, adverse effects were more common in the aspirin-treated than in the placebo patients [44]. In the VA study, however, which used a low dose of soluble buffered aspirin (325 mg/day), this was not the case, the rate of adverse effects in the aspirin-treated group being the same as in the control group [45].

These considerations support the use of the lowest dose of aspirin with established antithrombotic effects. Aspirin 325 mg (when given as a buffered preparation, as in Alka Seltzer) was shown to have no significant adverse effects in the VA study of 1266 patients with unstable angina [45]. The results of current studies testing lower doses should facilitate the choice of aspirin dose for the patient after aortocoronary vein grafting. Pending these results, 80–325 mg/day can be recommended. Even if lower doses are established as being effective in chronic use, doses adequate to suppress platelet cyclo-oxygenase completely should be given early in the postoperative phase, to ensure an adequate early antithrombotic effect.

Subgroups at high risk. Although all vein-graft patients develop some graft narrowing due to intimal hyperplasia, and virtually all develop graft atherosclerosis, some subgroups are at greater risk of thrombotic occlusion in the early postoperative months than others. Some patients may have lower fibrinolytic capacity than others [20], while grafts with low flow have a particular tendency to occlude. For example, in The Mayo Clinic study, 34% of grafts with flow rates of <40 ml/min were occluded in the placebo group at early angiogram [1]. Benefit in this study, where treatment was started before operation, was present in subgroups of patients at both high and low risk of graft occlusion. In the Wadsworth/VA study, however, in which treatment was started at least 48 hours after surgery, grafts at high risk of occlusion did not benefit from antiplatelet therapy [33]; here, in grafts without reactive hyperemia, i.e. grafts to regions in which native vessel or collateral flow had supplied the area well, platelet-inhibiting therapy was particularly efficacious in preventing graft closure.

These findings reaffirm the value of preoperative therapy and raise the issue of selecting or tailoring antithrombotic treatment to the individual patient's clinical condition. In the patient with a graft to a large coronary artery (>1.5 mm luminal diameter) in an area with no other blood supply, the risk of closure is low, and the use of more intensive antithrombotic therapy than aspirin plus dipyridamole may not be necessary. For the patient with higher-risk grafts, the combination of anticoagulants and platelet inhibitors may be of benefit, although this approach remains untested.

Approach to Non-Thrombotic Graft Disease

Intimal Hyperplasia
The results of the various published trials strongly support continuing therapy for one year [16,31,33]. During this time the pathology causing occlusion gradually alters, so that intimal hyperplasia is eventually a more important contributor to occlusion. The clinical trials offer few data on the specific role of aspirin and dipyridamole in preventing intimal hyperplasia; indeed, the benefit seen in The Mayo Clinic trial beyond one month, which may well have been due to the prevention of thrombosis rather than to a

reduction in intimal hyperplasia, was less than that in the first month [31].

Experimental studies in dogs suggest that the aspirin/dipyridamole combination reduces intimal hyperplasia, as assessed by measuring the diameter of the vein graft close to the distal anastomosis [27]. However, in clinical studies in man, there has been no effect on vein-graft diameter, as measured from spot films over a one-year period [16]. An explanation suggested for this is that in the dog studies intimal hyperplasia was largely consequent on organization of mural thrombus; considerably less thrombus formation occurs in man, thus reducing the potential contribution of this phenomenon.

In-vitro studies suggest that aspirin increases the area of a collagen-coated glass slide covered by a single layer of adherent platelets, while at the same time decreasing the number of platelet aggregates [46]. In a study in rabbits, intimal thickening in a vein graft placed in the carotid was significantly increased by aspirin and the aspirin/dipyridamole combination at aspirin doses of 0.5 mg/kg and 40 mg/kg, respectively [47]. Platelet deposition, as assessed by autoradiography one month after operation, covered a larger area of the graft in aspirin-treated animals (40 mg/kg) than it did in controls, or than in animals receiving low-dose (0.5 mg/kg) aspirin or dipyridamole alone [11]. Thus, aspirin may increase the area of the graft on which platelets are deposited and hence the extent of intimal hyperplasia; the contribution that intimal hyperplasia makes to early graft closure, however, is perhaps relatively minor. Although platelet aggregation is reduced by aspirin, it should be recalled that platelet adhesion alone may be enough to stimulate intimal hyperplasia [16], and that this is not reduced, and may even be enhanced, by platelet-inhibiting drug therapy.

Late Phase of Atherosclerosis

Following the year after surgery, vein grafts begin to develop changes similar to more advanced atherosclerosis, with identifiable intra- and extracellular lipid, insudation of blood and blood products, and calcium deposition in the vessel wall – this change appearing, pathologically at least, to be more common in patients with hyperlipidemia [10].

The role of platelet-inhibiting therapy in the prevention of this phenomenon is at present unclear. We know that aspirin protects against subsequent cardiac events in unstable angina, presumably by preventing thrombosis on ruptured plaque [44,45]. Mural thrombus was present on three-quarters of vein grafts examined pathologically up to 54 months after surgery [10]. However, the frequency of thrombotic events long after coronary artery grafting is low. Despite this, continued use of low-dose aspirin – where well-tolerated – is logical, although at present empirical. Some studies suggest that the incorporation of lipid into vein-graft wall is inhibited by platelet-inhibiting therapy. Aspirin and dipyridamole both together and separately inhibit lipid deposition in the wall of peripheral vein grafts of monkeys on both normal and high-fat diets [48]. If this phenomenon occurs in man, it may confer a benefit against atherogenesis. However, the interaction between lipid accumulation and platelet deposition, and intimal hyperplasia, needs to be clarified. Clinical studies show that high plasma lipid profiles are a major risk factor for graft closure after 10 years [15]. It seems likely that control of this and other risk factors, for example hypertension and glucose intolerance, will prove important in the long-term prevention of vein-graft disease.

Conclusions

Although several issues remain unanswered, platelet-inhibiting therapy, as outlined above, together with good surgical technique, achieves good patency rates at one year. However, there are no data to suggest how long platelet-inhibiting therapy should be continued, and several groups are currently attempting to define the optimal dose of aspirin.

Although antiplatelet drugs are efficacious in preventing closure during the first year after surgery, the long-term control of graft atherosclerosis remains a major challenge.

References

[1] Chesebro JH, Clements IP, Fuster V et al.
A platelet-inhibitor drug trial in coronary artery bypass operations: Benefit of perioperative dipyridamole and aspirin therapy on early post-operative vein-graft patency.
N Engl J Med 1982; 307: 73–8.

[2] Baur HR, Van Tassel RA, Pierach CA, Gobel FL.
Effects of sulfinpyrazone on early graft closure after myocardial revascularization.
Am J Cardiol 1982; 49: 420–4.

[3] Fitzgibbon GM, Burton JR, Leach AJ.
Coronary bypass graft fate: Angiographic grading of 1400 consecutive grafts early after operation and of 1132 after one year.
Circulation 1978; 57: 1070–4.

[4] Josa M, Lie JT, Bianco RL, Kaye MP.
Reduction of thrombosis in canine coronary bypass vein grafts with dipyridamole and aspirin.
Am J Cardiol 1981; 47: 1248–54.

[5] Unni KK, Kottke BA, Titus JL, Frye RL, Wallace RB, Brown AL.
Pathologic changes in aortocoronary saphenous vein grafts.
Am J Cardiol 1974; 34: 526–32.

[6] Fuster V, Dewanjee MK, Kaye MP, Josa M, Metke MP, Chesebro JH.
Noninvasive radioisotopic technique for detection of platelet deposition in coronary artery bypass grafts in dogs and its reduction with platelet inhibitors.
Circulation 1979; 60: 1508–12.

[7] Bulkley BH, Hutchins GM.
Pathology of coronary artery bypass graft surgery.
Arch Pathol Lab Med 1978; 102: 273–80.

[8] Slysh S, Goldberg S, Dervan QP, Zalewski A.
Unstable angina and evolving myocardial infarction following coronary bypass surgery: Pathogenesis and treatment with interventional catheterization.
Am Heart J 1985; 109: 744–52.

[9] Lowrie GM, Lie JT, Morris GC, Beazley HL.
Vein graft patency and intimal proliferation after aortocoronary bypass: Early and long-term angiopathologic correlations.
Am J Cardiol 1976; 38: 856–62.

[10] Lie JT, Lawrie GM, Morris GC Jr.
Aortocoronary bypass saphenous vein graft atherosclerosis: Anatomic study of 99 vein grafts from normal and hyperlipoproteinemic patients up to 75 months postoperatively.
Am J Cardiol 1977; 40: 906–14.

[11] Gershlick AH, Syndercombe-Court YD, Murday AJ, Lewis CT, Mills PG.
Adverse effects of high dose aspirin on platelet adhesion to experimental autogenous vein grafts.
Cardiovasc Res 1985; 19: 770–6.

[12] Metke MP, Lie JT, Fuster V, Josa M, Kaye MP.
Reduction of intimal thickening in canine coronary bypass vein grafts with dipyridamole and aspirin.
Am J Cardiol 1979; 43: 1144–8.

[13] Groves HM, Kinlough-Rathbone RL, Mustard JF.
Development of nonthrombogenicity of injured rabbit aortas despite inhibition of platelet adherence.
Arteriosclerosis 1986; 6: 189–95.

[14] Jørgensen L, Rowsell HC, Hovig T, Mustard JF.
Resolution and organization of platelet-rich mural thrombi in carotid arteries of swine.
Am J Pathol 1967; 51: 681–719.

[15] Campeau L, Enjalbert M, Lesperance J et al.
The relation of risk factors to the development of atherosclerosis in saphenous vein-bypass grafts and the progression of disease in the native circulation.
N Engl J Med 1984; 311: 1329–32.

[16] Fuster V, Chesebro JH.
Role of platelets and platelet inhibitors in aorto-coronary artery vein-graft disease.
Circulation 1986; 73: 227–32.

[17] Brooks N, Wright J, Sturridge M et al.
Randomized placebo controlled trial of aspirin and dipyridamole in the prevention of coronary vein graft occlusion.
Br Heart J 1985; 53: 201–7.

[18] Rajah SM, Salter MCP, Donaldson DR et al.
Acetylsalicylic acid and dipyridamole improve the early patency of aortocoronary bypass grafts: A double-blind, placebo-controlled, randomized trial.
J Thorac Cardiovasc Surg 1985; 90: 373–7.

[19] Loeliger EA.
Does dipyridamole have antithrombotic potential?
Thromb Haemost 1985; 54: 437.

[20] Verstraete M, Brown BG, Chesebro JH et al.
Evaluation of antiplatelet agents in the prevention of aorto-coronary bypass occlusion.
Eur Heart J 1986; 7: 4–13.

[21] Groves HM, Kinlough-Rathbone RL, Richardson M, Jørgensen L, Moore S, Mustard JF.
Thrombin generation and fibrin formation following injury to rabbit neointima: Studies of vessel wall reactivity and platelet survival.
Lab Invest 1982; 46: 605–12.

[22] Gohlke H, Gohlke-Bärwolf C, Sturzenhofecker P et al.
Improved graft patency with oral anticoagulant therapy after aortocoronary bypass surgery: A prospective randomized study.
Circulation 1981; 64 (Suppl 2): 22–7.

[23] Pantley GS, Goodnight SH Jr, Rahimtoola SH et al.
Failure of antiplatelet and anticoagulant therapy to improve patency of grafts after coronary-artery bypass: A controlled, randomized study.
N Engl J Med 1979; 301: 962–6.

[24] McEnany MT, Salzman EW, Mudth ED et al.
The effect of antithrombotic therapy on patency rates of saphenous vein coronary artery bypass grafts.
J Thorac Cardiovasc Surg 1982; 83: 81–9.

[25] Lubsen J.
Effect of anti-thrombotic therapy on bypass graft patency: Evidence from a non-randomized study [Abstract].
Eur Heart J 1984; 5 (Suppl 1): 1589.

[26] Torosian M, Michelson EL, Morganroth JL, MacVaugh H II.
Aspirin and Coumadin-related bleeding after coronary artery bypass graft surgery.
Ann Intern Med 1978; 89: 325–8.

[27] Dewanjee MK, Tago M, Josa M, Fuster V, Kaye MP.
Quantification of platelet retention in aortocoronary femoral vein bypass graft in dogs treated with dipyridamole and aspirin.
Circulation 1984; 69: 350–6.

[28] Chevigné M, David JL, Rigo P, Limet R.
Effect of ticlopidine on saphenous vein bypass patency rates: A double blind study.
Ann Thorac Surg 1984; 37: 371–9.

[29] Lorenz RL, Weber M, Kotzur J et al.
Improved aortocoronary bypass patency by low-dose aspirin (100 mg daily). Effects on platelet aggregation and thromboxane formation.
Lancet 1984; i: 261–4.

[30] Mayer JE Jr, Lindsay WG, Casteneda W, Nicoloff DM.
Influence of aspirin and dipyridamole on patency of coronary artery bypass grafts.
Ann Thorac Surg 1981; 31: 204–10.

[31] Chesebro JH, Fuster V, Elveback LR et al.
Effect of dipyridamole and aspirin on late vein graft patency.
N Engl J Med 1984; 310: 209–14.

[32] Sharma GVRK, Khuri SF, Josa M, Falland ED, Parisi AF.
The effect of antiplatelet therapy on saphenous vein coronary artery bypass grafts patency.
Circulation 1983; 68 (Suppl 2): 218–21.

[33] Brown BG, Cukingnan RA, Derouen T et al.
Improved graft patency in patients treated with platelet-inhibiting therapy after coronary bypass surgery.
Circulation 1985; 72: 138–46.

[34] Chesebro JH, Fuster V, Elveback LR et al.
Trial of combined warfarin plus dipyridamole or aspirin therapy in prosthetic heart valve replacement: Danger of aspirin compared with dipyridamole.
Am J Cardiol 1983; 51: 1537–41.

[35] Bousser MG, Eschwege E, Haguenau M et al.
"AICLA" controlled trial of aspirin and dipyridamole in the secondary prevention of atherothrombotic cerebral ischaemia.
Stroke 1983; 14: 5–14.

[36] American-Canadian Co-operative Study Group.
Persantine-aspirin trial in cerebral ischaemia: Endpoint results.
Stroke 1985; 16: 406–15.

[37] van den Dungen JJAM, Karliczek GF, Brenken U, Homan van der Heide JN, Wildevuur CRH.
Clinical study of blood trauma during perfusion with membrane and bubble oxygenators.
J Thorac Cardiovasc Surg 1982; **83**: 108–16.

[38] Harker LA, Malpass TW, Branson HE, Hessel EA II, Slichter SJ.
Mechanism of abnormal bleeding in patients undergoing cardiopulmonary bypass. Acquired transient platelet dysfunction associated with selective α-granule release.
Blood 1980; **56**: 824–34.

[39] Roth J, Stanford N, Majerus PW.
Acetylation of prostaglandin synthase by aspirin.
Proc Natl Acad Sci USA 1975; **72**: 3073–6.

[40] Patrignani P, Filabozzi P, Patrono C.
Selective cumulative inhibition of platelet thromboxane production by low-dose aspirin in healthy subjects.
J Clin Invest 1982; **69**: 1366–72.

[41] FitzGerald GA, Smith B, Pedersen AK, Brash AR.
Increased prostacyclin biosynthesis in patients with severe atherosclerosis and platelet activation.
N Engl J Med 1984; **310**: 1065–8.

[42] Pedersen AK, FitzGerald GA.
Dose-related kinetics of aspirin: Presystemic acetylation of platelet cyclooxygenase.
N Engl J Med 1984; **311**: 1206–11.

[43] Graham DY, Smith JL.
Aspirin and the stomach.
Ann Intern Med 1986: **104**: 390–8.

[44] Cairns JA, Gent M, Singer J et al.
Aspirin, sulfinpyrazone or both in unstable angina: Results of a Canadian Multicenter Trial.
N Engl J Med 1985; **313**: 1369–75.

[45] Lewis HD Jr, Davis JW, Archibald DG et al.
Protective effects of aspirin against acute myocardial infarction and death in men with unstable angina. Results of a Veterans Cooperative Study.
N Engl J Med 1983; **309**: 396–403.

[46] Baumgartner HR.
Effects of acetylsalicylic acid, sulfinpyrazone and dipyridamole on platelet adhesion and aggregation in flowing native and anticoagulated blood.
Haemostasis 1979; **8**: 340–52.

[47] Murday AJ, Gershlick AH, Syndercombe-Court YD, Mills PG, Lewis CT.
Intimal thickening in autogenous vein grafts in rabbits: Influence of aspirin and dipyridamole.
Thorax 1984; **39**: 457–61.

[48] Bonchek LI, Boerboom LE, Olinger GN et al.
Prevention of lipid accumulation in experimental vein bypass grafts by antiplatelet therapy.
Circulation 1982; **66**: 338–41.

ATHEROSCLEROSIS IN CORONARY BYPASS GRAFTS

[1] **The relative influence of arterial pressure versus intraoperative distention on lipid accumulation in primate vein bypass grafts.**
Boerboom LE, Olinger GN, Bonchek LI et al, Med Coll Wisconsin, Milwaukee, WI, USA.
J Thorac Cardiovasc Surg 1985; **90**: 756-64.

[2] **Coronary artery bypass graft failure — an autoimmune phenomenon?**
Morton KE, Gavaghan TP, Krillis SA et al, Univ New South Wales Sch Med, Sydney, NSW, Australia.
Lancet 1986; ii: 1353-7.

[3] **Atherosclerosis of coronary artery bypass grafts and smoking.**
FitzGibbon GM, Leach AJ, Kafka HP, Nat Defence Med Cent, Ottawa, Ontario, Canada.
Canad Med Assoc J 1987; **136**: 45-8.

[4] **Atherosclerosis in aortocoronary bypass grafts. Morphologic study and risk factor analysis 6 to 12 years after surgery.**
Neitzel GP, Barboriak JJ, Pintar K, Qureshi I, Clement J, Zablocki VA Med Cent, Milwaukee, WI, USA.
Arteriosclerosis 1986; **6**: 594-600.

Comment. The development of artherosclerosis in aortocoronary vein bypass grafts limits their long-term function. There are two possible factors that may influence atherogenesis: injury caused by graft distention during preparation for grafting, and chronic exposure to arterial pressures which exceed native venous pressure. Boerboom et al [1] investigated the relative influence of arterial pressure and high pressure of distention on cholesterol and apolipoprotein B accumulation in vein grafts inserted into an animal model. Before insertion, the veins were distended at 125 mmHg for one minute, and one half of the vein was distended for a further minute at 350 mmHg. After three months, it was found that cholesterol concentration in grafts distended at 125 mmHg was 213% of the concentration in ungrafted control vein, and the concentration of apolipoprotein B was 430% of control concentration; in grafts distended at 350 mmHg, cholesterol concentration was 250% that of normal, and apolipoprotein B was 925% that of normal. Although morphological differences were not as great as those observed biochemically, foam cells occurred more frequently in those grafts that had been distended at 350 mmHg. These results show that the chronic exposure of vein graft to arterial pressure has a significant effect on the accumulation of cholesterol; this effect is greater than that caused by intraoperative distention at moderate pressure, although the detrimental effects of excessive distention pressures should not be discounted.

Anticardiolipin antibody is thought to be related to the lupus anticoagulant, and high circulating levels of both have been shown to be associated with intravascular thrombosis. In young survivors of myocardial infarction, high anticardiolipin antibody levels are associated with an increased risk of recurrent cardiovascular events. Morton et al [2] correlated preoperative anticardiolipin antibody levels with graft patency in 83 patients who underwent aortocoronary bypass graft surgery; 76 completed the one-year-follow-up protocol. Preoperative anticardiolipin antibody was not related to the incidence of early graft occlusion, but it was very strongly associated with late occlusion — 8 of 15 patients whose maximum levels of anticardiolipin antibody exceeded 4 standard deviations above the mean of controls had a late occlusion. Moreover, there was a progressive increase in the frequency of graft occlusion according to the height of plasma anticardiolipin antibody. Most patients showed a rise in anticardiolipin antibody level during the 12 postoperative months; the highest levels were found in patients with a history of previous infarction. These interesting findings support the idea that anticardiolipin antibody production might be an immune response to myocardial injury and, if confirmed, this suggests that it is possible to define a group of patients at high risk for graft occlusion on whom special therapeutic efforts could be concentrated.

Angiographic studies have demonstrated that atherosclerotic lesions progress more rapidly in the coronary arteries of smokers when compared with lesions in non-smokers. FitzGibbon et al [3] performed follow-up angiography at one and five years in 340 men who had undergone coronary artery bypass grafting. At five-year follow-up,115 patients were smokers and 225 were not. Grafts were classified according to irregularities in graft outlines and patency. Disease-free grafts were found in 39% of smokers and 52% of non-smokers; moreover, the proportion of diseased or occluded grafts was found to be greater in the smokers than the non-smokers. These results indicate that men who continue to smoke following coronary artery bypass grafting are at a significantly increased risk of graft atherosclerosis or occlusion than non-smokers.

In another study investigating risk factors for late graft occlusion [4], saphenous vein aortocoronary bypass grafts from 42 patients were examined at autopsy 6–12 years after coronary artery bypass surgery. Complex atheromata, often associated with an acute thrombus, were found in 71% of the grafts; aneurysms of the atherosclerotic type were present in 14% of cases. Forty of these patients were compared with 535 patients who had undergone coronary artery bypass surgery but who did not require reoperation five or more years later. Those patients who required two bypass operations had significantly higher serum levels of triglyceride and cholesterol and lower levels of high density lipoprotein cholesterol than the control patients; upon examination of their medical history, it was found that more of the patients requiring two bypass operations were diabetic, smoked cigarettes or had abnormal lipoprotein phenotypes when compared with the control group. Hypertension was not identified as a significant risk factor. These results show that the factors involved in the development of atherosclerosis in coronary arteries are also those involved in the development of atherosclerosis in saphenous vein grafts. Therefore, those patients at greater risk of coronary atherosclerosis are also those at greatest risk of saphenous vein graft atherosclerosis and as such they should be considered as candidates for internal mammary artery grafting, which is much more resistant to the development of atherosclerosis than saphenous vein.

CORONARY SURGERY AT LIFE'S EXTREMES

[1] Young adults with coronary atherosclerosis: 10 year results of surgical myocardial revascularization.
Lytle BW, Kramer JR, Golding LR et al, Cleveland Clin Found, Cleveland, OH, USA.
J Am Coll Cardiol 1984; 4: 445–53.

[2] Coronary arteriography and coronary artery bypass surgery: morbidity and mortality in patients aged 65 years or older. A report from the Coronary Artery Surgery Study.
Gersh BJ, Kronmal RA, Frye RL et al, Univ Washington, Seattle, WA, USA.
Circulation 1983; 67: 483–90.

Comment. Papers from a collection of many on the same subject over the past three years review subsections of the population at the extremes of life. The criteria for what is young age are more specific than those for the elderly. Lytle et al [1] from The Cleveland Clinic reported 107 patients under the age of 35 years undergoing coronary artery surgery in the early period of 1971–1975. Early clinical events included one operative death and five non-fatal perioperative myocardial infarctions. Follow-up at a mean interval after operation of 115 months demonstrated actuarial survival rates of 94% at 5 years and 85% at 10 years. Analysis of the data showed that survival was decreased by multi vessel disease and impaired left-ventricular function; event-free survival was decreased by a family history of coronary disease and cigarette smoking. Both survival and event-free survival were decreased by diabetes and elevated serum cholesterol. Cardiac catheterization in 64 patients at a mean postoperative interval of 47 months demonstrated that mammary artery graft patency (25 of 27, 93%) exceeded vein graft patency (49 of 88, 56%, $P<0.01$). The authors conclude that use of internal mammary artery grafts may enhance the palliation of bypass surgery. It is unfortunate that this series is now somewhat dated, because the patient under 35 years old must account for only just over 5% of much Western coronary artery practice, whereas those over 65 now account for 25% of Western practice. In a small series by Gersh *et al* [2] on patients aged 65 years or over, the overall perioperative mortality was 5.2%, compared with 1.9% for patients under 65. Discriminant analysis identified five variables predictive of perioperative mortality, including the presence of a 70% or greater stenosis of the left main coronary artery and a dominant left circulation. Of less significance were an elevated left-ventricular diastolic pressure, a preoperative history of cigarette smoking, pulmonary rales and the presence of an associated medical disease.

LEFT MAIN STEM LESIONS

A life table and Cox regression analysis of patients with combined proximal left anterior descending and proximal left circumflex coronary artery disease: non-left main equivalent lesions (CASS).
Chaitman BR, Davis K, Fisher LD *et al*, St Louis Univ Med Cent, St Louis, MO, USA.
Circulation 1983; **68**: 1163–70.

Comment. Patients with pure left main stem lesions were excluded from CASS, although Chaitman *et al* compared survival rates of patients with left main stem equivalent lesions (combined proximal left anterior descending and proximal left circumflex artery stenoses >70%) with survival rates of patients with left main coronary artery stenoses >70%.

Stratified life-tables and a Cox regression model were used for this comparison. Patients with left main coronary artery disease had a poorer prognosis than patients with left main equivalent lesions. To determine whether the location of the left anterior descending stenosis influenced survival rates, patients with combined proximal left anterior descending stenosis and proximal left circumflex disease were compared with patients with combined stenoses >70% in the non-proximal left anterior descending and proximal circumflex coronary arteries. The survival rate was lower in patients with proximal left anterior descending artery disease (55% *vs* 70%). Therefore, combined proximal left anterior descending and proximal left circumflex disease identifies a high-risk patient subset, but it is not prognostically equivalent to left main coronary artery disease. However, it was noted that survival rates were poor for all these subsets when compared with surgically treated patients.

SIGNIFICANCE OF NEW Q WAVES AFTER BYPASS SURGERY

[1] Use of survival analysis to determine the clinical significance of Q waves after coronary bypass surgery.
Chaitman BR, Alderman EL, Sheffield LT *et al*, Montreal Heart Institute, Que, Canada.
Circulation 1983; **67**: 302–9.

[2] Detrimental effect of perioperative myocardial infarction on late survival after coronary artery bypass. Report from the Coronary Artery Surgery Study — CASS.
Schaff HV, Gersh BJ, Fisher LD *et al*, and participants in the Coronary Artery Surgery Study (Appendix 1), Coordinating Center for Collaborative Studies in Coronary Artery Surgery, Univ Washington, Seattle, WA, USA.
J Thorac Cardiovasc Surg 1984; **88**: 972–81.

Comment. Although the appearance of new 'Q' waves in a patient's electrocardiogram is only one criterion of myocardial infarction, its appearance after coronary artery surgery is effectively pathognomonic of perioperative infarction. Chaitman *et al* [1] found the incidence of perioperative 'Q' wave infarction to be 4.6% in a study of 1340 patients undergoing revascularization during 1978. Discriminant analysis of 44 clinical, angiographic and surgical variables showed that bypass time, topical cardiac hypothermia and cardiomegaly were significant. Hospital mortality was 9.7% in those with perioperative infarction and 1.0% in those without. In patients who survived to hospital discharge, the presence of new postoperative 'Q' waves did not adversely affect the three-year survival. These facts were only partially substantiated by CASS, in which the detrimental effect of perioperative myocardial infarction on the late survival of coronary artery bypass surgery was investigated. Working on the assumption that perioperative myocardial infarction was detrimental to patients in the long term, the criteria for perioperative myocardial infarction were tightened, so that by virtue of the size and completeness of the patient follow-up an unequivocal answer has been produced. Schaff *et al* [2] reported from CASS that definite or probable myocardial infarction occurred in 561 out of 9777 coronary bypass patients (5.7%). Diagnosis was based on new 'Q' waves in 51%, evolution of regional ST-segment changes in 63% and raised cardiac enzymes in 67%; 32% of patients had all three criteria, and 33% had two of three. Actuarial survival at 1, 3 and 5 years in these patients was 78%, 74% and 69%, respectively, compared with 96%, 94% and 90%, respectively, in those without perioperative infarction ($P<0.0001$). Multivariate analysis revealed that perioperative myocardial infarction was an independent factor predicting late mortality. The only predictive factors of any strength were impaired left-ventricular function, advancing age and a number of associated medical conditions.

VALVE SURGERY

MITRAL VALVE REPAIR

[1] Mitral regurgitation due to ruptured chordae tendinae. Early and late results of valve repair.
Orszulak TA, Schaff HV, Danielson GK et al, Mayo Clin and Mayo Found, Rochester, MN, USA.
J Thorac Cardiovasc Surg 1985; 89: 491–8.
[2] Experiences with the Carpentier techniques of mitral valve reconstruction in 103 patients (1980–1985).
Spencer FC, Colvin SB, Culliford AT, Isom OW, New York Univ Med Cent, New York, NY, USA.
J Thorac Cardiovasc Surg 1985; 90: 341–50.

Comment. It is difficult to evaluate papers on the usefulness of mitral valve repair for mitral regurgitation as a result of ruptured chordae tendinae because much depends on the surgeon's ability and experience of this procedure. Workers at the Mayo Clinic report on 131 patients who underwent repair of ruptured chordae tendinae of the mitral valve between 1958 and 1980 [1]. Various repair procedures were used, but 116 patients underwent leaflet plication without resection. Operative mortality (<30 days) was only 6.1% — an excellent result. The survival rate of those patients discharged from hospital was 92% at 5 years and 73% at 10 years. In contrast, patients who had undergone mitral valve replacement for ruptured chordae tendinae during the same time interval had a survival rate of 72% at 5 years. Moreover, the incidence of thrombo-embolism after repair was 1.8 episodes/100 patient-years, whereas after valve replacement it was 8 episodes/100 patient-years; the authors do not discuss the reasons for the discrepancy between these two figures.

Workers at the New York University Medical Center report on their experience of using Carpentier reconstruction techniques for mitral insufficiency in 103 patients [2]. The cause of mitral insufficiency was ruptured chordae tendinae in 52, mitral-valve prolapse in 13, rheumatic fever in 12, coronary disease in 8, congenital heart disease in 9 and endocarditis in 5. Multiple abnormalities were usually present. Four patients had severe calcification of the annulus. Repair was successful in all but one patient, who had moderate residual insufficiency. Two late hospital deaths occurred but these were not related to the mitral repair. After discharge from hospital, ring dehiscence occurred in one patient, who required a second operation. A minor neurologic deficit occurred in one patient which was the result of a thrombo-embolism. Three patients who had recurrent endocarditis had to have their mitral valves replaced. Late Doppler echocardiography was performed in 95 patients: the investigation revealed a trace of mitral insufficiency in 12 and moderate insufficiency in one. Patients appeared to fare better after mitral-valve repair than after mitral-valve replacement (although the two groups of patients are not identical), and the data from this well-documented series of patients suggest that mitral-valve repair can be successfully performed in 90% of patients with non-rheumatic non-calcified mitral valves.

RISKS OF MITRAL VALVE REPLACEMENT

[1] Operative risk of mitral valve replacement: discriminant analysis of 1329 procedures.
Scott WC, Miller DC, Haverich A *et al*, Stanford Univ Med Cent, Stanford, CA, USA.
Circulation 1985; **72** (Suppl II): 108–19.

[2] Morbidity and mortality in mitral valve surgery.
Christakis GT, Kormos RL, Weisel RD *et al*, Toronto Gen Hosp, Toronto, Ontario, Canada.
Circulation 1985; **72** (Suppl II): 120–8.

[3] Have the results of mitral valve replacement improved?
Ferrazzi P, McGiffin DC, Kirklin JW, Blackstone EH, Bourge RC, Univ Alabama at Birmingham, Birmingham, AL, USA.
J Thorac Cardiovasc Surg 1986; **92**: 186–97.

Comment. The operative mortality of patients undergoing mitral-valve replacement is higher than that of patients undergoing aortic-valve replacement. Attempts have been made to analyse factors determining operative risk, but they have been confounded by the interdependence of many factors. Scott *et al* [1] have investigated the independent preoperative and intraoperative predictors of operative mortality in 1329 isolated mitral-valve replacement procedures in 1300 patients undertaken between 1965 and 1981. The influence of 34 variables was assessed by univariate and multivariate analysis. Lesions were classified as mitral stenosis (20%), mitral regurgitation (44%) or mixed (34%); the operative mortality rates for these three groups were $8 \pm 1\%$, $13 \pm 2\%$ and $8 \pm 1\%$, respectively. Powerful clinical determinants of operative mortaity were found to be functional class (NYHA), previous myocardial infarction and hepatic dysfunction ($P<0.001$); age at operation and emergency operations were also significant determinants ($P=0.001$ and $P=0.04$, respectively). However, the following were not found to be significant independent determinants of operative risk: concomitant coronary artery bypass grafting or tricuspid annuloplasty, angina, ischemic etiology or physiologic lesion. Moreover, year of operation, prosthetic valve dysfunction and previous cardiac surgery did not have an important effect on operative mortality. Thus early operative risk for mitral-valve replacement is related to preoperative cardiac and hepatic function. Prior myocardial infarction was found to increase operative risk substantially even if the mitral-valve disease was not ischemic in origin. In the subgroup of patients with mitral regurgitation, increased operative mortality rate was related to advanced left ventricular failure and myocardial infarction rather than the etiology of mitral regurgitation. This paper makes a valuable contribution to the scant literature on early operative mortality for mitral-valve replacement and the authors are to be congratulated. The number of patients studied was large enough for Scott *et al* [1] to draw clear and simple conclusions in an area normally obfuscated by complexity.

Christakis *et al* [2] studied a much smaller group of patients ($n=214$) undergoing mitral-valve surgery in 1982 and 1983. They examined 38 preoperative and perioperative variables by univariate and multivariate analysis to determine risk factors for operative mortality and postoperative ventricular dysfunction. Overall operative mortality was 4.6%; however, those patients with coronary artery disease had a higher

ANTICOAGULATION AND MECHANICAL VALVES

operative mortality than those who did not. The following factors were found to be significant independent predictors of operative mortality or postoperative ventricular dysfunction: functional class (NYHA), age at operation, the presence of coronary artery disease or a mitral regurgitant lesion and tricuspid annuloplasty. Thus, the results of Christakis *et al* [2] are broadly similar to those of Scott *et al* [1]; any discrepancy is probably due to the differences in the number of patients studied and the length of time over which they were studied.

Ferrazzi *et al* [3] analysed the results of patients who had undergone isolated or combined mitral valve replacement between 1975 and 1979 ($n=478$) and those of patients who had been operated upon between 1979 and 1983 ($n=341$) at their center. The patients in the later period were older, had a higher left ventricular end-diastolic pressure and a higher prevalence of rheumatic mitral disease; they also underwent, on average, longer and more extensive operations. Although patients in the later period had a slightly lower survival rate at both 2 and 4 weeks, the difference was not significant. It was found that in the later era a higher proportion of deaths was caused by chronic heart failure. After multivariate analysis, neither the time-period nor the specific year in which a patient underwent operation was predictive of death. These results for mitral valve replacement contrast with the improvements seen in the results of surgery on patients with congenital or ischemic heart disease. They confirm that patients with mitral valve disease have a condition of progressive deterioration; delay in undertaking valve replacement, however imperfect the operative techniques and prostheses may be, has serious consequences for the patient. Although these results are humbling, it is important to publish such findings in order to gain perspective with respect to the improvements in surgical results.

ANTICOAGULATION AND MECHANICAL VALVES

[1] Risks of anticoagulant therapy in pregnant women with artificial heart valves.
Iturbe-Alessio I, del Carmen Fonseca M, Mutchinik O, Santos MA, Zajarias A, Salazar E, Inst Nat Cardiol Ignacio Chavez, Mexico, Mexico.
N Engl J Med 1986; *315*: 1390-3.
[2] Aspirin anticoagulation in children with mechanical aortic valves.
Verrier ED, Tranbaugh RF, Soifer SJ, Yee ES, Turley K, Ebert PA, Univ California, San Francisco, CA, USA.
J Thorac Cardiovasc Surg 1986; *92*: 1013-20.
[3] Effect of warfarin on calcification of spontaneously degenerated porcine bioprosthetic valves.
Stein PD, Riddle JM, Kemp SR, Lee MW, Lewis JW, Magilligan DJ Jr, Henry Ford Hosp, Detroit, MI, USA.
J Thorac Cardiovasc Surg 1985; *90*: 119-25.

Comment. Pregnany in patients with artificial heart valves poses a difficult therapeutic problem. Some form of anticoagulation is essential to protect the mother from thrombo-embolism (the tendency to which is increased during pregnancy); however, the coumarin derivatives are accompanied by a high risk of embryopathy if administered during the first trimester, and the efficacy of heparin in preventing valve thrombosis is unproven. In addition, long-term heparin use can be associated with osteoporosis, and as coumarin anticoagulants cross the placenta their use in pregnancy is likely to be complicated by hemorrhagic complications in the neonate. In a series of 72 pregnancies [1], those detected early were given subcutaneous heparin 5000 units 12 hourly from the 6th to the 12th week, or from the 7th to the 12th week, with resumption of the coumarin derivative thereafter. Pregnancies detected after the first trimester were maintained on the coumarin derivative throughout. In most patients, heparin was substituted for the oral anticoagulant after the 38th week. Three of 35 women had thrombosis of a tilting disc mitral prosthesis during heparin treatment, of whom two died. Coumarin embryopathy occurred in 25% of pregnancies in which heparin was started after the 7th week, and in 29.6% of those who did not have heparin during the first trimester. These findings emphasize the unacceptable risk to the fetus if coumarin anticoagulants are administered to the mother during the 6th to 12th weeks of pregnancy, and the ineffectiveness of the low-dose heparin regimen in protecting the mother from valvular thrombosis. It is clear that until a more effective regimen can be devised, women with artificial heart valves who require long-term anticoagulation should, if possible, be dissuaded from becoming pregnant.

Workers at the University of California, San Francisco [2] used aspirin, or aspirin and dipyridamole, as an anticoagulation agent in 51 children aged 1–23 years (mean 12.9 years) undergoing aortic valve replacement with a mechanical prosthesis between 1975 and 1986. Follow-up was for a mean of 36.5 months (range 3–100 months). Two patients were lost to follow-up, and four late deaths occurred but none of them were related to thrombosis or embolism. Although one minor neurologic event occurred perioperatively, it resolved spontaneously. No postoperative thromboembolic events occurred. Four patients had minor hemorrhagic complications, three of whom had nose bleeds and the remaining patient suffered an upper gastrointestinal hemorrhage. This patient was changed to warfarin, along with four others who had not experienced complications on aspirin but were referred by their physicians. Mechanical valve failure had not occurred, although one patient underwent reoperation at 9 months for perivalvular leak. During follow-up, all children have remained in normal sinus or paced rhythm. Magnetic resonance imaging or CT scanning of the brain was performed in 11 of the children; there was no evidence of silent cerebral thrombo-embolic defects. In conclusion, the authors maintain that aspirin alone or aspirin with dipyridamole is safe for the treatment of children with mechanical aortic valves, the associated risk of thrombo-embolic events being small; any hemorrhagic complications arising from treatment with aspirin were considered to be minor and could be treated easily.

As the synthesis of γ-carboxyglutamic acid, a calcium-binding amino acid, is a vitamin K-dependent enzymatic process inhibited by warfarin, it is possible that warfarin might diminish the calcification of porcine bioprosthetic valves. Stein et al [3] examined 40 explanted porcine bioprosthetic valves removed because of spontaneous degeneration; 17 of the patients had been treated with warfarin and 23 were untreated. Gross visualization revealed that there was no calcification or only one localized nodule in 11 of 17 valves (65%) in the warfarin-treated group and in only 5 of 23 valves (22%) in the untreated group. Histological examination showed that there was no calcium or only fine specks in 9 of 13 valves in the warfarin-treated group and in only 3 of 19 valves in the untreated group. Thus, it appears that warfarin diminished the calcification in spontaneously degenerated porcine bioprosthetic valves. It will be ironic if this finding is substantiated because bioprostheses were designed to reduce the need for anticoagulant therapy.

PERICARDIECTOMY

Early and late results of pericardiectomy for constrictive pericarditis.
McCaughan BC, Schaff HV, Piehler JM *et al*, Mayo Clin/Mayo Found, Rochester, MN, USA.
J Thorac Cardiovasc Surg 1985; **89**: 340–50.

Comment. McCaughan *et al* reviewed the results of operation for constrictive pericarditis in 231 patients seen at The Mayo Clinic from 1936 to 1982. All of the patients had hemodynamically significant pericardial constriction. Before operation, 69% of patients were in NYHA class III or IV, and 81% had peripheral edema or ascites. After operation, 28% of patients had evidence of low cardiac output; of 32 deaths that occurred within 30 days of operation, 70% were due to low cardiac output. Operative risk was found to be significantly related to preoperative status: 1% for classes I and II, 10% for class III and 46% for class IV ($P<0.001$).

Median follow-up was 9 years; the probability of survival for patients leaving hospital was 84% at 5 years, 71% at 15 years and 52% at 30 years. Long-term survival was not found to be significantly influenced by preoperative disability class or the development of a low cardiac output in the immediate postoperative period. The authors recommend early pericardiectomy once a diagnosis of constrictive pericarditis is made, because they found that a poor hemodynamic result after complete pericardiectomy relates to the degree of preoperative constriction and the resulting cardiomyopathy.

COMPLICATIONS OF CARDIAC SURGERY

CEREBRAL COMPLICATIONS OF CARDIAC SURGERY

Review: PAMELA J. SHAW

Neurologic morbidity has been a recognized risk of heart surgery since the earliest operations of the 1950s [1,2]. Cardiac surgery poses a much greater threat to the nervous system than major general surgical procedures, and this difference has been attributed largely to the use of cardiopulmonary bypass. There have been many improvements in bypass technology as well as in surgical and anesthetic methods in recent years, and these have undoubtedly reduced the incidence of serious complications. Operative mortality rates have steadily fallen [3], and the incidence of fatal cerebral damage has decreased to a level of 0.3%–2% [4–6]. Nevertheless, studies using clinical [7–9], neuropsychologic [10–12], electroencephalographic [13], neuropathologic [14,15], experimental [16,17], biochemical [18] and other methods of assessment [19,20] show that neurologic dysfunction following heart surgery remains a major cause of morbidity.

The reported incidence of neurologic complications is influenced by study design as well as by the sensitivity and specificity of the methods used. Retrospective studies have in general shown a low incidence of complications (of the order of 1%–5%) [21,22]. These studies are likely to detect only major neurologic disorders, such as postoperative coma or overt hemiplegia, and more subtle abnormalities will be missed [9]. Prospective studies in which patients have been evaluated by a neurologist have shown a higher incidence of neurologic morbidity, ranging from 30% [8,23] to 61% [7].

Clinical Aspects of Neurologic Complications
The neurologic disorders following cardiac surgery that have been described have varied in severity and affected all levels of the nervous system. The major clinical syndromes which may develop are discussed below.

Fatal Cerebral Damage
This still occurs after approximately 0.3%–2% of cardiac surgical procedures [6–8]. The neuropathologic changes occurring in patients who have died after open-heart surgery have been studied by several authors [14,15]. Brierley examined the brains of 11 patients who died within 11 days of cardiac operations [14]. He found that the majority of brains showed focal or multifocal ischemic lesions involving grey and white matter and varying in severity from minor perivascular cell loss to areas of frank infarction. Aguilar *et al* found neuropathologic abnormalities in 85% of 206 patients dying after cardiac surgery [15]. Focal hemorrhages, acute neuronal necrosis and embolic occlusion of small cerebral vessels were the principal features.

Impairment of Consciousness Level
One of the most frequent reasons for neurologic consultation after cardiac surgery is failure of the patient to awaken at the expected time after anesthesia. The problem may range from mild, protracted drowsiness to irreversible coma. In a study from Newcastle-upon-Tyne, UK, 10 out of 312 patients (3.2%) failed to recover a normal level of consciousness within 24 hours of coronary bypass surgery [7]; 9 of the 10 patients regained normal alertness by the 12th postoperative day. Furlan and Breuer concluded that frank non-metabolic coma is a rare complication of cardiac operations, occurring in less than 1% of patients [24]. They found the prognosis poor for patients in postoperative coma: 85% die, and 12% remain vegetative or with serious neurologic disability.

Stroke
This is the major cause of severe, persistent neurologic disability following heart surgery [25]. The incidence of stroke following coronary bypass surgery is of the order

of 5% in prospective studies [7,23]. Retrospective studies report a much lower stroke rate – of less than 1% [26,27]. The incidence of stroke appears to be higher following valve surgery than after coronary bypass. This probably reflects the potential for embolization of valve debris, and air embolism from cardiac chambers that have been opened to the atmosphere. In the prospective study of Sotaniemi, 24% of valve-surgery patients were found to have a postoperative hemiparesis [6].

Approximately 70% of strokes related to heart surgery develop perioperatively and 30% in the early postoperative period. Serious, persistent disability results in approximately 25% of patients sustaining a perioperative stroke [25].

Diffuse Encephalopathy
This may manifest itself as impairment of consciousness, behavioral changes ranging from mild confusion to frank psychosis and intellectual dysfunction. Impairment of consciousness has been discussed above. Postoperative delirium or psychosis was described in as many as 40%–57% of postoperative patients in early reports [28,29]. The exact incidence of these complications is difficult to define, because of the lack of consistent nosology and the variable diagnostic criteria used in different studies. In the Newcastle study, only 4 out of 312 coronary bypass patients developed postoperative psychosis [7].

Postoperative psychiatric dysfunction often presents as clouding of consciousness, confusion and agitation, together with perceptual distortions, which may have a para-noid flavor. This may develop immediately after recovery from anesthesia or after a lucid interval of several days. Factors other than hypoxic/ischemic cerebral injury may contribute to postoperative psychiatric derangement, including the cardiac and meta-bolic status of the patient [30] and environmental factors, such as sensory monotony and sleep deprivation in the intensive care unit [31,32].

Neuropsychologic testing is the best method available at present for assessing changes in intellectual function following heart surgery. Changes in psychometric scores after surgery have been found to correlate with biochemical markers of brain damage in the cerebrospinal fluid [18]. The reported incidence of postoperative cogni-tive dysfunction is variable, and depends on such factors as the sensitivity of the psychometric tests used, the timing of postoperative assessment and the criteria of abnormality employed. In general, the earlier and more extensively the patients have been tested, the higher the incidence and severity of observed deficit. Shaw *et al*, using a battery of 10 neuropsychologic tests and postoperative assessment one week after surgery, showed that 235 out of 298 coronary bypass patients (79%) deteriorated on one or more test scores after operation [33]. Of the patients with score deterioration, 52% were asymptomatic while in hospital, 38% had noticeable symptoms and 10% were considered to be overtly disabled in their everyday activities. Ellis *et al* found that 75% of 30 coronary bypass patients showed deterioration of cognitive function at one week after surgery, but that they had fully recovered by six months [34]. Savageau *et al*, using a small number of tests and postoperative testing at nine days and six months, showed that 30% of heart-surgery patients were neuropsychologically impaired in the early postoperative period and 5% were still abnormal in the long term [10,11]. Sotaniemi *et al*, in a study of valve-surgery patients, showed that intellectual dysfunction developed in 57% of patients with clinically evident cerebral complications and in 8% of those without clinical abnormalities [12].

The areas of intellectual function which most commonly deteriorate are attention span, psychomotor speed, short-term memory and new learning ability [12,33,35]. The impact of these changes on subsequent domestic life and employment status remains to be established. Several studies have indicated that considerable recovery of early intellectual deterioration can be expected to occur within six months [11,12,34,36].

A major question arising from the observed intellectual deterioration after heart surgery is whether this really reflects cardiopulmonary bypass-related brain injury. Could the observed changes merely reflect a non-specific effect of major surgery, i.e. a result of general tiredness, mood change or lack of motivation? Several studies have suggested that there is little change in psychometric scores following major general surgical procedures [37–39]. In the Newcastle study, 312 coronary bypass patients were compared with a control group of 50 patients undergoing major, non-cardiac vascular surgery. Minor neuropsychologic changes were observed in the control group, but these were significantly less frequent and severe than in the coronary bypass group [36].

Seizures

These may occur after heart surgery in isolation or together with other signs of central nervous system dysfunction. Late postoperative epilepsy may develop as a sequel to intraoperative cerebral injury [6,25].

Spinal Cord Injury

This is a rare complication of cardiac surgery. Sotaniemi reported postoperative hemi-paresis of suspected spinal origin in 2 out of 100 valve surgery patients [6], and Gonzales-Scarano and Hurtig discovered one case of spinal infarction in their re-trospective series of 1427 patients [27]. Patients requiring intra-aortic balloon counter-pulsation may develop spinal infarction, most commonly resulting from compromise of the spinal segmental arteries by the development of a subadventitial dissecting hemato-ma of the thoracic aorta [40].

Ophthalmologic Complications

The retina offers a unique opportunity to study microvascular events related to cardiopulmonary bypass. This is of particular interest, as similar changes presumably occur within vessels of a comparable size in the brain. Williams has reported on a study in which fundoscopy was performed during cardiac operations [41]. Refractile specks and plaques were observed to pass through the retinal arterioles, and in some cases white plugs formed *in situ* within the retinal vessels. The obstructing particles were shown to comprise aggregates of platelets, fibrin, red cells and leukocytes; or fragments of fat or silica [42].

Ophthalmologic complications are common, occurring in 25% of coronary bypass patients in the Newcastle study [7]. The abnormalities found include areas of retinal infarction, producing the appearance of cotton-wool spots, retinal emboli, isolated reduction of visual acuity, visual-field defects, Horner's syndrome and conjunctival petechiae [7,43].

Miscellaneous Minor Signs
Primitive reflexes and isolated extensor plantar responses may frequently be found if patients are examined in detail postoperatively [7,44].

Damage to the peripheral nervous system – particularly the brachial plexus [7,45] – may also occur as a result of heart surgery. Careful assessment may be required to distinguish these peripheral complications from disorders of the central nervous system.

Mechanisms of Cerebral Injury During Heart Surgery
Our understanding of the mechanisms of cerebral injury related to cardiopulmonary bypass is still far from complete. Clinical, neuropathologic and experimental studies have implicated three main mechanisms underlying central nervous system complications.

Macroembolization
This is particularly dangerous to the brain, which lacks a protective collateral circulation. Massive air embolism has been estimated to occur in 0.1%–0.2% of cardiopulmonary bypass operations [46,47]. This may result from the inadequate removal of air from cardiac chambers, unexpected resumption of heart beat, defects or detachment of the oxygenator or inadequate attention to the oxygenator reservoir level. Other potential sources of large cerebral emboli include atherosclerotic debris dislodged from the aortic arch [48] and left-ventricular thrombus or valve debris released during manipulation of the heart [49,50]. Macroemboli will produce major focal cerebral damage, presenting clinically as perioperative stroke.

Microembolization
All types of contemporary cardiopulmonary bypass apparatus produce microemboli which pass directly into the patient's arterial circulation. Gaseous microemboli may result from inadequate defoaming after bubble oxygenation or from temperature or pressure changes in the extracorporeal circuit. Adequate heparinization does not completely prevent the formation of platelet, leukocyte and fibrin aggregates [51,52]. Fat [53], silicone [54] and polyvinyl chloride tubing fragments [55] are other potential sources of particulate microemboli.

Experimental studies in animals have shown significant microembolic blockade of the microcirculation of the brain, persisting for 48 hours after bypass [17]. Microemboli have also been observed in the brains of humans dying after heart surgery [15]. Several authors have suggested that this microembolic cerebral insult may be reduced through the inclusion of arterial line filters in the extracorporeal circuit [16,56].

Inadequate Cerebral Perfusion
During bypass, inadequate perfusion has also been stressed as a potential cause of cerebral injury [20,57]. Hypoperfusion may result from low flow, loss of the pulsatile component of flow [58], hypotension [59], occlusive disease of the cerebrovascular system or incorrect placement of the aortic cannula. At present, there is insufficient knowledge of the patterns of change in human cerebral blood flow during extracorporeal circulation, and further work is needed so that safe thresholds for pressure, flow and pulsatility can be established.

Risk Factors for Cerebral Injury Associated with Heart Surgery
Preoperative Factors
Factors which have been found to influence postoperative neurologic outcome include age [10,60,61], a previous history of neurologic disease [6,44,61] and the type, severity and duration of heart disease prior to operation [6,10].

Intraoperative Factors
The duration of cardiopulmonary bypass seems to be an important determinant of cerebral outcome. There has been a dramatic increase reported in the incidence of cerebral complications with bypass times exceeding two hours [6,44]. This phenomenon may result from the cumulative effect of microembolism, and possibly from the accumulation of vasoconstrictor spasmogens [62].

Evidence for the importance of hypotension in the pathogenesis of cerebral injury is conflicting. Several authors have shown that sustained mean arterial pressure levels of less than 50 mmHg during bypass are associated with the development of postoperative cerebral dysfunction [44,59,63]. Others have considered that low pressure is not a major factor predisposing to cerebral dysfunction [34,64]. Ellis *et al* emphasized the potential advantage, in terms of myocardial preservation, in the employment of low flow and pressure during bypass [34].

The type of cardiac operation also appears to influence neurologic outcome. Cerebral complications are more common in patients having multiple- as opposed to single-valve operations [6,37], and in patients having mitral compared with aortic operations [6]. Coronary bypass appears to pose a smaller risk than valve operations, perhaps because air embolism is less likely when the cardiac chambers are not opened [64].

Unexpected intraoperative catastrophes, such as air embolism, aortic dissection or severe hypotension, occasionally occur which are frequently accompanied by brain injury [6,22].

Postoperative Factors
Most neurologic complications associated with heart surgery have been considered to develop intraoperatively, and postoperative factors have received scant attention. Stressful postoperative environmental factors, such as sleep deprivation and sensory monotony, have been considered to predispose to post-bypass psychiatric derangement [32,65]. Breuer *et al* found that the postoperative use of pressor agents or balloon-pump assistance (both markers for hemodynamically compromised patients) was associated with the development of diffuse encephalopathy [23].

Recent Developments and Prospects for the Future
Detection of Postoperative Neurologic Dysfunction
An important advance in recent years is the application of detailed clinical [6–8], neuropsychologic [10,33] and other neuroinvestigative methods such as EEG [13] and CT scanning [19] to detect not only major neurologic injury but also more subtle and even subclinical disorders. The application of these methods will be important in monitoring future refinements in cardiopulmonary bypass technology.

It would be useful to have a more objective and sensitive marker of cerebral damage. Biochemical markers of nerve-cell injury in the cerebrospinal fluid, such as adenylate kinase [18] and brain-specific creatine kinase [56], are potentially useful in this respect. The measurement of regional cerebral blood flow using xenon-133 single-photon emission computerized tomography may also prove a valuable method for assessing cerebral dysfunction objectively. Henriksen showed that 77% of patients developed a reduction in mean cerebral blood flow following cardiopulmonary bypass operations [20].

Intraoperative Neurophysiologic Monitoring of Cortical Function
The purpose of the intraoperative monitoring of cerebral function is to allow recognition of insults to the brain at the moment of occurrence, thus permitting possible therapeutic intervention. The EEG is a sensitive indicator of cerebral ischemia. Slowing of the EEG frequency in man occurs when regional cerebral blood flow drops to 16–22 ml/100 g/min, and severe voltage attenuation results if flow is further reduced [66]. Conventional EEG monitoring during cardiac surgery has not been widely adopted, largely because of the practical difficulties in recording and interpretation in the operating theatre. In skilled hands, EEG monitoring can be valuable in the immediate detection of compromise of the cerebral circulation during bypass [67]. Other instruments, such as the cerebral function monitor and the compressed spectral array, have been devised to provide simplified and compressed information from the raw EEG. There have been reports of the usefulness of these instruments in the early detection and prediction of severity of neurologic damage in individual patients [68,69]. Nevertheless, the detection of brain injury during bypass operations is at present unsatisfactory.

Management of Patients with Combined Cardiac and Cerebrovascular Disease
It has been suggested that extracranial carotid disease may be a potentially important factor predisposing to stroke during heart surgery. The rationale behind this hypothesis is that cerebral infarction may result from a critical decrease in perfusion pressure distal to a carotid stenosis. Several authors have concluded that the presence of an asymptomatic carotid bruit does not increase the risk of perioperative stroke during heart surgery [70–74]. In recent years, preoperative non-invasive test methods have been used to screen for hemodynamically significant carotid lesions. In several reports, the authors could not correlate abnormal preoperative Doppler studies with an increased risk of perioperative stroke [70,71]. Kartchner and McRae, however, concluded that hemodynamically significant carotid occlusive disease detected by oculoplethysmography is an important risk factor for stroke in cardiac surgery [75]. They found that patients with results indicative of an internal carotid stenosis of >60% had a 17% incidence of stroke, compared with a 1% incidence in those without flow-reducing carotid occlusive disease. In view of these conflicting reports, the best management policy for patients with asymptomatic carotid disease who require heart surgery remains to be elucidated.

There is a general impression that patients with recently symptomatic cerebrovascular disease have a substantially increased risk of perioperative stroke, although there are few firm data to support this view [76]. This group of patients with preoperative cerebral ischemic symptoms should probably have cerebral angiography prior to cardiac surgery.

The management of patients with combined symptomatic carotid and coronary disease remains a controversial issue, and firm guidelines are not yet available. The fundamental question is whether staged or combined cardiac and carotid operations effectively reduce the incidence of perioperative stroke in patients undergoing heart surgery. There are several problems in answering this question: (i) specific hemodynamic studies, detailing the effect of the institution of extracorporeal circulation on flow beyond significant carotid occlusive disease, are not yet available; (ii) the majority of strokes during bypass are probably of embolic origin and unrelated to low-flow states, i.e. many strokes associated with cardiac surgery are probably totally unrelated to the presence of cerebrovascular disease; and (iii) proof that carotid endarterectomy lowers the risk of cerebrovascular accident in cardiac surgery patients awaits the results of a randomized prospective study, in which patients with angiographically confirmed carotid stenosis are allocated to carotid surgery or no carotid surgery in addition to their cardiac operation.

The following information is available with regard to cerebrovascular disease in candidates for cardiac surgery.

1. The incidence of significant internal carotid or carotid bifurcation stenosis in patients selected for coronary bypass surgery has been reported at approximately 6%–16% [76,77].
2. Major stroke occurs in approximately 2% of coronary bypass operations [7,8], and this figure is likely to be higher in patients undergoing valve surgery [6]. The incidence of stroke is probably increased in cardiac-surgery patients with recently symptomatic cerebrovascular disease, although there is little clear information on this point. Jones *et al* found a perioperative stroke rate of 0.9% in coronary bypass patients without evidence of cerebrovascular disease, 3.3% in patients with an asymptomatic bruit and 8.6% in those with a previous stroke or transient ischemic attack [76].
3. Cardiac complications after carotid endarterectomy occur in 1%–17% of patients, the frequency depending on the severity of preoperative cardiac disease [76,78]. In experienced hands, the stroke rate after carotid endarterectomy should not exceed 2%–3% [78].

The first report of combined surgical management of carotid and coronary disease was by Bernhard *et al* in 1972 [79]. Since then, several authors have suggested that simultaneous unilateral carotid endarterectomy and coronary bypass can be undertaken with similar morbidity and mortality to that in patients undergoing coronary surgery alone [80–82]. However, other authors have found that stroke incidence and mortality were significantly greater with combined operations than with staged carotid–coronary procedures [83–86].

Further work is required to establish firm management guidelines, but several reports have suggested the following protocol.

1. Cardiac surgery alone for most patients with asymptomatic carotid bruit or mild-to-moderate asymptomatic carotid obstruction [70–74].

2. Staged carotid endarterectomy followed by cardiac surgery, in patients with symptomatic carotid lesions who have stable angina and are without left main or severe triple-vessel disease or left-ventricular failure [76,78].

3. Simultaneous operations for those with severe disease of either system, i.e. unstable angina, left main or triple-vessel disease, cardiac failure or symptomatic carotid occlusive disease which is high-grade or bilateral [76,78].

Non-invasive methods of screening for cerebrovascular disease are useful in skilled hands, but are inferior to angiography. Digital subtraction angiography is an important new technique, and could be used to visualize the degree and distribution of cerebrovascular atheroma prior to surgery with less risk than conventional angiography. Its use in the future will enable more accurate assessment of the relationship between the presence of cerebrovascular disease and the risk of post-bypass neurologic injury.

Relationship between Intraoperative Variables and Cerebral Outcome
There are many unresolved questions regarding the best techniques for protecting the brain during cardiopulmonary bypass.

The question of whether to use pulsatile or non-pulsatile perfusion during bypass surgery remains controversial. Animal studies suggest that more extensive cortical cellular necrosis and edema as well as increased cerebral lactate production occur in subjects undergoing non-pulsatile bypass [87,88]. Anderson has suggested that pulsation during bypass is beneficial, because it preserves the coupling between regional cerebral blood flow and metabolism [89]. Other studies suggest that pulsation is necessary for the maintenance of the vasomotor tone required for autoregulation [90,91]. Some authors, however, have failed to demonstrate a beneficial effect of pulsatile over non-pulsatile perfusion [92].

There is also conflicting evidence in the literature regarding the importance of hypotension in the pathogenesis of cerebral injury. Several studies have shown that sustained mean arterial pressure levels of <50 mmHg are significantly correlated with postoperative cerebral dysfunction [57,59,63]. Others have argued that mean arterial pressure during bypass is not a major determinant of neurologic injury, and have emphasized the potential advantage of low-flow, low-pressure bypass in myocardial preservation [34,64]. Further work is necessary to determine both the ideal and the acceptable minimum and maximum levels of mean arterial pressure needed to protect the brain during bypass, also to determine whether these values are different in elderly patients and in those with known cerebrovascular disease or hypertension.

Other factors requiring evaluation in terms of neurologic outcome are the use of arterial line filters and of membrane *versus* bubble oxygenators.

Pharmacologic Agents
There are various pharmacologic agents which may help protect the brain from hypoxic/ischemic injury during bypass. Barbiturates or calcium-blockers may help lessen the extent of cerebral damage resulting from a hypoxic or ischemic insult. The use of platelet antiaggregants, such as prostacyclin, may reduce the microembolic assault on the cerebral circulation. The potetial usefulness of these agents requires evaluation.

407

Menasche *et al* have recently demonstrated that an oxygenated fluorocarbon solution can reduce ischemic brain damage resulting from carotid arterial air embolism in rats [93]. Fluorocarbons are synthetic compounds with the ability to dissolve large amounts of various gases, particularly oxygen, carbon dioxide and nitrogen. The small size of fluorocarbon particles as well as the low viscosity of their emulsions enables effective gas exchange at microcirculatory level — i.e. in areas that may not be reached by red blood cells under ischemic conditions. The protective effect in cerebral air embolism is likely to result from increased oxygen availability for ischemic tissues and possibly from a reduction in the size of air bubbles through enhanced denitrogenation of blood [93]. The future development of stable, non-toxic and rapidly eliminated fluorocarbon emulsions may provide a useful therapeutic tool for the management of air embolism during cardiopulmonary bypass.

Prevention of Macroembolization
The use of echocardiography to detect air in the cardiac chambers during heart surgery has been the subject of several reports [94–96]. This represents a potentially valuable technique for the prevention of cerebral air embolism.

Atherosclerotic emboli resulting from manipulation of the ascending aorta during cardiac operations have increasingly been recognized as a potential threat to the brain [48,97]. Measures have been suggested to decrease the chance of dislodgement of atheromatous debris; these include attempting to cannulate and cross-clamp in areas free of significant atherosclerotic disease, the use of sequential anastomosis, Y grafts and the internal mammary artery graft to decrease the number of aortic anastomoses [97], the use of alternative methods of aortic occlusion [98].

Conclusions
The many improvements in surgical and anesthetic methods and cardiopulmonary bypass technology are reflected in the steady decrease in recent years in the mortality and serious morbidity associated with heart surgery. Nevertheless, current bypass techniques remain imperfect for the replacement of normal heart and lung functions, and it is not improbable that all patients undergoing extracorporeal perfusion suffer some degree of neurologic injury. Many of the neurologic complications are minor or recoverable. The detection of even minor and subclinical disorders is important, however, in relation to the assessment of future refinements in bypass technology. Major perioperative stroke is the chief cause of the severe, persistent neurologic disability which may nullify the overall clinical benefit of cardiac surgical repair. Our main effort should therefore be directed towards predicting and preventing this complication.

References

[1] Björk VO, Hultquist G.
Brain damage in children after deep hypothermia for open- heart surgery.
Thorax 1960; **15**: 284–91.

[2] Torres F, Frank GS, Cohen M, Lillehei CW, Kasper N.
Neurological and electroencephalographic studies in open-heart surgery.
Neurology 1959; **9**: 174–83.

[3] English TAH, Bailey AR, Dark JF, Williams WG.
The UK cardiac surgical register 1977–1982.
Br Med J 1984; **289**: 1205–8.

[4] Aberg T, Ronquist G, Tyden H *et al.*
Adverse effects on the brain in cardiac operations as assessed by biochemical, psychometric and radiologic methods.
J Thorac Cardiovasc Surg 1984; **87**: 99–105.

[5] Branthwaite MA.
Prevention of neurological damage during open-heart surgery.
Thorax 1975; **30**: 258–61.

[6] Sotaniemi KA.
Brain damage and neurological outcome after open-heart surgery.
J Neurol Neurosurg Psychiatr 1980; **43**: 127–35.

[7] Shaw PJ, Bates D, Cartlidge NEF, Heaviside D, Julian DG, Shaw DA.
Early neurological complications of coronary artery bypass surgery.
Br Med J 1985; **291**: 1384–7.

[8] Breuer AC, Furlan AJ, Hanson MR *et al.*
Neurologic complications of open-heart surgery.
Cleve Clin Q 1981; **48**: 205–6.

[9] Sotaniemi KA.
Cerebral outcome after extra-corporeal circulation. Comparison between prospective and retrospective evaluations.
Arch Neurol 1983; **40**: 75–7.

[10] Savageau JA, Stanton BA, Jenkins CD, Klein MD.
Neuropsychological dysfunction following elective cardiac operation. I: Early assessment.
J Thorac Cardiovasc Surg 1982; **84**: 585–94.

[11] Savageau JA, Stanton BA, Jenkins CD, Frater RWM.
Neuropsychological dysfunction following elective cardiac operation. II: A six month reassessment.
J Thorac Cardiovasc Surg 1982; **84**: 595–600.

[12] Sotaniemi KA, Juolasmaa A, Hokkanen ET.
Neuropsychologic outcome after open-heart surgery.
Arch Neurol 1981; **38**: 2–8.

[13] Witoska MM, Tamura H, Indeglia R, Hopkins RW, Simeone KA.
Electroencephalographic changes and cerebral complications in open-heart surgery.
J Thorac Cardiovasc Surg 1973; **6**: 855–64.

[14] Brierley JB.
Neuropathological findings in patients dying after open-heart surgery.
Thorax 1963; **18**: 291–304.

[15] Aguilar MJ, Gerbode F, Hill JD.
Neuropathologic of cardiac surgery.
J Thorac Cardiovasc Surg 1971; **61**: 676–85.

[16] Brennan RW, Patterson RH, Kessler J.
Cerebral blood flow and metabolism during cardiopulmonary bypass: Evidence of microembolic encephalopathy.
Neurology 1971; **21**: 665–72.

[17] Patterson RH, Rosenfeld L, Porro R.
Transient cerebral microvascular blockade after cardiopulmonary bypass.
Thorax 1976; **31**: 736–41.

[18] Åberg T, Tyden H, Ronquist G, Ahlund P, Bergstrom K.
Release of adenylate kinase into the cerebrospinal fluid during open-heart surgery and its relation to post-operative intellectual function.
Lancet 1982; **ii**: 1139–42.

[19] Muraoka R, Yokata M, Minoru A *et al.*
Subclinical changes in brain morphology following cardiac operations as reflected by computer tomographic scans of the brain.
J Thorac Cardiovasc Surg 1981; **81**: 364–9.

[20] Henriksen L.
Evidence suggestive of diffuse brain damage following cardiac operations.
Lancet 1984; **i**: 816–20.

[21] Bojar RM, Najafi H, Delaria GA, Serry C, Goldin MD.
Neurological complications of coronary revascularisation.
Ann Thorac Surg 1983; **36**: 427–32.

[22] Coffey CE, Massey W, Roberts KB, Curtis S, Jones RH, Pryor DB.
Natural history of cerebral complications of coronary artery bypass graft surgery.
Neurology 1983; **33**: 1416–21.

[23] Breuer AC, Furlan AJ, Hanson MR *et al.*
Central nervous system complications of coronary artery bypass graft surgery: Prospective analysis of 421 patients.
Stroke 1983; **14**: 682–7.

[24] Furlan AJ, Breuer AC.
Central nervous system complications of open-heart surgery.
Stroke 1984; **15**: 912–5.

[25] Shaw PJ, Bates D, Cartlidge NEF *et al.*
Natural history of neurological complications of coronary artery bypass graft surgery: A six month follow-up study.
Br Med J 1986; **293**: 165–7.

[26] Lee MC, Geiger J, Nicoloff D, Klassen AC, Resch JA.
Cerebrovascular complications associated with coronary artery bypass procedure.
Stroke 1979; **10**: 107.

[27] Gonzales-Scarano F, Hurtig HI.
Neurological complications of coronary artery bypass grafting: Case control study.
Neurology 1981; **31**: 1032–5.

[28] Blachly PH, Starr A.
Post-cardiotomy delirium.
Am J Psychiatry 1964; **121**: 371–5.

[29] Egerton N, Kay JH.
Psychological disturbances associated with open-heart surgery.
Br J Psychiatry 1964; **110**: 433–9.

[30] Dubin WR, Field HL, Gastfriend DR.
Postcardiotomy delirium: A critical review.
J Thorac Cardiovasc Surg 1979; **77**: 587–94.

[31] Kornfeld DS, Heller SS, Frank KA, Moskowitz R.
Personality and psychological factors in post-cardiotomy delerium.
Arch Gen Psychiatry 1974; **31**: 249–53.

[32] Sveinsson IS.
Post-operative psychosis after heart surgery.
J Thorac Cardiovasc Surg 1975; **70**: 717–26.

[33] Shaw PJ, Bates D, Cartlidge NEF *et al*.
Early intellectual dysfunction following coronary bypass surgery.
Q J Med 1986; **225**: 59–68.

[34] Ellis RJ, Wisniewski A, Potts R, Calhoun C, Loucks P, Wells MR.
Reduction of flow rate and arterial pressure at moderate hypothermia does not result in cerebral dysfunction.
J Thorac Cardiovasc Surg 1980; **79**: 173–80.

[35] Juolasmäa A, Outakoski J, Hirvenoja R, Tienari P, Sotaniemi K, Takkunen J.
Effect of open-heart surgery on intellectual performance.
J Clin Neuropsychol 1981; **3**: 181–97.

[36] Shaw PJ, Bates D, Cartlidge NEF *et al*.
Long-term intellectual dysfunction following coronary artery bypass graft surgery: a six month follow-up study.
Q J Med 1987; **62**: 259–68.

[37] Aberg T, Kihlgren M.
Effect of open-heart surgery on intellectual function.
Scand J Thorac Cardiovasc Surg 1974; Suppl 5: 1–63.

[38] Gruvstad M, Kebbon L, Lof B.
Changes in mental functions after induced hypotension.
Acta Psychiatr Scand 1962; **37** (Suppl 163).

[39] Raymond M, Conklin C, Schaeffer J, Newstadt G, Mattoff JM, Gray RJ.
Coping with transient intellectual dysfunction after coronary bypass surgery.
Heart Lung 1984; **13**: 531–9.

[40] Criado A, Agosti J, Horno R, Jimenez C.
Paraplegia balloon assistance after cardiac surgery.
Scand J Thorac Cardiovasc Surg 1981; **15**: 103–4.

[41] Williams IM.
Fundus oculi findings associated with cardiopulmonary bypass procedures.
Trans Asia-Pac Acad Ophthalmol 4th Congress 1972: 72–6.

[42] Williams IM.
Retinal vascular occlusions in open-heart surgery.
Br J Ophthalmol 1975; **59**: 81–91.

[43] Gutman FA, Zegarra H.
Ocular complications in cardiac surgery.
Surg Clin North Am 1971; **51**: 1095–103.

[44] Tufo HM, Ostfeld AM, Shekelle R.
Central nervous system dysfunction following open-heart surgery.
J Am Coll Cardiol 1970; **212**: 1333–40.

[45] Lederman RJ, Breuer AC, Hanson MR *et al*.
Peripheral nervous system complications of coronary artery bypass graft surgery.
Ann Neurol 1982; **12**: 297–301.

[46] Mills NL, Ochsner JL.
Massive air embolism during cardiopulmonary bypass.
J Thorac Cardiovasc Surg 1980; **80**: 708–17.

[47] Stoney WS, Alford WC, Burrus GR, Glassford DM, Thomas CS.
Air embolism and other accidents using pump oxygenators.
Ann Thorac Surg 1979; **29**: 336–40.

[48] McKibbon DW, Bulkley BH, Green WR, Gott UL, Hutchins GM.
Fatal cerebral atheromatous embolisation after cardiopulmonary bypass.
J Thorac Cardiovasc Surg 1976; **71**: 741–5.

[49] Breuer AC, Franco I, Marzewski D, Soto-Velasco J.
Left ventricular thrombi seen by ventriculography are a significant risk factor for stroke in open-heart surgery.
Ann Neurol 1981; **10**: 103–4.

[50] Gilman S.
Cerebral disorders after open-heart operations.
N Engl J Med 1965; **272**: 489–98.

[51] Guidoin RG, Awad JA, Laperche Y, Morin PJ, Harris GH.
Nature of deposits in a tubular membrane oxygenator after prolonged extracorporeal circulation: A scanning electronmicroscopy study.
J Thorac Cardiovasc Surg 1975; **69**: 479–91.

[52] Solis RT, Kennedy PS, Beall AC, Noon GP, Debakey ME.
Cardiopulmonary bypass. Microembolization and platelet aggregation.
Circulation 1975; **52**: 103–8.

[53] Caguin F, Carter MG.
Fat embolism with cardiotomy with use of cardiopulmonary bypass.
J Thorac Cardiovasc Surg 1963; **46**: 665–72.

[54] Lindberg DAB, Lucas FV, Sheagren J, Malm JR.
Silicone embolization during clinical and experimental heart surgery employing a bubble oxygenator.
Am J Pathol 1961; **31**: 129–35.

[55] Orenstein JM, Noriko S, Aaron B, Buchholz B, Bloom S.
Microemboli observed in deaths following cardiopulmonary bypass surgery. Silicone antifoam agents and polyvinyl chloride tubing as sources of emboli.
Hum Pathol 1982; **13**: 1082–90.

[56] Taylor KM, Durlin BJ, Mittra SM, Gillan JG, Brannan JJ, McKenna JM.
Assessment of cerebral damage during open-heart surgery. A new experimental model.
Scand J Thorac Cardiovasc Surg 1980; **14**: 197–203.

[57] Lee WH, Miller W, Rowe J, Havston P, Brady MP.
Effects of extracorporeal circulation on personality and cerebration
Ann Thorac Surg 1969; **7**: 562–9.

[58] De Paepe J, Pomerantzeff PMA, Nakiri K, Armeline E, Verginelli G, Zerbini EJ.
Observation of the microcirculation of the cerebral cortex of dogs subjected to pulsatile and nonpulsatile flow during extracorporeal circulation. In: *A propos du debit pulse*. Paris: Cobe Laboratories, 1979.

[59] Stockard JJ, Bickford RG, Schauble JF.
Pressure dependent cerebral ischaemia during cardiopulmonary bypass.
Neurology 1973; **23**: 521–9.

[60] Javid H, Tufo HM, Najafi H, Dye WS, Hunter JA, Julian OC.
Neurological abnormalities following open-heart surgery.
J Thorac Cardiovasc Surg 1969; **58**: 502–9.

[61] Branthwaite MA.
Neurological damage related to open-heart surgery.
Thorax 1972; **27**: 748–53.

[62] Chenoweth DE, Cooper SW, Hugli TE, Stewart RW, Blackstone EH, Kirklin JW.
Complement activation during cardiopulmonary bypass.
N Engl J Med 1981; **304**: 497–503.

[63] Henriksen L, Hjelms E, Lindeburgh T.
Brain hyperperfusion during cardiac operations.
J Thorac Cardiovasc Surg 1983; **86**: 202–8.

[64] Kolkka R, Hiberman M.
Neurologic dysfunction following cardiac operation with low- flow, low-pressure cardiopulmonary bypass.
J Thorac Cardiovasc Surg 1980; **79**: 432–7.

[65] Orr WC, Stahl ML.
Sleep disturbances after open-heart surgery.
Am J Cardiol 1977; **39**: 196–201.

[66] Trojaborg W, Boysen G.
Relation between EEG, regional cerebral blood flow and internal carotid artery pressure during carotid endarterectomy.
Electroenceph Clin Neurophysiol 1973; **34**: 61–9.

[67] Salerno TA, Lince DP, White DN, Lynn RB, Charrette EJP.
Monitoring of electroencephalogram during open-heart surgery. A prospective analysis of 118 cases.
J Thorac Cardiovasc Surg 1978; **76**: 97–100.

[68] Bolsin SNC.
Detection of neurological damage during cardiopulmonary bypass.
Anaesthesia 1986; **41**: 61–6.

[69] Kritikou PE, Branthwaite MA.
Significance of changes in cerebral electrical activity at onset of cardiopulmonary bypass.
Thorax 1977; **32**: 534–8.

[70] Barnes RW, Liebman PR, Marszalek PB, Kirk CL, Goldman MH.
The natural history of asymptomatic carotid disease in patients undergoing cardiovascular surgery.
Surgery 1981; **90**: 1075–83.

[71] Breslau PJ, Fell G, Ivey TB, Bailey WW, Miller DW, Strandness DE.
Carotid arterial disease in patients undergoing coronary bypass operations.
J Thorac Cardiovasc Surg 1981; **82**: 765–7.

[72] Ivey TB, Strandness DE, Williams DB, Langlois Y, Misbach GA, Kruse AP.
Management of patients with carotid bruit undergoing cardiopulmonary bypass.
J Thorac Cardiovasc Surg 1984; **87**: 183–9.

[73] Ropper AH, Wechsler LR, Wilson LS.
Carotid bruit and risk of stroke in elective surgery.
N Engl J Med 1982; **307**: 1388–90.

[74] Turnipseed WD, Berkoff HA, Belzer FD.
Post-operative stroke in cardiac and peripheral vascular disease.
Ann Surg 1980; **192**: 365–8.

[75] Kartchner MM, McRae LP.
Carotid occlusive disease as a risk factor in major cardiovascular surgery.
Arch Surg 1982; **117**: 1086–8.

[76] Jones EL, Craver JM, Michalik RA *et al.*
Combined carotid and coronary operations: When are they necessary?
J Thorac Cardiovasc Surg 1984; **87**: 7–16.

[77] Urschel HC, Razzuk MA, Gardner MA.
Management of concomitant occlusive disease of the carotid and coronary arteries.
J Thorac Cardiovasc Surg 1976; **72**: 829–34.

[78] Ennix CL, Lawrie GM, Morris GC *et al.*
Improved results of carotid endarterectomy in patients with symptomatic coronary disease. An analysis of 1546 consecutive carotid operations.
Stroke 1979; **10**: 122–5.

[79] Bernhard JM, Johnson WD, Peterson JJ.
Carotid artery stenosis: Association with surgery for coronary artery disease.
Arch Surg 1972; **105**: 837–40.

[80] Morris GC, Ennix CL, Lawrie GM, Crawford ES, Howell JF.
Management of coexistent carotid and coronary artery occlusive atherosclerosis.
Cleve Clin Q 1978; **45**: 125–7.

[81] Craver JM, Murphy DA, Jones EL *et al.*
Concomitant carotid and coronary artery revascularization.
Ann Surg 1982; **195**: 712–9.

[82] Emery RW, Cohn LH, Whittemore AD, Mannick JA, Couch NP, Collins JJ.
Coexistent carotid and coronary artery disease.
Arch Surg 1983; **118**: 1035–8.

[83] Hertzer NR, Loop FD, Taylor PC, Beven EG.
Staged and combined surgical approach to simultaneous carotid and coronary vascular disease.
Surgery 1978; **84**: 803–11.

[84] Hertzer NR, Loop FD, Taylor PL, Beven EG.
Combined myocardial revascularisation and carotid endarterectomy. Operative and late results in 331 patients.
J Thorac Cardiovasc Surg 1983; **85**: 577–89.

[85] Robertson JT, Fraser JC.
Evaluation of carotid endarterectomy with and without coronary artery bypass surgery. In: Moossy J, Reinmuth OM, eds. *Cerebrovascular Diseases*. New York: Raven Press, 1981; pp. 261–9.

[86] Ivey TD, Strandness E, Williams DB, Langlois Y, Misbach GA, Kruse AP.
Management of patients with carotid bruit undergoing cardiopulmonary bypass.
J Thorac Cardiovasc Surg 1984; **87**: 183–9.

[87] Mori A, Sono J, Nakashima M, Okada Y.
Application of pulsatile cardiopulmonary bypass for profound hypothermia in cardiac surgery.
Jpn Circ J 1981; **45**: 315–20.

[88] Matsumoto T, Wolferth CC, Perlman MH.
Effect of pulsatile and non-pulsatile perfusion upon cerebral and conjunctival microcirculation in dogs.
Arch Surg 1966; **93**: 730–40.

[89] Anderson K, Waaben J, Husum B *et al.*
Nonpulsatile cardiopulmonary bypass disrupts the flow–metabolism couple in the brain.
J Thorac Cardiovasc Surg 1985; **90**: 570–9.

[90] Grande PO, Borgstrom P, Mellander S.
On the nature of basal vascular tone in cat skeletal muscle and its dependence on transmural pressure stimuli.
Acta Physiol Scand 1979; **107**: 365–76.

[91] Portnay HD, Chopp M, Branch C, Shannon MB.
Cerebrospinal fluid pulse waveform as an indicator of cerebral autoregulation.
J Neurosurg 1982; **56**: 666–78.

[92] Geha AS, Salaymek MT, Abe T, Baue AE.
Effect of pulsatile cardiopulmonary bypass on cerebral metabolism.
J Surg Res 1972; **12**: 381–7.

[93] Menasché P, Pinard E, Desroches AM *et al.*
Fluorocarbons: A potential treatment of cerebral air embolism in open-heart surgery.
Ann Thorac Surg 1985; **40**: 494–7.

[94] Duff HJ, Buda AJ, Kramer R, Strauss HB, David TE, Berman MB.
Detection of entrapped intra-cardiac air with intra-operative echocardiography.
Am J Cardiol 1980; **46**: 255–60.

[95] Oka Y, Morivoki KM, Hong Y *et al.*
Detection of air emboli in the left heart by M-mode transesophageal echocardiography following cardiopulmonary bypass.
Anesthesiology 1985; **63**: 109–13.

[96] Furuya H, Suzuki T, Okumura F, Kishi Y, Vejugi T.
Detection of air embolism by transesophageal echocardiography.
Anesthesiology 1983; **58**: 124–9.
[97] Parker FB, Marvasti MA, Bove EL.
Neurologic complications following coronary artery bypass: The role of atherosclerotic emboli.
Thorac Cardiovasc Surg 1985; **33**: 207–9.

[98] Cosgrove DM.
Management of the calcified aorta: An alternative method of occlusion.
Ann Thorac Surg 1983; **36**: 718–9.

BLEEDING AFTER CARDIOPULMONARY BYPASS

[1] Treatment with desmopressin acetate to reduce blood loss after cardiac surgery. A double-blind randomized trial.
Salzman EW, Weinstein MJ, Weintraub RM *et al*, Beth Israel Hosp, Boston, MA, USA.
N Engl J Med 1986; **314**: 1402–6.
[2] Bleeding after cardiopulmonary bypass (Editorial).
Harker LA, Scripps Clin and Res Found, La Jolla, CA, USA.
N Engl J Med 1986; **314**: 1446–7.

Comment. Despite shorter cardiopulmonary bypass times and an improvement in both surgical technique and open-heart bypass technology which preserve clotting factors and platelets, hemorrhage following cardiopulmonary bypass continues to cause concern as a postoperative complication. Approximately 3% of patients who have undergone cardiac operations need to be re-explored for hemorrhage. In a small proportion of these cases, hemorrhage is due to hematologic problems. Desmopressin acetate is a synthetic vasopressin analogue used to improve hemostasis in patients with mild hemophilia or von Willebrand's disease by shortening bleeding time via the release of factor VIII. Salzman *et al* [1] prospectively studied the effect of intraoperative desmopressin acetate in 70 patients undergoing various cardiac operations that required cardiopulmonary bypass in a randomized double blind manner. (Patients undergoing uncomplicated coronary artery bypass grafting were excluded.) It was found that desmopressin significantly reduced the mean operative and early postoperative blood loss (1317 ±86 ml in the treated group *vs* 2210 ±1415 ml in the placebo group). Twenty-four-hour blood loss exceeded 2000 ml in 14 patients, 11 of whom were in the placebo group. Plasma levels of factor VIII were found to be higher in those receiving desmopressin than in those receiving placebo. It was also found that those patients who bled the most had relatively low levels of factor VIII before surgery. This result particularly indicates a role for factor VIII in the hemorrhagic tendency induced by extracorporeal circulation. The authors of this paper are to be commended. Not only do the results of their study contribute to our knowledge of the hematological diathesis following cardiopulmonary bypass, but they have found a cost-effective method of reducing hematological morbidity after cardiac surgery.

Harker [2] provides an excellent review of the factors contributing to hemostasis *post* bypass in his editorial. He also compares the results of Salzman *et al* [1] with those of another recent study (Czer *et al*) in which desmopressin acetate was given to patients who bled excessively after cardiopulmonary bypass. Harker examines their implications for other cardiac operations and different types of patient and concludes that, if these results are found to apply, therapy with desmopressin acetate could lead to substantial savings in blood supplies, a reduced risk of transfusion-transmitted disease and a reduced rate of reoperation for hemorrhagic complications. However, the possibility that preoperative desmopressin therapy could increase saphenous vein graft occlusion should be investigated, and a method of identifying those patients who are at particular risk of bleeding should be found.

TRANSPLANTATION

COMBINED HEART AND LUNG TRANSPLANTATION

Review: STUART W. JAMIESON

Transplantation of the combined heart and lung block is now considered rational therapy for end-stage pulmonary disease, or for cardiac disease where the presence of pulmonary hypertension (or Eisenmenger's syndrome) prevents simple cardiac transplantation. The first of these operations was carried out in 1967 [1], but success was finally achieved in 1981, with the fourth clinical attempt. The recipient in this case died recently, of unrelated causes, five years after her operation.

This relatively new therapy has been enthusiastically embraced by perhaps half a dozen centers, which have now performed a total of over 100 operations. The experience of some of these centers has confirmed the difficulty, both technical and in terms of postoperative management, of this undertaking. Extensive experience in cardiac transplantation would seem a requirement for success in this area, although some progress has been made since the subject was last presented in this series [2].

The Donor
The identification of suitable donors for heart–lung transplantation has emerged as the most significant restriction on the development of the operation.

The primary requirement for all donors is, of course, brain death. This concept is now widely recognized and accepted in most countries – although still with notable exceptions. The onset of brain death is most commonly the result of trauma, necessitating urgent intubation for the maintenance of cardiac function. Subsequent pulmonary function may be jeopardized, because in emergency situations: (i) intubation is often carried out under less-than-sterile conditions; (ii) the donor may have aspirated gastric contents; and (iii) management may not have been optimal if there was clearly no likelihood of survival. Early onset of pneumonia is common in potential donors, eliminating them from consideration for the purposes of pulmonary tissue transplantation. In addition, there is a tendency for brain-dead individuals to develop pulmonary edema; whether this is true 'neurogenic pulmonary edema' or whether it represents inadequate fluid management in patients with diabetes insipidus is not clear, and it may be a combination of both entities.

Matching of the donor is carried out by blood type and size. It is important to use a donor slightly smaller than the recipient. Difficulty has been experienced by at least two groups that have tried to place larger lungs into a smaller recipient, requiring a lobectomy in one case and resulting in the death of the patient in the other. Respiration requires that the lungs behave like bellows and, if the lungs cannot expand, pulmonary collapse, atelectasis, inadequate ventilation and infection are inevitable.

Until recently it was thought to be mandatory to bring the body of the donor to the recipient site, as techniques for preservation of the lungs were considered unreliable. The donor restriction that resulted from this requirement has precipitated the development of preservation methods, and long-distance procurement is currently used by all the major teams involved in heart–lung transplantation. However, this carries with it the problems of the timing of the recipient operation and of ensuring a good size-match, as well as the impossibility of a thorough screening of the donor before initiation of the recipient operation.

The lungs are unique in having both a dual blood supply (pulmonary and bronchial arteries) and a connection to the atmosphere (bronchial tree). Because of the alveolar structure, simple topical cooling is likely to be an ineffective method of cooling the body of the lungs. Cooling via the airways has been demonstrated to be detrimental [3]. Three methods of preservation have now been used clinically: flush perfusion of the pulmonary arteries with subsequent static cold immersion [4,5]; cooling of the donor systemically with cardiopulmonary bypass (bronchial artery and pulmonary artery cooling) and subsequent cold immersion; and the maintenance of a warm ventilated preparation (the 'Robicsek technique' [6]), where the heart continues to beat in a closed circuit, with coronary sinus return being provided to the lungs [7].

All of these methods have produced satisfactory preservation for four hours or more, although attempted preservation for much longer periods would probably be unwise. Continued effort will no doubt refine these techniques for the future, but simplicity is likely to be the key to the continued use of any given technique.

The Recipient

Recipients have to date fallen into many different categories, but generally they have been subjects with disease of both the lungs and the heart – patients with pulmonary hypertension, either due to Eisenmenger's syndrome or due to primary pulmonary hypertension [8]. Other potential candidates are those with primary lung disease; however, although good results have been obtained with the pulmonary fibroses, those with emphysema have fared badly. This may be due to the lack of compliance of the chest wall in these patients, with the consequent inability to produce full ventilatory excursion postoperatively, leading to failure of gas exchange and elimination of secretions.

Single-lung transplantation has recently achieved success for the first time [9]. This procedure has the disadvantage that one diseased lung will remain, but the advantage of an easier surgical technique and the avoidance of concomitant cardiac transplantation.

The Operation

The operative technique is now standard [10]. After early experience demonstrated that it was more difficult to ensure integrity of nervous structures if an attempt was made to remove the recipient's heart and lungs in one piece, the operation was modified to allow the separate removal of these structures, beginning with the heart, then removing first the left, then the right, lung. All the technical challenge of the operation lies in the removal of the old organs. Absolute hemostasis is a prerequisite – more especially since posterior structures become difficult to gain access to after the donor heart and lungs are in place. Hemostasis in general becomes less easy to achieve, because the patients present in varying degrees of hepatic failure; the time spent on bypass is longer than for standard cardiac operations; and patients with complex cyanotic heart disease may have multiple collateral bronchial vessels.

After the operation, respiration will depend upon diaphragmatic as well as chest-wall movement, and the cough reflex must be intact so as to clear secretions. Thus, the maintenance of integrity of the phrenic and recurrent laryngeal nerves is important. The vagus nerves are easily injured, since they course in the space between left atrium and esophagus, the former of which must be removed. The nerve is not always easily visible, and may be tented up during retraction. Transient lack of gastrointestinal motility is not uncommon after the operation, and, although this usually resolves, care must be taken to avoid inhalation of gastric contents. At least one patient has required a pyloroplasty several weeks after transplantation.

Patients who have had previous chest surgery present a greater problem during the operation. Adhesions from previous surgery may be vascular, and can make access from a median sternotomy difficult if they resulted from a lateral thoracotomy. Most active programs will regard patients with previous surgery with less favor than those without, and these patients certainly have a poorer overall survival.

Immunosuppression

Various immunosuppressive protocols have been used in combined heart–lung transplantation; at the present time, I favor a triple therapy, comprising steroids, cyclosporine and azathioprine. Immediate perioperative steroids are administered as for heart transplantation – in doses of 500 mg i.v. immediately, then 125 mg every 8 hours for three doses. Further steroid therapy is then withheld for two weeks, in order to allow full healing of the tracheal anastomosis. After this time, immunosuppression with steroids is reinstituted at a dose of 0.2 mg/kg given orally, and maintained indefinitely. Cyclosporine is given only orally, at an initial dose of 6 mg/kg; I monitor serum levels of the drug, and seek to maintain trough levels of 100–200 ng for the first two weeks, reducing this slightly if rejection has not been encountered. Intravenous administration of cyclosporine is not used at our center because of the potential added nephrotoxicity, more likely in these patients because of their pre-existing renal impairment as a result of venous congestion. Azathioprine is given orally at 2 mg/kg, although this dose may need modification if leukopenia results.

Results of Transplantation

Immediately after transplantation of both lungs and heart, lymphatic drainage is disrupted, afferent and efferent nerves are divided, and the bronchial arterial supply is lost. Surprisingly, little derangement in function results from this procedure.

Because of loss of lymphatic drainage, the lungs tend to develop edema readily, and a conscious effort must be made to minimize the administration of fluids until the patient has regained preoperative weight. These patients usually demonstrate renal impairment preoperatively, which is worsened postoperatively by cardiopulmonary bypass, limitation of fluid administration, and the toxic effects of cyclosporine. This may make fluid balance difficult to achieve, and plasma ultrafiltration with or without dialysis is often necessary early in the postoperative period.

In the first few days after operation, an impairment of gas exchange accompanied by diffuse radiologic opacity on chest X-ray may occur [11], often attributable to fluid overload and the loss of lymphatics. If pulmonary edema occurs, subsequent removal of fluid may still result in the manifestation of a continued capillary leak syndrome – similar in all respects to other types of adult respiratory distress, with the exception that it will resolve within a few days if supportive therapy can be maintained. Prolonged intubation and respiratory support will be necessary, administered with a positive end-expiratory pressure of less than 10 mmHg. High peak inspiratory pressures may be experienced, and these may be minimized (to help preserve the tracheal suture line) by rapid ventilation with lower tidal volumes. Extracorporeal membrane oxygenation might be helpful in severe respiratory distress, although the combination of pre-existing renal and hepatic failure with mechanical support would be unlikely to lead to success.

Patients are generally extubated on the first postoperative day and maintain satisfactory ventilation. Daily chest X-rays must be obtained, and any suggestion of pulmonary edema should be treated rapidly with diuresis or removal of fluid (as outlined above). The pulmonary lymphatics regenerate after about 10 days, and the need for rigorous fluid restriction then abates. Radiologic opacity after approximately one week is then more likely to be the result of rejection, usually accompanied by fevers and leukocytosis. Eosinophilia is common.

It is now well documented that the lungs are often rejected independently [12,13], and usually before the heart. Diagnosis of rejection is difficult because, unlike cardiac tissue, lung tissue cannot easily be obtained for histologic study: open-lung biopsy poses a substantial risk for the sick and immunosuppressed patient, and certainly cannot be performed repetitively; biopsy by bronchoscopy retrieves specimens that are generally too small to be helpful. A diagnosis of rejection is therefore made on the basis of the time of onset of diffuse, often fluffy radiologic opacity on chest X-ray, and after exclusion of infectious causes. Fortunately, marked changes on chest X-ray are usually accompanied by trivial clinical impairment. They may not appear until rejection is advanced.

Denervation of the heart has been shown to be fully compatible with normal exercise. Experience with combined heart and lung transplantation has now demonstrated that denervation of the lungs also appears to be without significance [14]: respiration continues in a normal pattern, and will increase in rate and depth with the demands of stress and activity. The regulation of respiration in humans apparently depends little on pulmonary afferent nerves.

The loss of bronchial arterial supply is also without apparent sequelae. The tracheal anastomosis heals well, this process probably being contributed to by the rich coronary artery–bronchial artery collateral circulation [8]; indeed, care must be taken to examine the donor pleural reflections after the aortic anastomosis is completed, because new bleeding sites may appear along these cut edges.

Patients who have survived the immediate perioperative hospitalization have usually returned to normal activity. In a small subgroup of these, however, late complications have developed [15,16], including bronchiolitis obliterans, pulmonary vascular disease, pulmonary fibrosis and coronary artery disease [17,18]. The precise etiology of these changes is unclear, but they are probably due to rejection. In my practice, immunosuppression has been achieved over the last two years by the triple therapy outlined earlier; although it is too early to make a definite statement, no late sequelae of the sort described above have been encountered since the change to triple therapy.

Survival

As of December 1986, the International Registry for Heart Transplantation shows a total of 101 combined heart-lung transplants performed worldwide [19]. Almost all of these have been performed within the last three years, so that any meaningful survival statistics are valid only for the first and second years, with an overall survival of 57% and 55%, respectively. However, superior figures have been published by individual centers [20]. The international figures clearly demonstrate that survival hinges on the immediate perioperative period. Data from the International Registry reveal 2560 heart transplants performed over the same period, with a one- and two-year survival of 77% and 74%, respectively, and a five-year survival of 73%. The marked disparity in numbers and survival between the two operations reflects the greater complexity of the combined procedure and the fact that suitable donors are very much more difficult to obtain.

The longest current survivor of this operation was transplanted about six years ago, and is unrestricted in activity. He embodies some of the learning process of the last five years, however, since progressive rejection resulted in his becoming dependent on a ventilator some three years after his original operation. He was subjected to retransplantation with success [21].

Conclusions

Heart–lung transplantation has been shown to be an effective therapy for prolonging life in end-stage heart and lung disease. The restriction on donors is likely to limit most programs involved in this endeavor, but combined heart–lung transplantation has established itself among the choices to be offered those with otherwise untreatable heart and lung disease.

References

[1] Cooley DA, Bloodwell RD, Hallman GL, Nora JJ, Harrison GM, Leachman RD.
Organ transplantation for advanced cardiopulmonary disease.
Ann Thorac Surg 1969; **8**: 30–42.

[2] Jamieson SW.
Cardiac transplantation in cardiovascular medicine. In: Sobel BE, Julian DG, Hugenholtz PG, eds. *Perspectives in Cardiology 1984*. London: Current Medical Literature, 1984; pp. 295–301.

[3] Haverich A, Scott WC, Jamieson SW.
Twenty years of lung preservation – A review.
Heart Transplant 1985; **4**: 234–40.

[4] Haverich A, Scott WC, Aziz S, Jamieson SW.
Influence of perfusate flow and volume on pre-servation of the lungs for transplantation.
Heart Transplant 1985; **4**: 129.

[5] Jamieson SW, Starkey T, Sakakibara N, Baldwin JC.
Procurement of organs for combined heart-lung transplantation.
Trans Proc 1986; **18**: 616–7.

[6] Robicsek F, Tam W, Dougherty HK, Robicsek M.
The stabilized autoperfusing heart–lung pre-paration as a vehicle for extracorporeal pre-servation.
Trans Proc 1969; **1**: 834–9.

[7] Ladowski JS, Kapelanski DP, Teodori MF, Stevenson WC, Hardesty RL, Griffith BP.
Use of autoperfusion for distant procurement of heart–lung allografts.
Heart Transplant 1985; **4**: 330–3.

[8] Jamieson SW, Stinson EB, Oyer PE *et al.*
Heart–lung transplantation for irreversible pul-monary hypertension.
Ann Thorac Surg 1984; **38**: 554–62.

[9] Cooper J.
Personal Communication, 1986.

[10] Jamieson SW, Stinson EB, Oyer PE, Baldwin JC, Shumway NE.
Operative technique for heart-lung trans-plantation.
J Thorac Cardiovasc Surg 1984; **87**: 930–5.

[11] Chiles C, Guthaner DF, Jamieson SW, Stinson EB, Oyer PE, Silverman JF.
Heart–lung transplantation: The post-operative chest radiograph.
Radiology 1985; **154**: 299–304.

[12] Scott WC, Haverich A, Billingham ME, Dawkins KD, Jamieson SW.
Lethal lung rejection without significant cardiac rejection in primate heart–lung allotransplanta-tion.
Heart Transplant 1984; **4**: 33–9.

[13] McGregor CGA, Baldwin JC, Jamieson SW *et al.*
Isolated pulmonary rejection after combined heart-lung transplantation.
J Thorac Cardiovasc Surg 1985; **90**: 623–30.

[14] Theodore J, Jamieson SW, Burke CM *et al.*
Physiological aspects of human heart-lung transplantation: Pulmonary status of the post-transplanted lung.
Chest 1984; **86**: 349.

[15] Jamieson SW, Dawkins KD, Burke C *et al.*
Late results of combined heart–lung trans-plantation.
Trans Proc 1985; **17**: 212–4.

[16] Dawkins KD, Jamieson SW, Hunt SA *et al.*
Long-term results, hemodynamics, and com-plications after combined heart and lung trans-plantation.
Circulation 1985; **1**: 919–26.

[17] Burke CM, Theodore J, Dawkins KD *et al.*
Post-transplant obliterative bronchiolitis and other late sequelae in human heart–lung trans-plantation.
Chest 1984; **86**: 824.

[18] Haverich A, Dawkins KD, Baldwin JC, Reitz BA, Billingham ME, Jamieson SW.
Long-term cardiac and pulmonary histology in primates following combined heart and lung transplantation.
Transplantation 1985; **39**: 356–60.

[19] Kaye MP (The Registry, International Society for Heart Transplantation).
Personal Communication, 1986.

[20] Jamieson SW, Baldwin JC, Reitz BA *et al.*
Combined heart and lung transplantation.
Lancet 1983; i: 1130–2.

[21] Jamieson SW.
Recent developments in heart and heart-lung transplantation.
Trans Proc 1985; **17**: 199–203.

PROSPECTS FOR THE ARTIFICIAL HEART

Review: CHRISTOPHER G.A. McGREGOR

The estimated incidence of congestive heart failure in the USA in 1983 was 394 000. Less than 50% of patients with this syndrome can be expected to survive five years after initial diagnosis. Furthermore, patients in functional class IV have a one-year survival rate of less than 50% [1]. A working group on mechanical circulatory support reported to the National Institutes of Health that 17–35 000 of these patients each year in the USA could be medically eligible for long-term circulatory support [2]. However, the number of potential donors of hearts available for transplantation in the USA is unlikely to exceed 1000 per year [3]. Thus, there is clearly a need for alternative effective, long term mechanical support systems. The US Congress, through the National Heart, Lung and Blood Institute, has supported, with additional private sector funding, the development of a spectrum of circulatory support systems over the last 20 years. Such systems can be considered as either ventricular assist devices that work in parallel with the patient's own heart or total artificial hearts that functionally replace the patient's heart entirely. During the last five years, the clinical application of a number of these mechanical circulatory support devices has increased following notable progress in technology, biocompatible materials, systems integration, and experimental animal research. Each of the two main categories of device (ventricular assist device and total artificial heart) can be pneumatically or electrically powered. The two will be discussed, as will the potential use of skeletal muscle-powered ventricular assist components. Intra-aortic balloon pumps and non-pulsatile centrifugal pumps are not considered to be applicable for long-term utilization and therefore will not be discussed here.

Air-Powered Ventricular Assist Devices

Most air-powered ventricular assist devices have the same overall design. They work in parallel with the patient's own heart and consist of a seamless polyurethane blood sac enclosed within a rigid metal case. Air is pulsed from an external drive unit, via a percutaneous drive line, between the metal case and blood sac with resultant pulsatile expulsion of blood from the device. Unidirectional flow is achieved by inlet and outlet prosthetic valves.

These pumps can be used on the left side of the circulation (left-ventricular assist device) or on the right side (right-ventricular assist device). When the device is used as a left-ventricular assist device, blood is drained from the left atrium and returned to the ascending or abdominal aorta; when used as a right-ventricular assist device, blood is drained from the right atrium and returned to the pulmonary artery. Two devices can be used together to provide biventricular support.

Examples of air-powered ventricular assist devices include the Pierce-Donachy pump manufactured by Thoratec and Pennsylvania State University, the air-driven Thermedics device described by Bernhard, and the Nimbus, Liotta and Abiomed air-driven systems.

Air-driven ventricular assist devices are suitable for temporary use only (i.e. for days to weeks). Indications for the use of a ventricular assist device include post-cardiotomy or post-myocardial infarct cardiogenic shock refractory to pharmacologic or intra-aortic balloon support. Physiologic criteria for the use of the left-ventricular and right-ventricular assist devices are shown in Table 1 and 2. Adequate physiologic monitoring, including the measurement of right-atrial pressure, pulmonary arterial wedge pressure, cardiac output and systemic arterial pressures is mandatory. Once a device is in place, ventricular assist device support is continued until recovery of the myocardium can be assumed to be complete. Experience indicates that right-ventricular functional recovery can take 3–5 days and left-ventricular recovery 7–10 days or more [4]. Weaning from the ventricular assist device is accomplished by intermittent cessation of the pump support, evaluation of cardiac action, and gradual reduction of pump output as tolerated, followed by removal of the pump.

TABLE I: Physiological Criteria for Use of Left-Ventricular Assist Device

Non-surgically correctable left-ventricular dysfunction
Systolic blood pressure <90 mmHg
Left-atrial pressure or pulmonary arterial wedge pressure >25 mmHg
Cardiac index <1.8 l/min/m^2

TABLE II: Physiological Criteria for Use of Right-Ventricular Assist Device

Systolic blood pressure <90 mmHg
Right-atrial pressure >20 mmHg
Left-atrial pressure or pulmonary arterial wedge pressure <12 mmHg
Cardiac index <1.8 l/min/m^2

Complications of the use of ventricular assist devices include hemorrhage, sepsis and multi-organ failure [5]. Many of these complications occur with late application of devices in severely compromised patients following prolonged cardiopulmonary bypass.

Patient survival following the use of ventricular assist devices has been reported as being 50% in an extremely high-risk group of patients [6]. A number of left-ventricular assist devices have been used recently as a temporary bridge to transplantation, supporting acutely deteriorating patients until a suitable donor heart can be obtained. A recent report provided encouraging early results in this situation with 68% of patients successfully supported prior to cardiac transplantation and 43% being discharged from hospital following successful transplantation [7].

Electrically Powered Ventricular Assist Devices
Electrically powered ventricular assist devices are designed to provide long-term circulatory support in those patients with terminal heart failure who do not meet the criteria for heart transplantation. These devices differ from air-powered ventricular assist devices in that the blood-pumps and energy convertors are designed to be totally implantable. Transcutaneous transmission of electrical power using primary and secondary induction belts will enable patients to be completely untethered during cir-

culatory support, obviating one of the fundamental draw-backs of air-powered systems. The absence of percutaneous lines or wires should provide a major improvement in quality of life and reduce the risk of infection. In addition, the patient's own heart may be able to provide temporary back-up if the device fails catastrophically.

One electrically powered left-ventricular assist device, the NOVACOR*, is currently in clinical use as a temporary bridge for transplantation or post-cardiotomy circulatory support. This system, developed and evaluated over the last 20 years at Stanford University, was the first left-ventricular assist device to be applied successfully, clinically, as a bridge to transplantation in man [8]. The NOVACOR left-ventricular assist device is a second-generation device designed for long-term use (Fig. 1). It consists of a dual pusher plate seamless sac blood-pump, a balanced pivoted solenoid energy convertor, a variable volume compensator, a micro processor control unit with standby back-up power, an intact skin built transformer and a primary power module with status monitor. The device is placed in the abdominal cavity in the preperitoneal position with inflow from the left-ventricular apex and outflow to the abdominal or ascending aorta. Porcine valves are used to produce unidirectional flow. To date, nine patients have been supported with the NOVACOR left-ventricular assist device as a bridge to transplantation. Six were supported sufficiently so that transplantation could be undertaken. There have been four long-term survivors for up to 30 months. One patient who received circulatory support for 90 days was ambulant and otherwise well in a general hospital ward for most of this interval [9].

Other electrically powered ventricular assist devices under development include the Thermedics, Nimbus, Ambiomed and Pennsylvania State University devices. None of these has yet been used clinically.

Air Powered Total Artificial Hearts
Most total artificial hearts at the present time are pneumatically powered. They are

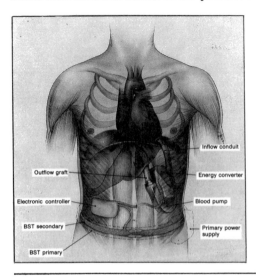

FIGURE 1. The NOVACOR LVAD.

---

* Novacor Medical Corporation, Oakland, California 94621.

essentially biventricular replacement devices. The best known and most commonly applied total artificial heart developed to date is the Jarvik 7, but similar devices are being developed in Pennsylvania State University, Phoenix, Berlin, Vienna, Tokyo and behind the Iron Curtain. Generally, total artificial hearts consist of two implantable pumps similar to ventricular assist devices each with a rigid case containing a seamless blood sac with inlet and outlet valves, two percutaneous drive lines, 'quick' connect prosthetic cuffs for anastomoses with the great vessels and recipient atria, and an external drive and control console. Pumping is achieved by driving the air between the rigid casing and the blood sac as for air-powered ventricular assist devices.

The first application of a long-term total artificial heart as part of a program of circulatory support for patients with end-stage cardiac failure who were not heart-transplant candidates occurred in 1982 when a Jarvik 7 was placed in Dr Barney Clark, who survived for 112 days [10]. Complications, particularly thromboembolism and sepsis in the first case and in later long-term implants, coupled with the need for a bulky external drive unit and percutaneous air lines, made this application of the device unacceptable to many so that the primary indication for insertion of an air-driven total artificial heart is now as a bridge to transplantation. By the end of 1986, 55 total artificial hearts had been implanted worldwide, 45 of which were either the Jarvik 7 or the smaller Jarvik 7/70 [11]. Forty of these 45 Jarvik implants were used as a bridge to transplantation; 6 of the 40 patients died before transplantation could be performed, and at the time of this writing four patients remain supported by the total artificial heart. Of the 30 patients who underwent cardiac transplantation, 22 are alive and 16 have been discharged from hospital [12]. The complete absence of cardiac rhythm or the presence of uncontrollable arrhythmias in a patient with profound biventricular failure who is unlikely to recover comprise indications for a total artificial heart as opposed to a ventricular assist device.

Electrically Powered Total Artificial Hearts
These devices are being developed for long-term circulatory support of patients with end-stage cardiac disease who are not candidates for heart transplantation. No such devices are available for clinical use at the present time. One advantage of an electrically powered total artificial heart compared with one that is air-driven is the absence of percutaneous drive lines and bulky external drive units. The electrical total artificial heart consists of two blood-pumps, an electrical motor, an energy convertor and primary and secondary electrical induction belts, one placed subcutaneously the other worn externally as a belt for percutaneous transmission of electricity across the intact skin. 'Quick' connect cuffs for attachment to the great vessels and atria, and two inlet and outlet valves are used as in pneumatically powered total artificial hearts. Results of early studies in animals at the Pennsylvania State University and the University of Utah have been encouraging, but clinical application is several years away.

A major disadvantage of the total artificial heart is the need to remove the patient's native heart with consequent loss of cardiovascular regulation via the autonomic nervous system and through responses to circulating catecholamines. The total artificial heart will be microchip controlled via a quasi Starling law or by fixed-rate pulsation which may not provide adequate long-term fine adjustment. In contrast, use of an electrical left-ventricular assist device can leave the normal control systems intact with the left-ventricular assist device being effectively 'slaved' to the natural heart.

Skeletal Muscle Ventricular Assist

Recent advances in the field of functional augmentation of the heart with autogenous skeletal muscle are based on the application of electrical conditioning described by Macoviak [13]. Both left-ventricular and right-ventricular assistance have been proposed and are currently under study in animals. Recently, selected patients have been treated with reinforcement myografts of latissimus dorsi muscle after ventricular resections [14,15]. Judging from the ability of skeletal muscle to become electrically conditioned and fatigue resistant, and the demonstration of functional assistance of latissimus dorsi muscle in human subjects, selected patients may benefit from functional myografts in the future, particularly for the lesser (pulmonary) circulation. The needs for a significant skeletal muscle mass, endogenous innervation and vascular supply all amenable to placement in the mediastinum without a tethering effect are major limitations. The thrombogenic nature of skeletal muscle exposed to circulating cavitary blood and the ill-defined long-term performance characteristics of electrically stimulated skeletal muscle in this context are potential limitations as well.

Conclusions

Ventricular assist devices and total artificial hearts have been shown to provide effective circulatory support for some patients, particularly when used as a bridge to transplantation. Patients with cardiogenic shock who cannot reasonably be expected to recover, who are considered as potential transplant candidates and fulfil several criteria are suitable candidates for insertion of a mechanical circulatory support device. The use of such devices should be restricted to centers with access to cardiac transplantation. For optimal results, the decision to use a mechanical circulatory support device must be acted upon before multi-organ failure has occurred. The implantation of such a device should not automatically give a specific patient priority over other cardiac-transplant candidates, but rather should be used to stabilize patients until a suitable donor can be found.

The marginal improvement of quality of life resulting from the use of pneumatic devices is unlikely to be deemed to be sufficient to justify their long-term use by patients or physicians. The electrical left-ventricular assist device will be available for long-term implantation perhaps within 2–3 years in patients who are not suitable candidates for heart transplantation. Clinical use of an electrical total artificial heart is unlikely to be feasible for 10 years or more. At present, the relative merits of a ventricular assist device system compared with a total artificial heart system remain unresolved, but early experience suggests that most patients can be supported adequately by a left-ventricular assist device and that many with biventricular failure can respond to left-ventricular assist only. Mechanical circulatory support systems are now available. Logistic, financial and ethical implications must be faced squarely.

References

[1] Smith WM.
Epidemiology of congestive heart failure.
Am J Cardiol 1985; **55**: 3A–8A.

[2] The Working Group on Mechanical Circulatory Support of the National Heart, Lung and Blood Institute.
Artificial Heart and Assist Devices: Direction, Needs, Costs, Societal and Ethical Issues.
Bethesda, Md: NHLBI; 1985.

[3] Evans RW, Manninen DL, Garrison LP, Maier AM.
Donor availability as the primary determinant of the future of heart transplantation.
J Am Med Assoc 1986; **255**: 1892–8.

[4] Pierce WS, Parr GVS, Myers JL.
Ventricular assist pumping in patients with cardiogenic shock after cardiac operations.
N Engl J Med 1981; **305**: 1606–10.

[5] Gaines WE, Pierce WS, Donachy JH *et al.*
The Pennsylvania State University paracorporeal ventricular assist pump: Optimal method of use.
World J Surg 1985; **9**: 47–53.

[6] Richenbacher WE, Pierce WS.
Clinical spectrum of mechanical circulatory assistance.
Heart Transplant 1985; **IV**: 481–8.

[7] Cardiac assist devices used as bridges to transplantation.
American Society for Artificial Internal Organs – International Society of Heart Transplantation Combined Registry Report for 1985 and 1986.

[8] Portner PM, Oyer PE, McGregor CGA *et al.*
First human use of an electrically powered implantable ventricular assist system.
Abst Proc Int Soc Artif Organs 1985

[9] Portner P.
Personal Communication.

[10] DeVries WC, Anderson JL, Joyce LD *et al.*
Clinical use of a total artificial heart.
N Engl J Med 1984; **310**: 273–8.

[11] Olsen DB.
Artificial Heart Registry: University of Utah Institute for Biomedical Engineering.
Salt Lake City, Utah 84112; 1987.

[12] Symbion Inc.
Clinical update: a current report on use of the Jarvik-7 (100 cc) and Jarvik-7 (70 cc's) as a bridge-to-transplant.
Salt Lake City, Utah 84103; 1987

[13] Macoviak J, Stephenson LW, Alavi A *et al.*
Effects of chronic stimulation of right ventricular diaphragmatic inlay grafts.
Surgery 1981; **90**: 271–7.

[14] Carpentier A, Chachques JC.
Myocardial substitution with a stimulated skeletal muscle: first successful clinical case (Letter to the editor).
Lancet 1985; **i**: 1267.

[15] Magovern JG, Park SB, Benckart DM *et al.*
Latissimus dorsi as a functioning synchronously paced muscle component in the repair of a left ventricular aneurysm (Letter to the editor).
Ann Thorac Surg 1986; **41**: 116.

CAROTID ENDARTERECTOMY

CAROTID ENDARTERECTOMY WITH AND WITHOUT CORONARY ARTERY BYPASS GRAFTING

Review: AVERIL O. MANSFIELD

Neurologic complications are among the most worrying problems that may occur following coronary artery bypass grafting (CABG). Discrete focal neurologic deficit can be detected in 4% of patients after CABG; less well-defined cerebral dysfunction is much more common, with around 40–60% of patients showing abnormalities on extensive and detailed testing [1]. The majority of the 312 patients in this series were not disabled in any way by these problems, and neurologic abnormalities accounted for one death (0.3%). However, four patients (1.3%) were severely disabled. A similar study had been carried out previously at the Cleveland Clinic and, in a prospective analysis of 421 patients, strokes were detected in 5.2% but were only observed to be severe in 2% [2]. Moreover, Smith *et al* found that abnormalities of a similar nature occurred after major vascular and thoracic surgery, albeit less frequently, and so they are not entirely attributable to cardiopulmonary bypass [3].

The important question is whether cerebrovascular disease, either symptomatic or occult, makes a contribution to this morbidity and, in particular, to the permanent stroke incidence. Further questions relate to whether detection and correction of accessible vascular lesions can lessen the risk of such complications. There is an established and close association between coronary artery disease and carotid artery disease. Myocardial infarction is the most common cause of postoperative death seen in the follow-up of patients who have had a carotid endarterectomy. Hertzer *et al* have documented this association by the use of coronary angiography in patients with carotid disease [4].

Hence, there are two major questions to be answered. First, should the patient who requires CABG have routine investigation of his carotid arteries, on the assumption that part of the stroke morbidity of CABG surgery will be the result of preexisting carotid artery disease. Second, should the patient who has undergone carotid artery surgery have routine investigation of his coronary arteries in the hope of preventing some of the late deaths from myocardial infarction?

Subsidiary questions relate to the relative timing of these procedures. Which operation should come first? Should the two operations take place under the same anesthetic and, if so, should they be consecutive or simultaneous?

The recent greater awareness of these two problems is undoubtedly related to advances in the availability and safety of the investigations. This is particularly true of carotid investigations, where invasive and dangerous angiography has been replaced by the use of duplex Doppler scanning and digital subtraction angiography, often via the intravenous route.

The Role of Surgery

Although there is fairly general acceptance of the value of carotid endarterectomy in the symptomatic patient, in the asymptomatic patient the controversy is large and unresolved. This is mainly due to the lack of convincing data on the natural history of the asymptomatic carotid stenosis. The risk of the abnormality must be seen to exceed that of the corrective surgery; overall, evidence for this is doubtful. The benefit of the operation should be reasonably durable with minimal restenosis; again this is uncertain. It is probably wrong to place all carotid stenoses in the same bracket of management because some patients may be at greater risk than others. It is, for example, currently being suggested that very tight stenoses pose a greater hazard then lesser stenoses.

Combined Coronary and Carotid Surgery

If the patient is known to require both coronary and carotid surgery, the nature of the coronary disease will influence the planning. For example, the patient with left main stem coronary disease or unstable angina probably should not have a staged procedure with the carotid surgery first because there is a risk of death due to myocardial infarction with the first operation.

The situation was greatly advanced by Hertzer *et al* in 1983, with the publication of the results of combined myocardial revascularization and carotid endarterectomy [5]. A total of 331 patients underwent combined operations between 1973 and 1981; 173 patients had had no symptoms attributable to their carotid stenosis, and they were detected because of a bruit and confirmed by angiography. There were 19 deaths (5.7%) and 30 patients had neurologic complications (9%), of which half were permanent and three of these were fatal. This is a high complication rate in an admittedly high-risk population. Although the survivors appear to fare reasonably well in comparison with an age-matched population, the initial death rate cannot be ignored and the illustrative graphs give a biased view because of the emphasis on survivors. A disease-matched control population is greatly needed.

Two years later from the same institution, Furland and Craciun identified a group of patients who were known to have carotid disease at the time of their coronary surgery and whose carotid lesions had been documented angiographically [6]. The study suffers from being retrospective and from the fact that the majority of the patients studied (115 out of 144) had had the opposite carotid operated upon at the time of the CABG. However, there did not appear to be any increased stroke risk from the stenosed carotid which was managed conservatively, although judgement was reserved in the patients with >90% stenosis. There were only 16 such lesions in the study, and one of these patients had a postoperative stroke. The overall stroke rate was 2%.

Diagnosis of Cardiovascular Disease
In many of the published series, it is difficult to differentiate between the symptomatic and the asymptomatic patients. It is also often difficult to achieve the very basic distinction between stenosis and bruit; this is particularly important because cervical bruits are common and not necessarily the result of internal carotid artery stenosis. Bruits can be expected in around 5% of the population aged over 45 years, and the incidence rises with age [7].

There seems little doubt that the presence of a bruit over the carotid bifurcation is an indicator of some stroke risk [8], and more importantly it is an indicator of cardiovascular disease in general. Kuller and Sutton review the topic very well, and provocatively question the safety of auscultation of the neck [9]: "Perhaps the patients should be advised and required to sign informed consent prior to auscultation of the neck."

In the absence of symptoms, the cervical bruit is likely to be the starting point in determining treatment in the patient awaiting CABG. Thus, it would seem to be entirely reasonable to make a policy decision prior to auscultation, and to pursue that bruit only if there is convincing evidence that further steps are desirable or if it is necessary as part of an investigation to acquire that evidence.

Even the incidence of severe carotid artery disease in association with coronary artery disease is uncertain. It may depend on the technique used for detection and on the definition of severe. The incidence ranges from 2% to 54% in different series [10–16].

Several uncontrolled studies, employing a range of screening tests including occuloplethysmography, duplex Doppler scanning and angiography, have each attempted to add to our knowledge [10,17]. However, the reverse has been achieved as there is no way of knowing whether the patients would have fared better or worse without surgery.

427

Risks from Surgery

The case against surgery for the asymptomatic carotid stenosis is well made by Chambers and Norris, and essentially revolves around the complication rate of the carotid endarterectomy [18]. The results vary widely and range from 2% to 20% complications for carotid endarterectomy alone. In a review of the results of carotid endarterectomy from a large metropolitan area, Brott and Thalinger looked at results from 16 hospitals and found an overall stroke rate of 8.6% and an operative death rate of 2.8% [19]. The stroke rate was lower in the asymptomatic patients at 5.6% compared with 11.6% in the symptomatic patients. However, one vascular surgeon in the area had a combined stroke and death rate of 1.9%, indicating that a knowledge of the particular surgeon's 'track record' is very important.

Carotid occlusion certainly appears to be worth detecting prior to cardiac surgery because it appears to carry a high risk of stroke. In Brener's series, preoperative evaluation of the carotids was undertaken in 2026 patients undergoing cardiac surgery [20]. Five strokes were suffered by 18 patients who were known to have one or both carotids occluded. Hertzer's series also emphasized the high risk in the patient with a contralateral occlusion or very high-grade stenosis >90%. The neurologic deficit rate reached 20% in those patients. Although occlusion of the carotid is usually inoperable, the increased risk for these patients needs to be considered when deciding whether to offer cardiac surgery.

The risks of cardiac surgery are changing and one of the changing factors is the incidence of stroke. Gardner *et al* reported the results from Johns Hopkins and looked at 3816 patients who underwent CABG [21]. The stroke rate varied but was 2.4% in 1982, 1983 and 1984. It was less than 1.5% in those aged under 60 and over 5% in those over 70. In this study, they found that age and previous cerebrovascular symptoms were important risk factors.

Course of Action

Most authors are in favor of intervention if the carotid artery lesion is symptomatic. The only question then is whether to combine the operations or to stage them. If the carotid endarterectomy is carried out first, there is a risk of perioperative or interval myocardial infarction. A combined operation would appear to be the most logical option, but it carries a substantial morbidity.

In the asymptomatic patient, Ivey recommends a conservative approach [15]. He reports a prospective study of 818 patients undergoing CABG with a stroke rate of 0.7%. Only one event might have been prevented by prophylactic carotid endarterectomy in an asymptomatic patient. His advice is to carry out preliminary carotid endarterectomy if the carotid is symptomatic. However, if the carotid stenosis is not producing symptoms then the cardiac surgery should be performed first, followed by the carotid if the stenosis is >80%. A combined operation is recommended if the patient has unstable angina and has carotid symptoms.

Generally, therefore, combined operations are likely to be undertaken in a particularly high-risk group from both the carotid and the cardiac viewpoint. Cosgrove [22] and Babu [10] have reviewed the complications reported in the literature from combined simultaneous surgery, and they range as follows:

Myocardial infarction 0 – 6.8%
Stroke 0 – 6.2%
Mortality 0 – 9.5%

Perler reported a small series of high-risk combined operations with a more optimistic outcome [23]. There were 37 combined operations and 70% of the patients had either unstable angina, left main stem disease or both; 73% had had previous myocardial infarction. Over half the carotids were asymptomatic, but all had >50% stenosis on at least one side. There were no fatal strokes and no permanent deficits. One transient deficit occurred in a patient with one stenosed and one occluded carotid. There were three deaths from cardiac causes, none of whom had neurologic complications.

It would seem, therefore, that some conclusions can be drawn although a greater number of questions have yet to be answered.

Summary
The patient with symptomatic carotid disease should be directed to a surgeon with a good 'track record'. The carotid surgery should take place before the coronary surgery, provided that the patient does not have left main stem disease or its equivalent or unstable angina. In these circumstances, a combined operation is advisable.

A plan of campaign must be drawn up for the asymptomatic stenosis, because if surgery is not to be contemplated then no investigations are needed except as part of a prospective study.

If the investigations reveal an occluded carotid, then reconsideration of the need for CABG in the light of the potentially high stroke risk is necessary.

If the stenosis is thought to be >80%, then there are no clear guidelines to be obtained from the literature and nothing to substantiate my belief that carotid endarterectomy should be carried out first, except in the severe cardiac risk case when a combined approach is needed.

If the stenosis is <80% and asymptomatic, then no carotid operation is needed and the patient can be followed up in the expectation that warning symptoms are likely to occur before a stroke.

In the group of patients requiring carotid surgery only, the opposite questions need to be addressed. Should the carotid disease be regarded as a pointer to the myocardium and should all such patients have investigations of their coronary arteries? Certainly the highest cause of mortality in the follow-up of patients after carotid endarterectomy is myocardial infarction. Perhaps the best option here is non-invasive cardiac assessment by exercise testing or thallium scanning, with confirmation of detected disease by angiography.

Collection of data is clearly difficult in this group of patients, but objective evidence needs to be obtained to support one or other method of management.

References

[1] Shaw PJ, Bates D, Cartlidge NEF, Heaviside D, Julian DG, Shaw DA.
Early neurological complications of coronary artery bypass surgery.
Br Med J 1985; **291**: 1384–7.

[2] Breuer AC, Furlan AJ, Hanson MR et al.
Central nervous system complications of coronary artery bypass graft surgery: prospective analysis of 421 patients.
Stroke 1983; **14**: 682–7.

[3] Smith PLC, Treasure T, Newman SP et al.
Cerebral consequences of cardiopulmonary bypass.
Lancet 1986; i: 823.

[4] Hertzer NR, Young JR, Beven EG et al.
Coronary angiography in 506 patients with extracranial cerebrovascular disease.
Arch Intern Med 1985; **145**: 849–52.

[5] Hertzer NR, Loop FD, Taylot PC, Beven EG.
Combined myocardial revascularisation and carotid endarterectomy.
J Thorac Cardiovasc Surg 1983; **85**: 577–89.

[6] Furlan AJ, Craciun AR.
Risk of stroke during coronary artery bypass graft surgery in patients with internal carotid artery disease documented by angiography.
Stroke 1985; **16**: 767–99.

[7] Wolf PA, Kannel WB, Sorlie P, McNamara P.
Asymptomatic carotid bruit and risk of stroke.
J Am Med Assoc 1981; **245**: 442–5.

[8] Heyman A, Wilkinson W, Heyden S.
Risk of stroke in asymptomatic persons with cervical arterial bruits.
N Engl J Med 1980; **302**: 838–41.

[9] Kuller LH, Sutton KC.
Carotid artery bruit: is it safe and effective to auscultate the neck?
Stroke 1984; **15**: 944–7.

[10] Babu SC, Shah PM, Singh BM, Semel L, Clauss RH, Reed GR.
Coexisting carotid stenosis in patients undergoing cardiac surgery: indications and guidelines for simultaneous operations.
Am J Surg 1985; **150**: 207–11.

[11] Mehigan JT, Buch WS, Pipkin RD, Fogarty TJ.
A planned approach to coexistent cerebrovascular disease in coronary artery bypass candidates.
Arch Surg 1977; **112**: 1403–9.

[12] Balderman SC, Gutierrez IZ, Makala P Bhayana JN, Gage AA.
Non invasive screening for asymptomatic carotid artery disease prior to cardiac operation. Experience with 500 patients.
J Thorac Cardiovasc Surg 1983; **85**: 427–33.

[13] Turnipseed WD, Berkoss HA, Belzer FO.
Post operative stroke in cardiac and peripheral vascular disease.
Ann Surg 1980; **192**: 365–8.

[14] Barnes RW, Marszalak PB.
Asymptomatic carotid disease in the cardiovascular surgical patient: is prophylactic endarterectomy necessary?
Stroke 1981; **12**: 497–500.

[15] Ivey TD.
Combined carotid and coronary disease – a conservative strategy.
J Vascular Surg 1986; **3**: 687–9.

[16] Breslau PJ, Fell G, Ivey TD, Bailey WW, Miller DW, Strandness Jr DE.
Carotid arterial disease in patients undergoing coronary artery bypass operations.
J Thorac Cardiovasc Surg 1981; **82**: 765–7.

[17] Rosenthal D, Caudill Dr, Lamis PA, Logan W, Stanton PE.
Carotid and coronary arterial disease. A rational approach.
Am Surg 1984; **50**: 233–5.

[18] Chambers BR, Norris JW.
The case against surgery for asymptomatic carotid stenosis.
Stroke 1984; **15**: 964–7.

[19] Brott T, Thalinger K.
The practice of carotid endarterectomy in a large metropolitan area.
Stroke 1984; **15**: 950–5.

[20] Brener BJ, Brief DK, Alpert J.
A four year experience with preoperative non invasive carotid evaluation of 2026 patients undergoing cardiac surgery.
J Vasc Surg 1984; **1**: 326–37.

[21] Gardner TJ, Horneffer PJ, Manolio TA, Hoff SJ, Pearson TA.
Major stroke after coronary artery bypass surgery: Changing magnitude of the problem.
J Vasc Surg 1986; **3**: 684–7.

[22] Cosgrove DM, Hertzer NR, Loop FD.
Surgical management of synchronous carotid and coronary artery disease.
J Vasc Surg 1986; **3**: 690–2.

[23] Perler BA, Burdick JF, Melville Williams G.
The safety of carotid endarterectomy at the time of coronary artery bypass surgery: analysis of results in a high risk population.
J Vasc Surg 1985; **2**: 558–63.

9. Physiology

ATRIAL NATRIURETIC PEPTIDE: PHARMACOLOGY, PHYSIOLOGY AND CLINICAL SIGNIFICANCE IN MAN

Review: JOHN McMURRAY, ALLAN D. STRUTHERS

In 1981, de Bold *et al* showed that the injection of atrial, but not ventricular, extract into intact rats produced a marked diuresis and natriuresis [1]. Within three years, the molecular structure of the major circulating form of atrial natriuretic peptide (α-hANP1-28) in man had been elucidated [2], and since then a vast literature on the biological role of atrial natriuretic peptide has appeared.

Pharmacologic Action

Until very recently, most of the published studies on the effects of α-hANP in man used relatively large doses, given by bolus injection or short-term infusion and achieving plasma levels far in excess of those achieved physiologically (although often approaching those seen in certain disease states). Such experiments have, however, clearly shown pronounced hemodynamic, renal and hormonal effects of α-hANP at these doses.

Hemodynamic Effects

Dose-dependent falls in systolic, diastolic and mean blood pressures with a rise in heart rate have been observed in most studies [3–6]. In addition, Cody *et al* found a significant fall in pulmonary capillary wedge pressure after a short infusion of atrial natriuretic peptide at a dose of 0.1 µg/kg/min (40 pmol/kg/min) [7]. Lower-dose infusions over longer periods (2–4 hours) produced increases in skin and forearm blood flow, but a reduction in hepatic blood flow [6,8]. The mechanism of the vasodilator effect of atrial natriuretic peptide is uncertain. Prostaglandins do not seem to be involved, and dopamine$_1$- receptor blockade does not prevent forearm arterial dilatation due to atrial natriuretic peptide [9,10]. More interestingly, bolus injections of atrial natriuretic peptide antagonize the pressor effects of infused norepinephrine in man [11]. Atrial natriuretic peptide has, however, a lesser effect on the pressor response to angiotensin II in man [11,12].

Renal Effects

Pharmacologic doses of atrial natriuretic peptide have profound and reproducible diuretic and natriuretic effects [3,5,13]. These effects can occur at doses of atrial natriuretic peptide lower than those required to produce systemic hemodynamic changes [13]. Although there is no evidence, as yet, in man, it is assumed that the above responses are due to a direct action within the kidney. Recent postmortem studies have identified glomerular and collecting duct atrial natriuretic peptide receptors within the human kidney [14]. Apart from its effects on electrolyte excretion, atrial natriuretic peptide consistently reduces renal plasma flow – or at least aminohippuric acid clearance. The effects on glomerular filtration rate are more controversial; most studies show a trend towards increased glomerular filtration rate that is not statistically significant [4,6,7,13]. Because renal plasma flow decreases and glomerular filtration rate remains unchanged or increases, filtration fraction rises. How these changes relate to the increases in sodium (and other electrolyte) excretion is unclear. It is even less clear, especially in man, whether atrial natriuretic peptide has direct, or indirect, tubular actions. Two initial reports, however, do raise the possibility of a proximal tubular effect in the human kidney. First, Brown has shown that atrial natriuretic peptide-induced natriuresis is associated with an increase in fractional lithium clearance [15]. Second, Cody *et al* [7] and our group [16] have found significant increase in fractional free water clearance after administration of atrial natriuretic peptide to maximally hydrated subjects. Although increases in these two indices suggest a proximal site of action, it should be noted that atrial natriuretic peptide receptors have not been found in this part of the kidney [14].

Endocrine Effects
The homeostatic mechanisms maintaining salt balance in man would appear to be complex. The renin–angiotensin–aldosterone system, the sympathetic nervous system, the renal dopaminergic system, and now atrial natriuretic peptide play important roles. In the finer control of sodium balance, it seems that there may be several interactions between the renin–angiotensin–aldosterone system and atrial natriuretic peptide: (i) basal renin release is inhibited by lower doses of atrial natriuretic peptide, although the opposite occurs with higher doses which cause vasodilatation and reflex sympathetic activation [4,5,7]; (ii) atrial natriuretic peptide suppresses both basal and angiotensin II-stimulated aldosterone release [5,7,12,17]; (iii) pressor infusions of angiotensin II increase circulating levels of atrial natriuretic peptide, though this does not occur with doses of angiotensin II that do not alter blood pressure [11,16]; and (iv) we have recently found that low-dose, non-pressor infusions of angiotensin II also reduce the absolute natriuresis due to atrial natriuretic peptide in man [16]. Activation of the renin–angiotensin–aldosterone system, with elevated angiotensin II levels, may therefore explain the reduced natriuretic effect of atrial natriuretic peptide seen in sodium-depleted subjects and in patients with cardiac failure (see below) [15]. Thus, there is evidence for interactions at several sites between atrial natriuretic peptide and the antinatriuretic renin–angiotensin–aldosterone system. Our current knowledge is summarized in Figure 1.

So far, there is little to suggest any significant interaction with the sympathetic nervous system in man. Norepinephrine may rise following infusion of atrial natriuretic peptide, but this is almost certainly due to vasodilatation with reflex sympathetic activation [4,5].

In rats, pretreatment with dopamine$_1$-receptor blocking drugs inhibits the natriuretic response to atrial natriuretic peptide [18–20], but there is very little evidence to support an interaction between the renal dopamine natriuretic system and atrial natriuretic peptide in man. Urinary dopamine levels do not increase following infusion of atrial natriuretic peptide, although this may not be a sensitive enough index to detect

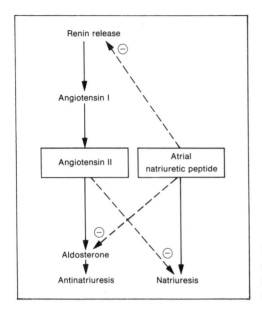

FIGURE 1: Diagram of the interactions at several sites between atrial natriuretic peptide and the anti-natriuretic renin-angiotensin-aldosterone. system.

changes in intrarenal dopamine production [21]. Similarly, dopamine$_2$-receptor block-ade in man has no effect on the natriuretic and diuretic actions of atrial natriuretic peptide [22]. Premedication with carbidopa, a dopamine decarboxylase inhibitor, however, does seem to attenuate the natriuretic response to atrial natriuretic peptide in man [23]. Further study of this area is clearly necessary, although the lack of specific dopamine receptor blocking drugs for use in man greatly hampers such research. Several studies have now shown that atrial natriuretic peptide significantly depresses basal plasma cortisol levels [5,24]. In-vitro evidence suggests that atrial natriuretic peptide also inhibits ACTH-stimulated cortisol and aldosterone release, but whether this occurs in man is not known.

Hypothyroidism is associated with depressed atrial natriuretic peptide levels and thyrotoxicosis with elevated levels [25,26]. However, these conditions are associated with the confounding influences of pericardial effusion and tachycardia, respectively.

Physiology
Animal evidence now strongly suggests that atrial natriuretic peptide is a circulating peptide released from the heart in response to volume/pressure stimuli, and that this results in enhanced sodium and water excretion. Experiments using pharmacologic doses of atrial natriuretic peptide certainly suggest that the 'efferent' end of this system exists in man. However, it has only very recently been shown that physiologic stimuli can increase circulating levels of atrial natriuretic peptide (the 'afferent' end) and the administration of doses of atrial natriuretic peptide that achieve similar physiologic concentrations of atrial natriuretic peptide can produce natriuresis in man.

Maneuvers that increase central blood volume/right-atrial pressure, such as exer-cise, changing from the erect to supine position and head-out-of-water immersion, are all associated with rises in the circulating concentration of atrial natriuretic peptide [27–29]. The last two procedures are also associated with increased sodium and water

434

excretion. Similarly, lowering right-atrial pressure/central venous volume by rising from the supine to erect position, or by applying lower-body negative pressure, is associated with a fall in circulating atrial natriuretic peptide levels; in the former case, this can be partially inhibited by preventing venous pooling in the lower limbs [28,30]. These facts suggest, but do not prove, that physiologic stimuli can elevate endogenous atrial natriuretic peptide levels which then enhance urinary sodium excretion. Perhaps the most significant recent report in this context is the demonstration by Anderson *et al* that prolonged, low-dose infusions of atrial natriuretic peptide, which elevate plasma concentrations within the physiologic range, are associated with significant increases in urinary sodium loss [31]. These acute changes in urinary sodium excretion, although small, could have a major impact on total body sodium status if they are maintained in the long term.

Further evidence to support the hypothesis that atrial natriuretic peptide is a circulating hormone involved in sodium homeostasis comes from studies undertaken during different dietary salt intakes. Sagnella *et al* have shown that, with increased intake, atrial natriuretic peptide levels rise significantly within 2–3 days and remain elevated until dietary sodium is reduced [32]. Similarly, a sustained reduction in salt intake is associated with a sustained fall in plasma atrial natriuretic peptide. Each of these changes is associated with a similar change in sodium excretion and a reciprocal change in the activity of the renin–angiotensin–aldosterone system.

Taken together, all these findings strongly support the notion that atrial natriuretic peptide is a circulating hormone responding to physiologic stimuli and influencing body sodium and volume homeostasis.

Cardiovascular Disease
Chronic Heart Failure
Perhaps the area of greatest interest and advance concerning the role of atrial natriuretic peptide in cardiovascular disease has been in the field of chronic heart failure. It has become clear that both acute and chronic heart failure are accompanied by elevated circulating concentrations of atrial natriuretic peptide [7,33,34], and, in general, more severe clinical grades of chronic heart failure are associated with higher plasma concentrations of atrial natriuretic peptide [35,36]. Similarly, there are strong positive correlations between hemodynamic indices of severity and circulating atrial natriuretic peptide concentrations [35,37,38]. Relationships with right-atrial, left-atrial and pulmonary capillary wedge pressures have been found in patients with chronic heart failure from a variety of causes [37,38]. Reciprocal relationships with cardiac index and left-ventricular ejection fraction have also been reported [39,40]. These hemodynamic parameters are all interrelated, and it is difficult to be sure which is the major determinant of atrial natriuretic peptide release. In valvar disease, left-ventricular function may be normal, and left-atrial pressure rather than right-atrial pressure may be the main hemodynamic correlate of plasma atrial natriuretic peptide [41]. In most forms of chronic heart failure, left-atrial pressure may be at least as important a stimulus to atrial natriuretic peptide release as right-atrial pressure [37,41]. (It is worth noting here that the left-atrial venous drainage is into the coronary sinus, which opens into the right atrium.)

Since the more advanced degrees of chronic heart failure are associated with higher levels of atrial natriuretic peptide, it would initially appear that the mechanisms governing atrial natriuretic peptide release do not undergo desensitization, and that myocardial atrial natriuretic peptide content is not depleted with chronic stimulation. Two recent observations make this view less certain. As in normal subjects, exercise in patients with chronic heart failure is associated with a rise in atrial natriuretic peptide levels. This increase is, however, much less than would be expected considering the exaggerated rises in right- and left-side filling pressures that occur in these patients [37]. Thus, the endocrine response to exercise may be 'relatively attenuated' in chronic heart failure, in the same way that the sympathetic nervous system response is impaired in these patients. An impaired atrial natriuretic peptide response may then fail to prevent the excessive increases in preload that limit exercise in patients with chronic heart failure. A further relevant observation (requiring confirmation) is that at least a proportion of the increased circulating atrial natriuretic peptide in patients with chronic heart failure may be of a different molecular form than α-hANP [41]. The presence of this molecular weight polypeptide may reflect disordered synthesis or release in chronic heart failure.

Treatment associated with clinical improvement of both acute and chronic heart failure coincides with a reduction in circulating atrial natriuretic peptide concentrations [34]. Intravenous furosemide and digoxin do not alter atrial natriuretic peptide levels in normal subjects, and any fall in atrial natriuretic peptide in treated heart failure probably reflects hemodynamic improvement [41]. Angiotensin converting enzyme inhibitors also reduce circulating atrial natriuretic peptide in chronic heart failure, although here the multiple neurohormonal actions of these drugs may suggest other than hemodynamic mechanisms for the reduction in atrial natriuretic peptide after treatment [40]. Also of some note in this context is a report that, in rats, intravenous morphine is associated with a fiftyfold rise in atrial natriuretic peptide levels, perhaps explaining this drug's therapeutic effect in chronic heart failure [42].

The area of greatest interest in chronic heart failure must be in explaining the apparent paradox of a salt-retaining state despite increased endogenous levels of atrial natriuretic peptide. One possibility is that some of the molecular forms of atrial natriuretic peptide secreted in chronic heart failure are less active than α-hANP [40]. However, ample evidence exists to show that in most patients α-hANP reaches levels associated with natriuresis in normal individuals [34–38]. This suggests a resistance to the natriuretic effect of atrial natriuretic peptide in chronic heart failure. Furthermore, two major studies have shown that exogenous administration of pharmacologic doses of atrial natriuretic peptide, while still associated with hemodynamic changes, fails to cause either diuresis or natriuresis [7,33].

Several other factors could account for the apparent attenuation of the renal effects of atrial natriuretic peptide in congestive heart failure. First, hemodynamic changes in chronic heart failure (e.g. low renal perfusion pressure) could reduce the response to atrial natriuretic peptide. Second, activation of the sympathetic nervous system and renin–angiotensin–aldosterone system also occurs in chronic heart failure, and it is attractive to suggest that these neuroendocrine changes may outweigh any benefit from increased circulating concentrations of atrial natriuretic peptide. There is some evidence supporting this view from our own observation that when circulating levels of angiotensin II are increased the natriuretic effect of atrial natriuretic peptide is diminished [16]. The converse also appears to be true, in that the natriuretic action of atrial natriuretic peptide is enhanced by pretreatment with angiotensin converting enzyme inhibitors in experimental animals and in man [43,44]. Third, 'down-regulation' of atrial natriuretic peptide receptors could occur in chronic heart failure. The recent identification of platelet atrial natriuretic peptide receptors may shed some light on this matter, if they prove to be as useful as peripheral blood cell receptors have been in the study of adrenergic receptor responses to chronic stimulation [45]. Finally, one (as yet unconfirmed) report has shown that very large (450 µg bolus injections followed by an infusion of 20 µg/min for 30 min) doses of atrial natriuretic peptide given over a short period *can* increase urinary sodium and water excretion in patients with chronic heart failure [46]. This would support the possiblility of end-organ hyporesponsiveness due to receptor change, or may suggest that high enough levels of atrial natriuretic peptide can overcome the antinatriuretic effect of excessive sympathetic nervous system and renin–angiotensin–aldosterone system activity. The latter seems more likely since, if down-regulation were to be the explanation, it would have to be limited to the renal and not the vascular receptors, as atrial natriuretic peptide retains its hemodynamic effects in chronic heart failure. These latter effects include sustained reductions in pulmonary capillary wedge pressure and systemic vascular resistance and elevations in cardiac index [7,33]. Such beneficial hemodynamic effects occur in the absence of any neurohumoral activation (which usually complicates diuretic and vasodilator treatment) and with the suppression of circulating aldosterone. Obviously this profile of action is extremely attractive from a therapeutic viewpoint.

Arrhythmias
Spontaneous and induced supraventricular arrhythmias are associated with rises in circulating atrial natriuretic peptide, this perhaps explaining their long-observed relationship with polyuria [34]. Termination of these arrhythmias is associated with a rapid return of atrial natriuretic peptide to normal levels. A rise in atrial pressure, rather than the rate or rhythm *per se*, is thought to be the stimulus to atrial natriuretic peptide release. If pressure is the main determinant of release, then atrial natriuretic peptide levels should also rise during ventricular tachycardia. So far this has not been studied in man. It is, however, often forgotten that in Wood's original description of this phenomenon up to 40% of cases of ventricular tachycardia were associated with polyuria [47].

Hypertension
Several groups have found atrial natriuretic peptide levels to be elevated in patients with essential hypertension [48–52]. However, even when compared with age-matched controls, there is a considerable overlap with the levels found in normal subjects [48]. It has long been suggested that, in some individuals at least, the basic abnormality in essential hypertension is a renal inability to excrete sodium. The consequent rise in blood pressure is thought to compensate by enhancing sodium loss through the pressure/natriuresis mechanism. Elevated atrial natriuretic peptide levels may also indicate a further compensatory response to any underlying renal hyporesponsiveness. It is interesting that 'low-renin' hypertensives seem to have higher atrial natriuretic peptide levels than other hypertensives, because it is in this group that blood pressure is

most dependent on sodium-volume status [50,51]. There are, however, several confounding influences in assessing the significance of circulating atrial natriuretic peptide concentrations in hypertensives. Atrial natriuretic peptide levels rise with age and renal impairment, and these variables have not been allowed for in all studies. In addition, subclinical hypertensive heart disease may have been present in some of the reported cases.

Administration of atrial natriuretic peptide to hypertensive subjects, on the other hand, has similar, or greater, renal and hemodynamic effects to those seen in normal subjects [53,54]. Diminished responsiveness to atrial natriuretic peptide, like that seen in chronic heart failure, does not seem to occur in hypertensives (at least at pharmacologic doses in the short term). Further studies with lower doses over longer periods of time are required to assess fully the role of atrial natriuretic peptide in essential hypertension.

Atrial natriuretic peptide levels are elevated in primary hyperaldosteronism and fall after treatment with spironolactone, dexamethasone or surgical removal of the causative lesion [50]. Atrial natriuretic peptide levels rise during mineralocorticoid administration in man, and may account for the natriuretic escape that occurs after the initial period of intense sodium and water retention [55].

Coronary Artery Disease
There is one preliminary report that atrial natriuretic peptide levels are higher in patients with chest pain and significant obstructive coronary artery disease than in those with normal coronary arteries [56]. This presumably reflects the likelihood of pump impairment in the former group. Whether such findings will have diagnostic utility is not clear.

Other Conditions
Studies in patients undergoing intensive care and studies of experimental pericardial disease have shed light on the exact nature of the stimulus for the cardiac release of atrial natriuretic peptide. Patients undergoing positive end-expiratory pressure ventilation have long been known to retain sodium and water and, as a consequence, to develop edema. Positive end-expiratory pressure also causes increases in right-atrial pressure and pulmonary capillary wedge pressure. It is somewhat surprising, therefore, that atrial natriuretic peptide levels are depressed in these patients [57]. However, Edwards *et al* have shown in studies of experimental pericardial tamponade that net transmural pressure, rather than intra-atrial (cavity) pressure, is probably the more important stimulus to atrial natriuretic peptide release [58]. This interpretation would explain the seemingly paradoxical findings in patients ventilated with positive end-expiratory pressure.

The Future
Much more needs to be learnt about the role of atrial natriuretic peptide in other cardiovascular disorders. For example, the normal pulmonary vasculature must be exposed to the highest circulating concentrations of atrial natriuretic peptide, and the possible etiologic and therapeutic significance of atrial natriuretic peptide in primary pulmonary hypertension deserves attention. It is also possible that a primary disorder of

synthesis or secretion of atrial natriuretic peptide is the underlying cause of certain dilated cardiomyopathies. Currently, however, the two main hopes for atrial natriuretic peptide are that its measurement may allow us to monitor disease progress, and that atrial natriuretic peptide may itself become a therapeutic tool. As a marker of disease activity, plasma atrial natriuretic peptide levels may be used to optimize therapy in chronic heart failure. In chronic renal failure, there is already evidence that the concentration of circulating atrial natriuretic peptide may be the most sensitive indicator of fluid balance in hemodialysis patients [59]. Clearly, any similar objective indicator of a patient's status in chronic heart failure would be welcomed.

More importantly, the powerful and beneficial hemodynamic effects of atrial natriuretic peptide in chronic heart failure suggest great therapeutic potential if stable oral analogs can be developed. These benefits will become even more important if it can be confirmed that higher doses of atrial natriuretic peptide will also enhance urinary sodim and water excretion. Furthermore, from what is known so far, atrial natriuretic peptide seems able to act as both a vasodilator and diuretic without causing the neurohumoral activation and metabolic derangement that limit the use of currently available drugs of this type. This profile of action would be equally useful in the treatment of hypertension.

References

[1] de Bold AJ, Borenstein HB, Veress AT, Sonnenberg H.
A rapid and potent natriuretic response to intravenous injection of atrial myocardial extract in rats.
Life Sci 1981; **28**: 89–94.

[2] Kangawa K, Matsuo H.
Purification and complete amino acid sequence of α-human atrial natriuretic polypeptide (α-hANP).
Biochem Biophys Res Commun 1984; **118**: 131–9.

[3] Richards AM, Nicholls MG, Ikram H, Webster MWI, Yandle TG, Espiner EA.
Renal, haemodynamic, and hormonal effects of human alpha atrial natriuretic peptide in healthy volunteers.
Lancet 1985; i: 545–8.

[4] Ishii M, Sugimoto T, Hiroaki M *et al.*
Hemodynamic, renal and endocrine responses to α-human atrial natriuretic polypeptide (α-hANP) in healthy volunteers.
Circulation 1985; **72** (Suppl 3): III–294.

[5] Weidmann P, Hellmueller B, Uehlinger DE *et al.*
Plasma levels and cardiovascular, endocrine and excretory effects of atrial natriuretic peptide during different sodium intakes in man.
J Clin Endocrinol Metab 1986; **62**: 1027–36.

[6] Biollaz J, Nussberger J, Waeber B, Brunner HR.
Clinical pharmacology of atrial natriuretic (3-28) eicosahexapeptide.
J Hypertens 1986; **4** (Suppl 2): S101–8.

[7] Cody RJ, Atlas SA, Laragh JH *et al.*
Atrial natriuretic factor in normal subjects and heart failure patients.
J Clin Invest 1986; **78**: 1362–74.

[8] Muller FB, Erne P, Raine AEG *et al.*
Atrial antipressor natriuretic peptide: Release mechanisms and vascular actions in man.
J Hypertens 1986; **4** (Suppl 2): S109–14.

[9] Brown J, Dollery CT, Ritter J, Valdes G.
Prostaglandins do not mediate the hypotensive effect of human and atrial natriuretic peptide in man. In: *Proceedings of the British Pharmacological Society, London, 17–19 December 1986.*

[10] Hughes A, Goldberg P, Sever P.
Dopamine does not mediate forearm vasodilation due to atrial natriuretic peptide. In: *Proceedings of the British Pharmacological Society, London, 17–19 December 1986.*

[11] Uehlinger DE, Weidmann P, Gnaedinger MP, Shaw S, Lang RE.
Depressor effects and release of atrial natriuretic peptide during norepinephrine or angiotension II infusion in man.
J Clin Endocrinol Metab 1986; **63**: 669–74.

[12] Vierhapper H.
Effect of human atrial natriuretic peptide on angiotensin II-induced secretion of aldosterone in man.
Klin Wochenschr 1986; **64** (Suppl 6): 50–2.

[13] Anderson J, Struthers A, Christofides N, Bloom S.
Atrial natriuretic peptide: An endogenous factor enhancing sodium excretion in man.
Clin Sci 1986; **70**: 327–31.

[14] Mantyh CR, Kruger L, Brecha NC, Mantyh PW.
Localisation of specific binding sites for atrial natriuretic factor in peripheral tissues of the guinea pig, rat and human.
Hypertension 1986; **8**: 712–21.

[15] Brown J.
Effect of atrial natriuretic peptide on the excretion of lithium in man.
J Physiol 1986; **379**: 45P.

[16] McMurray J, Struthers AD.
The effect of angiotension II on sodium excretion due to atrial natriuretic peptide in man. In: *Proceedings of the British Pharmacological Society, Cambridge, 1987.*

[17] Anderson JV, Struthers AD, Payne NN, Slater JDH, Bloom SR.
Atrial natriuretic peptide inhibits the aldosterone response to angiotensin II in man.
Clin Sci 1986; **70**: 507–12.

[18] Marin-Grez M, Briggs JP, Schubert G, Schnermann J.
Dopamine receptor antagonists inhibit the natriuretic response to atrial natriuretic factor.
Life Sci 1985; **36**: 2171–6.

[19] Pettersson A, Hedner J, Hedner T.
The diuretic effect of atrial natriuretic peptide (atrial natriuretic peptide) is dependent on dopaminergic activation.
Acta Physiol Scand 1986; **126**: 619–21.

[20] Webb RL, Puca RD, Manniello J, Robson RD, Zimmerman MB, Ghai RD.
Dopaminergic mediation of the diuretic and natriuretic effects of ANF in the rat.
Life Sci 1986; **38**: 2319–27.

[21] Struthers AD, Anderson JV, Payne N, Causon RC, Slater JDH, Bloom SR.
The effect of atrial natriuretic peptide on plasma renin activity, plasma aldosterone and urinary dopamine in man.
Eur J Clin Pharmacol 1986; **31**: 223–6.

[22] Jungman N, Haak T, Schwab N, Fassbinder W, Althoff PH, Schoffling K.
In-vivo evidence that human atrial natriuretic peptide (hANP) does not interact with dopaminergic D_2-receptor function. In: *11th Scientific Meeting of the Internaltional Society of Hypertension, Heidelberg; 1986.*

[23] Wilkins MR, Kendall MJ, Lote CJ, West MJ, Wood JA.
Partial inhibition of renal response to high dose α-hANP infusion by carbidopa. In: *World Conference of Clinical Pharmacology and Therapeutics, Stockholm, 1986.*

[24] Ohashi M, Fujio N, Kato K, Nawata H, Ibayashi H, Matsuo H.
Effect of human α-atrial polypeptide on adrenocortical function in man.
J Endocrinol 1986; **110**: 287–92.

[25] Weissel M, Punzengruber C, Hartter E, Lupuik B, Noloszczuk W.
Thyroid hormones and pericardial effusion may influence plasma levels of atrial natriuretic peptide (ANP) in humans.
Klin Wochenschr 1986; **64** (Suppl 6): 93–6.

[26] Zimmerman RS, Gharib H, Zimmerman D, Heublein DM, Burnett JC.
Hypothyroidism: The first metabolic abnormality associated with decreased atrial natriuretic peptide.
Circulation 1986; **74** (Suppl 2): II–463.

[27] Richards AM, Tonolo G, Cleland JGF *et al.*
Plasma atrial natriuretic peptide concentrations during exercise in sodium replete and deplete normal man.
Clin Sci 1987; **72**: 159–64.

[28] Solomon LR, Atherton JC, Bobinski H, Green R.
Effect of posture on plasma immunoreactive atrial natriuretic peptide concentrations in man.
Clin Sci 1986; **71**: 299–305.

[29] Anderson JV, Millar ND, O'Hare JP, Mackenzie JC, Corrall RJ, Bloom SR.
Atrial natriuretic peptide: Physiological release associated with natriuresis during water immersion in man.
Clin Sci 1986; **71**: 319–22.

[30] Mohanty PK, Thames MD, Sowers JR, Walsh M.
Influence of lower body negative pressure (LBNP) on plasma atrial natriuretic factor (ANF) in heart failure.
Circulation 1986; **74** (Suppl 2) II–463.

[31] Anderson JV, Donckier J, Bloom SR.
Evidence supporting the hypothesis that atrial natriuretic peptide (ANP) is a natriuretic hormone in normal man.
J Physiol 1986; **380**: 46P.

[32] Sangella GA, Markandu ND, Shore AC, Forsling ML, MacGregor GA.
Plasma atrial natriuretic peptide: Its relationship to changes in sodium intake, plasma renin activity and aldosterone in man.
Clin Sci 1987; **72**: 25–30.

[33] Crozier IG, Nicholls MG, Ikram H, Espiner EA, Gomez HJ, Warner NJ.
Haemodynamic effects of atrial peptide infusion in heart failure.
Lancet 1986; ii: 1242–5.

[34] Anderson JV, Gibbs JSR, Woodruff PWR, Greco C, Rowland E, Bloom SR.
The plasma atrial natriuretic peptide response to treatment of acute cardiac failure, spontaneous supraventricular tachycardia and induced re-entrant tachycardia in man.
J Hypertens 1986; **4** (Suppl 2): S137–41.

[35] Tikkanen I, Fyhrquist F, Metsarinne K, Leidenius R.
Plasma atrial natriuretic peptide in cardiac disease and during infusion in healthy volunteers.
Lancet 1985; ii: 66–9.

[36] Nakaoka H, Imataka K, Amano M, Fujii J, Ishibashi M, Yamaji T.
Plasma levels of atrial natriuretic factor in patients with congestive heart failure.
N Engl J Med 1985; **313**: 892–3.

[37] Raine AEG, Erne P, Burgisser E *et al*.
Atrial natriuretic peptide and atrial pressure in patients with congestive heart failure.
N Engl J Med 1986; **315**: 533–7.

[38] Richards AM, Cleland JGF, Tonolo G *et al*.
Plasma natriuretic peptide in cardiac impairment.
Br Med J 1986; **293**: 409–12.

[39] Schiffrin EL, Taillefer R.
Correlation of left ventricular ejection fraction and plasma atrial natriuretic peptide in congestive heart failure.
N Engl J Med 1986; **315**: 765–6.

[40] Arendt RM, Gerbes AL, Ritter D, Stangl E.
Molecular weight heterogenicity of plasma ANF in cardiovascular disease.
Klin Wochenschr 1986; **64** (Suppl 6): 97–102.

[41] Dietz R, Purgaj J, Lang RE, Schomig A.
Pressure dependent release of atrial natriuretic peptide (ANP) in patients with chronic cardiac diseases: Does it reset?
Klin Wochenschr 1986; **64** (Suppl 6): 42–6.

[42] Horky K, Gutkowska J, Garcia R, Thibault G, Genest J, Cantin M.
Effect of different anaesthetics on immunoreactive atrial natriuretic factor concentrations in rat plasma.
Biochem Biophys Res Commun 1985; **129**: 651–7.

[43] Agabati-Rosei E, Castellano M, Beschi M, Muiesan ML, Rowanelli G, Muiesan G.
Effects of infusing α-atrial natriuretic peptide in essential hypertension during converting enzyme inhibition. In: *11th Scientific Meeting of the International Society of Hypertension, Heidelberg, 1986.*

[44] Wang SL, Gilmore JP.
Renal responses to atrial natriuretic factor during converting enzyme inhibition.
Can J Physiol Pharmacol 1985; **63**: 220–3.

[45] Gerzer R, Weil J, Strom T, Muller T.
Mechanisms of action of atrial natriuretic factor: Clinical consequences.
Klin Wochenschr 1986; **64** (Suppl 6): 21–6.

[46] Reigger AJG, Kromer EP, Kochsiek K.
Atrial natriuretic peptide in patients with severe heart failure.
Klin Wochenschr 1986; **64** (Suppl 6): 89–92.

[47] Wood P.
Paroxysmal tachycardia and paroxysmal atrial flutter and fibrillation.
Br Heart J 1963; **25**: 273–82.

[48] Sagnella G, Markandu ND, Shore AC, MacGregor GA.
Raised circulating levels of atrial natriuretic peptides in essential hypertension.
Lancet 1986; i: 179–81.

[49] Sugawara A, Nakao K, Sakamoto M *et al*.
Plasma concentrations of atrial natriuretic polypeptide in essential hypertension.
Lancet 1985; ii: 1426–7.

[50] Yamaji T, Ishibashi M, Sekihara H, Takaku F, Nakaka H, Fujii J.
Plasma levels of atrial natriuretic peptide in primary aldosteronism and essential hypertension.
J Clin Endocrinol Metab 1986; **63**: 815–8.

[51] Sugawara A, Nakao K, Morri N *et al*.
Plasma atrial natriuretic polypeptide (ANP) in essential hypertension.
Circulation 1986; **74** (Suppl 2): II–22.

[52] Arendt RM, Gerbes AL, Ritter D, Stangl E, Bach P, Zahringer J.
Atrial natriuretic factor in plasma of patients with arterial hypertension, heart failure or cirrhosis of the liver.
J Hypertens 1986; **4** (Suppl 2): S131–6.

[53] Richards AM, Nicholls MG, Espiner EH et al.
Effects of α-human atrial natriuretic peptide in
essential hypertension.
Hypertension 1985; **7**: 812–7.

[54] Weidmann P, Gnaedinger MP, Ziswiler HR et
al.
Cardiovascular, endocrine and renal effects of
atrial natriuretic peptide in essential hypertension.
J Hypertens 1986; **4** (Suppl 2): S71–83.

[55] Zimmerman RS, Edwards BS, Schwab TR,
Heublein DM, Burnett JC.
Atrial natriuretic peptide (ANP) is increased
during mineralocorticoid escape in the human.
Circulation 1986; **74** (Suppl 2): II–21.

[56] Genest J.
The atrial natriuretic factor.
Br Heart J 1986; **56**: 302–16.

[57] Pacher R, Frass M, Hartter E, Woloszczuk W,
Leithner C.
The role of α-atrial natriuretic peptide in fluid
retention during mechanical ventilation with
positive end-expiratory pressure.
Klin Wochenschr 1986; **64** (Suppl 6): 64–7.

[58] Edwards BS, Schwab TR, Zimmerman RS, Burnett JC.
Increased transmural but not intra-atrial pressure stimulates atrial natriuretic peptide (ANP)
release.
Circulation 1986; **74** (Suppl 2): II–462.

[59] Eisenhauer T, Talartschik J, Scheler F.
Detection of fluid overload by plasma concen-
tration of human atrial natriuretic peptide (h-
ANP) in patients with renal failure.
Klin Wochenschr 1986; **64** (Suppl 6): 68–72.

DOPAMINE IN CARDIOVASCULAR MEDICINE

Review: STEPHEN G. BALL

Many comprehensive reviews have already been undertaken on the subject of dopamine in cardiovascular medicine, illustrating an increasing awareness of the potential importance of this agent [1–5].

Dopamine, a catecholamine, is the immediate precursor of norepinephrine. It is distributed widely through the brain and peripheral tissues [1–3]. In its free uncon-jugated form, dopamine is found in the circulation of man in pico- to nanomolar con-centrations, similar to those of epinephrine in the resting state [3,6,7]. Undoubtedly an important neurotransmitter in the central nervous system [8], its function in peripheral tissue as a transmitter or local hormone, or merely as precursor, is less clear. When infused in large amounts, dopamine has marked cardiovascular effects, some of which may be through its action at a specific dopamine receptor, others through stimulation of α- or β-receptors. A number of drugs that mimic or antagonize its action are available and have found clinical use [2].

Dopamine Receptors

An understanding of dopamine receptors is essential to an appreciation of dopamine's actions. Receptors are classified and defined in different ways. Ideally, one should be able to identify (i) a 'binding site' of known structure linked to (ii) a par-ticular second-messenger system and (iii) subsequent biologic response. Our understanding of dopamine falls far short of this.

Only two receptor sites are currently thought to exist: in peripheral vascular smooth muscle, the DA_1 receptor linked to cAMP formation mediates vasodilatation; the DA_2 receptor sited presynaptically on nerve terminals inhibits transmitter release. The physiologic roles of these two receptors remain obsure [2–4], although their potential for pharmacologic manipulation has been well exploited [2].

Presynaptic dopamine receptors occur also in the central nervous system, on dopaminergic and other nerves. They are usually termed D_2 and are, pharmacologically at least, similar to the DA_2 receptors of the periphery; but they also are found postsynaptically. Indeed, in the central nervous system as an axon from one neuron may terminate on another axon, dendrite or cell body, the simple concept of pre-and postsynaptic sites becomes less firm. Stimulation of DA_2 or D_2 receptors may reduce cAMP formation, although other second-messenger systems have been implicated. This confusing area of receptor subtypes is reviewed for the central nervous system by Creese [8] and for the periphery by Goldberg [1,2,9].

Dopamine agonists and antagonists with central actions may have cardiovascular effects — for example, bromocriptine, predominantly a D_2 agonist, will reduce blood pressure [10,11] — but their precise site and mode of action remain unclear. Certainly, there is little direct evidence to implicate dopamine in the central pathways thought to control blood pressure. Even so, intracerebral injection of dopamine lowered blood pressure in the spontaneously hypertensive rat [12], and dopamine acting centrally has been implicated in the control of aldosterone [13].

Dopamine: A Physiologic Function in the Regulation of the Cardiovascular System?
The existence of specific dopamine receptors throughout the cardiovascular system, particularly in the cardiac, celiac, mesenteric and renal vascular beds, has been established [1,2]. However, it is not clear whether these receptors serve a physiologic role. Circulating concentrations of free dopamine are low, lying close to the detection limit of most assays currently available. Dopamine also exists conjugated with sulfuric or glucuronic acid, the proportions varying between species. Only the free form seems biologically active [14,15]. Indeed, conjugation was originally thought to be the major pathway for metabolism of the catecholamines before the discovery of catecholamine-*O*-methyltransferase and monoamine oxidase. Kuchel and colleagues have suggested important functions for the seemingly inert conjugates [14,16,17].

Nanomolar, or smaller, concentrations of free dopamine normally in circulation might act at DA_2 sites, but they are far below the micromolar amounts needed to stimulate the D_1 receptor. Dopamine seems to have little to offer as a circulating hormone.

On the other hand, dopamine released at nerve endings or formed locally within a particular tissue could reach its receptors in much greater concentration. In contrast to the situation in the central nervous system, it has proved difficult to provide convincing evidence of the release of dopamine by peripheral neurons.

Are There Specific Dopamine-Containing Nerves Regulating the Cardiovascular System?
An obvious starting point is to look for dopamine within a tissue; however, since dopamine is the immediate precursor of norepinephrine, and as noradrenergic innervation is so extensive, interpretation of the findings is difficult.

Concentrations of dopamine as a simple precursor would not be expected to exceed 10% of the total catecholamine content [18,19]. Measurement of the total tissue dopamine cannot detect a proportionately small dopaminergic supply, nor give any information as to release, nor locate the catecholamine in a nerve ending. Similarly,

443

histochemical techniques lack sensitivity, as they cannot readily separate norad-renergic from dopaminergic neurons. A more direct approach is to seek evidence of the release of dopamine during nerve stimulation, although again a specific dopaminergic neuronal source cannot be established with certainty.

Dopamine and the Heart
The heart is richly innervated by the autonomic nervous system. Overall the concentration of dopamine in cardiac tissue is in keeping with its presence simply as a precursor [18]. However, Drake and Stanford made the interesting observation that, after denervation of the dog heart, norepinephrine concentrations decreased markedly as expected while the dopamine content of the cardiac tissue was little altered [20]. More recently, Mohanty *et al* produced effective denervation by cardiac transplantation in the dog, and found cardiac tissue concentrations of norepinephrine reduced to less than 5% of control, whereas dopamine concentration was only halved [21] — again suggesting a non-neuronal site of dopamine formation.

Further support for a non-neuronal source of dopamine comes from the observations of Ilebekk *et al*, who sampled blood simultaneously from the coronary sinus and arterial circulation of the pig. They found a relatively constant net secretion of dopamine from the heart whether norepinephrine was being secreted or extracted [22]; the change from a negative to positive arteriovenous norepinephrine gradient presumably reflects the degree of activity of the sympathetic nerves supplying the heart at the time of blood sampling.

Irrespective of whether the heart normally has a dopaminergic supply or can form dopamine extraneuronally, interesting changes in cardiac catecholamine content occur in heart failure. Pierpont *et al* studied the catecholamine content of hearts removed from three patients undergoing cardiac transplantation for intractable heart failure [23]. As reported previously by other workers, the norepinephrine content of cardiac tissue in the setting of heart failure was much reduced, but (unexpectedly) tissue dopamine concentrations were high. A likely explanation is the failure of nerves 'exhausted' by continued stimulation to form norepinephrine in adequate amounts [24]. Perhaps in this situation dopamine is released in much greater proportion than occurs normally (usually <10%). An increase in non-neuronal dopamine could also partly explain these findings.

Dopamine and the Kidney [3]
Human urine contains a disproportionate amount of dopamine compared with norepinephrine and epinephrine [7]. The kidney is the major source, probably converting dopa to dopamine in the tubules [25–27]. Histochemical studies [28] and other work in animals [19] also suggests the presence of a specific dopaminergic nerve supply to this organ. However, experiments in the anesthetized dog in my own laboratory do not support the idea of an important dopaminergic innervation of the kidney in this species [29]. Our work indicates both a non-neuronal source of dopamine in the kidney and a neuronal release, in keeping with the expected small amount co-released with norepinephrine at the noradrenergic nerve ending. Other workers would not agree [19,30,31].

Dopamine formed within the kidney may be important in determining sodium excretion, and it has been suggested that the atrial natriuretic peptide might act through this system [32]. Failure to generate adequate amounts of dopamine could then result in elevation of blood pressure [3].

Dopaminergic Regulation of Aldosterone [4,5]

Corticosteroidogenesis is regulated by circulating adrenocorticotrophin, angiotensin II and plasma potassium concentrations [33]. In 1975, Edwards *et al* observed that the response of plasma aldosterone concentration to stimulation by intravenous furosemide was blunted by administration of the dopamine agonist, bromocriptine [34]. From this and subsequent work emerged the idea that aldosterone secretion was under a maximal tonic inhibition by dopamine — an attractive hypothesis to complement dopamine's putative role in the kidney. Much of the early support for this concept depended on the effects of various antagonists and agonists of dopamine, with all the attendant problems of lack of drug specificity and physiologic relevance of the findings. More recently, however, Holland *et al* claimed that dopamine inhibited basal aldosterone secretion in patients with low-renin hypertension [35], and Drake and Carey suggested that the increased sensitivity of aldosterone response to infused angiotensin II in sodium-depleted subjects could be explained by the removal of the negative effect of dopamine [36]. Our own studies, using physiologically relevant concentrations of dopamine [37,38], favor an action of dopamine outside the adrenal gland in increasing renal clearance of circulating angiotensin II [39], and perhaps in increasing extra-adrenal formation of 11-deoxycorticosteroids [40].

A major difficulty with the hypothesis that dopamine is important in controlling steroidogenesis within the adrenal gland seems to be in identifying the source of the dopamine acting on the adrenal tissue: is it from the circulation, locally formed, or neuronally released in the adrenal cortex? Although dopamine does seem to have effects within the adrenal cortex, the physiologic relevance of these effects remains open to serious doubt.

Whatever the physiologic role of the dopamine receptor, it has proved possible to exploit it therapeutically in cardiovascular medicine.

Dopamine in Clinical Medicine

A major use has been found for dopamine in the treatment of patients with circulatory failure [2]. For the physician, this is often in the treatment of patients with cardiac failure secondary to acute myocardial infarction or sudden worsening of chronic heart failure. The majority of such patients respond well to diuretic therapy, and are managed without invasive hemodynamic monitoring. Management of the more severely ill is made easier with measurements of right-atrial, wedge and arterial pressures, cardiac output, and regular monitoring of urine output.

To find out where dopamine fits into the treatment regimen, it is necessary to understand its mode of action.

Actions of Dopamine at Its Own Receptor Site [1,2,6,9,41,42]

Infusion of dopamine, even in 'so-called' low doses (0.5–1.0 µg/kg/min), produces circulating dopamine concentrations 50–100 or more times those normally found in the circulation — close to the micromolar concentrations needed to stimulate the DA_1

receptors but well into the range to affect the DA_2 receptor, assuming adequate access to these sites from the circulation. With a failing circulation, there will be intense vasoconstriction, induced in large part by sympathetic activity but also by pressor hormone systems like the renin-angiotensin system. Stimulation of the presynaptic DA_2 receptors would be expected to diminish the release of norepinephrine at peripheral sites (an obvious site would be the renal nerves) and perhaps reduce the sympathetically mediated release of renin. Certainly, low infusion rates of dopamine do not seem to stimulate renin release. As infusion rates rise (1–5 µg/kg/min), direct vasodilatation would be anticipated through activation of the DA_1 receptors, particularly in the renal, but also in the mesenteric, coronary and perhaps other peripheral vessels, leading to a decrease in overall peripheral resistance.

β-*Adrenergic Stimulation: Loss of Selectivity*
As rates of infusion (~5 µg/kg/min and above) and circulating levels of dopamine rise further, selectivity is lost and $β_1$-adrenergic effects begin to appear, giving direct intropic and chronotropic effects. Initially, these may be supportive, increasing cardiac output, but later they can lead to a worsening situation, with an unacceptable increase in heart rate and eventually the appearance of serious dysrhythmias. Renin release would now be stimulated.

Stimulation of α-Adrenoceptors
At higher rates, α-effects predominate, adding to the vasoconstriction and afterload and increasing the occurrence of dysrhythmias, perhaps in part through a direct action at the recently recognized cardiac α-adrenoceptors.

Treatment of Acute Heart Failure
Current therapy for acute heart failure is based on the premise that cardiac output and arterial pressure are to be maintained only to the extent that the tissue requirements for perfusion can be met. Reduction of 'preload' or 'afterload' is often the main aim, rather than simply stimulation of cardiac contractility. On this basis, other agents like nitroprusside, nitrates or converting enzyme inhibitors might offer more powerful vasodilatory effects than dopamine. If an inotropic action were needed, dobutamine [42–46], a synthetic catecholamine resembling isoproterenol, or pirbuterol [47], a derivative of isoproterenol but with modifications both in ring structure and side-chain, might be more appropriate. These drugs exhibit marked β-actions, but without the unwanted stimulation of α-adrenoceptors found with high-dose dopamine infusion. Similarly, newer agents like dopexamine may give inotropic support without α-stimulation but with added vasodilatation via their agonist action at the $β_2$-adrenoceptor site [48–50]. Dopamine's attraction appears to lie predominantly with its selective renal effects. A combination of low-dose dopamine for this attribute with other agents for their particular profiles of action might allow the physician to tailor therapy to the individual patient.

Propylbutyl Dopamine
This derivative of dopamine acts at both DA_1 and DA_2 sites but lacks important activity at the $β_1$ site, thus giving it an interesting profile to exploit in the treatment of

heart failure [51]. When administered intravenously it was found to increase cardiac index and decrease systemic vascular resistance, without any increase in heart rate; blood pressure was reduced. Its effects on renal function were not studied here, but would be expected to be similar to those reported by others in a different setting [2].

Treatment of Chronic Heart Failure

Dopamine must be given intravenously, and therefore, except in unusual circumstances, it is unlikely to have much of a role in the management of chronic heart failure. However, Goldberg and others reported recently that the oral administration of levodopa was effective in the treatment of heart failure through its conversion to dopamine [52]. Both acute and long-term hemodynamic improvement were found: there was an increase in cardiac index and decrease in systemic vascular resistance, with little change in either blood pressure or heart rate. The study was not controlled adequately and the findings, while encouraging, must be regarded as preliminary. Furthermore, objective evidence that such hemodynamic improvement results in increased exercise tolerance and reduced symptomatology is required: of interest here was the observation that infusion of dobutamine improved hemodynamic status at rest in patients with heart failure but did not increase their maximum exercise tolerance [53]. In addition, cardiac dysrhythmias may be induced with levodopa treatment, suggesting actions at sites other than the dopamine receptor and dictating caution with its use. Nevertheless, dopamine's unique profile, in particular its selective renal effect, might offer distinct advantages; being a natural agonist, less tolerance to prolonged infusion might be expected than with partial agonist drugs [54].

Ibopamine [2,42,55–58]
Ibopamine is the diisobutyric ester of *N*-methyldopamine. After absorption, it is converted to its *N*-methyl derivative by esterases in plasma. *N*-methyldopamine, or epinine, resembles dopamine pharmacologically [59]. Hemodynamic improvement has been claimed after its use in heart failure.

Fenoldopam
This relatively specific DA_1 agonist has essentially no inotropic or adrenergic activity (action at α- or β-receptor sites), but can reduce, at least acutely, vascular resistance in patients with heart failure [60]. Longer-term controlled studies are awaited.

Dopamine and the Treatment of Hypertension

Infusion of dopamine has little effect on blood pressure until selectivity is lost when pressure tends to rise. Small reductions in pressure may occur with the acute infusion of dopamine in patients with essential hypertension, presumably through reduction of peripheral resistance [61]. If, as stated earlier, failure to mobilize renal dopamine underlies a subset of patients with raised pressure [61], then longer-term infusion of dopamine in selected patients might be expected to cause blood pressure to fall. Orally active dopaminergic agents would be more appropriate to testing this hypothesis. Unfortunately, as with all pharmacologic agents, they lack specificity, which complicates interpretation. Compounds like gamma-glutamyl dopa converted preferentially to dopamine in the kidney could prove of special interest [3].

Oral Dopaminergic Agents and Hypertension

The D_2 agonist, bromocriptine, reduced blood pressure when administered to patients with hypertension [10,11]. Its mode of action remains obscure, but a reduction of sympathetic activity through presynaptic inhibition of transmitter release, either centrally or peripherally, could be responsible [11]. D_2 agonists, which penetrate the central nervous system, would be expected to produce nausea — a side-effect found with this drug, which does not bode well for the development of centrally acting D_2 agonists as therapeutic agents for hypertension. The vomiting 'center' lies close to the area postrema, and may be accessible even to agents which do not readily cross the blood–brain barrier. Dopamine itself can induce vomiting at high intravenous dosing.

A more productive approach to the development of effective antihypertensive agents may be through the DA_1 receptor. Fenoldopam, a selective agonist at the DA_1 site, reduces blood pressure through a reduction in peripheral resistance [62]. Reflex tachycardia in response to the initial pressure reduction did not appear to be a problem with long-term use in this study.

Conclusions

Dopamine has emerged from the shadow of the other catecholamines. Its physiologic importance in the central nervous system is beyond doubt, but questions remain over its peripheral role. An understanding of dopamine's unique profile has allowed its rational use in clinical medicine, and has led to the continuing development of new drugs with major therapeutic potential in the field of cardiovascular medicine.

References

[1] Goldberg LI.
Cardiovascular and renal actions of dopamine: Potential clinical applications.
Pharmacol Rev 1972; **24**: 1–29.

[2] Goldberg LI.
Dopamine receptors and hypertension: Physiologic and pharmacologic implications.
Am J Med 1984; **77**: 37–44.

[3] Lee MR.
Dopamine and the kidney.
Clin Sci 1982; **62**: 439–48.

[4] Ganguly A.
Dopaminergic regulation of aldosterone secretion: How credible?
Clin Sci 1984; **66**: 631–7.

[5] Campbell DJ, Mendelsohn FAO, Adam WR, Funder JW.
Is aldosterone secretion under dopaminergic control?
Circ Res 1981; **49**: 1217–27.

[6] Ball SG, Tree M, Morton JJ, Inglis GC, Fraser R.
Circulating dopamine: Its effect on the plasma concentrations of catecholamines, renin, angiotensin, aldosterone and vasopressin in the conscious dog.
Clin Sci 1981; **61**: 417–22.

[7] Ball SG, Oates NS, Lee MR.
Urinary dopamine in man and rat. The effects of inorganic salts on dopamine excretion.
Clin Sci Mol Med 1978; **55**: 167–73.

[8] Creese I.
Dopamine receptors explained. In: Bousfield D, ed. *Neurotransmitters in Action.* Amsterdam: Elsevier Biomedical Press, 1985; pp. 242–51.

[9] Goldberg LI, Glock D, Kohli J, Barnett A.
Separation of peripheral dopamine receptors by a selective DA_1 antagonist. SCH23390.
Hypertension 1984; **6** (Suppl 1): 125–30.

[10] Stumpe KO, Kolloch R, Higuchi M, Kruck F, Vetter H.
Hyperprolactinaemia and antihypertensive effect of bromocriptine in essential hypertension.
Lancet 1977; ii: 211–4.

[11] Kolloch R, Kobayashi K, De Quattro U.
Dopaminergic control of sympathetic tone and blood pressure. Evidence in primary hypertension.
Hypertension 1980; **2**: 390–4.

[12] Kawabe H, Kondo K, Saruta T.
Effect of the intracerebroventricular injection of dopamine on blood pressure in the spontaneously hypertensive rat.
Clin Exp Hypertens [A] 1983; **A5**: 1703–16.

[13] Huang B-S, Malvin RL, Grekin RJ.
Central effects of angiotensin II and dopamine in sodium-depleted sheep.
Am J Physiol 1985; **248**: R541–8.

[14] Unger T, Buu NT, Kuchel O.
Conjugated dopamine: Peripheral origin, distribution and response to acute stress in the dog.
Can J Physiol Pharmacol 1980; **58**: 22–7.

[15] Van Loon GR, Sole MJ.
Plasma dopamine: Source, regulation, and significance.
Metabolism 1980; **29** (Suppl 1): 1119.

[16] Snider SR, Kuchel O.
Dopamine: An important neurohormone of the sympathoadrenal system. Significance of increased peripheral dopamine release for the human stress response and hypertension.
Endocrinol Rev 1983; **4**: 291.

[17] Kuchel O, Buu NT, Roy P, Hamet P, Larochelle P, Genest J.
Regional sources of free and sulfoconjugated catecholamines in hypertension.
Hypertension 1984; **6** (Suppl 1): 151–5.

[18] Anton AH, Sayre DF.
The distribution of dopamine and dopa in various animals and a method for their determination in diverse biological material.
J Pharmacol Exp Ther 1964; **145**: 326–34.

[19] Bell C, Lang WJ, Laska J.
Dopamine containing vasomotor nerves in the dog kidney.
J Neurochem 1978; **31**: 77–83.

[20] Drake AJ, Stanford C.
Effect of cardiac denervation on catecholamine levels in dog heart.
J Physiol 1982; **324**: 14P.

[21] Mohanty PK, Sowers JR, Thames MD, Beck FWJ, Kawaguchi A, Lower RR.
Myocardial norepinephrine, epinephrine and dopamine concentrations after cardiac autotransplantation in dogs.
J Am Coll Cardiol 1986; **7**: 419–24.

[22] Ilebekk A, Anderson FR, Kjeldsen SE, Eide I.
Dopamine release from the porcine myocardium.
Acta Physiol Scand 1983; **119**: 197–201.

[23] Pierpont GL, Francis GS, DeMaster EG, Levine TB, Bolman RM, Cohn JN.
Elevated left ventricular myocardial dopamine in preterminal idiopathic dilated cardiomyopathy.
Am J Cardiol 1983; **52**: 1033–5.

[24] Sole MJ, Helke CJ, Jacobowitz DM.
Increased dopamine in failing hampster heart: Transvesicular transport of dopamine limits rate of norepinephrine synthesis.
Am J Cardiol 1982; **49**: 1652–90.

[25] Chan YL.
Cellular mechanisms of renal tubular transport of L-dopa and its derivatives in the rat: Microperfusion studies.
J Pharmacol Exp Ther 1976; **199**: 17–24.

[26] Baines AD, Chan W.
Production of urine free dopamine from DOPA: A micropuncture study.
Life Sci 1980; **26**: 253–9.

[27] Ball SG, Gunn IG, Douglas IHS.
Renal handling of dopa: Dopamine, noradrenaline and epinephrine in the dog.
Am J Physiol 1982; **242**: F56–62.

[28] Dinerstein RJ, Vannice J, Henderson RC, Roth LJ, Goldberg LI, Hoffmann PC.
Histofluorescence techniques provide evidence for dopamine containing neuronal elements in canine kidney.
Science 1979; **205**: 497–9.

[29] Ball SG, Gunn IG, McArthur KJD, Inglis GC, Douglas IHS.
The renal nerves in dogs: Noradrenergic and dopaminergic?
Clin Sci 1983; **63**: 297S–9S.

[30] Kopp U, Bradley T, Hjemdahl P.
Renal venous outflow and urinary excretion of norepinephrine, epinephrine, and dopamine during graded renal nerve stimulation.
Am J Physiol 1983; **44**: E52–60.

[31] Bell C, Lang WJ.
Neural dopaminergic vasodilator control in the kidney.
Nature 1973; **246**: 27–9.

[32] Marin-Grez M, Briggs JP, Schubert G, Schnermann J.
Dopamine receptor antagonists inhibit the natriuretic response to atrial natriuretic factor (ANF).
Life Sci 1985; **36**: 2171–6.

[33] Fraser R, Brown JJ, Lever AF, Mason PA, Robertson JIS.
Control of aldosterone secretion.
Clin Sci 1979; **56**: 389–99.

[34] Edwards CRW, Thorner MO, Miall PR, Al-Dujaili EAS, Hanker JP, Besser GM.
Inhibition of the plasma aldosterone response to frusemide by bromocriptine.
Lancet 1975; **ii**: 903–4.

[35] Holland OB, Thomas C, Brown M, Schindewolf D, Hillier Y, Gomez-Sanchez C.
Aldosterone suppression with dopamine in low renin hypertension.
J Clin Invest 1983; **72**: 754–66.

[36] Drake CR, Carey RM.
Dopamine modulates sodium dependent aldosterone response to angiotensin II in humans.
Hypertension 1984; **6** (Suppl 1): 119–23.

[37] Connell JMC, Padfield PL, Bunting EA, Ball SG *et al.*
Inhibition of prolactin secretion by low-dose dopamine infusion in patients with hyperprolactinaemia.
Clin Endocrinol (Oxford) 1983; **18**: 527–32.

[38] Connell JMC, Ball SG, Inglis GC, Beastall GH, Davies DL.
The effect of low-dose dopamine infusion on anterior pituitary hormone secretion in normal female subjects.
Clin Sci 1984; **67**: 219–23.

[39] Connell JMC, Tonolo G, Davies DL, Finlayson J, Ball SG, Fraser R.
Dopamine affects adrenal response to angiotensin II infusion by altering angiotensin II clearance in sodium deplete man.
J Endocrinol (Oxford) 1985; **107** (Suppl): 37.

[40] Connell JMC, Kenyon CJ, Ball SG, Davies DL, Fraser R.
Dopamine effects on adrenocorticotrophin-stimulated aldosterone, cortisol, corticosterone and 11-deoxycorticosteroid concentrations in sodium-replete and sodium-deplete man.
J Endocrinol (Oxford) 1986; **109**: 339–44.

[41] Levinson PD, Goldstein DS, Munson PJ, Gill JR, Keiser HR.
Endocrine, renal and haemodynamic responses to graded dopamine infusions in normal man.
J Clin Endocrinol Metab 1985; **60** (Suppl): 821–6.

[42] Goldberg LI, Rajfer SI.
Dopamine receptors: Application in clinical cardiology.
Circulation 1985; **72**: 245–7.

[43] Leier CV, Heban PT, Huss P, Bush CA, Lewis RP.
Comparative systemic and regional hemodynamic effects of dopamine and dobutamine in patients with cardiomyopathic heart failure.
Circulation 1978; **58**: 466–75.

[44] Uretsky BF, Generalovich T, Verbalis JE, Valdes AM, Reddy PS.
Comparative hemodynamic and hormonal response of encoramine and dobutamine in severe congestive heart failure.
Am J Cardiol 1986; **58**: 110–6.

[45] Wilson JR, Martin JL, Ferraro N.
Impaired skeletal muscle nutritive flow during exercise in patients with congestive heart failure: Role of cardiac pump dysfunction as determined by effects of dobutamine.
Am J Cardiol 1984; **53**: 1308–75.

[46] Benotti JR.
Comparative vasoactive therapy for heart failure.
Am J Cardiol 1985; **56**: 19B–24B.

[47] Awan NA, Needham K, Evenson MK, Mason DT.
Comparison of hemodynamic actions of pirbuterol and dobutamine on cardiac function in severe congestive heart failure.
Am J Cardiol 1982; **47**: 665.

[48] Brown RA, Dixon J, Farmer JB *et al.*
The effects of dobutamine on cardiovascular system of the dog.
Br J Pharmacol 1985; **85**: 609–19.

[49] Brown RA, Dixon J, Farmer JB *et al.*
Dopexamine: A novel agonist at peripheral DA receptors and β_2-adrenoceptors.
Br J Pharmacol 1985; **85**: 599–608.

[50] Dawson JR, Thompson DS, Signy M *et al.*
Acute hemodynamic and metabolic effects of dopexamine, a new dopaminergic receptor agonist, in patients with chronic heart failure.
Br Heart J 1985; **54**: 313–20.

[51] Fennell WH, Taylor AA, Young JB *et al.*
Propylbutyldopamine: Hemodynamic effects in conscious dogs, normal human volunteers and patients with heart failure.
Circulation 1983; **67**: 829–36.

[52] Rajfer SI, Anton AH, Rossen J, Goldberg LI.
Beneficial haemodynamic effects of oral levodopa in heart failure: Relationship to generation of dopamine.
N Engl J Med 1984; **310**: 1357.

[53] Maskin CS, Ocken S, Chadwick B, Le Jemtel TH.
Acute inotropic stimulation with DA in severe congestive heart failure: Beneficial hemodynamic effect at rest but not during maximal exercise.
Am J Cardiol 1983; **52**: 1028–32.

[54] Unverferth DV, Blanford M, Kates RE, Leier CV.
Tolerance to dobutamine after 72 h continuous infusion.
Am J Med 1980; **69**: 262–6.

[55] Ghirardi P, Brusoni B, Mangiovacchi M *et al.*
Acute haemodynamic effects of dopamine in patients with severe congestive heart failure.
Br J Clin Pharmacol 1985; **19** (Suppl): 613–8.

[56] Dei Cas L, Fappani A, Riva S *et al.*
Hemodynamic advantage of combined administration or oral ibopamine and nitroprusside in patients with ischaemic and idiopathic congestive cardiomyopathy.
Clin Cardiol 1985; **8**: 427–32.

[57] Ren JH, Unverferth DV, Leier CV.
The dopamine congener, ibopamine, in congestive heart failure.
J Cardiovasc Pharmacol 1984; **6**: 748.

[58] Ren JH, Unverferth DV, Leier CV.
The dopamine congener, ibopamine, in congestive heart failure.
J Cardiovasc Pharmacol 1984; **6**: 748–55.

[59] Itoh H, Kohli JD, Rajfer SI, Goldberg LI.
Comparison of cardiovascular actions of dopamine and epinine in the dog.
J Pharmacol Exp Ther 1985; **233**: 87–93.

[60] Young JB, Leon CA, Pratt CM, Suarez JM, Aronoff RD, Roberts R.
Hemodynamic effects of an oral dopamine receptor agonist (fenoldopam) in patients with congestive heart failure.
J Am Coll Cardiol 1985; **6**: 792–6.

[61] Lee MR.
The kidney fault in essential hypertension may be a failure to mobilise renal dopamine when dietary sodium chloride is increased.
Cardiovasc Rev Rep 1981; **2**: 785–9.

[62] Carey RM, Stote RM, Dubb JW, Townsend LH, Rose CE, Kaiser DL.
Selective peripheral dopamine-1 receptor stimulation with fenoldopam in human essential hypertension.
J Clin Invest 1984; **74**: 2198–207.

CARDIOVASCULAR PEPTIDES

[1] Renal, haemodynamic, and hormonal effects of human alpha atrial natriuretic peptide in healthy volunteers.
Richards AM, Nicholls MG, Ikram H, Webster MWI, Yandle TG, Espiner EA, Princess Margaret Hosp, Christchurch, New Zealand.
Lancet 1985; i: 545–8.

[2] Specific membrane receptors for atrial natriuretic factor in renal and vascular tissues.
Napier MA, Vandlen RL, Albers-Schonberg G *et al*, Merck Sharp & Dohme Res Labs, Rahway, NJ, USA.
Proc Natl Acad Sci USA 1984; **81**: 5946–50.

[3] Atrial natriuretic factor inhibits the stimulation of aldosterone secretion by angiotensin II, ACTH and potassium in vitro and II-induced steroidogenesis in vivo.
Chartier L, Schiffrin E, Thibault G, Garcia R, Clin Res Inst Montreal, Montreal, Que, Canada.
Endocrinology 1984; **115**: 2026–7.

[4] Haemodynamic effects of atrial peptide infusion in heart failure.
Crozier IG, Nicholls MG, Ikram H, Espiner EA, Gomez HJ, Warner NJ, Princess Margaret Hosp, Christchurch, New Zealand.
Lancet 1986; ii: 1242–5.

[5] Calcitonin gene-related peptide is a potent vasodilator.
Brain SD, Williams TJ, Tippins JR, Morris HR, MacIntyre I, Royal Coll Surgeons England, London, UK.
Nature 1985; **313**: 54–6.

[6] Calcitonin gene-related peptide: potent vasodilator and major product of calcitonin gene.
Girgis SI, Macdonald DWR, Stevenson JC *et al*, Royal Postgrad Med Sch, London, UK.
Lancet 1985; ii: 14–60.

[7] Calcitonin gene-related peptide (Editorial).
Lancet 1985; ii: 25–6.

[8] Human calcitonin gene related peptide: a potent endogenous vasodilator in man.
Struthers AD, Brown MJ, Macdonald DWR *et al*, Royal Postgrad Med Sch, London, UK.
Clin Sci 1986; **70**: 389–93.

Comment. Atrial natriuretic peptide has recently emerged as a major new factor in cardiovascular medicine. Richards *et al* [1] were the first to show that atrial natriuretic peptide causes natriuresis and vasodilatation when given as a bolus to normal volunteers. Animal data have shown that, as might be expected, there are specific membrane receptors for atrial natriuretic peptide in both renal and vascular tissue [2]. Curiously, atrial natriuretic peptide has been found in adrenal glomerulosa cells to inhibit aldosterone release as stimulated by either angiotensin II, ACTH or potassium [3]. This suggests an interaction between atrial natriuretic peptide and the other salt-regulating mechanisms, in the form of the renin-angiotensin-aldosterone system.

The natriuresis and vasodilatation of atrial natriuretic peptide would theoretically be of benefit in patients suffering from heart failure. In a study of seven patients with chronic congestive heart failure [4], placebo or a synthetic analog of plasma atrial natriuretic peptide (5 µg/minute) was given in random order for 4 hours on two separate occasions at least one week apart. Hemodynamic, hormonal and electrolyte indices were measured. It was found that atrial natriuretic peptide caused significant decreases in mean systemic arterial pressure, mean pulmonary artery pressure, pulmonary diastolic pressure and right atrial pressure for at least 2 hours after the infusion when compared with placebo. It also caused an increase in cardiac output. However, significant natriuresis or diuresis did not occur with the infusion, and plasma renin activity, angiotensin, arginine vasopressin, aldosterone and cortisol volumes did not change significantly.

Calcitonin gene-related peptide is another new endogenous peptide of cardiovascular interest. It appears to be a very potent vasodilator, and it is possible that it is a major determinant of peripheral vascular tone [5–8].

INTRACELLULAR CALCIUM

[1] Correlation of platelet calcium with blood pressure. Effect of antihypertensive therapy.
Erne P, Bolli P, Burgisser E, Buhler FR, Univ Hosp, Basel, Switzerland.
N Engl J Med 1984; **310**: 1084–8.

[2] Cytoplasmic free [Ca^{2+}] is increased in the platelets of spontaneously hypertensive rats and essential hypertensive patients.
Bruschi G, Bruschi ME, Caroppo M, Orlandini G, Spaggiari M, Cavatorta A, Univ Parma, Parma, Italy.
Clin Sci 1985; **68**: 179–84.

[3] Mononuclear leucocyte intracellular free calcium — does it correlate with blood pressure?
Shore AC, Beynon GW, Jones JC, Markandu ND, Sagnella GA, MacGregor GA, Charing Cross and Westminster Med Sch, London, UK.
J Hypertens 1985; **3**: 183–7.

Comment. Interest has focused recently on the relationship between calcium and blood pressure. Erne *et al* [1] reported a very close correlation between blood pressure and cytosolic free calcium in platelets. Bruschi *et al* [2] agreed that intracellular calcium in platelets was higher in hypertensive than in normotensive subjects, and found this difference to be more obvious in platelets than in lymphocytes. This tissue difference may partly explain why Shore *et al* [3] found no difference between hypertensives and normotensives in the intracellular calcium concentrations in mononuclear leukocytes.

PROSTAGLANDINS

[1] Drug-induced inhibition of platelet function delays progression of peripheral occlusive arterial disease. A prospective double-blind arteriographically controlled trial.
Hess H, Mietaschk A, Deichsel G, Univ Munich, Munich, FRG.
Lancet 1985; i: 415–8.

[2] Prolonged infusion of prostacyclin in patients with advanced stages of peripheral vascular disease: a placebo-controlled cross-over study.
Hossmann V, Auel H, Rucker W, Schror K, Univ Cologne, Cologne, FRG.
Klin Wochenschr 1984; **62**: 1108–14.

[3] Double-blind trial of CL115,347, a transdermally absorbed prostaglandin E$_2$ analogue, in treatment of Raynaud's phenomenon.
Belch JJF, Madhok R, Shaw B, Leiberman P, Sturrock RD, Forbes CD, Royal Infirm, Glasgow, UK.
Lancet 1985; i: 1180–4.

Comment. The therapeutic potential of prostanoids in peripheral vascular disease has continued to attract attention. In a large comprehensive study of 240 patients with peripheral vascular disease [1], arteriography was used to assess progression of the disease in three different treatment groups. Aspirin in combination wtih dipyridamole was found to be better than aspirin alone, which in turn was superior to placebo. Hossmann *et al* [2] showed that a seven-day infusion of prostacyclin reduced platelet aggregation during its infusion, but that there was a rebound increase in platelet aggregation and thromboxane B$_2$ seven days after the infusion was stopped. Belch *et al* [3] investigated a novel transdermal preparation of a prostaglandin E$_2$ analog (CL115,347), and found favorable results in a double-blind clinical trial in patients with Raynaud's phenomenon.

ANGIOTENSIN II RESPONSIVENESS IN HYPERTENSION

[1] Defect in the sodium-modulated tissue responsiveness to angiotensin II in essential hypertension.
Shoback DM, Williams GH, Moore TJ, Dluhy RG, Podolsky S, Hollenberg NK, Brigham and Women's Hosp, Harvard Med Sch, Boston, MA, USA.
J Clin Invest 1983; **72**: 2115–24.

[2] Converting-enzyme inhibition corrects the altered adrenal response to angiotensin II in essential hypertension.
Taylor T, Moore TJ, Hollenberg NK, Williams GH, Brigham and Women's Hosp, Boston, MA, USA.
Hypertension 1984; **6**: 92–9.

[3] Correction of abnormal renal blood response to angiotensin II by converting enzyme inhibition in essential hypertensives.
Redgrave J, Rabinowe S, Hollenberg NK, Williams GH, Brigham and Women's Hosp, Boston, MA, USA.
J Clin Invest 1985; **7**: 1285–90.

Comment. In normal subjects, dietary sodium intake modulates the renovascular and aldosterone responses to infused angiotensin II. Shoback *et al* [1] have shown that 40% of patients with essential hypertension (defined as non-modulators) are not able to modulate the above responses to a high-sodium diet. Workers have now shown that angiotensin converting enzyme inhibitors are able to correct the aldosterone and renovascular responses to angiotensin II in these non-modulators [2,3]. Consequently, angiotensin converting enzyme inhibitors may be more effective as antihypertensive agents in this subset of hypertensive patients.

10. Hypertension

ION TRANSPORT AND HYPERTENSION

Review: J.D. SWALES, A.M. HEAGERTY

The study of ion fluxes across cell membranes in patients with hypertension continues to be a focus of intense scientific activity and controversy. The explanation is not difficult to discern. Several transmembrane transport processes have been characterized; in some cases, their contributions to intracellular electrolyte homeostasis, even in such an accessible and well-investigated cell as the erythrocyte, remain uncertain. Our knowledge of transmembrane fluxes in the tissue most relevant to hypertension, the resistance vessel wall, was until recently only primitive (see below). Further, the kinetics of ion movement through the various transmembrane pathways are undoubtedly influenced by a variety of intrinsic and blood-borne factors.

Early studies of human erythrocytes alluded to decreased sodium/potassium co-transport and increased lithium/sodium countertransport (see review [1]). Unfortunately, however, conflict with regard to the important transporter – the sodium/potassium pump – was rampant, with some workers reporting increased activity and others a decrease (see Parker and Berkowitz [2]). Rather more consistent findings were reported in studies of the leukocyte: here the sodium pump appeared to be less active, as assessed by a reduction in the rate constant for ouabain-sensitive sodium efflux [3].

These findings could have at least one of several explanations: the variable relationship between the abnormality and blood pressure in the various reports could be fortuitous, reflecting a failure to recognize a common determining factor of blood pressure and ion transport; this would result from poor matching of patients and controls. Alternatively, the blood-cell abnormality could reflect a disturbance in ion transport which contributed to the elevation in blood pressure. This in turn could occur in two ways: either the transport abnormality could be attributable to a circulating factor which influences ion fluxes as well as blood pressure; or the blood-cell abnormality could be a marker for a global disturbance in cell membrane function which gives rise to elevated blood pressure through involvement of other tissues.

Is the Association of Altered Ion Fluxes with Hypertension a Real One?
Initial studies of sodium/potassium co-transport and lithium/sodium countertransport indicated a dramatic difference between values obtained from hypertensive and normotensive subjects, with little overlap between the two. More recent reports, even when generally consistent with the initial reports, have shown less marked disturbances. This could be attributed to the greater care taken in matching populations to be studied for such factors as weight, race, age and sex. The optimal approach is probably to obtain all individuals to be studied from the same population.

In a careful report on erythrocyte maximal lithium/sodium countertransport, Cooper *et al* characterized certain selected populations, such as black schoolchildren and adults recruited from routine health-screening programs [4]. In three of these populations, blood pressure and countertransport appeared to correlate significantly. However, neither passive sodium leak nor erythrocyte sodium content correlated with blood pressure. Despite the gross correlation between countertransport and blood pressure in a group of 448 individuals, statistical significance was absent when age and weight were included in a step-wise linear regression analysis. (Weight is of particular importance, since hypertensive patients tend to be heavier than normotensive controls unless careful attention is paid to matching.) Weder *et al* examined the effect of weight reduction upon erythrocyte sodium content and fluxes [5]. Although lithium/sodium countertransport did not change with weight reduction, both maximal sodium/potassium co-transport and intracellular sodium rose. The authors believe that a decrease in body fat is associated with an increase in cell sodium.

Two other large-scale studies have looked at the relationship between blood pressure and lithium/sodium countertransport. In one, samples of blood from 238 randomly selected healthy donors were examined [6]. There was a highly significant positive association between the two, even when moderately and severely hypertensive patients were excluded (weight made a modest contribution to this association and in women only). In addition, there was an apparent bimodal distribution of values. Hunt *et al* obtained samples from 2091 healthy individuals in Utah [7]. A weak positive association between sodium/lithium countertransport and both weight and blood pressure was observed. The most striking finding was an association between plasma lipids and sodium/lithium countertransport. Triglycerides were positively associated, while total, HDL_2 and HDL_3 cholesterol were negatively correlated. When multivariate analysis was performed on lipids, weight and blood pressure, the association between triglycerides and total HDL cholesterol on the one hand and countertransport on the other persisted, as did the association between weight and countertransport. However, a relationship between mean blood pressure and countertransport was no longer apparent. Higher plasma triglyceride levels and lower HDL_2 and HDL_3 cholesterol were significantly associated with the presence of hypertension.

In an intervention study, results were similar. A group of normotensive and hypertensive subjects were put through a three-month exercise training program [8]. Sodium/lithium countertransport declined and HDL cholesterol increased, although there was no change in blood pressure. Thus, exercise-induced changes in membrane lipids may have occurred and altered ion fluxes.

Results of these studies emphasize the need for consideration of lipids and bodyweight when comparing between-population differences in erythrocyte ion transport. The influence of lipids is difficult to discern from plasma lipid values, which may not reflect altered concentrations of membrane lipids *per se*.

Other potentially confounding factors may be of importance. Countertransport is reported as being slightly higher in women [6]. However, black hypertensive subjects do not show the increased sodium/lithium countertransport repeatedly demonstrated in white hypertensives [9,10]. Stress may influence results when outpatients are compared with laboratory staff who are more familiar with the venepuncture procedure. For example, when red and white cell ion fluxes were measured before and after a cold-pressor test [11], the rate constant for ouabain-sensitive erythrocyte sodium efflux fell from 0.23 to 0.16. Although mean leukocyte ouabain-sensitive sodium efflux did not change, a negative correlation was seen among individual subjects between pre- and post-stress test plasma norepinephrine and the change in the ouabain-sensitive sodium efflux rate constant.

In conclusion, there appears to be a real association between hypertension and lithium/sodium countertransport. However, the association probably reflects effects of determinants common to both, rather than cause and effect.

Is a Circulating Humoral Factor a Determinant of Ion-Flux Abnormalities?

One hypothesis attributes a causal role in hypertension to ion-transport abnormalities [12,13]. It is proposed that the ouabain-like inhibitor of the sodium pump is released as a result of sodium retention, with consequent peripheral vasoconstriction mediated by reduced calcium efflux and increased influx attributable to the sodium/calcium exchange system in vascular smooth muscle. This hypothesis has been tested in several ways since it was first put forward. The difficulty has been in demonstrating that inhibition of the sodium pump is a feature of essential hypertension in man. In an extensive review of the literature up to 1983 on erythrocyte transport, Parker and Berkowitz conclude that the results reported are 'disparate and conflicting', although the majority of studies in the red cell demonstrate increased rather than decreased Na^+/K^+-ATPase activity and ouabain binding [2]. As they point out, most studies were carried out in synthetic media from which the putative inhibitor may have been removed. However, it is noteworthy that the reduced rate constant for ouabain-sensitive leukocyte sodium efflux, which has been demonstrated in several studies of hypertensive patients, is detectable in synthetic media [3]. Two groups have reported that either boiled or untreated plasma from hypertensive patients inhibits binding of ouabain by erythrocytes [14,15]. By contrast, another group was unable to demonstrate any differential effect upon ouabain binding when plasma from hypertensive and normotensive subjects was added to human leucokytes [16].

The role of a putative inhibitor can be assessed more directly by measuring the effect of plasma upon erythrocyte or leukocyte sodium fluxes. Two early studies reported inhibition by plasma from hypertensive patients [17,18]. A more recent report from the St Thomas' group has described a correlation between the capacity of serum from hypertensives to inhibit active sodium transport and diastolic blood pressure [19]. A study by Boon et al adopts a novel in-vivo approach [20]. Rubidium was given orally to hypertensive patients, and plasma and red cell concentrations of rubidium were measured. (Since cell membranes handle rubidium as they do potassium, the influx of rubidium would provide a measure of sodium-pump activity.) Boon et al were able to validate the method by demonstrating inhibition of erythrocyte rubidium uptake both by ouabain and in chronic renal failure, in which in-vitro studies have indicated that the sodium pump is inhibited. By contrast, erythrocyte rubidium uptake was *enhanced* in hypertensive subjects, as was erythrocyte uptake of ^{42}K. In experimental animals, the results are equally conflicting. Although rubidium uptake by large arteries is reduced by plasma from volume-expanded animals with hypertension, no such inhibition could be demonstrated in the spontaneously hypertensive rat [21]. Cross-incubation experiments have likewise failed to demonstrate an inhibitor of erythrocyte sodium pumping in the spontaneously hypertensive rat [22].

Na^+/K^+-ATPase is susceptible to a variety of influences. Thus, the rate constants for ouabain-sensitive sodium efflux are considerably greater when leukocytes are incubated in plasma or serum than when synthetic media are used. The same non-specific effects of plasma constituents are encountered with other tissues. When resistance vessels are incubated in plasma after preliminary incubation in synthetic media, the total sodium efflux rate constant increases [23].

Both stimulation and inhibition of the sodium pump may occur simultaneously. Usually plasma electrolyte concentrations are measured in studies of cross-incubation, but other factors may be more relevant to alterations in electrolyte fluxes: thus, free fatty acids inhibit Na^+/K^+-ATPase [24]. Linoleic and oleic acids in particular have been implicated in inhibition of the sodium pump with volume expansion in dogs [25]. In addition, these fatty acids inhibit the binding of ouabain to its membrane receptor [25]. Inhibition of sodium-pump activity may be produced by elevated levels of bile acids and phenolic acids [26] and by raised circulating thyroxine levels [27]. By contrast, insulin stimulates sodium-pump activity in adipocytes [28]: increased pH and bicarbonate levels increase erythrocyte permeability and active sodium pumping [29]. While one study reported inhibition of leukocyte sodium pumping by norepinephrine when cells were incubated in plasma [30], another described increased sodium pumping as a result of the addition of epinephrine to leukocytes suspended in synthetic media [31]. These observations may be of particular relevance where the level of stress differs between patients and laboratory controls.

In conclusion, the specificity and relationship to hypertension of activators or inhibitors of the Na^+/K^+-ATPase pump remains obscure.

Ion Fluxes in Relation to Sodium Balance

Another key issue in the interpretation of ion-transport abnormalities in hypertension is the relationship between changes in sodium balance and changes in the cellular handling of electrolytes. Several groups have tried to characterize the effects of changes in sodium balance on erythrocyte sodium content and fluxes. Stokes *et al* could detect no change in pump activity, although there was a decrease in cell sodium concentration and passive sodium influx in cells from normotensive subjects subjected to severe salt depletion [32]. Cells from hypertensive subjects exhibited no specific features. Modest salt restriction had no effect upon either the intracellular sodium or sodium/lithium countertransport of normotensive individuals [33]. Gudmundsson *et al* observed decreased intracellular sodium and an increase in pump activity with salt-loading of normotensive subjects with a family history of hypertension [34]. Subjects without a family history showed no increase. Myers *et al* reported that erythrocytes from hypertensive patients given a high-salt diet showed no change in sodium-pump activity [35]. However, when erythrocytes were incubated in plasma from such subjects, ouabain-sensitive sodium transport was reduced compared with sodium transport of erythrocytes incubated in plasma from salt-restricted subjects. Weissberg *et al* incubated erythrocytes in plasma, and observed a fall in the ouabain-sensitive sodium efflux rate constant when subjects were changed from a salt-restricted to a salt-loaded diet [36]; however, there was no change in measurable intraerythrocytic sodium content, and no inhibitor of Na^+/K^+-ATPase could be detected in the plasma of salt-loaded subjects by chemical assay. By contrast, salt restriction produced a small reduction in ouabain-sensitive human leukocyte sodium pumping, with no change in intracellular sodium [37]. Similar studies using rat thymocytes produced a remarkably similar response: in this report, no inhibitor could be detected on cross-incubation of thymocytes with plasma from salt-loaded rats [38].

These disparate results emphasize perhaps that intracellular sodium changes remarkably little in response to alterations in sodium balance. Alterations in sodium balance produce a number of metabolic and humoral responses, and it seems likely that the diverse implications of published data on electrolyte transport reflect this fact. Changes in salt intake in some studies were accompanied by changes in other dietary factors, e.g. lipids, that may be of relevance. The presence of a specific inhibitor of sodium transport released in response to salt-loading and increasing intracellular sodium certainly cannot be regarded as proven at present, although it remains a possibility. The role of such an inhibitor in the pathogenesis of essential hypertension is speculative.

What is the Membrane Abnormality in Essential Hypertension?

One problem in this, as in so many other areas of hypertension research, is not only that an abnormality is difficult to detect but that multiple abnormalities have been reported. Individual investigators usually focus upon highly selective aspects of electrolyte transport which they are studying as pathogenetic. The confusion has been compounded by poor matching of patient and control populations — a factor of critical importance because transport systems are influenced by heterogeneous factors, most of which are ill understood [39]. Nevertheless, the evidence would seem to point strongly to an abnormality in the cell membrane which influences electrolyte transport and which is (modestly, perhaps) associated with blood pressure.

The concept of an intrinsic abnormality in red cell membranes was supported by an imaginative study carried out by Bianchi and co-workers in Milan [40]. This group transplanted bone marrow between irradiated Milan hypertensive rats and their normotensive controls. Erythrocytes circulating after the transplant retained the ion-transport characteristics of the donor strain, despite persistent hypertension. Levy *et al* studied the temperature dependence of lithium/sodium countertransport [41]. Arrhenius plots showed a change in slope in erythrocytes from normotensive subjects at about 30°C, indicating a substantial influence of the physical state of membrane lipids at this temperature. These results are consistent with many others, indicating a substantial influence of the physical state of membrane lipids on several ion transport processes. However, in addition, Levy *et al* demonstrated that the corresponding break in the Arrhenius line in hypertensive patients was significantly lower. The same abnormality could be demonstrated in normotensive offspring of hypertensive subjects, indicating a genetic origin for the abnormality.

Alterations in membrane lipoproteins may influence more than one transport system, as has been shown by an in-vitro study by Brand and Whittam [42]. The erythrocyte membrane is more permeable to the nitrate anion than to chloride. Substituting nitrate for chloride increases passive permeability of the erythrocyte to monovalent cations, probably as a result of the rearrangement of membrane lipids: thus nitrate reproduces one of the flux abnormalities most commonly reported in hypertension, i.e. an increase in passive sodium fluxes [2]. This induced change in membrane properties also gives rise to a reduction in outward sodium and potassium co-transport and a failure of active sodium pumping to respond to the increased intracellular sodium load. Modification of the lipid component of semipurified preparations of Na^+/K^+ATPase modifies its activity, while sodium and potassium co-transport can be altered both *in vitro* and *in vivo* by changing the erythrocyte lipid membrane composition (see review [11]). It is perhaps relevant that modification of the ratio of saturated to unsaturated dietary lipids produces biologically significant alterations in indices of cardiovascular sympathetic nervous system activity [43,44].

The Nature of Potential Associations between Blood Pressure and Cellular Membrane Transport Abnormalities

The cell membrane plays a central role in the activity of excitable tissues: variability in cell-membrane characteristics could therefore influence blood pressure in a variety of ways. Interest has focused on altered calcium transport as a determinant of smooth-muscle tone, although changes in the neurogenic control of vascular tone might be primary. Erne *et al* reported a close correlation between platelet-free calcium and blood pressure in a group of normotensive and hypertensive subjects [45]. The closeness of the association was surprising, and raises the possibility of a systematic artefact perhaps related to enhanced platelet activation in hypertensives. Thus, even if platelet calcium were to reflect smooth-muscle free calcium and, therefore, vascular tone, the superimposition of such other important determinants of vascular reactivity as structural changes in resistance vessel including hypertrophy would be expected to modify this relationship substantially in hypertensive patients. While recent studies of platelet calcium have shown slightly higher values in hypertensives, the original reported close correlation has not been confirmed and the differences between groups — although statistically significant —have been small [46,47].

The hypothesis that, in essential hypertension, vascular smooth muscle or neuronal calcium handling is abnormal is attractive. Thus, ion-transport abnormalities in circulating cells might serve as markers for the disorder. Altered calcium handling in membrane preparations of tissues from spontaneously hypertensive rats has been observed, including decreased calmodulin-stimulated, ATP-dependent calcium transport and decreased calcium binding to the inner surface of the cell membrane (see reviews [48,49]).

Within the last few years another intriguing possibility has been raised. The hydrolysis of the inner lamellar lipid phosphoinositol to water-soluble inositol triphosphate provides an important second messenger for the control of intracellular calcium, and probably mediates the calcium response to such stimuli as angiotensin II and vasopressin in vascular tissue [50–52]. In addition, the other product of phosphoinositol hydrolysis, diacylglycerol, performs another role as an activator of the transmembrane Na^+/H^+ exchange transport system [53]: regulation of intracellular pH by this system is probably of importance in cell differentiation and growth [54]. The phosphoinositol cycle also regulates basal aortic membrane sodium pumping [55]. Thus, a single component of cell-membrane lipids acts as a common factor in the regulation of smooth-muscle contractility and neurotransmitter release (through intracellular calcium), and also in the development of hyperplasia and in the control

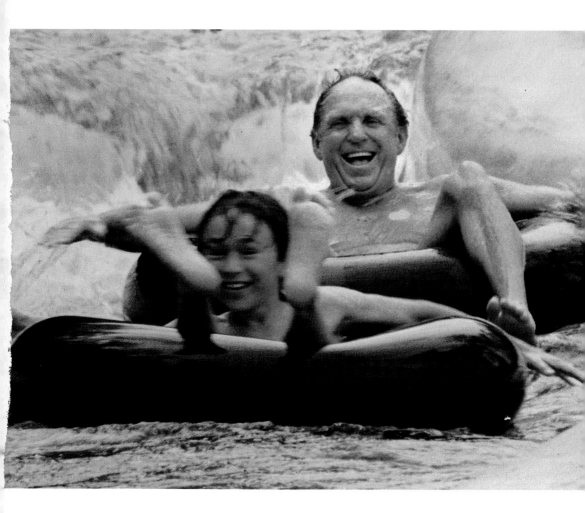

Transiderm®-Nitro

glyceryl trinitrate

Winning the hearts of patients everywhere

Presentation Transdermal therapeutic system containing glyceryl trinitrate, available in 2 strengths: Transiderm-Nitro 5 patches containing a drug reservoir of 25mg glyceryl trinitrate (average amount of glyceryl trinitrate absorbed per patch in 24 hours is 5mg). Transiderm-Nitro 10 patches containing 50mg glyceryl trinitrate (average of 10mg absorbed per patch in 24 hours).
Indications Prophylactic treatment of attacks of angina pectoris.
Dosage Individually variable: 1 Transiderm-Nitro 5 or 1 Transiderm-Nitro 10 daily. Tolerance: see full prescribing information.
Contra-indications Known hypersensitivity to nitrates, severe

hypotension, increased intracranial pressure, myocardial insufficiency due to obstruction.
Precautions Pregnancy and lactation. Recent myocardial infarction, arterial hypoxaemia due to severe anaemia, acute heart failure. Withdraw gradually when discontinuing treatment. Remove before cardioversion or DC defibrillation. Concomitant use of blood pressure lowering agents.
Side-effects Mostly mild and transient: e.g. headache, reflex-tachycardia. Occasionally skin reactions. Rarely after high doses: postural hypotension, dizziness, nausea and vomiting.

Packs and prices Boxes of 30 patches. Transiderm-Nitro 5 (PL0001/0094), basic NHS price 64.4p per day; Transiderm-Nitro 10 (PL0001/0095) 70.9p per day.
® denotes registered trademark. Full prescribing information is available on request from Ciba Laboratories, Horsham, West Sussex.

Ciba

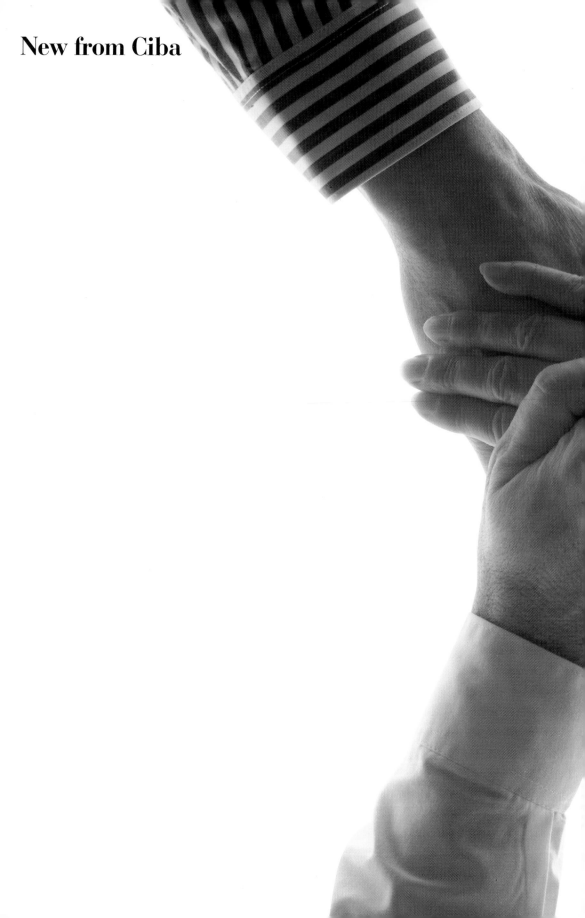

New from Ciba

of sodium-pump activity. Recent reports have described abnormalities of phosphoinositide turnover in erythrocytes of spontaneously hypertensive rats and of hypertensive patients [56,57]. Whether these abnormalities extend to vascular tissue has still to be established.

Changes in Resistance Vessels

In most studies, it has been assumed that abnormalities in other tissues (the circulating cells or the large arteries) reflect changes at the level of resistance vessel. This assumption has been difficult to test directly. Recently, however, a myographic method has been developed for the measurement of resistance-vessel contractility and ion fluxes using dissected rat or human resistance vessels [58]. Results with this method suggest that the extrapolation of data from other tissues to vascular smooth muscle may not be justified. A number of abnormalities of membrane ion flux have been described in the red cells, thymocytes and large arteries of the spontaneously hypertensive rat. However, Aalkjaer *et al* could find no abnormality of intracellular sodium, total or ouabain-sensitive sodium efflux, nor in the concentration of ouabain-binding sites in resistance-vessel smooth muscle [59]. This would suggest that one relevant area for exploration may be the sympathetic innervation of these vessels. By contrast, in the first study of this type in man, a correlation between total and ouabain-sensitive sodium pumping by leukocytes and omental resistance vessels from the same individual was noted [60]. There was no correlation, on the other hand, between ouabain-resistant pumping in leukocytes and resistance vessels. These subjects were normotensive; whether hypertensive patients would show a common divergence from normality in the two tissues remains to be determined.

References

[1] Swales JD.
Abnormal ion transport by cell membranes in hypertension. In: Robertson JIS, ed. *Handbook of Hypertension, Vol 1.* Amsterdam: Elsevier, 1983; pp. 239–66.

[2] Parker JC, Berkowitz LR.
Physiologically instructive genetic variants involving the human red cell membrane.
Physiol Rev 1983; 63: 261–313.

[3] Edmondson RPS, Thomas RD, Hilton PJ, Patrick J, Jones NF.
Abnormal leucocyte composition and sodium transport in essential hypertension.
Lancet 1975; i: 1003–5.

[4] Cooper R, Trevisan M, Ostrow D, Sempos C, Stamler J.
Blood pressure and sodium–lithium countertransport: Findings in population-based surveys.
J Hypertens 1984; 2: 467–71.

[5] Weder AB, Torreth BA, Katch VL, Rocchini AP.
The antihypertensive effect of calorie restriction in obese adolescents: Dissociation of effects on erythrocyte countertransport and cotransport.
J Hypertens 1984; 2: 507–14.

[6] Turner ST, Johnson M, Boerwinkle E, Richelson E, Taswell HF, Sing CF.
Sodium–lithium counter-transport and blood pressure in healthy blood donors.
Hypertension 1985; 7: 955–62.

[7] Hunt SC, Williams RR, Smith JB, Ash KO.
Associations of three erythrocyte cation transport systems with plasma lipids in Utah subjects.
Hypertension 1986; 8: 30–6.

[8] Adragna NC, Chang JL, Morey MC, Williams RS.
Effect of exercise on cation transport in human red cells.
Hypertension 1985; 7: 132–9.

[9] Canessa M, Spalvins A, Adragna N, Falkner B.
Red cell sodium counter-transport and co-transport in normotensive and hypertensive blacks.
Hypertension 1984; **6**: 344–51.

[10] Weder AB, Torretti BA, Julius S.
Racial differences in erythrocyte cation transport.
Hypertension 1984; **6**: 115–23.

[11] Heagerty AM, Riozzi A, Brand SC, Bing RF, Thurston H, Swales JD.
Membrane transport of ions in hypertension: A review.
Scand J Clin Lab Invest 1986; **46** (Suppl 180): 54–64.

[12] Blaustein MP.
Sodium ions, calcium ions, blood pressure regulation, and hypertension: A reassessment and a hypothesis.
Am J Physiol 1977; **232**: C165–73.

[13] de Wardener HE, MacGregor GA.
The natriuretic hormone and essential hypertension.
Lancet 1982; i: 1450–4.

[14] Devynck MA, Pernollet MG, Rosenfeld JB, Meyer P.
Measurement of digitalis-like compound in plasma: Application in studies of essential hypertension.
Br Med J 1983; **187**: 631–4.

[15] Sagnella GA, Jones JC, Shore AC, Markandu ND, MacGregor GA.
Evidence for increased levels of a circulating ouabain-like factor in essential hypertension.
Hypertension 1986; **8**: 433–7.

[16] Boon NA, Harper C, Aronson JK, Grahame-Smith DG.
Cation transport functions in vitro in patients with untreated essential hypertension.
Clin Sci 1985; **68**: 511–5.

[17] Poston L, Sewell RB, Wilkinson SP *et al.*
Evidence for a circulating sodium transport inhibitor in essential hypertension.
Br Med J 1981; **282**: 847–9.

[18] Hamlyn JM, Ringel R, Schaeffer J *et al.*
A circulating inhibitor of (Na^+-K^+)ATPase associated with essential hypertension.
Nature 1982; **300**: 650–2.

[19] Gray HH, Hilton PJ, Richardson PJ.
Effect of serum from patients with essential hypertension on sodium transport in normal leucocytes.
Clin Sci 1986; **70**: 583–6.

[20] Boon NA, Aronson JK, Hallis KF, Grahame-Smith DG.
Cation transport abnormalites in vivo in untreated essential hypertension.
Clin Sci 1986; **70**: 611–6.

[21] Haddy FJ.
The role of a humoral Na^+K^+-ATPase inhibitor in regulating precapillary vessel tone.
J Cardiovasc Pharmacol 1984; **6**: S439–6.

[22] Feig PU, Mitchell PP, Boylan JW.
Erythrocyte membrane transport in hypertensive humans and rats: Effect of sodium depletion and excess.
Hypertension 1985; **7**: 423–9.

[23] Aalkjaer C, Mulvaney MJ.
Sodium transport in vascular smooth muscle cells from resistance vessels.
Scand J Clin Lab Invest 1986; **46**: 49–53.

[24] Dahl DR.
Short-chain fatty acid inhibition of rat brain Na^+K^+ adenosine triphosphatase.
J Neurochem 1968; **15**: 815–9.

[25] Tamura M, Kuwano H, Kinoshita T, Inagami T.
Identification of linoleic and oleic acids as endogenous Na^+,K^+-ATPase inhibitors from acute volume-expanded dog plasma.
J Biol Chem 1985; **260**: 9672–7.

[26] Seda HWM, Gove CD, Hughes RD, Williams R.
Inhibition of partially purified rat brain Na^+K^+-dependent ATPase by bile acids, phenolic acids and endotoxin.
Clin Sci 1984; **66**: 415–20.

[27] Smith EKM, Samuel PD.
Abnormalities in the sodium pump of erythrocytes from patients with hyperthyroidism.
Clin Sci 1970; **38**: 49–61.

[28] Resh MD, Nemenoff RA, Guidotti G.
Insulin stimulation of (Na^+K^+)-adenosine triphosphatase-dependent 6Rb uptake in rat adipocytes.
J Biol Chem 1980; **255**: 10938–45.

[29] Funder J, Wieth JO.
Effect of some monovalent anions on fluxes of Na and K and on glucose metabolism of ouabain treated human red cells.
Acta Physiol Scand 1967; **71**: 168–95.

[30] Riozzi A, Heagerty AM, Bing RF, Thurston H, Swales JD.
Noradrenaline: A circulating inhibitor of renal transport.
Br Med J 1984; **289**: 1025–7.

[31] Baron DN, Green RJ, Khan FA.
Adrenaline and ion flux in isolated human leucocytes.
Clin Sci 1985; **68**: 517–21.

[32] Stokes GS, Monaghan JC, Middleston AT, Shirlow M, Marwood JF.
Effects of dietary sodium deprivation on erythrocyte sodium concentration and cation transport in normotensive and untreated hypertensive subjects.
J Hypertens 1986; **4**: 35–8.

[33] Cooper R, Trevisan M, Van Horn L *et al.*
Effect of dietary sodium reduction on red blood cell sodium concentration and sodium-lithium countertransport.
Hypertension 1984; **6**: 731–5.

[34] Gudmundsson O, Berglund G, Herlitz H, Andersson O, Jonsson O.
Influence of age on the response to increased salt intake: Effects on blood pressure and sodium in erythrocytes.
J Hypertens 1983; 1 (Suppl 2): 15–7.

[35] Myers JB, Fitzgibbon WR, Morgan TO.
Effect of acute and chronic salt loading on erythrocyte ^{22}Na efflux in males with essential hypertension.
Clin Sci 1981; **61**: 37s–9s.

[36] Weissberg PL, West MJ, Kendall MJ, Ingram M, Woods KL.
Effect of changes in dietary sodium and potassium on blood pressure and cellular electrolyte handling in young normotensive subjects.
J Hypertens 1985; **3**: 475–80.

[37] Swales JD, Bing RF, Bradlaugh R *et al.*
Cell membrane handling of sodium, sodium balance and blood pressure.
J Cardiovasc Pharmacol 1984; **6**: S42–8.

[38] Bradlaugh R, Heagerty AM, Bing RF, Swales JD, Thurston H.
Rat thymocyte sodium transport.
Hypertension 1984; **6**: 454–9.

[39] Swales JD.
Interpreting ion transport studies in hypertension: Methods, myths and hypotheses.
J Hypertens 1983; 1 (Suppl 2): 391–4.

[40] Bianchi G, Ferrari P, Trizio D *et al.*
Red blood cell abnormalities and spontaneous hypertension in the rat: A genetically determined link.
Hypertension 1985; **7**: 319–25.

[41] Levy R, Paran E, Keynan A, Livne A.
Essential hypertension: Improved differentiation by the temperature dependence of Li efflux in erythrocytes.
Hypertension 1983; **5**: 821–7.

[42] Brand SC, Whittam R.
The change from symmetry to asymmetry of a sodium transport system in red cell membranes.
Proc Roy Soc B 1985; **223**: 449–57.

[43] Schwartz JH, Young JB, Landsberg L.
Effect of dietary fat on sympathetic nervous system activity in the rat.
J Clin Invest 1983; **72**: 361–70.

[44] Panek RL, Dixon WR, Rutledge CO.
Modification of sympathetic neuronal function in the rat tail artery by dietary lipid treatment.
J Pharmacol Exp Ther 1985; **233**: 578–83.

[45] Erne P, Bolli P, Burgisser E, Buhler F.
Correlation of platelet calcium with blood pressure: Effect of antihypertensive therapy.
N Engl J Med 1984; **310**: 1084–8.

[46] Bruschi G, Bruschi ME, Caroppo M, Orlandini G, Spaggiari M, Cavatorta A.
Cytoplasmic free [Ca^{2+}] is increased in the platelets of spontaneously hypertensive rats and essential hypertensive patients.
Clin Sci 1985; **68**: 179–84.

[47] Lenz T, Haller H, Ludersdorf M *et al.*
Free intracellular calcium in essential hypertension. Effects of nifedipine and captopril.
J Hypertens 1985; **3** (Suppl 3): S13–5.

[48] Postnov YV, Orlow SN.
Cell membrane alteration as a source of primary hypertension.
J Hypertens 1984; **2**: 1–6.

[49] Robinson BF.
Altered calcium handling as a cause of primary hypertension.
J Hypertens 1984; **2**: 453–60.

[50] Schoepp DD, Rutledge CD.
Relationship between developmental changes in angiotensin II induced contractions and stimulation of phosphatidyl inositol labelling of rat aorta.
J Pharmacol Exp Ther 1984; **229**: 880–6.

[51] Berridge MJ, Irvine RF.
Inositol trisphosphate, a novel second messenger in cellular signal transduction.
Nature 1984; **312**: 315–21.

[52] Alexander RW, Brock TA, Gimbrone MA, Rittenhouse SE.
Angiotensin increases inositol triphosphate and calcium in vascular smooth muscle.
Hypertension 1985; **7**: 447–51.

[53] Moolenaar WH, Tertoolen LGJ, de Laat SW.
Phorbol ester and diacylglycerol mimic growth factors in raising cytoplasmic pH.
Nature 1984; **312**: 371–4.

[54] Hahnensmith RL, Aronsen PD.
The plasma membrane sodium–hydrogen exchanger and its role in physiological and pathophysiological processes.
Circ Res 1985; **56**: 773–88.

[55] Simmons DA, Kern EFO, Winegrad AI, Martin DB.
Basal phosphatidylinositol turnover controls aortic NA^+/K^+ ATPase activity.
J Clin Invest 1986; **77**: 503–13.

[56] Koutouzov S, Marche P, Cloix JF, Meyer P.
Phospholipid phosphorylation in erythrocytes of spontaneously hypertensive rats.
Am J Physiol 1982; **243**: H590–7.

[57] Marche P, Koutouzov S, Girard A, Elghozi JL, Meyer P, Ben-Ishay D.
Phosphoinositide turnover in erythrocyte membranes in human and experimental hypertension.
J Hypertens 1985; **3**: 25–30.

[58] Aalkjaer C, Mulvaney MJ.
Sodium metabolism in rat resistance vessels.
J Physiol 1983; **343**: 105–16.

[59] Aalkjaer C, Kjeldsen K, Norgaard A, Clausen T, Mulvaney MJ.
Ouabain binding and Na^+ content in resistance vessels and skeletal muscles of spontaneously hypertensive rats and K^+ depleted rats.
Hypertension 1985; **7**: 277–86.

[60] Aalkjaer C, Heagerty AM, Parvin SD, Bell PRF, Bing RF, Swales JD.
Cell membrane sodium transport: A correlation between human resistance vessels and leucocytes.
Lancet 1986; **i**: 649–51.

THE SYMPATHETIC NERVOUS SYSTEM AND ESSENTIAL HYPERTENSION

Review: JOHN L. REID, KENNEDY R. LEES

The contribution of the nervous system to hypertension has been a source of speculation and controversy for over 50 years. Sir George Pickering wrote [1]: "the information available up to 1955 ... led to no conclusive answer as to which mental factors ... participate in the pathogenesis of essential hypertension ... ". Thirty years later we have a much clearer understanding of the role of 'mental factors' in general and the sympathetic nervous system in particular in the regulation of the circulation and the maintenance of arterial blood pressure, but we have not yet reached a firm conclusion about the part played by the sympathetic nervous system in human essential hypertension.

The role of the sympathetic nervous system in short-term blood pressure control has been amply confirmed, and a role in long-term blood-pressure regulation can reasonably be proposed on the basis of long-term responses to sympatholytic drugs of various groups. It is now clear that a sympathetic contribution to blood-pressure control can be identified in normotensive as well as hypertensive subjects. Although quantitative differences between the two can easily be shown, there is little good evidence of qualitative differences between those arbitrarily classified as normotensive or hypertensive. Although there have been claims that subgroups of hyperadrenergic hypertensives could be identified [2], this has not been confirmed in larger-scale studies, and the observed differences could have been related to differences in anxiety or stress, and not directly to the level of blood pressure. More recent findings favor Pickering's view of blood pressure and its regulation as a continuous distribution, with no clearcut divisions between normotensives and hypertensives.

What has become increasingly apparent is the close interrelationship between the sympathetic nervous system and other neurogenic and endocrine pressor and depressor mechanisms [3,4]. This is exemplified by the contribution of renal sympathetic nerves (via their neurotransmitter, norepinephrine) and beta-adrenoceptors to the control of release of renin from the kidney, and by the multiple and complex interactions between angiotensin II and adrenal medullary, peripheral sympathetic and central nervous function [4].

The sympathetic nervous system's role in essential hypertension thus cannot be defined simply with respect to pathogenicity or etiology, or to the proportion of patients manifesting abnormalities. Its participation can be understood only in the context of a complex series of interactions between the sympathetic nervous system and other circulatory controls. This may be of some pathogenic importance, but is much more relevant to the therapeutics and long-term drug management of hypertension and the avoidance of vascular disease.

Three main questions are considered in this necessarily selective review.

1. What are the implications of analytical and technical improvements for the role of sympathetic mechanisms in hypertension?
2. What are the implications of better epidemiologic approaches with improved study design and greater sample size?
3. What are the implications of recently identified non-adrenergic peripheral autonomic transmitters and co-transmitters?

Implications of Technical and Analytical Developments

Direct Nerve Recording
A major problem in evaluating the role of the sympathetic nervous system lies in the difficulty of assessing sympathetic function. The disadvantages of using measurements of plasma norepinephrine as an index of sympathetic activity have been well documented [5,6]. Direct measurement of nerve traffic in a sympathetic nerve in the upper or lower limb was reported several years ago. Muscle nerve discharges are correlated with plasma norepinephrine [7], but there are no differences between hypertensives and controls [8]. There is a limitation on direct recording: only accessible nerves can be used, and there may be limitations on the duration and repetition of the procedure.

Spillover, Release and Clearance
An important development has been the study of plasma norepinephrine kinetics, which distinguishes between norepinephrine clearance and the apparent release or spillover of the neurotransmitter from the sympathetic nerve endings. This spillover is the amount of norepinephrine that escapes local uptake or metabolism and reaches the systemic circulation. Early studies used subpressor steady-state infusions of norepinephrine but the use of tracer doses of [3H]norepinephrine has since been pioneered by Esler and his group in Australia [9]. They found no change in the clearance of norepinephrine in most hypertensives, although they suggested that in one subgroup there might be a change in the early phase of elimination [10]. Calculated whole-body release rates did not differ between hypertensives and normotensives. In a recent refinement, the Australian group has studied the contribution

of individual organs to whole-body or total spillover in man [11]. Lung contributes a substantial proportion, while heart makes only a small contribution; the combined renal and hepatomesenteric vascular beds make up about 32% of the total. It is therefore not surprising that changes in plasma norepinephrine measured in forearm venous blood do not always correlate directly with changes in sympathetic activity -let alone blood pressure.

In addition to the above developments, analytical improvements have been introduced to improve the specificity and accuracy of this approach and to eliminate the contribution of deaminated radiolabeled metabolites [12].

Measurement of Plasma Catecholamines
Two principal methods are currently used for assay of plasma epinephrine and norepinephrine: radioenzymatic assay, or high-performance liquid chromatography with electrochemical detection (HPLC/ECD). The former is expensive to perform but requires little special equipment; the latter is less expensive. Both are subject to large and unacceptable inter- and intra-assay variation; this was highlighted in a recent inter-laboratory study, which suggested that HPLC/ECD may be preferable [13], although other workers claim to have overcome the problem by use of a second [^{14}C]-radiolabeled internal standard [14]. Sensitive, reliable and reproducible analytical methods are clearly essential to any study, and previous reports including little or no information on these points should be interpreted with caution and not used as 'pivotal' or key studies.

It has been suggested that the plasma levels of the intraneuronally formed dihydroxy metabolite of norepinephrine, dihydroxyphenylethylene glycol, might provide a better index for overall sympathetic activity than norepinephrine itself [15,16]. While plasma dihydroxyphenylethylene glycol may be helpful in the diagnosis of pheochromocytoma [15], it does not appear to offer any advantages over plasma norepinephrine and indeed might be misleading in some circumstances [17].

The use of urinary catecholamine measurement is discussed below. In general, urinary free catecholamines make up only a small and variable proportion of the total catecholamines released. Unless an elaborate, balanced study is undertaken, with quantitative assay of several methoxy derivatives, deaminated compounds and their conjugates, it is unlikely that reliable and readily interpretable results will be obtained.

Implications of Epidemiologic Studies for Large-Scale Trials
Studies in the 1970s which appeared to show substantial increases in plasma norepinephrine in hypertensives were generally undertaken in small groups of selected patients [2,18]. The importance of the choice of control reference group was highlighted by studies showing that normotensive *patients* differed from normotensive laboratory staff but not from hypertensive patients [19], and revealing an independent effect of age on plasma norepinephrine [20]. Goldstein, in his classic reviews in 1981 and 1983, pointed up the lack of information about controls and the paucity of analytical details [21,22]. However, from a compilation of 70 published studies including over 1500 patients, he reported a small but significant increase in plasma norepinephrine in young hypertensives under 40 years compared to age-matched controls [22].

A study of Dutch adolescents lent support to the view that plasma norepinephrine is raised in young people with mild hypertension and/or a family history of hypertension [23]; this was a well-designed attempt to study a defined population and to avoid selection bias in either hypertensive or control groups. A later study of a population under controlled circumstances did not lead to such clear conclusions.

Brown *et al* examined urinary norepinephrine and epinephrine in an untreated cohort of participants in the Medical Research Council of Great Britain (MRC) trial of mild hypertension [24]. They found no difference between hypertensives and normotensives in excretion of either amine. However, few of the subjects were under 40 years (age range, 35–65), and the limitations of urinary catecholamine measurement have already been mentioned. In addition to failing to provide evidence for a role of the sympathetic nervous system in essential hypertension, this study also failed to provide support for the 'epinephrine hypothesis' [25], that the increase in epinephrine release from the adrenal medulla, via an action on a putative prejunctional facilitatory beta-receptor, was a trigger to increase sympathetic activity in early hypertension [25,26]. As the MRC trial found no differences in epinephrine excretion between 'hypertensives' and 'controls' [24], it is unlikely that epinephrine from the adrenal medulla is the link between the sympathetic nervous system and essential hypertension.

If any further useful information is to be obtained in this area (and the limitations of plasma or urine catecholamine measurements must be borne in mind), large-scale, defined populations should be examined. A longitudinal component with adequate controls would be a further advantage.

Non-Adrenergic Sympathetic Transmitters and Co-Transmitters

In recent years, it has been recognized not only that other transmitters may be co-localized and co-released with norepinephrine at sympathetic nerve endings [27], but that there are many non-adrenergic sympathetic nerves to the heart and blood vessels [28]. Established methods for their study explain the previous preoccupation with catecholamines; however, non-adrenergic sympathetic mechanisms must now be considered as an alternative explanation for the contribution of sympathetic tone to blood-pressure control in hypertension.

Neuropeptide Y is a 32-amino acid peptide which has been co-localized in noradrenergic neurons of the periphery and the brain. It has only a modest pressor action in its own right, but it potentiates the effects of other pressor stimuli, including norepinephrine [29]. This peptide's role in circulatory regulation remains to be determined.

The purines adenosine and ATP have been proposed as neurotransmitters in non-adrenergic nerves, and are also thought to be co-localized and released from sympathetic nerve terminals in peripheral tissues, including blood vessels [28,30]. Specific receptors for both adenosine and ATP have been identified, which appear to be located pre- and post-junctionally, respectively. Relatively selective agonists and antagonists for these receptors have been described. ATP has been proposed to have a pressor role and to be responsible for the prazosin-resistant phasic contractions and excitatory-junctional potentials induced by sympathetic nerve stimulation of vascular preparations [28,30].

467

Although not part of the sympathetic nervous system, atrial natriuretic factor is proving to have an interesting role in the control of blood pressure and plasma volume. It comprises a series of peptides, which are stored in granules within cells of the atria; release occurs in response to stretching of the atrial wall. Atrial natriuretic factor causes potent natriuresis and diuresis, relaxes smooth muscle, inhibits the release of aldosterone and modifies the release of vasopressin. There is still controversy regarding the levels of circulating atrial natriuretic factor in human essential hypertension. Current knowledge of atrial natriuretic factor has recently been reviewed [31,32].

Characterization of the interactions between purines, catecholamines and peptide transmitters and modulators at the vascular neuroeffector junction should present an exciting challenge over the next few years.

Conclusions

The sympathetic nervous system is undoubtedly a major factor in the short-term regulation of blood pressure; it can probably modify blood pressure in the long term also. It is, however, increasingly unlikely that a global increase in sympathetic nervous activity is an important factor in the causation or maintenance of human essential hypertension, although there are pointers that sympathetic tone may be inappropriately increased in young, genetically predisposed hypertensives. Disturbances of autonomic-activity regulation may well interact with other humoral/ionic/membrane effects to initiate the increase in blood pressure.

References

[1] Pickering GW.
The Nature of Essential Hypertension. Edinburgh: J&A Churchill, 1961.

[2] de Champlain J, Cousineau D, Lapointe L.
Evidence supporting an increased sympathetic tone and reactivity in a subgroup of patients with essential hypertension.
Clin Exp Hypertens 1980; 2: 359-67.

[3] Keeton TK, Campbell WB.
The pharmacodynamic alteration of renin release.
Pharmacol Rev 1980; 31: 81-227.

[4] Zimmerman BG, Sybertz EJ, Wong PC.
Interaction between sympathetic and renin-angiotensin system.
J Hypertens 1984; 2: 581-7.

[5] Lake CR, Ziegler MG, Kopin IJ.
Use of plasma norepinephrine for evaluation of sympathetic neuronal function in man.
Life Sci 1976; 18: 1315-26.

[6] Folkow B, Dibona GF, Hjelmdahl P, Thoren PH, Wallin BG.
Measurement of plasma norepinephrine concentrations in human primary hypertension: A word of caution on their applicability for assessing neurogenic contributions.
Hypertension 1983; 5: 399-403.

[7] Wallin BG.
Muscle sympathetic activity and plasma concentrations of noradrenaline.
Acta Physiol Scand 1984; Suppl 527: 21-9.

[8] Morlin C, Wallin BG, Eriksson BM.
Muscle sympathetic activity and plasma noradrenaline in normotensive and hypertensive man.
Acta Physiol Scand 1983; 119: 117-21.

[9] Esler M, Jackman G, Bobik A et al.
Determination of norepinephrine apparent release rate and clearance in humans.
Life Sci 1979; 25: 1461-70.

[10] Esler M, Jackman G, Bobik A et al.
Norepinephrine kinetics in essential hypertension: Defective neuronal uptake in some patients.
Hypertension 1981; 3: 149-56.

[11] Esler M, Jennings G, Leonard P et al.
Contribution of individual organs to total noradrenaline release in humans.
Acta Physiol Scand 1984; Suppl 527: 11-26.

[12] Howes LG, MacGilchrist A, Hawksby C, Sumner D, Reid JL.
An improved approach for the determination of plasma [³H]noradrenaline kinetics using high performance liquid chromatography.
Clin Sci 1986; **71**: 211-5.

[13] Hjelmdahl P.
Inter-laboratory comparison of plasma catecholamine determination using several different assays.
Acta Physiol Scand 1984; Suppl 527: 43-54.

[14] Brown MJ, Jenner DA.
A novel double isotope technique for the enzymatic assay of plasma catecholamines permitting high precision, sensitivity and single capacity.
Clin Sci 1981; **61**: 591-8.

[15] Brown MJ.
Simultaneous assay of noradrenaline and its deaminated metabolite dihydroxyphenylglycol in plasma.
Eur J Clin Invest 1984; **14**: 67-72.

[16] Howes LG, Miller S, Reid JL.
Simultaneous assay of 3,4-dihydroxyphenylethylene glycol and norepinephrine in human plasma by high performance liquid chromatography with electrochemical detection.
J Chromatogr 1985; **228**: 401-3.

[17] Howes LG, Hawksby CC, Reid JL.
Comparison of plasma 3,4-dihydroxyphenylethylene glycol (DHPG) and norepinephrine levels as indices of sympathetic activity in man.
Eur J Clin Invest 1986; **16**: 18-21.

[18] Engelman K, Portnoy B, Sjoerdsma A.
Plasma catecholamine concentrations in patients with essential hypertension.
Circ Res 1970; **27** (Suppl 1): 405-11.

[19] Jones DH, Hamilton CA, Reid JL.
Choice of control groups in the appraisal of sympathetic nervous activity in essential hypertension.
Clin Sci 1979; **57**: 339-44.

[20] Lake CR, Zeigler MG, Coleman MD, Kopin IJ.
Age adjusted plasma norepinephrine levels are similar in normotensives and hypertensive subjects.
N Engl J Med 1977; **296**: 208-9.

[21] Goldstein DS.
Plasma norepinephrine in essential hypertension: A study of the studies.
Hypertension 1981; **3**: 48-52.

[22] Goldstein DS.
Plasma catecholamines and essential hypertension: An analytical review.
Hypertension 1983; **5**: 86-9.

[23] Hofman A, Boomsma F, Schalekamp MADH, Valkenburg HA.
Raised blood pressure and plasma noradrenaline concentrations in teenagers and young adults selected from an open population.
Br Med J 1979; **i**: 1536-8.

[24] Brown MJ, Causon RC, Barnes VF, Brennan P, Barnes G, Greenberg G.
Urinary catecholamines in essential hypertension.
Q J Med 1985; **57**: 637-52.

[25] Majewski H, Tung LH, Rand MJ.
Adrenaline induced hypertension in rats.
J Cardiovasc Pharmacol 1981; **3**: 179-85.

[26] Brown MJ, Macquin I.
Is adrenaline the cause of essential hypertension?
Lancet 1981; **ii**: 1079-82.

[27] Lundberg L, Hokfelt T.
Coexistence of peptides and classical neurotransmitters.
Trends Neurosci 1983; **6**: 325-33.

[28] Burnstock G, Sneddon P.
Evidence for ATP and noradrenaline as cotransmitters in sympathetic nerves.
Clin Sci 1985; **68** (Suppl 10): 89-92.

[29] Lundberg JM, Savia A, Anggard A, Hokfelt T, Terenius L.
Neuropeptide Y and noradrenaline interaction in peripheral cardiovascular control.
Clin Exp Hypertens 1984; **A6**: 1961-72.

[30] Sneddon P, Burnstock G.
ATP as a cotransmitter in rat tail artery.
Eur J Pharmacol 1985; **106**: 149--52.

[31] Thibault G, Garcia R, Gutkowska J, Genest J, Cantin M.
Atrial natiuretic factor: A newly discovered hormone with significant clinical implications.
Drugs 1986; **31**: 369-75.

[32] Palluk R, Gaida W, Hoefke W.
Minireview: Atrial natriuretic factor.
Life Sci 1985; **36**: 1415-25.

THE TREATMENT OF MILD HYPERTENSION

Review: PETER SLEIGHT

Recent years have been very important for all those concerned with the treatment of mild hypertension, with the publication of the UK Medical Research Council (MRC) trial of mild hypertension [1], the Swiss-based International Prospective Primary Prevention Study of Hypertension (IPPPSH) [2], and the report of the European Working Party on High Blood Pressure in the Elderly (EWPHE) [3]. Results of another trial comparing beta-blockade and diuretic treatment, the Heart Attack Primary Prevention in Hypertension trial (HAPPHY), were presented in September 1986 at the International Society of Hypertension (ISH) meeting in Heidelberg [4]. An updated version of the WHO/ISH guidelines for the treatment of mild hypertension has recently been published [5].

The Trials

Definition of 'Mild Hypertension'
Despite the very good epidemiologic data showing that systolic pressure is as good as, if not better than, diastolic pressure in determining future risk for cardiovascular disease, most of the major trials base their classification of hypertension on diastolic pressure. Mild hypertension is generally defined as a diastolic pressure of between 90 and 109 mmHg, but this disguises a number of differences in screening methods and patient selection. Such a definition also tends to throw together subjects with great differences in prognosis based on sex, age, diabetes, cholesterol levels and ECG, and subjects with initial signs of target-organ damage are excluded from some trials. It is also clear that when diastolic pressures of 100–104 mmHg are compared with those of 105–109 mmHg there is a steep increase in risk, so that the overall small benefit from treatment seen in the MRC trial disguises a much greater benefit in higher-risk subgroups.

The very large multicenter studies have produced results that are at first sight a little disappointing, since they have (not surprisingly) yielded very little new information. Furthermore, trial treatment is generally out of date because of the inevitable delays inherent in the design, recruitment and execution of such large studies. The MRC trial, comprising about 18 000 patients treated for 5 years, confirmed that stroke could be reduced, but only at considerable cost not only in terms of drug expenses but also of side-effects for the vast majority of participants who would not have had any complications from their mild hypertension. Overall, the MRC trial showed that about 850 patients needed to be treated for one year to save one stroke.

Perhaps the most important lesson to be learned from these studies is that the prognosis of mild hypertension is very good indeed, and any proposed new treatment has to involve few or no drug-related deaths.

Treatment of 'Mild Hypertension'
The MRC and, to a lesser extent, the IPPPSH trials compared beta-blockade with diuretic treatment. Because of their 'protection' against sudden death and reinfarction

after myocardial infarction (which was seen in the Norwegian and US trials of long-term treatment with these agents after infarction), beta-blockers were previously thought to be preferable to diuretics, which lower serum potassium and perhaps even increase the risk of arrhythmia and sudden death. Diuretics were perhaps more effective overall than propranolol in the MRC trial, particularly for women, in whom they appeared slightly more effective in lowering blood pressure and in preventing stroke [1]. In non-smoking men, propranolol had a significantly better effect than the diuretic. It has been postulated that results might have been better still with cardioselective beta-blockade, using more modern drugs such as atenolol or metoprolol. There also appeared to be fewer coronary events in men on beta-blockade.

These results need to be viewed with caution, however, as the subgroup analyses were not prospective. Data-dredging increases the possibility that a chance difference will be observed. Nevertheless, the IPPPSH trial results support the superiority of beta-blocking agents in the treatment of mild hypertension in non-smoking men [2]. It has been argued that the lack of such a benefit in smoking men is due to the fact that smoking raises blood pressure by stimulation of the sympathetic nervous system, with release of norepinephrine and epinephrine, and that the rise in blood pressure in this setting will be less well controlled by non-selective (β_1 plus β_2) compared with cardioselective (β_1) beta-blockade because of blockade of the β_2-mediated vasodilatation. Thus, catechol-induced alpha-mediated vasoconstriction will predominate in the presence of non-selective drugs, propranolol (MRC) and oxprenolol (IPPPSH). It therefore remained unproven whether more modern treatment with cardioselective agents, such as atenolol or metoprolol, might have been more effective than diuretic treatment in both smoking and non-smoking subjects with hypertension, until reports of the HAPPHY trial were published [4].

The HAPPHY trial randomized 6569 patients with a diastolic blood pressure of between 100 and 130 mmHg, to receive either a diuretic (bendrofluazide 5 mg/day or hydrochlorothiazide 50 mg/day) or a cardioselective beta-blocker (atenolol 100 mg/day or metoprolol 100 mg twice daily) as first-line treatment [4]. Additional treatment, if necessary, was with hydralazine or spironolactone. Significantly more patients withdrew from diuretic treatment. There were 83 deaths in the diuretic group and 77 in the beta-blocker group (not significant). There were significantly more strokes in the diuretic group ($n = 10$) than in the beta-blocker group ($n = 2$).

This trial supported the tentative explanation for the smoker/non-smoker differences outlined above. With these cardioselective beta-blockers, there was *no* evidence that beta-blockade was inferior to diuretics in smokers. In non-smokers, there were 51 deaths in the diuretic group and 55 in the beta-blocker group; in smokers, the figures were 140 and 121, respectively. There were 4234 non-smokers and 2263 smokers, confirming a two- to threefold increase in risk for smokers. There was no evidence for 'cardioprotection' in the group given beta-blockade.

Implications of the Trials
A disappointing feature of many of the hypertension trials is that it has been easy to demonstrate a reduction in cerebrovascular accidents, but not in coronary events. Pooling of results of all available trials does suggest that coronary events are reduced by about 20% after two years of antihypertensive treatment [6]; it may be that the trials

are of inadequate size and length to show a decisive influence on such a chronic process.

The results of the placebo-controlled EWPHE trial were a striking exception [3]: it *did* show a 38% reduction in mortality from cardiovascular disease by active treatment (hydrochlorothiazide plus triamterene, with methyldopa added if necessary). This trial was conducted in patients over the age of 60 years. It was somewhat of a marathon effort — taking about 12 years to recruit 840 patients from many different hospitals and clinics. The low recruitment rate from any individual center has raised doubts about the general applicability of the results to elderly hypertensive patients. Nevertheless, two crucial points should be noted: first, the length of treatment — an average of 4.7 years; second, the fall in blood pressure achieved was greater than in the other trials (~20 mmHg systolic and >5 mmHg diastolic). These two factors may have led to the trial's unusually positive findings for cardiac deaths (reduced by 47%). Surprisingly, stroke was reduced by 43% (not significant), and 'study-terminating events' were reduced by 60%. Once again, however, the overall mortality reduction (9%) was not significant [3].

An important message from these trials is that we should be very much more reluctant to begin treatment in women, because they tolerate mild hypertension so well and experience a high dropout rate from side-effects (particularly from cold extremities when on beta-blockade [1]).

The role of smoking and the value of its elimination is more clear. It should be discouraged in all patients, particularly in those with hypertension. The benefits of giving up smoking far outweigh any effect of drugs in reducing mortality and morbidity.

The financial cost of saving one life in these trials of mild hypertension is considerable — of the order of tens of thousands of dollars for each death avoided — a fact which focuses attention on the non-drug treatment of mild hypertension. Other non-drug treatment could include increased physical exercise, weight reduction, a reduction in alcohol intake and dietary saturated fat, and perhaps a trial of salt restriction. This approach becomes even more attractive when the side-effects and reduction in the quality of life caused by drug treatment are taken into account.

The recent emphasis on 'quality of life' comparisons —which particularly favor the angiotensin-converting enzyme inhibitors [7] — is important but not all-important. Most mildly hypertensive subjects feel well; indeed, there is some evidence that they feel even better than normal subjects [8]. Treatment is therefore usually instigated with a view to a reduction in morbidity or mortality. There is little doubt that angiotensin-converting enzyme inhibition lowers pressure with fewer side-effects than beta-blockade or diuretic treatment [6], but it is, perhaps, too early to recommend these agents preferentially as first-line treatment unless there is some contraindication to beta-blockers, diuretics or calcium-blocking agents — a not uncommon occurrence — or if side-effects with the more traditional agents impair the patient's quality of life.

Individual Treatment

The difficulty in conducting trials and in mustering sufficient numbers to spot small but worthwhile effects means that the number of agents tested rigorously in trials is limited. Clinical reality entails a much wider choice of agents. Instead of relying on the rather old-fashioned concept of rigid, stepped care, factors such as gender, age, race and certain disorders can provide important guides to the ideal treatment regimen. Several salient considerations follow.

Gender

Female patients tolerate beta-blockers less well than males [1], and I would therefore generally begin with a diuretic. In the MRC trial, male patients experienced a fivefold greater incidence of impotence on diuretics [1], so I start men on a cardioselective beta-blocker — usually atenolol (50 mg, increasing the dose to 100 mg if necessary). If the first drug is ineffective for either men or women, I change to the alternative, and use both together only if necessary. If a beta-blocker alone is not sufficiently effective, then the addition of the retard preparation form of nifedipine often provides a more satisfactory combination than a diuretic, particularly in counteracting the cold extremities often seen with beta-blockade [1].

Age

Beta-blockade is less effective in older patients [9]. Diuretics are preferable as first-line agents. Thiazides are inexpensive and effective; potassium-sparing diuretics such as amiloride may be helpful. Indapamide is a newer alternative, with some claim to vasodilator properties [10]. Beta-blockers may be helpful in combination with any of these agents.

Race

Blacks respond better than whites to diuretics [11], as they often have low-renin hypertension [12]. Calcium-channel blockers are another alternative.

Peripheral Vascular Disease

Calcium-channel blockade or vasodilatation with prazosin is often useful when peripheral vascular disease is present.

Angina

Beta-blockade or, if this is contraindicated, verapamil or diltiazem, should be used before diuretics in patients with angina pectoris. If verapamil is used as monotherapy, the dose may be raised to 120 mg every eight hours. At this dose, constipation may be a problem, and this effect should be counteracted by increasing the amount of fiber in the diet. Beta-blockade plus a calcium-channel blocker (nifedipine or nicardipine) is an attractive combination. Beta-blockade plus verapamil should be used with caution because of the risk of heart block or heart failure [13].

Diabetes

The use of thiazide diuretics should be avoided in diabetic patients. The recent trials have largely exonerated these drugs from short-term risk [1–4]. Nevertheless, there remain long-term risks associated with metabolic effects.

Obstructive Airways Disease

Beta-blockade is contraindicated in patients with obstructive airways disease. Diuretics and/or calcium-channel agents are preferable. If these are unsuccessful, angiotensin converting enzyme inhibitors, of which captopril is the best-established agent, may be useful. Angiotensin converting enzyme inhibition alone controls pressure in perhaps one-third to one-half of patients [14]; if monotherapy is not fully effective, a thiazide diuretic is a natural and effective second agent. Nifedipine or nicardipine are also well tolerated.

Conclusions

Results of recent trials of treatment of mild hypertension have underscored the need for caution with respect to the initiation of drug therapy. Changes in diet, smoking, exercise and lifestyle should be emphasized first. This requires a team effort involving general practitioners, nutritionists, paramedical personnel and public education. Drug treatment, despite the implementation of non-pharmacologic measures, is indicated generally only when pressures remain above 160/100 mmHg.

References

[1] Medical Research Council Working Party. MRC trial of treatment of mild hypertension: Principal results.
Br Med J 1985; **291**: 97–104.

[2] The IPPPSH Collaborative Group.
Cardiovascular risk and risk factors in a randomized trial of treatment based on the beta-blocker oxprenolol: The International Prospective Primary Prevention Study in Hypertension (IPPPSH).
J Hypertens 1985; **3**: 379–92.

[3] Amery A, Birkenhager W, Brixko P *et al.*
Mortality and morbidity result from the European Working Party on high blood pressure in the elderly trial.
Lancet 1985; i: 1349–54.

[4] Wilhemsen L, for the HAPPHY trial research group.
Beta-blockers versus saluretics in hypertension – results of the HAPPHY trial. In: *Proceedings of the 11th Scientific Meeting of the International Society of Hypertension* 1986; p. 398.

[5] World Health Organization and the International Society of Hypertension.
Guidelines for the treatment of mild hypertension.
J Hypertens 1986; **4**: 383–6.

[6] Collins R, Peto R.
Unpublished findings.

[7] Croog SH, Levine S, Testa MA *et al.*
The effects of anti-hypertensive therapy on the quality of life.
N Engl J Med 1986; **314**: 1657–64.

[8] Robinson JO.
Symptoms and the discovery of high blood pressure.
J Psychosom Res 1969; **13**: 157–61.

[9] Buhler FR, Burkhart F, Lutold BE, Kung M, Marbert G, Pfisterer M.
Antihypertensive betablocking action as related to renin and age.
Am J Cardiol 1975; **36**: 653–9.

[10] Burgess CD, McKee CEL, Wilson CA, Warren DJ.
The effect of indapamide on muscle blood flow in hypertensive patients.
Postgrad Med J 1981; **57** (Suppl 2): 23.

[11] Weber MA, Priest RT, Ricci MS, Ettorai MI, Brewer DD.
Low dose diuretic and beta adrenoceptor blocker in essential hypertension.
Clin Pharmacol Ther 1980; **28**: 149–58.

[12] Holland OB, Gomez-Sanchez C, Fairchild C, Kaplan NM.
Role of renin classification for diuretic treatment of black hypertensive patients.
Arch Intern Med 1979; **139**: 1365–70.

[13] Seabia-Gomes R, Richards A, Sutton R.
Hemodynamic effects of verapamil and practolol.
Eur J Cardiol 1976; **4**: 79.

[14] Stumpe KO, Overlack A, Kolloch R, Schreyer S.
Long term efficacy of angiotensin converting enzyme inhibition with captopril in mild to moderate hypertension.
Br J Clin Pharmacol 1982; **14**: 121S–6S.

ANGIOTENSIN CONVERTING ENZYME INHIBITORS IN HYPERTENSION: RECENT DEVELOPMENTS

Review: MAARTEN A.D.H. SCHALEKAMP

Angiotensin converting enzyme (ACE) inhibitors have been used in clinical practice since 1975, and there is now little doubt that they provide a valuable addition to the list of antihypertensive drugs. As with any relatively new drug, it is important to clarify their position with respect to alternative treatments; and since many hypotensive patients are treated concomitantly for other diseases, possible drug interactions must be considered. Because of the complex actions of ACE, the precise mechanism of the hypotensive effect of ACE inhibitors is still a matter of some debate. ACE is necessary for the conversion of angiotensin I to angiotensin II, the biologically active end-product of the renin–angiotensin system. Angiotensin II is formed in the circulation as well as in the tissues, and there is growing evidence for the presence of a complete renin–angiotensin system in certain cells, which may serve important physiological functions. ACE inhibitors may lower blood pressure not only by lowering the concentration of angiotensin II in the blood, but also by inhibiting angiotensin II formation in certain tissues, particularly blood vessels, the kidneys and brain. ACE is also involved in the degradation of bradykinin, a peptide with potent hypotensive actions. Local accumulation of this peptide may contribute to the hypotensive effect of ACE inhibitors.

The Place of ACE Inhibitors in the Management of Hypertension

ACE Inhibitors and Plasma Renin

Initially, it was thought that the ACE inhibitors would be particularly effective in hypertension associated with high circulating renin levels, such as in renovascular hypertension and accelerated or malignant hypertension. However, a positive correlation between the pretreatment plasma level of renin and the fall in blood pressure after treatment has not been uniformaly observed. Most authors agree that the decrease in arterial pressure and peripheral vascular resistance following acute ACE inhibition is greater when plasma renin is high than when it is normal or low, but this correlation is rather weak [1,2]. Furthermore, several studies of chronic ACE inhibition have shown no correlation at all [3,4]. Measurement of plasma renin is therefore of little value as a guideline for selecting patients for treatment with ACE inhibitors. Many patients with mild and moderate uncomplicated essential hypertension and normal or even low plasma renin respond well to these agents.

Angiotensin II influences tubular reabsorption both directly and by an aldosterone-dependent mechanism. It has a biphasic action on proximal tubular sodium reabsorption; at low doses it increases reabsorption, but at high doses it causes natriuresis. In careful balance studies, ACE inhibition has been shown to have a weak natriuretic effect, which may contribute to the antihypertensive action of these drugs [5].

Renovascular Hypertension

Angiotension II has a range of actions on the kidney. It acts on the renal vasculature both by systemic delivery and probably also by local formation causing contraction of the afferent and efferent glomerular arterioles. It is probably by being more potent on the efferent arteriole that it is involved in the maintenance of glomerular capillary pressure and thereby glomerular filtration, when renal perfusion pressure and flow are decreased, for instance, in the case of renal artery stenosis or severe sodium depletion. Under these conditions, the glomerular filtration rate may fall after ACE inhibition. In patients with bilateral renal artery stenosis and in cases with unilateral stenosis, in whom only the kidney with the stenosis is functioning, ACE inhibition may induce overt renal failure [6,8]. This will not occur in unilateral stenosis when the contralateral kindey is unaffected, because the unaffected kidney can compensate for the loss of function on the affected side. Isotope renography has shown that, if treatment is discontinued within two months, the return glomerular filtration rate returns to pre-treatment levels. It is possible, however, that long-term impairment of renal function will lead to irreversible damage. It would seem to be a wise precaution in this situation to perform renography in the first weeks of treatment [9].

Hypertension in the Elderly
In essential hypertension, the two most widely used ACE inhibitors, captopril and enalapril, reduce blood pressure without serious side-effects, such as postural hypotension, cerebral ischemia, deteriorating renal function or mental change. There-fore, they must be seriously considered for long-term treatment of elderly hyperten-sives. In a study of a large group of patients 65 years or older, of whom almost half received captopril for at least one year, a significant reduction in both systolic and diastolic blood pressure was achieved [10]. Side-effects were infrequent and renal function was undisturbed in the majority of patients. There was no increase in hypoten-sive periods and, although some antihypertensive drugs are associated with mood depression and psychological impairment, this does not seem to be the case with captopril and enalapril.

Studies in spontaneously hypertensive rats and in normotensive control rats have shown that, during captopril-induced hypotension, cerebral blood flow is maintained at its resting level. This contrasts with the expected decrease in cerebral blood flow following hemorrhagic hypotension [11] and suggests that autoregulation of cerebral blood flow was maintained at a lower level of blood pressure. Observations in patients with severe cardiac failure and in normotensive young volunteers also indicate that ACE inhibitors lower the limit of autoregulation [12]. Such a mechanism may explain why hypotensive symptoms have rarely occurred during ACE inhibitor treatment in patients with congestive heart failure, despite a rapid, and sometimes very pronounced, fall of blood pressure. It has been speculated that the beneficial effect of ACE inhibition on cerebral blood flow autoregulation can be attributed to these agents choosing the blood–brain barrier. However, blood–brain barrier permeability for these agents is minimal and, furthermore, inhibition of the brain renin–angiotensin system appears to have no effect on global cerebral blood flow [13]. The effect of ACE inhibitors on cerebral blood flow autoregulation can probably be explained by the inhibition of ACE on the luminal surface of the cerebral vessels.

Diabetes
The prevalence of hypertension is higher in patients with diabetes mellitus, particularly non-insulin-dependent disease, than in age-matched controls. In insulin-dependent

diabetes, the occurrence of hypertension appears to be associated with the development of nephropathy detectable by the presence of small quantities of protein in the urine (microalbuminuria) [14,15]. In non-insulin-dependent diabetes, hypertension frequently occurs when there are no signs of nephropathy. The pathogenesis of diabetic nephropathy is still obscure but there may be a stage of hyperfiltration and microalbuminuria before the development of gross nephropathy. It has been postulated that hyperfiltration in this early stage is responsible for glomerular damage, which eventually leads to diabetic glomerulosclerosis [16].

Decrease in glomerular blood flow and glomerular capillary pressure by ACE inhibition may favorably influence the progression of diabetic nephropathy. Studies in patients with early diabetic nephropathy have indeed provided evidence for such an effect [17,18]. ACE inhibitors may also have a protective role in the development of progressive renal failure associated with hyperfiltration of the remaining glomeruli in pathological states other than diabetes mellitus. ACE inhibitors may lower intraglomerular capillary pressure and flow by removing the vasoconstrictor effect of angiotensin II on the efferent glomerular arteriole. ACE inhibitors appear to slow the progression of experimental renal disease [19].

Although experience is still limited, ACE inhibitors appear to have no adverse effects on metabolic control either in insulin-treated or non-insulin-treated diabetic patients [20,21].

Quality Of Life
The most comprehensive study on the effect of antihypertensive therapy on the quality of life compared the effects of monotherapy with standard doses of either captopril, methyldopa or propranolol [22]. Of 626 white patients with mild-to-moderate hypertension who took part in the study, 486 were followed for 24 weeks of active treatment. If blood pressure control was unsatisfactory after eight weeks, hydrochlorothiazide was added as a secondary therapy. Quality of life was assessed at baseline and after 24 weeks using scales relating to general well-being, physical symptoms, sleep dysfunction, sexual function, work performance satisfaction and cognitive function. With regard to general well-being, physical symptoms, sexual function, work performance and satisfaction with life, scores of the captopril group were better than those of the methyldopa group. Scores in the captopril group were also better than those of the propanolol group for general well-being, physical symptoms and sexual functioning. Patients receiving captopril were least likely to withdraw from treatment because of adverse effects. In a less comprehensive study, it was found that the complaint rate was higher with methyldopa than with captopril [23]. A small pilot study comparing enalapril and atenolol suggested that atenolol, but not enalapril, may be associated with mild memory impairment [24].

Interactions with Other Drugs
Some important drug interactions with the ACE inhibitors have been identified, the most important being those with thiazide and loop diuretics. Reactive hyper-reninemia following diuretic therapy may limit their antihypertensive effect. ACE inhibition would reduce the effect of this hyper-reninemia, and this could explain the well-established potentiating hypotensive effect of combining diuretics with ACE inhibitors.

The response rate of hypertensive patients to ACE inhibitors has been reported to be increased from under 60% to over 80% by the addition of a diuretic or the introduction of a low-salt diet. Whether this results from rendering the hypertension more renin dependent is not known. Although the increased response to ACE inhibitors when combined with a diuretic is usually advantageous, it may have an adverse effect, particularly in salt-depleted subjects who sometimes respond with serious hypotension. Therefore, care should be taken in patients who have received intensive diuretic treatment prior to the administration of an ACE inhibitor.

ACE inhibitors prevent the occurrence of secondary hyperaldosteronism and the resultant hypokalemia produced by diuretic therapy. Patients on a combined ACE inhibitor–diuretic treatment usually do not require potassium supplementation. This is particularly important in patients receiving digitalis for congestive heart failure. Because ACE inhibitors lower the secretion rate and plasma concentration of aldosterone, combination with potassium-sparing diuretics, such as spironolactone and amiloride, may lead to hyperkalemia, particularly when renal function is compromised. This danger should be bourne in mind. Futhermore, caution should be exercised when ACE inhibitors are given together with potassium supplements in hypokalemic patients with impaired renal function.

Both captopril and enalapril have been reported to blunt the hyperuricemic and hyperglycemic effects of thiazide diuretics [25,26]. It is theoretically possible that ACE inhibitors potentiate the natriuretic and diuretic effects of thiazides and loop diuretics. ACE inhibitors may convert a patient with congestive heart failure who is diuretic resistant into one who responds with marked natriuresis and diuresis with clinical improvement. A detailed account of such an effect in a well-controlled study is still lacking.

Theoretically, ACE inhibitors could interfere with adrenergic transmission and baroreflex function, because angiotensin II is known to facilitate adrenergic transmission. In practice, ACE inhibitors can safely be combined with alpha$_1$-, beta$_1$-, and beta$_2$-blocking agents. ACE inhibitors seem to have a small additional antihypertensive effect when given to patients on a beta-blocker [27] and beta-blockers are useful in the occasional patient who develops tachycardia when treated with combined ACE inhibitor–diuretic treatment.

Because ACE inhibitors block the rise of renin in response to vasodilators, such as nitroprusside, minoxidil and hydralazine, they can potentiate the hypotensive effect of vasodilator drugs. They have also been reported to potentiate the hypotensive effect of the calcium-entry blocker, nifedipine [28].

The prostaglandins may be involved in the hypotensive effect of ACE inhibitors, particularly in patients with low plasma renin. Indomethacin and other non-steroidal anti-inflammatory drugs with similar actions on prostaglandin production probably blunt the hypotensive effect of ACE inhibitors, while ACE inhibitors may prevent the fluid retention in response to non-steroidal anti-inflammatory drugs.

Possible Future Developments
Although the exact place of ACE inhibitors in relation to other antihypertensive drugs is still not clear, captopril and enalapril are now widely used in so-called refractory hypertension and as a first-choice drug. It is clear that, in mild hypertension, treatment

is justified only if it can be demonstrated that adverse effects on the quality of life are minimal. Research into the effects of antihypertensive drugs aspects such as memory function and alertness are still at an early stage. ACE inhibitors, and in particular captopril, were among the first drugs that have been systematically subjected to quality-of-life research, and thus far they have fared well. This confirms the clinical impression of high patient acceptability. However, their possible psychological advantages have still to be carefully compared with other new classes of drugs, such as the calcium-entry blockers.

If it is true that part of the antihypertensive effect of ACE inhibitors depends on their action on the renin–angiotensin system in tissues rather than in the circulation, it might be of interest to compare ACE inhibitors that penetrate the tissues and cells easily with those that do not. It will also be of interest to compare the effects of ACE inhibitors with those of renin inhibitors, which may become available for clinical use in the near future. Finally, it is still a matter of debate as to whether there are several forms of ACE which differ in enzyme kinetic properties and substrate specificity. If this is so, it could be the basis for developing ACE inhibitors with different therapeutic profiles.

References

[1] Atkinson AB, Robertson JIS.
Captopril in the treatment of clinical hypertension and cardiac failure.
Lancet 1979; ii: 836–9.

[2] Heel RC, Brogden RN, Speight TM, Avery GS.
Captopril. A preliminary review of its pharmacological properties and therapeutic efficacy.
Drugs 1980; **20**: 409–52.

[3] Gavras H, Brunner HR, Turini GA *et al.*
Antihypertensive effect of the oral converting enzyme inhibitor SQ 14225 in man.
N Engl J Med 1978; **298**: 991–5.

[4] Wenting GJ, De Bruyn JHB, Man in't Veld AJ, Woittiez AJJ, Derkx FHM, Schalekamp MADH.
Hemodynamic effects of captopril in essential hypertension, renovascular hypertension and cardiac failure. Correlations of short-term and long-term effects with plasma renin.
Am J Cardiol 1982; **49**: 1453–9.

[5] De Zeeuw D, Navis GJ, Donker AJM, De Jong P.
The angiotensin converting inhibitor enalapril and its effects on renal function.
J Hypertens 1983; **1** (Suppl 1): 93–7.

[6] Curtis JJ, Luke RG, Whelchel JD, Diethelm AG, Jones P, Dustan HP.
Inhibition of angiotensin-converting enzyme in renal transplant recipients with hypertension.
N Engl J Med 1983; **308**: 377–81.

[7] Hricik DE, Browning PJ, Kopelman R, Goorno WE, Madia NE, Dzau VJ.
Captopril-induced functional renal insufficiency in patients with bilateral renal-artery stenosis or renal-artery stenosis in a solitary kidney.
N Engl J Med 1983; **308**: 373–6.

[8] Silas JH, Klenka Z, Solomon SA, Bone JM.
Captopril-induced reversible renal failure: a marker of renal artery stenosis affecting a solitary kidney.
Br Med J 1983; **286**: 1702–3.

[9] Wenting GJ, Tan-Tjiong HL, Derkx FHM, De Bruyn JHB, Man in 't Veld AJ, Schalekamp MADH.
Split renal function after captopril in unilateral renal artery stenosis.
Br Med J 1984; **288**: 886–90.

[10] Jenkins AC, Knill JR, Dreslinski GR.
Captopril in the treatment of the elderly patient.
Arch Intern Med 1985; **145**: 2029–31.

[11] Barry DI, Jarden JO, Paulson OB, Graham DI, Strandgaard S.
Cerebrovascular aspects of convering enzyme inhibition, I. Effects of intravenous captopril in spontaneously hypertensive and normotensive rats.
J Hypertens 1984; **2**: 589–97.

[12] Paulson OB, Vorstrup S, Andersen AR, Smith J, Godtfredsen J.
Converting enzyme inhibition resets cerebral autoregulation at lower blood pressure.
J Hypertens 1985; **3** (Suppl 3): 487–8.

[13] Jarden JO, Barry DI, Juhler M, Graham DI, Strandgaard S, Paulson OB.
Cerebrovascular aspects of converting enzyme inhibition, II. Blood-brain barrier permeability and effect on intracerebrovascular administration of captopril.
J Hypertens 1984; **2**: 599–604.

[14] Parving HH, Andersen AR, Smidt UM, Oxenboll B, Edsberg B, Sandahl Christiansen J.
Diabetic nephropathy and arterial hypertension.
Diabetologia 1983; **24**: 10–2.

[15] Feldt-Rasmussen B, Borch-Johnsen K, Mathiesen ER.
Hypertension in diabetes as related to nephropathy. Early blood pressure changes.
Hypertension 1985; **7** II 8–II: 20.

[16] Hostetter TH, Rennke HG, Brenner BM.
The case for intrarenal hypertension in the initiation and progression of diabetic and other glomerulopathies.
Am J Med 1982; **72**: 375–8.

[17] Hommel E, Parving HH, Mathiesen E, Edsberg B, Damkjaer Nielsen M, Giese J.
Effect of captopril on kidney function in insulin-dependent diabetic patients with nephropathy.
Br Med J 1986; **293**: 457–70.

[18] Bjorck S, Nijberg G, Mulec H, Granerus G, Herlitz H, Aurell M.
Beneficial effects of angiotensin converting enzyme inhibition on renal function in patients with diabetic nephropathy.
Br Med J 1986; **293**: 471–4.

[19] Meyer TW, Andersen S, Raenke HG, Brenner BM.
Converting enzyme inhibitor therapy limits progressive glomerular injury in rats with renal insufficiency.
Am J Med 1985; **79** (Suppl 3c): 31–6.

[20] Vidt DG, Bravo EL, Fouad FM.
Captopril.
N Engl J Med 1982; **306**: 214–9.

[21] Lanza G, Barbara R, Fontana S.
Treatment of hypertension in the diabetic with captopril.
Minerva Med 1985; **11**: 183–4.

[22] Croog SH, Levine S, Testa MA *et al.*
The effect of antihypertensive therapy on quality of life.
N Engl J Med 1986; **1214**: 1657–64.

[23] Hill JF, Bulpitt CJ, Fletcher AE.
Angiotensin converting enzyme inhibitors and quality of life: the European Trial.
J Hypertens 1985; **3** (Suppl 2): S91–4.

[24] Lichter I, Richardson PJ, Wijke MA.
Differential effects of atenolol and enalapril on tests of memory during treatment for essential hypertension.
J Hypertens 1984; **2**: 560.

[25] Lant AF, McNabb RW, Noormohamed FH.
Kinetic and metabolic aspects of enalapril action.
J Hypertens 1984; **2** (Suppl 2): 37–42.

[26] Weinberger MH.
Comparison of captopril and hydrochlorothiazide alone and in combination in mild to moderate hypertension.
Br J Clin Pharmacol 1982; **14**: 127–131.

[27] Staessen J, Fagart R, Lynen P, Verschueren LJ, Amery A.
Double blind comparison between propanolol and bendroflumethazide in captopril treated resistant hypertensive patients.
Am Heart J 1983; **106**: 321–8.

[28] Brouwer RML, Bolllik P, Erne P, Conen D, Kiowski W, Buhler FR.
Antihypertensive therapy using calcium antagonists in combination with captopril rather than diuretics.
J Cardiovasc Pharmacol 1985; **7**: S88–91.

TREATMENT OF HYPERTENSION

DIETARY MANIPULATION

[1] Evaluation of the effectiveness of a low sodium diet in the treatment of mild to moderate hypertension.
Silman AJ, Locke C, Mitchell P, Humpherson P, London Hosp Med Coll, London, UK.
Lancet 1983; **i**: 1179–82.

[2] Blood-pressure response to moderate sodium restriction and to potassium supplementation in mild essential hypertension.
Richards AM, Nicholls MG, Espinker EA *et al*, Princess Margaret Hosp, Christchurch, New Zealand.
Lancet 1984; i: 757–60.

[3] Potassium supplementation in hypertensive patients with diuretic-induced hypokalemia.
Kaplan NM, Carnegie A, Raskin P, Heller JA, Simmons M, Univ Texas Hlth Sci Cent, Southwestern Med Sch, Dallas, TX, USA.
N Engl J Med 1985; **312**: 746–9.

[4] Moderate potassium chloride supplementation in essential hypertension: is it additive to moderate sodium restriction?
Smith SJ, Markandu ND, Sagnella GA, MacGregor GA, Charing Cross Hosp Med Sch, London, UK.
Br Med J 1985; **290**: 110–2.

[5] Effect of magnesium on blood pressure.
Dyckner T, Wester PO, Univ Hosp, Umea, Sweden.
Br Med J 1983; **286**: 1847–9.

[6] Lack of effect of oral magnesium on high blood pressure: a double blind study.
Cappuccio FP, Markandu ND, Beynon GW, Shore AC, Sampson B, MacGregor GA, Charing Cross and Westminster Med Sch, London UK.
Br Med J 1985; **291**: 235–9.

Comment. Over the years, conflicting data have been produced on the effect of low-sodium diets on blood pressure in hypertensive patients. Silman *et al* [1] found no hypotensive effect of a low-sodium diet. Richards *et al* [2] found that neither sodium restriction nor potassium supplementation produced any consistent effect on blood pressure. Potassium supplementation did produce a small hypotensive effect in patients with diuretic-induced hypokalemia [3], but not in patients already on a low intake of dietary sodium [4]. Finally, magnesium supplementation of the diet may produce a hypotensive effect without causing any other biochemical derangement [5], although there is conflicting evidence [6].

DIURETICS

[1] Ventricular extrasystoles during thiazide treatment: substudy of MRC mild hypertension trial.
Medical Research Council Working Party on Mild to Moderate Hypertension, Northwick Park Hosp, Harrow, UK.
Br Med J 1983; **287**: 1249–54.

[2] Nonarrhythmogenicity of diuretic-induced hypokalemia. Its evidence in patients with uncomplicated hypertension.
Madias JE, Madias NE, Gavras HP, Mount Sinai-Sinai-City Hosp Cent, Elmhurst, NY, USA.
Arch Intern Med 1984; **144**: 2171–6.

[3] Diuretic-induced hypokalemia in uncomplicated systemic hypertension: effect of plasma potassium correction on cardiac arrhythmias.
Papademetriou V, Fletcher R, Khatri M, Freis D, VA Med Cent, Washington, DC, USA.
Am J Cardiol 1983; **52**: 1017–22.

Comment. There is a great deal of interest in the possible relationship between diuretic-induced hypokalemia and the incidence of cardiac arrhythmias. In the largest study yet to address this question — the MRC study of mild hypertension [1] — it was shown that ventricular extrasystoles were commoner in patients receiving long-term thiazide treatment, and that their incidence correlated with serum potassium level. A smaller study of 20 patients was unable to confirm these observations [2], while Papademetriou *et al* [3] made the important observation that normalizing the serum potassium in patients with thiazide-induced hypokalemia does not significantly reduce ectopic activity. This suggests that either potassium is not the mediator of the arrhythmogenic effect of thiazides or intracellular rather than extracellular potassium is the crucial factor.

ALCOHOL REDUCTION

[1] Evidence for a direct effect of alcohol consumption on blood pressure in normotensive men. A randomized controlled trial.
Puddey IB, Beilin LJ, Vandongen R, Rouse IL, Rogers P, Royal Perth Hosp, Perth, Western Australia, Australia.
Hypertension 1985; **7**: 707–13.
[2] Regular alcohol use raises blood pressure in treated hypertensive subjects. A randomised controlled trial.
Puddey IB, Beilin LJ, Vandongen R, Royal Perth Hosp, Perth, Western Australia, Australia.
Lancet 1987; **i**: 647–51.

Comment. The results of a study by Puddey *et al* [1] provide evidence for a direct association between alcohol consumption and blood pressure. The authors conducted a randomized controlled crossover trial of the effects of varying alcohol intake on the blood pressure of 46 healthy male drinkers. Alcohol consumption was reduced by 80% over 6 weeks from an average of 336 ml ethanol per week. This reduction in alcohol consumption was associated with a significant decrease in both systolic and diastolic blood pressure and bodyweight. However, after an adjustment was made for the change in weight, an independent effect of alcohol was observed on systolic blood pressure only; a 3.1-mmHg fall in systolic blood pressure is predicted with a decrease in alcohol consumption from 350 to 70 ml ethanol per week. When the subjects resumed their normal drinking habits, their systolic blood pressure rose. Although these results demonstrate that alcohol consumption and blood pressure are directly related, the changes in systolic blood pressure that were observed are small.

In a randomized controlled crossover trial from the same workers [2], the effects of alcohol intake on blood pressure were studied in 44 men who were receiving treatment for essential hypertension and were classified as moderate to heavy drinkers. Subjects consumed their normal alcohol intake for six weeks and drank only low-alcohol beer for six weeks. Usual antihypertensive therapy was continued throughout the study period. The mean ($\pm$SEM) change in alcohol consumption fell from 452 ± 30 ml/week on the normal drinking pattern to 64 ± 8 ml/week whilst on low-alcohol beer. It was found that mean systolic and diastolic blood pressures were significantly lower during the last two weeks of the low alcohol intake study period when compared with the normal alcohol intake study period — the mean differences in supine readings were 5 ± 1.4 and 3 ± 0.9 mmHg, respectively. Following regression analysis, these changes in blood pressure were found to be independent of bodyweight.

OTHER TREATMENT STRATEGIES

[1] Single-agent and combination therapy of essential hypertension.
Weber MA, Drayer JIM, VA Med Cent, Long Beach, CA, USA.
Am Heart J 1984; **108**: 311-5.

[2] Lack of effect of beta-blocker on flat dose response to thiazide in hypertension: efficacy of low dose thiazide combined with beta-blocker.
MacGregor GA, Banks RA, Markandu ND, Bayliss J, Roulston J, Charing Cross Hosp Med Sch, London, UK.
Br Med J 1983; **286**: 1535-9.

[3] Influence of angiotensin converting-enzyme inhibitor on diuretic-induced metabolic effects in hypertension.
Weinberger MH, Indiana Univ Sch Med, Indianapolis, IN, USA.
Hypertension 1983; **5**(Suppl III): 132-8.

[4] Crossover comparison of captopril and propranolol as step 2 agents in hypertension.
Oren A, Rotmensch HH, Vlasses PH *et al*, Thomas Jefferson Univ, Philadelphia, PA, USA.
Am Heart J 1985; **109**: 554-7.

[5] "Third drug" trial: comparative study of antihypertensive agents added to treatment when blood pressure remains uncontrolled by a beta blocker plus thiazide diuretic.
McAreavey D, Ramsey LE, Latham L *et al*, Western Infirm, Glasgow, UK.
Br Med J 1984; **288**: 106-10.

[6] Hydralazine and prazosin in the treatment of hypertension.
Vandenburg MJ, Sharman VL, Wright P, Drew PJ, Barnes JN, London Hosp, UK.
Br J Clin Pharmacol 1983; **16**: 537-42.

[7] Transdermal continuous antihypertensive therapy.
Weber MA, Drayer JM, Brewer DD, Lipson JL, VA Med Cent, Long Beach, CA, USA.
Lancet 1984; i: 9-10.

Comment. Stepped-care therapy for essential hypertension remains the best-accepted regimen. Weber and Drayer [1] challenged part of this by suggesting that, if a patient responded poorly to either a thiazide or a beta-blocker as initial therapy, they should be tried on the other drug first, and should not be put on dual therapy at this stage. The effect of adding a beta-blocker to a thiazide was further studied by

MacGregor *et al* [2], who showed that the flat dose-response curve of thiazide diuretics was unaltered by the addition of a beta-blocker; this is in contrast to their previous work with captopril, which did abolish the flat dose-response curve of thiazide diuretics. Indeed, Weinberger [3] showed that captopril was able to block all the adverse metabolic effects of thiazides, including changes in serum potassium, uric acid, glucose and cholesterol. Oren *et al* [4] showed, however, that in terms of efficacy and side-effects there was little to choose between captopril and propranolol as step-2 drugs in hypertension.

Important data were presented by McAreavey *et al* [5] to answer the question of which is the best step-3 drug to add to thiazides and beta-blockers. In practice, hydralazine followed closely by prazosin proved superior to methyldopa, minoxidil, labetolol or placebo. However, the stepped-care regimen was challenged by Vandenburg *et al* [6], who showed that a combination of both prazosin and hydralazine at low dose reduced blood pressure more than did either drug at high dose.

A novel preparation of transdermal clonidine, containing a seven-day supply of the drug, has been studied and appears to be both efficacious and well tolerated by the patients [7].

HYPERTENSION IN PREGNANCY

[1] Low-dose aspirin prevents pregnancy-induced hypertension and pre-eclampsia in angiotensin-sensitive primigravidae.
Wallenburg HCS, Dekker GA, Makovitz JW, Rotmans P, Erasmus Univ Med Sch, Rotterdam, The Netherlands.
Lancet 1986; i: 1–3

[2] Aspirin and pre-eclampsia (Editorial).
Lancet 1986; i: 18–20.

[3] Antihypertensive treatment in pregnancy: analysis of different responses to oxprenolol and methyldopa.
Gallery EDM, Ross MR, Gyory AZ, Royal North Shore Hosp, St Leonards, NSW, Australia.
Br Med J 1985; **291**: 563–7.

[4] Antihypertensive drugs in pregnancy (Leading article).
de Swiet M, Queen Charlotte's Maternity Hosp, London, UK.
Br Med J 1985; **291**: 365–6.

Comment. Wallenburg *et al* investigated the possibility of preventing pregnancy-induced hypertension and pre-eclampsia with low-dose aspirin in 46 normotensive women at 28 weeks' gestation who were thought to be at risk of developing these conditions because of an increased blood-pressure response to intravenous angiotensin II [1]. Twenty-three women received 60 mg aspirin per day until delivery; the remaining 23 received matching placebo. Two women in the treatment group developed mild pregnancy-induced hypertension, whereas pregnancy-induced hypertension developed in four of the placebo group. Moreover, pre-eclampsia developed in seven of the placebo group and one of them developed eclampsia. The authors suggest that low-dose aspirin may restore the prostacyclin-thromboxane imbalance which has been put forward as important in the etiology of pregnancy-induced hypertension and pre-eclampsia. The accompanying editorial [2] contains a discussion on the role of platelets in the etiology of pre-eclamptic hypertension and the place of therapy with low-dose aspirin.

Gallery, Ross and Gyory [3] conducted a randomized trial of oxprenolol and methyldopa in hypertensive pregnant women; 96 women received oxprenolol and 87 received methyldopa. The control of hypertension was found to be equivalent in both treatment groups; hydralazine had to be added to the regimen in 64 cases in order to achieve the therapeutic aim. One perinatal death occurred in the oxprenolol-treated group; four occurred in the methyldopa-treated group. Detailed analysis revealed greater fetal growth in the oxprenolol-treated group, irrespective of the severity of hypertension or parity. However, after 10 weeks of treatment this difference was no longer apparent.

De Swiet [4] discusses the use of beta-adrenergic blocking drugs in the treatment of pregnancy-associated hypertension, and raises the question of beta-blockers replacing methyldopa as the agent of first choice in this condition. He concludes, having reviewed the published trials, that when treatment is initiated primarily for the benefit of the fetus, methyldopa should remain the drug of choice. He does not discuss the work of Gallery, Ross and Gyory [3] which was published after his leading article [4].

RENOVASCULAR HYPERTENSION

[1] Enalapril in the treatment of hypertension with renal artery stenosis.
     Hodsman GP, Brown JJ, Cumming AMM et al, Western Infirm, Glasgow, UK.
     Br Med J 1983; 287: 1413-7.
[2] Split renal function after captopril in unilateral renal artery stenosis.
     Wenting GJ, Tan-Tjiong HL, Derkx FHM, de Bruyn JHB, Man in 't Veld AJ, Schalekamp MADH, Univ Hosp Dijkzigt, Erasmus Univ, Rotterdam, The Netherlands.
     Br Med J 1984; 288: 886-90.
[3] Long-term converting-enzyme inhibition as a guide to surgical curability of hypertension associated with renovascular disease.
     Staessen J, Bulpitt C, Fagard R, Lijnen P, Amery A, Univ Hosp Saint Rafael, Leuven, Belgium.
     Am J Cardiol 1983; 51: 1317-22.
[4] The decision on surgery in renal artery stenosis.
     Mackay A, Boyle P, Brown JJ et al, Western Infirm, Glasgow, UK.
     Q J Med 1983; 52: 363-81.
[5] Percutaneous transluminal renal angioplasty in renovascular hypertension due to atheroma or fibromuscular dysplasia.
     Sos TA, Pickering TG, Sniderman K et al, New York Hosp-Cornell Univ Med Cent, USA.
     N Engl J Med 1983; 309: 274-9.

[6] Follow up study of 70 patients with renal artery stenosis treated by percutaneous tran-
sluminal dilatation.
Geyskes GG, Puylaert CBAJ, Oei HY, Dorhout Mees EJ, Univ Hosp, Utrecht, The
Netherlands.
Br Med J 1983; **287**: 333–7.

[7] Percutaneous transluminal angioplasty vs. surgery for renovascular hypertension.
Miller GA, Ford KK, Braun SD *et al*, Duke Univ Med Cent, Durham, NC, USA.
Am J Roentgenol 1985; **144**: 447–50.

[8] Renal revascularization in the azotemic hypertensive patient resistant to therapy.
Ying CY, Tifft CP, Gavras H, Chobanian AV, Boston Univ Sch Med, Boston, MA, USA.
N Engl J Med 1984; **311**: 1070–5.

[9] Renovascular hypertension and azotemia [Editorial].
Dustan HP, Univ Alabama Med Cent, Birmingham, AL, USA.
N Engl J Med 1984; **311**: 1114–5.

Comment. In renal artery stenosis, the choice of treatment is between surgery, percutaneous renal angioplasty and medical therapy, usually with angiotensin converting enzyme inhibitors. Enalapril was found to control blood pressure well in a group
of 20 such patients [1], although, in another study [2], long-term captopril caused a
marked deterioration in renal function in 50% of affected kidneys. Staessen *et al* [3]
suggested that the preoperative response to chronic captopril therapy predicted fairly
well the postoperative blood-pressure response to renal revascularization. Mackay *et
al* [4] also examined the factors which help predict a successful blood-pressure response to surgery, and found that no single investigation or combination of investigations was an accurate predictor, although a renal vein renin ratio >2.0 was the best
available predictor.

Percutaneous angioplasty is the latest therapy available, and its long-term effects
are only just becoming known. Two studies [5,6] have shown that the short-term
results are better in fibromuscular dysplasia than in atheromatous disease, and that
the long-term results are encouraging, with a 12% average increase in kidney size over
two years. In fact, Miller *et al* [7] have compared percutaneous angioplasty with surgical revascularization and found them to be equally beneficial in fibromuscular dysplasia and in atheromatous disease involving the origin of the renal artery.
Angioplasty was more successful than surgery in atheromatous disease not involving
the origin of the renal artery. These authors therefore conclude that angioplasty is the
treatment of choice for all renal artery lesions.

In patients with renovascular disease and renal impairment, medical therapy normally causes a further deterioration in renal function. Two papers [8,9] attest to the
fact that revascularization either by angioplasty or surgery causes a stabilization or
even an improvement in renal function.

Overall, it would appear that percutaneous angioplasty is beginning to emerge as
the treatment of choice for renovascular hypertension.

PULMONARY HYPERTENSION

[1] Primary pulmonary hypertension: Natural history and the importance of thrombosis.
Fuster V, Steele PM, Edwards WD *et al*, Mayo Clinic, Rochester, MN, USA.
Circulation 1984; **70**: 580–7.

[2] Magnitude and implications of spontaneous hemodynamic variability in primary pulmonary hypertension.
Rich S, D'Alonzo GE, Dantzker DR, Levy PS, Univ Illinois Coll Med, Chicago, IL, USA.
Am J Cardiol 1985; **55**: 159–63.

[3] Treatment of primary pulmonary hypertension with intravenous epoprostenol (prostacyclin).
Jones DK, Higenbottam TW, Wallwork J, Papworth Hosp, Cambridge, UK.
Br Heart J 1987; **57**: 270–8.

Comment. A paper from The Mayo Clinic [1] describes a retrospective study of 120 patients in whom a diagnosis of primary pulmonary hypertension was made, using strict clinical and cardiac catheterization criteria, between 1955 and 1977. Most of the findings confirm familiar features of the disease: low average age at presentation, female preponderance, the advanced state by the time symptoms develop and poor prognosis. There was no particular evidence to support a role of either pregnancy or oral contraceptive use in the pathogenesis, although the initial symptoms did occur shortly after pregnancy in 14 patients. Two brothers in two families were affected.

Two observations stand out as of clinical importance: lung tissue was obtained from 56 patients at autopsy, and 32 specimens showed the features of thromboembolic pulmonary hypertension; in those with the characteristic pathologic changes of primary pulmonary hypertension, there was frequent evidence of fresh fibrin-platelet thrombosis. Multivariate analysis showed a significant association between anticoagulant therapy and longer survival, although this data-derived conclusion should be accepted cautiously. Thus, the diagnosis of thromboembolic pulmonary hypertension cannot be excluded without a lung biopsy, and the findings of this study support the use of anticoagulant treatment for all affected patients.

The inexorable progression of primary pulmonary hypertension has defied effective therapy, but some patients appear to respond to a variety of vasodilators, and it has been recommended that measurements of pulmonary artery pressure and vascular resistance should be made before and after drug administration in order to select the most suitable agent for long-term therapy. Rich and colleagues [2] advise caution in the interpretation of such studies: they found that pulmonary artery pressure and vascular resistance varied spontaneously in 12 patients with primary pulmonary hypertension who were studied over a six-month period. The coefficient of variation was greatest in the patients with the highest pulmonary resistances. There was no relation between degree of spontaneous variability and responses to hydralazine and nifedipine. The authors calculated that for a change to be ascribed to a drug effect (with 95% confidence) it would have to exceed 37% for pulmonary vascular resistance, or 22% for pulmonary artery pressure.

Intravenous prostacyclin can induce short-term pulmonary vasodilatation in patients with primary pulmonary hypertension and workers in Cambridge [3] have described their experience with continuous intravenous infusion over 1–25 months in

10 patients. The drug was delivered through a cannula inserted into the subclavian vein, via a subcutaneous tunnel, using a syringe connected to a battery-driven system so that patients could live at home. The acute effects of prostacyclin, documented by cardiac catheterization, were favorable in all patients, with an increase in cardiac output and, generally, a fall in pulmonary vascular resistance, although the pulmonary artery pressure rose in two cases. Continued intravenous infusion was associated with subjective and clinical improvement in all but one of the patients, and exercise tolerance and the maximum rate of oxygen consumption increased. In some patients, the symptomatic improvement was dramatic, but there was no evidence to suggest a significant alteration in the prognosis of the disease; two died on treatment and three have undergone heart-lung transplantation. The major complications were septicemia and ascites. The authors suggest that the principal role of this treatment may be in the management of patients who are awaiting heart-lung transplantation.

11. Thrombosis and Embolism

ATRIAL FIBRILLATION AND STROKE

[1] Duration of atrial fibrillation and imminence of stroke: The Framingham Study.
Wolf PA, Kannel WB, McGee DL, Meeds SL, Bharucha NE, McNamara PM, Boston Univ Sch Med, Boston, MA, USA.
Stroke 1983; **14**: 664-7.

[2] Early recurrent embolism associated with nonvalvular atrial fibrillation: A retrospective study.
Hart RG, Coull BM, Hart D, Univ Texas Health Sci Cent, San Antonio, TX, USA.
Stroke 1983; **14**: 688-93.

Comment. Atrial fibrillation from any cause is accompanied by an increased risk of stroke. In the Framingham Study the incidence of stroke following the development of chronic non-rheumatic atrial fibrillation was increased more than fivefold, and this association was independent of other cardiovascular risk factors. A more recent analysis [1] paid particular attention to the time-course of the threat of stroke in relation to the onset and duration of atrial fibrillation. During the 30-year follow-up period, 501 strokes occurred, of which 59 were in association with non-rheumatic atrial fibrillation. The fivefold increased risk of stroke accompanying atrial fibrillation was independent of cardiac failure and coronary heart disease, both of which were frequently associated with the arrhythmia. There was a distinct clustering of strokes around the time of onset of atrial fibrillation. Mortality rates at 30 days were similar in patients with and without atrial fibrillation, and early recurrences were also of similar frequency. However, recurrence in the first six months was more than twice as common in patients with atrial fibrillation (47%, as against 20% in patients without atrial fibrillation).

These data are complemented by a retrospective study of 56 patients with acute cerebral infarction associated with non-valvar atrial fibrillation [2]. Thirty-five (63%) of the strokes were judged, on the basis of a standardized clinical algorithm, to be embolic, 13 (23%) were thought to be non-embolic, and in 8 (14%) the pathogenesis was indeterminate. Of the 35 patients presumed to have had an embolic infarct, 12 received immediate anticoagulation without complications, and none developed evidence of recurrent embolism. Of the 23 patients who were not immediately anticoagulated, 3 had recurrent systemic emboli within 10 days; 5 additional patients had had a probable systemic embolus within 11 days of the marker stroke event, so that, by including these patients, 8 out of 40 (20%) of all non-valvar atrial fibrillation patients who presented with a systemic embolism, and who were not immediately anticoagulated, experienced a recurrence.

These findings, albeit in a relatively small number of patients, suggest that immediate anticoagulation should be given to patients with a clinical diagnosis of cardiogenic brain embolism. However, this approach is not without its risks, particularly if the etiology of the stroke is based on clinical criteria; the problem is discussed in more detail below.

ANTICOAGULATION FOR EMBOLIC STROKE

[1] Immediate anticoagulation of embolic stroke: Brain hemorrhage and management options.
Cerebral Embolism Study Group, Hart RG (Co-ordinator), Univ Texas Health Sci Cent, San Antonio, TX, USA.
Stroke 1984; **15**: 779–89.

[2] Anticoagulation and hemorrhagic infarction in cerebral embolism secondary to rheumatic heart disease.
Calandre L, Ortega JF, Bermejo F, '1 de Octobre' Univ Hosp, Madrid, Spain.
Arch Neurol 1984; **41**: 1152–4.

Comment. The therapeutic dilemma, when confronted by a patient who is thought to have had a cerebral embolus arising from the heart, is that of balancing the risk of hemorrhagic cerebral infarction caused by anticoagulant therapy against the risk of recurrent embolism (which is likely to occur in approximately 12% of patients within the first two weeks) if such treatment is withheld. A report from the Cerebral Embolism Study Group [1] describes observations on 30 patients with cardiogenic brain embolism in whom hemorrhagic infarction or intracerebral hematoma was demonstrated by computerized tomography. At the time the hemorrhage was iden-tified, 19 patients were receiving anticoagulants and 11 were not; 11 patients (8 anticoagulated, 3 not) developed late hemorrhagic transformation unassociated with clinical deterioration (this was particularly liable to occur with large initial infarcts); 8 patients (7 anticoagulated, 1 not) developed hemorrhage accompanied by abrupt clinical worsening (these patients also tended to have had large infarcts); in 4 of 5 of those receiving heparin, either this therapy or acute hypertension was thought to have contributed to the complication. These observations suggest that computerized tomography is an essential investigation for the optimal management of such patients, and the authors conclude that, in patients with extensive embolic infarcts, early large bolus doses of heparin should be avoided.

This cautious conclusion is supported by the results of a study from Madrid [2], in which the clinical course of 42 patients with cerebral embolism secondary to rheumatic mitral valve disease was analyzed. All had CT scans. In 25 patients, immediate anticoagulant therapy was initiated with heparin. There was only one inci-dent of recurrent embolism (which occurred despite anticoagulation), but seven patients developed hemorrhagic infarction, of whom five showed signs of recurrent stroke and three (all receiving anticoagulant therapy) died.

None of these data, from relatively small numbers of selected patients, permits com-prehensive recommendations to be made, but in general they support a cautious approach to cardiogenic brain embolism, with computerized tomography as an essential prerequisite to anticoagulant therapy, which, if initiated, should probably exclude the use of heparin.

VENOUS THROMBOSIS

[1] Continuous intravenous heparin compared with intermittent subcutaneous heparin in the initial treatment of proximal-vein thrombosis.
Hull RD, Raskob GE, Hirsh J *et al*, Chedoke-McMaster Hosp, Hamilton, Ontario, Canada.
N Engl J Med 1986; **315**: 1109–14.

[2] Need for long-term anticoagulant treatment in symptomatic calf-vein thrombosis.
Lagerstedt CI, Olsson C-G, Fagher BO, Oqvist BW, Albrechtsson U, Univ Hosp, Lund, Sweden.
Lancet 1985; ii: 515–8.

Comment. It has been suggested that subcutaneous heparin would be more suitable than intravenous heparin for the initial treatment of proximal vein thrombosis because it is simpler and would allow the earlier mobilization of patients. Hull *et al* [1] conducted a randomized double-blind trial of 115 patients with deep venous thrombosis to compare the efficacy of intermittent subcutaneous heparin ($n=57$) with that of continuous intravenous heparin ($n=58$) during the initial treatment period. It was found that intermittent subcutaneous heparin was inferior to continuous intravenous heparin in preventing the recurrence of venous thrombo-embolism (19.3% *vs* 5.2% recurrence rate, $P=0.024$). Also, the subcutaneous regimen resulted in an anti-coagulant response below the therapeutic range in the majority of patients. Recurrence of deep venous thrombo-embolism was confined to those patients in whom there had been an initial subtherapeutic anticoagulant response. These results demonstrate the efficacy of intravenous heparin as the initial treatment for patients with deep venous thrombosis, and they suggest a relation between the efficacy of heparin and the level of anticoagulation achieved which would explain the ineffectiveness of the subcutaneous regimen.

In a study of 51 patients with calf-vein thrombosis, 23 were randomized to treatment with warfarin for 3 months [2]. All patients received an initial course of heparin and all wore compression stockings. During the first 3 months of the trial, 8 patients in the non-warfarin-treated group experienced recurrence of symptoms, whereas there were no recurrences in the warfarin-treated group ($P<0.01$). After one year of the trial, only one patient in the warfarin-treated group experienced a recurrence, whereas recurrences had occurred in 9 of the non-warfarin-treated group ($P<0.02$).

ORAL CONTRACEPTIVES

Oral contraceptives and venous thromboembolism: findings in a large prospective study.
Vessey M, Mant D, Smith A, Yeates D, Radcliffe Infirm, Oxford, UK.
Br Med J 1986; **292**: 526.

Comment. This short report is a summary of the latest findings of the Oxford Family Planning Association contraceptive study with respect to oral contraceptives and venous thrombo-embolism. Over 17 000 women were recruited between 1968 and 1974; data were collected on subsequent hospital referrals and deaths. A first attack of venous thrombo-embolism unassociated with pregnancy or the puerperium occurred in 105 women; in 34 the disease occurred within three months of a surgical operation. Three diagnostic categories were considered: certain or probable deep vein thrombosis or pulmonary embolism, possible deep vein thrombosis or pulmonary embolism, and superficial venous thrombosis. There was a strong association between oral contraceptive use and certain or probable venous thrombo-embolism (relative risk 3.1) and little or no association with superficial venous thrombosis (relative risk 1.4, not significant). The risk was confined to current users of the pill, and there was no association with duration of use. For postoperative thrombo-embolism, those taking oral contraceptives had nearly twice the risk of non-users, but the overall number was small, and the difference was not satistically significant. It is worth noting that although the relative risk of postoperative venous thrombosis is only about 2, the incidence of the disease is much higher than that of spontaneous thrombosis, and so the attributable risk, which is what matters in clinical practice, is considerable; therefore combined oral contraceptives should always be withdrawn at least one month before elective surgery. Finally, the risk of venous thrombo-embolism was lower among women taking a pill that contained less than 50 μg oestrogen than among those on a higher dose. These findings are consistent with those of the other major studies of oral contraceptives from Britain, North America and Scandinavia.

Index

Note: page numbers in italics refer to figures and tables

Abiomed ventricular assist devices 420, 422
acebutolol 90
acquired long QT syndrome 312
acute heart failure 446-7
adenosine
  formation during ischemia 56
  mediator of anginal pain 68
  as neurotransmitter 467
adenosine triphosphate
  effect of nitroglycerin in cardioplegia 368
  as neurotransmitter 467
  in oxygenated crystalloid cardioplegia 370
adenylate kinase 405
beta-adrenergic receptor blockers see beta-blockers
adrenergic vasoconstriction 38
afterload 245-6
alcohol
  consumption 21-2, 339
  coronary spasm induction 44
aldosterone
  biochemical marker of heart failure 249
  control and dopamine 443, 445
  inhibition of release by atrial natriuretic peptide 452
alpha-blockers 48, 75
alpha$_2$-macroglobulin 135
ambulatory ECG monitoring 69, 247
  and amiodarone therapy 311
  predictive power of 288
  in silent ischemia 247
  in ventricular arrhythmia 270
amiloride 253
aminohippuric acid clearance 433
aminophylline 56
  in stress testing with dipyridamole 63
amiodarone 48, 311
  in arrhythmia 224
  in hypertrophic cardiomyopathy 237, 239
  intravenous infusion 311
  oral therapy 311
  in pediatric practice 311-12
  prevention of sustained ventricular tachycardia 289-90
  toxicity 311
anemia in cardiac failure 245
angina pectoris
  adenosine release 56
  ambulatory ST-segment monitoring 61-2
  aortocoronary venous bypass grafting 379
  beta-blockade 473
  beta-blockers 72-7
  calcium antagonists 47, 72-7
  l-carnitine in 98-9
  coronary artery bypass surgery 111, 372
  and coronary artery spasm 45
  diagnosis and assessment 57-67
  diltiazem therapy 76
  effects of cigarettes and coffee 67
  exercise testing 62-7
  Holter monitoring 69
  incidence after internal thoracic artery grafts 375, 376, 377
  left-ventricular function 58-60
  and mental stress 18
  nicardipine therapy 77
  nifedipine therapy 75
  nitrates 77-83
  nocturnal 55
  pacemakers 337
  pacing-induced 60
  pain 46, 68
  pathophysiology 55-7
  plasma viscosity in 17
  prognosis 150-8
  prophylaxis 77
  psychological traits 68
  and Syndrome X 113-14
  treatment 77
  variant 43, 44, 46, 48 see also coronary artery spasm
  vasospastic 44
angina, Prinzmetal's 58, 89
  beta-blockade in 90
  calcium antagonists in 91
angina, unstable 56-7, 83-98
  anticoagulants 89
  aspirin therapy 95, 386
  beta-blocking agents 90
  calcium antagonists 91-3
  classification of patients 85, 86, 87
  coronary obstruction 86
  management of patient 88
  mechanical recanalization 93
  mortality rate 84
  and myocardial infarction 83
  nifedipine with beta-blocker therapy 91-2
  pain 84, 86
  pathophysiology 84-8
  plaque fissuring 123
  restenosis 102
  survival rate 153
  therapy-resistant cases 93
  thrombolytic therapy 89
angiography 41
  in carotid investigations 426
  digital subtraction 407, 426
  wall motion abnormalities 129
angioplasty 163-7
  during cardiac catheterization 163
  laser 106-9
  percutaneous in renovascular hypertension 486
  in thrombolysis 144
angioscopy, fiberoptic 108
angiotensin converting enzyme (ACE) inhibitors 244, 248, 249
  addition to conventional therapy 250
  and atrial natriuretic peptide levels 436, 437
  and beta-blockers 478
  combination with diuretics 256-7
  in diabetic nephropathy 477
  effect on renal function 256
  glomerular filtration rate 476
  in heart failure 254-6
  in hypertension 454, 475-80
  and indomethacin 478
  interactions with other drugs 477-8
  in mild hypertension 472
  and non-steroidal anti-inflammatory drugs 478
  and plasma renin 475
  and prostaglandins 478
  in renal artery stenosis 486
  and renal function 249
  and vasodilators 478

angiotensin II
  -mediated vasoconstriction 248
  action on kidney 475-6
  biochemical marker of heart failure 249
  formation 475
  in hypertension 454
anisoylated plasminogen streptokinase activator
complex (APSAC) 137
α-hANP1-28 432
anterior descending artery 377
antiarrhythmic drugs 272, 276
  combination with beta-blockers 312
  deleterious effects 290-1
  dosage 290
  efficacy 289-90
  and late potentials 327
  and QRS duration 327
  therapy 308-13
  in ventricular arrhythmia 286, 288-91
  in ventricular ectopy 281
anticardiolipin antibody
  and intravascular thrombosis 391
  levels in aortocoronary bypass graft surgery 391
  and myocardial infarction 391
anticholinergic drugs 48
anticoagulants
  aspirin/dipyridamole in children 398
  and mechanical valves 397-9
  in unstable angina 89
  in vein grafts 381-2
alpha₂-antiplasmin 135, 136
antiplatelet agents 102-3
antitachycardia pacemakers 301
aortic aneurysms 348
aortic coarctation 166-7, 180, 213-18
  balloon dilatation techniques 214, 215-16
  Dacron tube graft 215
  hypertension after repair 216
  incidence 222
  left ventricular function 217
  onlay patch 215
  pathogenesis 217-18
  propanolol prior to repair of complications 216
  pulmonary trunk banding 215
  resection and end-to-end anastomosis 215
  restenosis 166-7
  subclavian flap procedure 215
aortic cross-clamping 367
aortic stenosis 203-4
  in children 359
  Doppler ultrasound 359
  valvotomy 204
aortic valve
  prosthesis 230-1
  replacement 233, 398
  site of infection in infective endocarditis 242
  stenosis 165-6, 222
aortic valvuloplasty 227-8
aortocoronary
  artery vein-graft disease 111
  bypass graft surgery 379, 391
aorto-pulmonary shunt 208
apolipoprotein B 391
apoprotein 22
arginine 249
  vasopressin 255
argon laser 107-8, 307, 319
Arrhenius line 459
arrhythmia see also ventricular arrhythmia

amiodarone therapy 224
  atrial 193
  atrial natriuretic peptide in 437
  cardiac 91
  catheter ablation 313
  and diuretic-induced hypokalemia 482
  in ergonovine provocative testing 43
  implantable devices 301
  intraoperative mapping 301-2
  lasers in therapy 319
  in left-ventricular dysfunction 247
  and polyuria 437
  postoperative 193
  reperfusion 45-6
  supraventricular 311, 312, 313
  surgical treatment 301-8
arrhythmogenic right-ventricular dysplasia 340-1
arterial
  lesions 28
  pressure during bypass 407
arterial ducts 188-90
  closure 163, 167
  closure with indomethacin 190, 191
  persistent patency 189-90
  prostaglandin administration 189
  surgical closure 190
arterial switch operation 170, 171, 172, 173
  for complete transposition 177-8
  survival rate 175, 177
arteriovenous fistulae 245
artificial heart 420-5
  air powered total 422-3
  electrically powered total 423-4
aspirin 49
  anticoagulation in children 398
  in aortic valve replacement 398
  blood loss 384
  and coronary artery disease 112
  dipyridamole combination 382, 384, 387, 453
  dosage 385
  effect on graft atheroma 112
  gastric adverse effects 385-6
  in hypertension in pregnancy 484
  inhibition of prostaglandin system 189
  in intimal hyperplasia 387
  lipid deposition inhibition in vein grafts 387
  in peripheral vascular disease 453
  and platelet aggregation 387
  and platelet deposition 382
  in restenosis 102
  in thromboxane A2 generation 385
  timing of therapy 384-5
  in unstable angina 95
  and vein grafts 379-90
Aspirin Myocardial Infarction Study 18
atenolol
  and beta-blocker combination 74
  efficacy and smoking 67
  in mild hypertension 471
  in unstable angina 90
atheroma
  graft 111, 112
  and vascular endothelial injury 33
atheromatous plaque *124*
atheronecrosis 123
atherosclerosis
  angiographic studies of lesions 391
  in coronary bypass grafts 390-2
  development 33

and development of coronary artery spasm 42, 43
emboli and threat to brain 408
following vein grafts 380, 387, 392
heart rate lowering 34–5
incidence in internal thoracic artery grafts 374
interferon-inducing agents 35
late phase after vein grafts 387
nutritional/metabolic causes 19
progression 34
prostacyclin production in 33
in unstable angina 88
atherosclerotic plaque 108
atrial
    arrhythmia 193
    fibrillation 338–40, 489
    pacing 332
    redirection 176
    septostomy 207
    shunt 224
    switch operation 171–2, 173
    synchronous ventricular pacing 337
    systole 364
    tachycardia 305
atrial natriuretic peptide 248, 432–42
    attenuation of renal effects in congestive heart failure
    436
    biochemical marker of heart failure 249
    blood pressure control 468
    in cardiovascular disease 435–8
    in chronic heart failure 435–7
    and coronary artery disease 438
    and dopamine 433–4
    effect of changes in central blood volume/right-atrial
    pressure 434
    effect of exercise 436
    endocrine effects 433–4
    hemodynamic effects 432
    and hypertension 437–8
    inhibition of aldosterone release 452
    interaction with renin-angiotensin-aldosterone system
    433, 434
    levels in hyperaldosteronism 438
    pharmacologic action 432–4
    physiology 434–5
    plasma volume control 468
    receptors in chronic heart failure 437
    receptors in kidney 432–3
    release and transmural pressure 438
    renal effects 432–3
    sodium homeostasis 435
    stimulus for cardiac release 438
    thyroid effects 434
    vasodilation effects 452
atrial septal defects 163, 191–6
    age of subject 193
    bidirectional shunting 193
    hemodynamics 192–3
    incidence 222
    magnetic resonance imaging 347
atrioventricular
    block 313, 336
    canal malformations 194
    conduction 193
    junction 318
    node re-entry tachycardia 304–5
    valve atresia 224–5
    valve orifice 195
atrioventricular septal defects 191–6
    Down's syndrome 195

morphology 194
mortality rate 195
prognosis 195–6
surgical closure 194–5
atropine, in coronary artery spasm 48
Australia
    CHD mortality rate 9
    dietary changes 9
automatic atrial tachycardia 305
AV sequential pacemakers see dual-chamber
pacemakers
    azathioprine 416

balloon
    angioplasty 163–4
    dilatation techniques in aortic coarctation 214, 215–16
    valvuloplasty 227, 228, 229
balloon atrial septostomy 163, 171, 172, 173
    in complete transposition 175
    echo-controlled 175
balloon catheter
    developments 104
    dilatation of valvar stenosis 203–4
    mounted 163
    in percutaneous transluminal coronary angioplasty
    (PTCA) 101, 103
    pressure and restenosis 103
balloon dilatation
    aneurysms 216
    in aortic valvuloplasty 227–8
    or calcific aortic stenosis 228
    in congenital stenosis of pulmonary veins 224
balloon-pump support, intra-aortic 94
barbed active fixation electrode 317
barbiturates 407
behavior, type A 18
Belgian Heart Disease Prevention Project 14
Bernouilli equation 180, 181, 182
    for valve gradients 360–1
Beta-Blocker Heart Attack Trial 157
beta-blockers
    and ACE inhibitors 478
    age of patients 473
    in angina 72–7
    in cardiac failure 244
    cold extremities 472, 473
    combination with antiarrhythmics 312
    combination with diltiazem 76
    in coronary artery spasm 45, 47–8
    effect on mortality 90
    in hypertensive pregnant women 485
    in mild hypertension 470–1
    in myocardial infarction 90
    in myocardial salvage 142
    protective effect before coronary artery bypass surgery
    269
    side effects 74
    tolerance by females 473
    in unstable angina 90
Björk-Shiley
    disc prostheses 231
    valve 360
Blalock-Taussig procedure 198
blood
    cardioplegia 365
    clotting 16–17
    -flow mapping 181–2
    flow velocity 246
    regional cerebral flow 405
    viscosity 16–17

blood pressure *see also* hypertension
  atherosclerosis aggravation 19
  in CHD mortality 10
  in coronary artery spasm 42
  identification of high risk men 15
bradyarrhythmia 89
bradykinin 249
  degradation by ACE inhibitors 475
brain
  death 414
  magnetic resonance imaging 344
British Regional Heart Study 15
Brock operation 198, 203
bromocriptine 443, 448
bruit, cervical 427

calcific aortic stenosis
  balloon aortic valvoplasty 166
  balloon dilatation 228
calcitonin, gene-related peptide 452
calcium
  channel blockade 473
  handling in hypertension 460
  intracellular 452-3
  platelet-free and blood pressure 460
calcium antagonists
  in angina 72-7
  combined therapy 91
  in coronary artery spasm 47
  mechanism of action 91
  prevention of re-infarction in patients with non-Q wave infarction 134
  in PTCA 103
  in small-vessel coronary artery spasm 46
  in unstable angina 91-3
  withdrawal 75-6
calcium blockers
  protection against cerebral damage during cardiac surgery 407
  response of patients with coronary artery spasm 45
captopril 248
  catecholamine levels in heart failure patients 255
  combination with diuretics 256-7
  effect on renal function 256
  in hypertension in the elderly 476
  interaction with thiazide diuretics 478
  and quality of life in hypertensives 477
  in renal artery stenosis 486
  and thiazide adverse metabolic effects 484
  vasopressin levels 255
carbidopa 434
cardiac
  arrhythmia 91
  catheterization in thrombolysis 144
  and cerebrovascular combined disease 405-7
  death in survivors of myocardial infarction 283-4, 285
  function 245
  output 246
  pacemakers 197
  physiology 364
  transplant rejection 352
  valve replacement and Doppler echocardiography 360
Cardiac Arrhythmia Pilot Study 293
cardiac failure 244-52
  causes 245
  diagnosis 246-7
  drug therapy 248-50
  fluid retention 244
  hemodynamic considerations 245-6

  inotropic effect drugs 249
  neuroendocrine axis 248, 253-4
  plasma arginine vasopressin 255
  prognosis 250-1
  vasodilator therapy 255
cardiac surgery
  cerebral complications 399-413
  and cerebrovascular disease 406
  complications 399-414
  detection of postoperative neurologic dysfunction 404-5
  hemorrhage after 413-14
  inadequate cerebral perfusion 403
  intellectual deterioration 402
  intraoperative neurophysiologic monitoring of cortical function 405
  macroemboli 403
  mechanisms of cerebral injury 403
  microemboli 403
  neurologic complications 400-3
  neuropsychologic testing 401-2
  ophthalmologic complications 402
  postoperative coma 400
  postoperative epilepsy 402
  risk factors for cerebral injury 404
  seizures 402
  spinal cord injury 371, 402
  and stroke 405
cardiogenic shock 363-4
cardiomyopathy, hypertrophic *see* hypertrophic cardiomyopathy
cardioplegia
  blood-containing solutions 366
  in cardiopulmonary bypass 368-9
  crystalloid 366, 370
  intramyocardial pH 367
  lactate extraction from myocardium 365
  in left-ventricular end-diastolic pressure 366
  myocardial preservation 365, 365-7
  nitroglycerin during 368
  in pediatric cardiac surgery 367
cardiopulmonary bypass
  air embolism management 408
  in aortic valve stenosis 204
  bleeding after 413-14
  cardioplegia in 368-9
  duration and cerebral outcome 404
  mannitol in 369
cardiovascular disease
  atrial natriuretic peptide in 435-8
  diagnosis 427
cardiovascular peptides 451-2
cardioversion 340
cardioverter-defibrillator 337-8
cardioverters, internal 301
l-carnitine 98-9
carotid and coronary combined artery disease 406-7, 427, 429
carotid endarterectomy 425-31
  cardiac complications 406
  combined with myocardial revascularization 427
  and coronary artery bypass grafting 425-9
  intraluminal shunts 431
  myocardial infarction following 426
  neurologic deficits 431
  risks from surgery 428
  simultaneous with coronary bypass 406-7
Carpentier reconstruction techniques 395
Carpentier-Edwards bioprosthesis 232

catecholamines
  levels in heart failure after ACE inhibitor therapy 255
  measurement for epidemiological studies 466-7
catheter
  bail-out 104
  dielectric breakdown voltage 316
  electrode pitting in catheter ablation 315, 316-17
  flow-directed cardiac 244, 248
  flow-through 104
  multipolar 316
  standard electrode 314
  steerable 93-4
catheter ablation 313-23
  acute complications 314
  barotrauma 318
  breakdown of dielectric insulation in multipolar
    catheters 316
  catheter effects 316-17
  contraindication in coronary sinus 314
  defibrillator as power source 318-19
  electrical characteristics in vivo 317-18
  electrode pitting 315, 316-17
  gas analysis 316
  high energy anodal shock 315-16
  high-intensity short-duration discharge 320
  high temperature electric arc 315
  in vivo histology 318
  microbubble formation with laser energy 319
  modified defibrillator 320
  persistent complete block 313
  physical effects in vitro 315-16
  power sources 318-20
  radio-frequency energy 319-20
  radiographic black hole around electrode 315
  shock-wave formation 315
catheter-tip flow velocity measurement 37
catheterization
  interventional 163
  pediatric 192
  pre-operative 185-6
cell membrane transport abnormalities 460-1
cerebral
  damage in cardiac surgery 400
  embolism 408, 490
  function and intraoperative monitoring 405
  injury and risk factors in cardiac surgery 404
  ischemia 405
Cerebral Embolism Study Group 490
cerebrovascular
  accident see stroke
  disease 407
chest pain 57-8, 62
cholesterol
  accumulation in vein grafts 391
  and atherosclerosis induction 26
  and CHD risk 15
  and coffee consumption 21
  correlation with sodium/lithium countertransport 456
  dietary 9, 26
  effect of polyunsaturated fatty acids 26
  high-density lipoprotein (HDL) 15, 20, 26, 27, 456
  levels in Eskimos 25
  low density lipoprotein (LDL) level and fish
    consumption 27
  and monounsaturated fatty acids 26
  and plaque fissuring 123
  serum total 13, 14, 15, 21
cholestyramine 13, 28
chordae tendinae rupture 395

chronic heart failure 447
  atrial natriuretic peptide in 435-7, 452
cigarettes see smoking
circulatory support, mechanical 420
clotting factors 135
coarctation see aortic coarctation
co-enzyme Q10 99
coffee 21, 67
cold stimulation testing 44
color flow mapping 181-2
complete atrioventricular canal defect see
  atrioventricular valve orifice
complete transposition 174-8
  repair time and cognitive function 178
  surgical correction 175-8
complex
  dextrocardia 222
  ventricular ectopy 281
computerized tomography see also positron emission
  tomography
  in detection of postoperative neurologic dysfunction
    405
  in silent ischemia 69
  X-ray 348
congenital heart disease 159-225
  arrhythmias 341-3
  catheter treatment 163-70
  cost of care 223
  prevalence 331-2
  preventative health care 222
congenitally complete heart block 223
congenitally malformed heart
  alpha-numeric classification 160-1
  anatomy 161-2
  embryology 159-63
  terminology 160
congestive cardiomyopathy 286
congestive heart failure
  dopamine in 363
  levodopa in 363
  survival rate 420
consciousness level impairment 400
contraceptive pill 17
contraction band necrosis 318
converting enzyme inhibitors 446
coronal spin echo image 352
coronary
  angioplasty 142
  atheroma 122
  autoregulation 38
  and carotid combined disease 406-7
  obstruction in unstable angina 86
  occlusion and Q wave infarction 133
  pressure reduction and adaptation to 38
  resistance and smoking 67
  stenosis 56
  surgery 392-3
  thrombosis 56
  tone and effect of beta-blockers 74
  vascular resistance in Syndrome X 115
coronary arteries
  normal and chest pain 57-8
  resistance to intimal thickening and plaque
    development 33-4
coronary arteriography 114, 118, 354
  interpretation 36-7
  quantitative 36
coronary artery bypass grafting 34, 93-4
  in angina 111
  cardioplegia 365

laser therapy 108
magnetic resonance imaging 352, 353
in mild angina 372
neurologic complications 425
oral anticoagulant therapy 381
positron emission tomography 361
and smoking 391
stroke incidence 426
stroke risk 428
coronary artery disease
aspirin therapy 112
in association with carotid artery disease 427
atherosclerotic and vein grafts 377
and atrial natriuretic peptide 438
CoQ10 therapy 99
effect on myocardium 155
multi-vessel 100, 101
pacemakers 337
prognosis for smokers 157
silent 68
ST-segment depression 61
surgery 109-13
survival rate 153
ventricular aneurysm 154
coronary artery spasm 42-54
angiography 43
cold stimulation testing 44
etiology 43
exercise testing 44
heart rate response 42
myocardial oxygen demand 45
pathology 42
pre-existing organic lesions 43
prognosis 46-7
provocative testing 43-4
small vessel 46
surgery for 49-50
treatment 47-8
coronary artery stenosis
angiographic severity 41
assessment of functional significance 41
effect on myocardium 155
hemodynamic significance 40-1
myocardial infarction incidence 46
pressure gradient 41
and reactive hyperemia 41
coronary artery surgery 109-13
choice of conduit 111
internal thoracic (mammary) artery grafts 372-9
management 111
myocardial protection 366
significance of new Q waves 394
survival rate 110
Coronary Artery Surgery Study (CASS) 109-11, 372
coronary bypass surgery
arterial pressure and protection of brain 407
atherosclerosis in 390-2
and percutaneous transluminal coronary angioplasty (PTCA) 100
pharmacologic agents and protection of brain 407-8
stroke incidence 401, 406
coronary care unit
access to 156
mobile 155
coronary disease
ambulatory ST-segment monitoring 61
atrial contribution to stroke volume 364
coronary flow 37-8
and aortic pressure 37

and effective resistance of stenosis 35
in nocturnal angina 55
and Q wave infarction 134
reduction and adaptation to 38
and regional cardiac wall motion 361
reserve measurement 41
reserve in Syndrome X 115
in silent ischemia 70
coronary heart disease
identification with heart rate corrected ST-segment depression 65
nutritional/metabolic causes 19
coronary heart disease mortality 1-12
blood pressure and 10
case-fatality rate 5-6
and hormone replacement therapy 17
identification of high risk men 15
incidence 5-6
international trends 1-5
male/female ratios 5
physical activity and 10-11, 19
prevention trials 13-15
risk factors 12
seasonal incidence 17
smoking and 7-8
coronary heart disease risk factors 12-24
alcohol consumption 21
coffee intake 21
family history 17
hypertension 16
lipids 15-16
overweight and obesity 19
physical exercise 18-19
psychologic factors 18
sex hormones 17
smoking 16
strategy for identification 15
coronary sinus
ablation contraindication 314
blood flow during coronary artery spasm 42
blood flow and smoking 67
effects of high energy shocks in ablation 318
oxygen content 45
coronary spasm
calcium antagonists in 91
induction 44
in unstable angina 56
Coronary Surgery Study 157
Coumadin 102
coumarin 398-9
counselling, genetic 222
creatine kinase
brain-specific 405
elevation in catheter ablation 314
level in reciprocal ST-segment changes 128-9
marker of reperfusion 144
in myocardial reperfusion 144
cross-sectional echocardiogrpahy 184-8
in hypertrophic cardiomyopathy 240
sensitivity of machines 225
in septal defect diagnosis 192
cryosurgery ablation 304
cyclic guanosine monophosphate see cGMP
cyclo-oxygenase 49
cyclosporin 416
cystic medial necrosis 216

Danes
ischemic heart disease rate 28

plasma HDL cholesterol 27
DDD pacemaker 331-2
defibrillation 155, 340
defibrillator
    automatic 301
    automatic implantable 260
    high energy pulse 315
    modified for catheter ablation 320
delerium, postoperative 401
desmopressin acetate 413, 414
dexamethasone 438
dextran in restenosis 103
diabetes mellitus
    hypertension and 476
    identification of high risk men 15
diabetics
    ACE inhibition in 477
    carotid endarterectomy in 431
    hypertension in 476-7
    with mild hypertension 473
    nephropathy 477
    thiazide diuretics 473
diastolic relaxation 42
diet
    atherosclerosis and 19
    and CHD 8-10, 19-22
    fish 20, 27
    optimal fatty acid composition 28
diethylene triamine penta-acetic acid (DTPA) 352
DiGeorge syndrome 218
digitalis 301
digoxin 339, 340
dihydropyridine vascular calcium antagonists 249
dilatation, mechanical 94
diltiazem 76
    in atrial fibrillation 339
    in coronary artery spasm 47
    mechanism of action 91
    in myocardial salvage 142
    prevention of re-infarction in patients with non-Q
    wave infarction 134
dipyridamole 37, 56
    in antiplatelet agents 102
    in coronary artery surgery 112
    lipid deposition inhibition in vein grafts 387
    and platelet deposition 382, 384
    timing of therapy 384, 385
    vein graft closure 381
disc-valve in mitral-valve replacement 231
disopyramide 276
dissecting hemorrhage 122
distal coronary bed 37
diuretics
    in cardiac failure 249, 253
    and diabetes 473
    in hypertension treatment 481-2
    induction of hypokalemia and cardiac arrhythmia 482
    interaction with ACE inhibitors 477-8
    in mild hypertension 471
    response of different races 473
    stimulation of neuroendocrine mechanisms in heart
    failure 248
    thiazide 482, 483
dobutamine 363-4
    inotropic action 446
    postoperative in tetralogy of Fallot 200
dopamine
    agonists and antagonists 443
    and atrial natriuretic peptide 433-4

beta-adrenergic stimulation 446
    in cardiogenic shock 363-4
    in cardiovascular medicine 442-51
    in congestive heart failure 363
    and control of aldosterone 443, 445
    in denervated heart tissue 444
    and the heart 444
    induction of vomiting 448
    and the kidney 444-5
    measurement in tissues 443-4
    neuronal and non-neuronal source 444
    presynaptic 443
    receptors 442-3
    in regulation of cardiovascular system 443
    route of administration 447
    in treatment of hypertension 447-8
    in vasodilatation 446
dopexamine 249, 446
Doppler echocardiography 179-84, 246, 359-61
    in carotid investigations 426
    flow velocity probe 37
    in mitral valve repair 395
    prosthetic function of bioprosthetic valves 360-1
    pulsed 187-8
    qualitative 179
    quantitative 179-80
Down's syndrome 195
dual-chamber
    pacemakers 332, 337
    rate-response pacing 331-2

Ebstein's anomaly 342
echocardiography see also Doppler echocardiography
and cross-sectional echocardiography
    in cardiac failure 246
    in exercise testing 64-5
    mitral valve prolapse 226
    in myocardial infarction 126
    right-ventricular tachycardia 341
Eisenmenger's syndrome 414, 415
electrocardiogram
    diagnostic function of signal-averaged 327
    signal-averaged 325-6
electroencephalogram see also ambulatory ECG
monitoring
    patient activated transtelephonic monitors 281
    signal-averaged 294-6
electrophysiologic studies 258-64
    aims 258-9
    current strength 261
    extrastimuli 262
    interelectrode distance 262-3
    mode of stimulation 262-3
    patient response 263
    reasons for performing 259
    site of stimulation 262
    stimulus 260-2
    successful endpoints 259
    tachycardia initiation 265
    termination regimen 263-4
electrophysiology
    after myocardial infarction 272-80
    with amiodarone 311
    and exercise testing 275
    inducibility of arrhythmia 269-70
    rationale for testing 272-3
    reproducibility of ventricular tachycardia 269
    tilt table 271
    value of testing 268-71

variable results 276-7
in ventricular arrhythmia 269-70
and ventricular late potentials 275
embolism
atherosclerotic 408
carotid arterial 408
embolization 167
during cardiac catheterization 163
of vascular abnormalities 163
enalapril 248
combination with diuretics 256-7
effect on renal function 256
in hypertension in the elderly 476
interaction with thiazide diuretics 478
in renal artery stenosis 486
encainide 289, 290, 312
encephalopathy, diffuse 401-2
endocardial
cryoablation 306
cushion defects 194
resection 306
ventriculotomy 306
England, CHD mortality rate 1, 3, 5
enoximone 249
epilepsy, postoperative 402
epinephrine 44, 466
equilibrium radionuclide ventriculography 349
ergonivine 43-4
erythrocytes
ion transport 455-6, 457
lipid membrane composition 460
transplant from hypersensitive rats 459
erythromycin 243
Eskimos
CHD incidence 20
cholesterol and triglyceride levels 25
fish diet 27
ischemic heart disease 28
plasma HDL cholesterol 27
esophageal disease 57-8
estrogen for postmenopausal symptoms 17
European Coronary Artery Surgery Study 109, 110
European Working Party on High Blood Pressure in the
Elderly 470
even-echo rephasing 353
exercise
capacity 247
effect on atrial natriuretic peptide 436
exercise testing 44
in angina pectoris 62-7
echocardiography 64-5
and electrophysiology 275
predictive value in asymptomatic subjects 69
scores 63
in silent ischemia 68-9
ST-segment changes 62

factor VIII 413
false tendons 225
fast CT flow measurement 37
fast-Fourier transform 324, 327
fat
animal 25
dietary 8-10
marine polyunsaturated 20, 25
plant 25
saturated and ischemic heart disease 27
fatty acids
composition of adipose tissue 20

consumption 10
dietary 25-31
effect on blood lipids 28
effect on ischemic heart disease 28
effect on lipoproteins 28
essential:saturated 9
monounsaturated 25, 26
optimal composition of diet 29
polyunsaturated 20, 25, 26-7
in red cell membranes and plasma 22
saturated 20, 25, 26
felodipine 249-50
fenoldopam 447, 448
fetal
arrhythmias 187
echocardiography 186-7
flow patterns and aortic coarctation 217
heart 182
fiberoptic angioscopy 108
fibrillation
and atrial-demand pacing 332
induction in catheter ablation 314
refractive atrial and amiodarone 311
ventricular and late potentials 328
fibrin
on clot surface 136
specificity 138
and thrombi with vein grafts 380, 381
fibrinogen 16
degradation products 135
fibrinogenolysis by urokinase 137
fibrinolysis 135
intracoronary 121
fibrinolytic system activators 136
fibrinopeptide A 33
Finland
adipose tissue composition 20
CHD mortality rate 1
Finnish Mental Hospitals Trial 28
first-pass radionuclide ventriculography 349
fish
consumption 27, 28
oils 20-1, 25-31
flecainide 261, 289, 290
and arrhythmia 312
fluorine-18-deoxyglucose 361
fluorocarbon solution, oxygenated 408
flow measurement techniques 37
flow-directed cardiac catheters 244, 248
Fontan procedure 207, 208-9
left ventricular dysfunction 213
modifications 211-12
performance of right atrium after 212
survival rate 210
in tricuspid atresia 210-11, 213
Framingham Study 68, 156, 339, 489
France, CHD mortality rate 1, 3, 5
Frank-Starling mechanism 246
furosemide 253

gadolinium 352
gamma-glutamyl dopa 447
gas bubble nucleation 315
gated magnetic resonance imaging 223
genetic counselling 239, 240-1
GISSI trial 139, 143
Glenn shunt 210, 211
glomerular filtration rate 433

c-GMP 80
graft
    atheroma 111, 112
    non-thrombotic disease 386-7

Hancock valves 360
headache from nitrate handling 77
heart
    attack 15
    block by catheter ablation 313
    failure *see* cardiac failure
    transplantation 421-2
Heart Attack Primary Pevention in Hypertension trial
470
heart rate
    in angina pectoris 55
    changes in ischemic episodes 62
    in coronary artery spasm 42
    corrected ST-segment depression 65
    lowering in atherosclerosis 34-5
    in nifedipine treated angina 75
heart-lung transplantation 414-19
    denervation of heart and lungs 417
    donors 414-15
    gastrointestinal motility 416
    hemostasis 416
    immunosuppression 416
    lymphatic drainage loss 417
    maintenance of nerve integrity 416
    operation 416
    preservation methods for tissues 415
    pulmonary edema 417
    recipients 415
    removal of old organs 416
    renal impairment 417
    results 416-18
    size of lungs 415
hemoglobin oxygen dissociation curve 114
hemophilia 413
heparin
    in cerebral embolism 490
    during vein grafts 381
    perioperative 384-5
    post-PTCA 103
    in pregnancy 398
    in restenosis 103
    in venous thrombosis 491
high density lipoprotein *see* cholesterol, high density
lipoprotein
His bundle ablation 304-5, 314
    and microbubbles 315
    and peak current 317
    with unipolar Helifix permanent pacing electrode 317
His-Purkinje disease 237
histamine coronary spasm induction 44
Holter monitoring
    in angina pectoris 69
    in ischemia 70
hormone replacement therapy 17
hydralazine
    in cardiac failure 248, 255
    continued efficacy on cardiac function 250
hydralazine-isosorbide dinitrate 255
hydrochlorothiazide
    in control of hypertension 477
    /triamterene in mild hypertension 472
hyperplasia, intimal 386-7
    aspirin/dipyridamole combination 387
    in vein grafts 380

hypertension
    alcohol consumption 482-3
    altered calcium handling 460
    angiotensin converting enzyme inhibitors in 454, 475-
    80
    angiotensin II in 454
    Arrhenius line 459
    atrial natriuretic peptide in 437-8
    body weight and 456
    cellular membrane transport abnormalities 460
    in CHD mortality 13
    and coronary events 471-2
    death rate 3, 4
    dietary manipulation 480-1
    dietary salt 458-9
    diuretic treatment 471, 481-2
    dopamine in treatment 447-8
    effect of bromocriptine 448
    in the elderly 476
    epidemiological studies 466-7
    erythrocyte ion uptake 457
    ion fluxes in relation to sodium balance 458-9
    ion transport 455-64
    lithium/sodium countertransport 455-7
    magnesium supplementation 481
    membrane abnormality 459
    mild and individual treatment 472-4
    mild and obstructive airways disease 474
    non-adrenergic sympathetic transmitters 467-8
    non-drug treatment 472
    norepinephrine in 465-7
    potassium supplementation 481
    in pregnancy 484-5
    pulmonary 487-8
    renovascular 475-6, 485-6
    role of calcium 453
    sodium pump inhibition 457, 458
    sodium restriction 481
    stepped-care therapy 483
    sympathetic nervous system 464-9
    tolerance of mild by women 472
    treatment 470-4, 477, 480-4
    treatment of patients with angina 473
hypertrophic cardiomyopathy 235-41
    arrhythmias 236-7
    in childhood 240-1
    drug therapy 238
    inheritance 239-40
    intramural coronary artery abnormalities 236
    pathophysiology 235-6
hyperventilation and coronary spasm induction 44
hypotension
    in nitrate therapy 89
    and pathogenesis of cerebral injury 404, 407

ibopamine 447
immunofibrinolytic mechanisms 137
immunosuppression in heart-lung transplants 416
increased motor tone *see* coronary artery spasm
Indians, CHD mortality rate 1
indomethacin 49
    and ACE inhibitors 478
    arterial duct closure 190, 191
    inhibition of prostaglandin system 189
indoramin 75
infective endocarditis 241-3
    antibiotic prophylaxis 242-3
    incidence and etiology 241-2
insulin stimulation of sodium pump activity 458

intact ventricular septum 176, 177
interferon and atherosclerosis 35
internal mammary artery grafts 111–12, 392–3
internal thoracic artery grafts 372–9
    atherosclerosis incidence 374
    contraindications 377
    nutritive perfusion 374
    patency 373–5
    perioperative risk 377
    regional myocardial perfusion 374
    survival rate 375–7
    xenon washout studies 374
International Classification of Diseases (ICD) 1, 3
International Prospective Primary Prevention Study of
    Hypertension 470
International Registry for Heart Transplantation 418
ion transport in hypertension 455–64
Ionescu-Shiley valve 232, 360
ischemia see also myocardial ischemia
    adenosine formation and release 56
    effect of exercise 64
    and heart rate changes 62
    myocardial in reciprocal ST-segment depression 129–
        30
    nifedipine therapy 75
    propanolol in 90
    silent 68–72
    wall-motion abnormalities 64
ischemic heart disease
    ambulatory electrocardiographic monitoring 247
    in cardiac failure 245
    effect of different fatty acids 28
    exercise testing 247
    myocardial metabolism 362
    and saturated fat intake 27
    ST-segment depression 247
    thrombin production in 33
isoprenaline 263
isoproterenol 200
isosorbide dinitrate 77, 78
    hemodynamic tolerance 80
    ointment 79, 89
    oral 80
    therapeutic strategies 81
    tolerance to transdermal 80
Israel, CHD mortality and dietary changes 9–10
Italy
    adipose tissue composition 20
    CHD mortality rate 1, 3

Japan
    blood pressure and mortality from strokes 10
    CHD mortality rate 1, 3, 5
    dietary changes 9
    ischemic heart disease rate 28
Jarvik 7 total artificial heart 423

ketanserin 49
kidney
    in cardiac failure 248
    dopamine in 444–5
    effect of ACE inhibitors 256
    function in cardiac failure 244, 246

labetalol
    in coronary artery spasm 48
    therapy in angina 75
lactate extraction from myocardium 365
laser

ablation 306–7, 319
angioplasty 106–9
argon 107–8, 307, 319
carbon dioxide 307
Nd-YAG 107–8, 307, 319
perforation 108
photoablation 307
thermal injury 107
transcatheter use of energy 319
late potentials 323–31
    origin 326
    predictive value 327–8
    recording 323–4
    signal averaging 323–4
    and surgical control of ventricular tachycardia 326–7
    ventricular 324
Lecompte manoever 178
left main stem lesions 393
left-atrial pressure wave 193
left-ventricular
    ejection fraction 74
    end-diastolic pressure 366
left-ventricular function 59–60
    in acute myocardial infarction prognosis 154
    in angina prognosis 154
    in aortic coarctation 217
    in arrhythmia 247
    in cardiac failure 245
    magnetic resonance imaging 348–9
    in pulmonary vascular disease 218–19
    relationship with atrial contribution to stroke volume
        364
    and survival after coronary bypass 394
Leiden Intervention Trial 27, 29
levodopa 363
lidocaine
    self-injection 313
    in ventricular fibrillation 312
linoleic acid 8–9, 25
    in adipose tissue 20
    sodium pump inhibition 458
Liotta air-driven ventricular assist device 420
Lipid Research Clinics Primary Prevention Trial 13–14,
    28, 63, 69
lipids
    effect of different fatty acids 28
    in ischemic heart disease 25–31
    risk factors in CHD 15–16
lipoprotein 28
lithium/sodium countertransport 455–6
lorcainide 289
Los Angeles Trial 28
lung
    cancer and smoking 7–8
    denervation 417
    preservation methods 415
    rejection 417
    transplantation 415
lupus anticoagulant 391
lymphatic drainage loss in heart-lung transplant 417

macroemboli 403
    prevention during heart surgery 408
magnetic resonance imaging 344–58
    angiography 352–4
    aortic aneurysms 348, 349
    blood flow 350, 352–4
    cardiac anatomy 346–8
    cardiac pathology 346–8

cardiac-transplant rejection 352
congenital disease 347–8
coronary artery bypass grafts 352, 353
cost of scanner 355
even-echo rephasing 353
heart valves 348
myocardial infarction 352
nuclear magnetism 344
paramagnetic contrast agents 352
pericardium 351
physical principles 344–6
prosthetic valves 348
pulmonary vessels 350
pulsatile arterial flow 353
regional function 349
relaxation 345
spectroscopy 345–6
thrombi in heart 351
tissue characterization 349–52
tumors 351
ventricular function 348–9
wall motion 349
malnutrition and cardiac surgery 230
mammary artery grafts 111–12
mannitol 369
marital status and survival in acute myocardial
infarction 158
mechanical valves 230–2, 397–9
metaprolol 92
methacholine 58
provocative testing 44
methyldopa
in hypertensive pregnant women 485
and quality of life in hypertensives 477
metoprolol
in mild hypertension 471
in unstable angina 90
mexiletine 276, 289
microemboli 403
in sudden ischemic death 120
milrinone 249
mineralocorticoids 438
mitral
regurgitation 395
stenosis 229
valve repair 395
valvuloplasty 229
mitral valve prolapse 226–7
echocardiography 226
in infective endocarditis 243
prognosis 226–7
ventricular ectopy in 286
mitral valve replacement 231, 232, 396–7
anticoagulant related hemorrhage 233
operative risk 396–7
thromboembolism following 233
molsidomin 90
Monitoring Trends and Determinants in Cardiovascular
Diseases (MONICA) 11, 13
morphine 436
multi-vessel disease 130–1
Multiple Risk Factor Intervention Trial (MRFIT) 14, 15,
62, 69
Mustard's procedure 175, 176, 178
arrhythmia 343
myocardial infarction
anticardiolipin antibody levels and recurrent
cardiovascular events 391
arrhythmia 272

beta-blockers in 90
coronary artery spasm in 45, 46
development of sustained ventricular arrhythmia 283
diagnosis techniques 126–7
echocardiography 126
electrophysiologic studies after 272–80
exercise testing 275
following carotid endarterectomy 426
hospital admission 156
incidence in coronary artery stenosis 46
intracoronary streptokinase 138
left ventriculograms during 59
lidocaine therapy 312
magnetic resonance imaging 352
marital status and survival rate 158
mortality 272
myocardial oxygen consumption after 60
nifedipine therapy 93
non-Q wave 133–4
nuclear magnetic resonance 126
perioperative 394
predictive value of late potentials 327–8
prevalence of unrecognized 68
prognosis 134, 150–8
PTCA and thrombolysis 103–4
rate after coronary artery surgery 110
signal-averaged ECG 325–6
silent 18, 156
size 130, 131, 134
ST–segment depression 127–33
stress and 157
subendocardial scarring 273
survival rate 153
and unstable angina 83
myocardial infarction, acute
arterial spasm 122–3
focal necrosis 122
necrosis 120
pathology 118–26
plaque fissuring 122, 123
postmortem angiograms 121
Q waves 119
subtending artery occlusion 121
total occlusion 122
myocardial ischemia see also ischemia
beta blockade 369–70
in hypertrophic cardiomyopathy 236
propanolol 370
recording during sleep 55–6
in Syndrome X 114–5
myocardial preservation 365–70
cardioplegia 365–70
experimental 367–70
nitroglycerin 368
in pediatric cardiac surgery 367
myocardium
effect of left anterior descending coronary artery
stenosis 155
hypoperfusion 155
lactate 114
necrosis 46
oxygen consumption 60
oxygen demand 35, 45, 75
perfusion 114, 374
reperfusion injury 369
salvage 141–2

naloxone 68
National Heart, Lung and Blood Institute 420

National Institutes of Health Consensus Department Conference 14
Nd-YAG laser 107–8, 307, 319
necrosis, focal in acute myocardial infarction 122
neonates
    aortic valve stenosis correction 204
    balloon aortic valvoplasty 166
    cross-sectional echocardiography 185
    intact ventricular septum 172–3
    pulmonary vascular disease 218
    selection for correction of congenital heart disease 223
    transposition of the great arteries 171–3
Netherlands Interuniversity Cardiology Institute study 139, 143
neuropeptide Y 467
neuropsychologic testing 401–2
New York Heart Association functional classification 94, 244–5
nicardipine 76–7, 250
    as calcium-channel blocker 473
nifedipine
    and beta-blocker combination 74
    as calcium-channel blocker 473
    in coronary artery spasm 47
    efficacy and smoking 67
    mechanism of action 91
    in severe heart failure 255–6
    side effects 76
    in unstable angina 92
    withdrawal 76, 92
Nimbus ventricular assist devices 420, 422
nisoldipine 91, 250
nitrates
    in angina pectoris 77–83
    and cardiac function 250
    in coronary artery spasm 47
    effect on platelet aggregation 89
    mechanism of action 80–1
    metabolism 77
    side effects 77,89
    sublingual 78, 116
    tolerance 77, 78, 79, 81
    transdermal 78–9
    vasodilatory effects 77, 446
nitrogen-13-ammonia 361
nitroglycerin 43, 47, 77
    consumption with calcium antagonists 74–5
    infusion 80
    ointment 78–9, 89
    patches 78, 79
    sublingual 89
    tablets 89
    transdermal 80,81
nitroprusside 446
nitrosothiol 80
non-pulsatile perfusion during bypass 407
non-rheumatic heart disease 3, 4
non-steroidal anti-inflammatory drugs 478
norepinephrine 44
    assay 466
    clearance 465
    effect of atrial natriuretic peptide on pressor effect 432
    in hypertension 465–7
North American Society of Pacing Electrophysiology (NASPE) 259
Northern Ireland, CHD mortality rate 1, 5
NOVACOR electrically powered left-ventricular assist device 422
nuclear magnetic resonance 126, 344–5
nutritional status and cardiac surgery 230

O.K.Y.-046 49
obesity and CHD incidence 19
oleic acid 25
    sodium pump inhibition 458
ophthalmologic complications of cardiac surgery 402
opioid peptides 68
    oral contraceptives 491–2
    ouabain-sensitive leukocyte sodium efflux 457, 458, 459
overweight and CHD incidence 19
Oxford Family Planning Association contraceptive study 491–2
oximetry 224, 349
oxprenolol 485
oxygen consumption measurement 247

pacemakers 331–2
    antitachycardia 301
    in atrioventricular block 336
    costs 332
    permanent implantation 336
pacing 334–8
    atrial 337
    impaired fatty acid metabolism 362
Paget's disease 245
pain
    chest and arm prior to sudden ischemic death 120
    chest and normal coronary arteries 113
    in Syndrome X 115
    ^{11}C-palmitate clearance kinetics 362
palmitic acid 25
paraplegia 371
patient-activated transtelephonic ECG monitors 281
pediatric cardiac surgery 367
penicillin 243
percutaneous balloon mitral commisurotomy 229
percutaneous transluminal coronary angioplasty (PTCA) 93–5, 99–106
    acute closure of dilated artery 101
    calcium antagonists in 103
    complications 101
    heparin in 103
    long-term results 102, 103
    mortality rate 100, 101–2
    in multi-vessel disease 100, 101
    selection of patients 99–100
    and thrombolysis 103–4
    training and performance 100–1
pericardiectomy 399
peripheral vascular disease 453
persantine 112
persistent fetal circulation 218
personality and CHD incidence 18
pharmacologic agents, hemodynamics 363–4
phenoxybenzamine 48
phentolamine 48
phosphoinositol cycle 460
phosphorus-31 spectroscopy 346
physical
    activity in CHD mortality 11–12
    exercise 18–19
physiologic rate-responsive testing 331–4
Pierce-Donachy pump 420
pirbuterol 446
plaque fissuring
    in acute myocardial infarction 122, 123, 124
    and cholesterol 123
plasma renin activity 254
plasmin
    circulating 135, 136

on clot surface 136
proteolysis 135
plasminemia, circulating 136
plasminogen 136-7
plasminogen activator (t-PA)
    binary complex with fibrin 136
    clot selectivity 138
    intravenous in thrombolysis 145
    pharmacodynamics and pharmacokinetics 141
    release 136
    and reocclusion 143
    synthesis 136
    thrombolysis 135, 140-1
    tissue-type 140-1
platelet
    activation 385
    aggregation 45, 89, 453
    antiaggregants in bypass surgery 407
    cyclo-oxygenase acetylation 385
    deposition 380, 382
    function modifying drugs 49
    monolayer 38
Poiseuille's equation 371
porcine valve 231, 360
positron emission tomography 361-2
    coronary artery bypass surgery 361
    glucose uptake in myocardium 361
    ^{11}C-palmitate clearance kinetics 362
positron-tomographic flow measurement 37
prazosin 48
    in cardiac failure 248
    effect on epinephrine and norepinephrine concentrations 255
    effect on renal function 256
    in mild hypertension 473
pre-eclampsia 484
pregnancy 397, 398-9, 484-5
    mechanical valves 397
preload 245
Prinzmetal's angina 58, 89, 90, 91
procainamide
    deleterious effects 291
    induction of ventricular tachycardia 292
    prevention of sustained ventricular tachycardia 289, 290
progestogen 17
propranolol
    in complications of aortic coarctation repair 216
    efficacy and smoking 67
    in hypertension 484
    in ischemia 90
    in mild hypertension 471
    and quality of life in hypertensives 477
propantheline bromide 271
propylbutyl dopamine 446-7
prostacyclin 49
    deficiency in variant angina 49
    during bypass surgery 407
    effect on platelet aggregation 453
    production 33
    in pulmonary hypertension 487-8
prostaglandin
    and ACE inhibitors 478
    E2 453
    infusion in neonates 173
    nitrate mechanism of action 81
    in peripheral vascular disease 453
    system in venous and arterial ducts 189
prostheses
    porcine heterograft 231

valve 230-2, 260
protein-calorie malnutrition 230
psychiatric dysfunction, postoperative 401
psychosis, postoperative 401
pulmonary
    artery 180, 202
    edema 414, 417
    hypertension 218-19, 414, 415
    outflow tract patch reconstruction 197
    regurgitant jet 181, 182
    stenosis 203-4
    to systemic flow ratio 224
    trunk banding 207-8, 209, 215
    valve stenosis 164-5
    vascular disease 218-19
pulsatile arterial flow 353

Q wave
    in acute myocardial infarction 119
    infarction 153-4
    myocardial infarction 134
    significance after bypass surgery 394
QRS
    complex 325, 326, 327
    frequency analysis 294-6
QT interval 311
QT-sensing pacemaker 332-3
quinidine 276, 312

radio signal in magnetic resonance imaging 344
Rastelli concept 202
Raynaud's phenomenon 453
recanalization
    laser 107
    mechanical 93-4
red-cell deformity and nifedipine 75
regional non-transmural infarction 122
renal function
    angiotensin converting enzyme (ACE) inhibitors 249
    effect of ACE inhibitors in heart failure 256
    in heart failure 249
    impairment after heart-lung transplantation 417
renal plasma flow 433
renin
    activity 254
    biochemical marker of heart failure 249
    inhibitors 248
renin-angiotensin-aldosterone system
    activation 249, 253
    anti-natriuretic 434
    and atrial natriuretic peptide 433, 436
    in cardiac failure 248, 254
resistance vessel contractility 461
restenosis 102
    coarctation 166-7
    modification 102-3
rheumatic fever 234
right-atrial
    myxoma 351
    pressure wave 192
right-ventricular
    dysplasia 341
    postoperative function in neonates 173
    tachycardia 341
rubidium-82 69

saphenous vein 112
    aortocoronary bypass grafts 392

Scotland
    adipose tissue composition 20
    CHD mortality rate 1, 3, 5
Seattle Heart Watch 63
secundum atrial septal defect 343
septal fibroma *351*
serotonergic receptors 42
serotonin inhibitors 49
Seven Countries Study 26, 27–8
shunt magnitude 181
sick-sinus syndrome 237, 332
    and pacemakers 336, 337
signal-averaged ECG 294–6
simple ventricular ectopy 281
single-chamber
    pacing device 331
    rate-responsive pacemakers 332–3
single ventricle heart 206
smoking 67
    atherosclerosis aggravation 19
    and CHD 7–8, 16
    cholesterol content in aorta 34
    collagen content of coronary endarterectomy
    specimens 34
    and coronary artery bypass grafting 391
    and coronary surgery survival rate 392–3
    effect on acute myocardial infarction prognosis 156
    effect on angina prognosis 156
    and estrogen administration 17
    identification of high risk men 15
    and plasma fibrinogen levels 16
    and treatment of mild hypertension 471, 472
sodium
    balance and ion fluxes 458–9
    excretion 434
    /potassium pump 455, 457–8
sodium pump
    and high-salt diet 458
    inhibition 458
    ouabain-like inhibitor 457
    and phosphoinositol cycle 460–1
    rubidium studies of activity 457
    stimulation 458
South Africa, CHD mortality rate 1
spark erosion 108
spin-lattice relaxation time 345, 349–50
spin-spin relaxation time 349–50
spinal cord
    injury 402
    magnetic resonance imaging 344
    preservation 370–1
spironolactone 438
ST-segment
    ambulatory monitoring 61–2
    analysis and time course patterns 64
    changes in coronary artery spasm 44, 45
    computer classification of changes 62–3
    effect of combination therapy 74
    frequency analysis 294–6
ST-segment depression 18
    and abnormal ejection fraction 64
    CoQ10 therapy 99
    effect of l-carnitine 98
    heart rate corrected 65
    in ischemia 247
    in nocturnal angina 55
    and regional wall-motion abnormalities 64
    in silent ischemia 68–9
    in Syndrome X 114

ST-segment depression, reciprocal
    complications 131
    during myocardial infarction 127–33
    incidence 127–33
    and infarct size 128–9, 130, 131
    infarct zone necrosis 129
    magnitude 128
    mechanisms of change 127
    mortality rate 131
    multi-vessel disease 130–1
    myocardial ischemia 129
    as prognostic indicator after myocardial infarction 131
Starr-Edwards
    non-cloth-covered silicone ball 230–1
    valves 360
stenosis *see also* coronary artery stenosis
    in acute myocardial infarction 121
    in angina 118
    aortic 203–4, 359
    aortic valve 165–6, 222
    and autoregulatory vasodilatation 37
    cardioplegia in 368
    carotid 428, 429
    congenital of pulmonary veins 224
    effect on coronary flow 37
    energy loss across 35–6
    flow separation 35
    functional severity 36, 37
    and limitation of coronary reserve 38
    mitral 229
    pressure-gradient across 36
    pulmonary 203–4
    pulmonary artery 167
    pulmonary valve 164–5
    renal and ACE inhibitors 476
    renal artery 486
    semilunar valve 180
    valvar and balloon dilatation 203
    viscous loss 35
stenotic gradient 180
steroids 416
Still's murmur 225
Streptococcus viridans 242
streptokinase
    activation of circulating plasminogen 136
    acylated 137
    allergic reactions 136
    coronary thrombolysis 135
    intracoronary 89, 138, 142
    intravenous 139, 143
    plasminogen activation 136
stress 11–12
and myocardial infarction 157
and silent myocardial ischemia 18
testing 61, 63–4
stroke 16–17
    and atrial fibrillation 339, 489
    bruit as indication of risk 427
    after cardiac surgery 400–1, 405, 406
    in carotid endarterectomy 428, 429, 431
    carotid occlusion 428
    and cerebrovascular disease 405
    in coronary artery bypass grafting 426, 428, 429
    embolic and anticoagulation 490
    fibrinogen and 16
    and mild hypertension 470, 471
    and mitral valve prolapse 227
    mortality and hormone replacement therapy 17
    mortality rate 10

perioperative 403, 406
seasonal incidence 17
volume 246
subendocardial flow 38
subvalvar outflow obstruction 178
suction electrode catheter 317
sudden ischemic death 118-26
Sweden
blood pressure and mortality from strokes 10
CHD mortality and dietary changes 9-10
dietary changes 9
sympathetic nervous system
direct nerve recording 465
in essential hypertension 464-9
and neurogenic and endocrine pressor and depressor mechanisms 465
plasma catecholamine measurement 466
syncope 271
Syndrome X 113-18
myocardial ischemia in 114-15
natural history 115-16
pain threshold 115
systemic vascular resistance 246

telemetry monitoring 285
tetralogy of Fallot 196-201
age for correction 199
arrhythmias 342
cross circulation technique 197
effect of catecholamines postoperatively 200
late deaths after surgical correction 199
palliation for young patients 198
postoperative ventricular arrhythmia 200
thallium
exercise scintigraphy 69
myocardial perfusion scan 37
scintigraphy 41
Thermedics device 420, 422
thoracic aortic interruption and paraplegia 371
thrombin production 33
thromboembolism
following mitral valve replacement 233
protection of pregnant mothers 397
thrombolysis 134-50
clinical trials 138-41
fibrin specificity 138
myocardial salvage augmentation 141-2
non-invasive markers of reperfusion and reocclusion 144
pharmacology 135-6
plasminogen activation 136-7
and PTCA for acute myocardial infarction 103-4
reocclusion 143
return of myocardial oxygen supply 134
in unstable angina 89
thrombosis
antiplatelet agents 382
and coronary artery spasm 45
deep-vein 89
elicited by arterial spasm 122
intravascular and anticardiolipin levels 391
mural 120
pulmonary artery 89
rate of change 118
risk in pregnancy 398-9
in sudden ischemic death 119
venous 491-2
thromboxane A_2 385
inhibitors 49

thromboxane B_2 385
thrombus
in acute myocardial infarction 122
formation with vein grafts 379-80
magnetic resonance imaging 351
occlusion and infarction 123
thyrotoxicosis 245
tilt, head-up 271
tissue plasminogen activator (t-PA) 16, 135-45
tocainide 289
torsade de pointes 312
tracheal compression 225
transplantation, combined heart and lung 414-19
transposition of the great arteries 170-4
transthoracic impedance 340
treadmill exercise 247
tricuspid atresia 206, 207
atriopulmonary *versus* atrioventricular connection 210, 211
Fontan procedure 209, 210-11, 212, 213
survival rate 209
tricuspid-valve replacement 231
triglycerides 456
truncal valve
insufficiency 202
replacement 202
truncus arteriosus see common arterial trunk

UK Medical Research Council (MRC) trial of mild hypertension 470
ultrasound imaging 179-84
unipolar Helifix permanent pacing electrode 317
univentricular atrioventricular connection 204-13
atrial septostomy 207
banding 207, 208, 209
Fontan procedure 207-13
septation 207
shunt procedure 207
urokinase 136, 137
USA
blood pressure and mortality from strokes 10
case-fatality rate in CHD 5-6
CHD mortality rate 1, 3, 5
dietary fat 8-9
USCI temporary pacing catheter 316

vagus nerve 416
valve surgery 395-9
valvoplasty 163-7, 203-4
valvotomy, closed mitral 234
valvuloplasty
aortic 227-8
mitral 229
percutaneous transluminal 228
vascular endothelial injury 33
vasoconstrictors 43
vasodilatation
calcitonin gene-related peptide 452
improvement of heart function 244
in pulmonary hypertension 487
in stenosis 37
vasodilator
and ACE inhibitors 478
in cardiac failure 248, 249
coronary reserve 37
loss and coronary artery spasm 43
reserve and coronary flow 37
vasopressin 248, 249

vasospasm 45
vegetable oils 26
vein graft
  angiography 380
  anticoagulant treatment 381-2
  antithrombotic treatment 380-6
  and arterial pressure 391
  and aspirin 379-90
  closure and anticoagulants 381
  degeneration 373
  early thrombotic occlusion 379-80
  high risk groups 386
  inhibition of lipid deposition 387
  intimal hyperplasia 380
  late phase atherosclerosis 380, 387
  mechanism of closure 379
  platelet deposition 382
  survival rate 375
venous ducts 188-90
ventricle
  double inlet 206, 207, 208
  surgical isolation of right 306
ventricular
  aneurysm 154
  ectopy 286
  hypertrophy 207
  late potentials 275
  outlet obstruction 180
  premature complex (VPC) 272
  programmed stimulation 288, 293-4
  stroke volume 60
  tachyarrhythmia 250
  volume 246
ventricular arrhythmia 311, 312
  ambulatory ECG monitoring 270
  antiarrhythmic drugs 286, 288-91
  assessment of value of drug therapy 258
  definition 259
  drug prophylaxis 272, 276
  electrophysiologic stimulation 258-68, 269-70
  indications for treatment 281-300
  induction by electrophysiologic stimulation 261-2,
    269-70
  and left-ventricular dysfunction 342
  mortality with sustained 282
  as predictor of mortality 250
  prevention of sustained 281-91
  reproducibility of inducing 265
  stimulation protocols 264, 265
  stimulation site 262
  termination 263-4
  therapy 258
  treatment with ventricular ectopy 281
ventricular assist devices 420-2
  air powered 420-1
  electrically powered 421-2
  skeletal muscle 242
ventricular ectopy 272, 281
  antiarrhythmic drugs 281, 289, 292-3
  asymptomatic 281-2, 291-3
  and sudden cardiac death 283
  suppression 286-9
  and sustained ventricular arrhythmia 283
ventricular fibrillation 258, 259, 282
  and abnormal signal-averaged ECG 327
  identification of patients at risk 293-6
  lidocaine therapy 312
  mobile coronary care unit 155-6
  mortality rate 134, 154

  prevention of sustained 286-9
  in sudden ischemic death 120
ventricular septal defect 192
  and aortic coarctation 218
  cross-sectional echocardiography 196
  magnetic resonance imaging 347
  surgical closure 193-4
ventricular septum, intact 171
ventricular tachycardia 258
  and abnormal signal-averaged ECG 327
  catheter ablation success rate 314
  definition 259
  electrogram mapping 326
  in hypertrophic cardiomyopathy 236-7
  identification by electrogram 270
  induction in catheter ablation 314
  intraoperative mapping 301-2
  laser ablation 306-7
  late potentials with signal averaging 326
  left bundle branch block configuration 341
  non-ischemic 306
  and polyuria 437
  predictive value of late potentials 328
  prevention of sustained 286-9
  secondary to ischemia 306-7
  surgery for 301, 306-7
  surgical control and signal-averaged ECG 326
  sustained 282, 293-6
ventriculography, radionuclide 246-7, 349
verapamil 35
  in atrial fibrillation 339
  and beta-blocker combination 74
  in coronary artery spasm 47
  in hypertrophic cardiomyopathy 238-9
  mechanism of action 91
  in spinal cord ischemia 371
Veterans Administration trial 110
videodensitometry 36-7
volumetric flow 181
von Willebrand's disease 413
VVI pacemaker 331-2, 337

Wales, CHD mortality rate 1, 3, 5
warfarin
  anticoagulation in restenosis 102
  and calcification of porcine bioprosthetic valves 398
  with dipyridamole 382
  in venous thrombosis 491
water excretion 434
Wenckebach conduction patterns 326
Wessex porcine valves 360
Western Electric Study 28
Western Washington trial 139
WHO MONICA studies 11, 13
WHO myocardial infarction registry 5
Wolff-Parkinson-White syndrome 301, 302
  cryosurgery 304
  intraoperative mapping for 303
  postoperative recurrence 302-3
  surgery 302-4

X-ray computed tomography 348
xamoterol 249
xenografts 231, 232
xenon-133 single-photon emission computerized
tomography 405

Zutphen Study 28